Otolaryngology–Head and Neck Surgery

Rapid Clinical and Board Review

Matthew L. Carlson, MD
Assistant Professor
Department of Otorhinolaryngology–Head and Neck Surgery
Mayo Clinic
Rochester, Minnesota

Kathryn M. Van Abel, MD
Clinical Instructor
Department of Otorhinolaryngology–Head and Neck Surgery
Mayo Clinic
Rochester, Minnesota

David J. Archibald, MD
Founder, Center for Plastic Surgery at Castle Rock
Castle Rock, Colorado

Daniel L. Price, MD
Assistant Professor
Department of Otorhinolaryngology–Head and Neck Surgery
Mayo Clinic
Rochester, Minnesota

Thieme
New York • Stuttgart • Delhi • Rio de Janiero

Thieme Medical Publishers, Inc.
333 Seventh Ave.
New York, NY 10001

Executive Editor: Timothy Y. Hiscock
Managing Editor: J. Owen Zurhellen, IV
Editorial Assistant: Kate Barron
Senior Vice President, Editorial and Electronic Product Development: Cornelia Schulze
Production Editor: Sean Woznicki
International Production Director: Andreas Schabert
International Marketing Director: Fiona Henderson
Director of Sales, North America: Mike Roseman
International Sales Director: Louisa Turrell
Vice President, Finance and Accounts: Sarah Vanderbilt
President: Brian D. Scanlan
Printer: CPI Books, Leck

Library of Congress Cataloging-in-Publication Data

Carlson, Matthew L. (Assistant professor of otolaryngology), author.
  Otolaryngology–head and neck surgery: rapid clinical and board review / Matthew L. Carlson, Kathryn M. Van Abel, David J. Archibald, Daniel L. Price.
      p. ; cm.
  Summary: "This publication will provide residents and practicing otolaryngologists a well-organized and concise resource for rapid examination review. It contains succinct and high-yield facts using simple one to two phrase questions and answers. Over 9,100 Q&A are included, half in the book and half online as part of WinkingSkull.com. We will include drawings to illustrate important points when needed. Chapters will be divided based on the various subspecialties in the field (rhinology, facial plastics, otology etc)"–Provided by publisher.
  ISBN 978-1-60406-768-2 (paperback) – ISBN 978-1-60406-769-9 (eISBN)
  I. Abel, Kathryn M. Van (Kathryn Mckinna Van), author. II. Archibald, David J., author. III. Price, Daniel L., author. IV. Title.
  [DNLM: 1. Otorhinolaryngologic Diseases–Examination Questions. 2. Head–surgery–Examination Questions. 3. Neck–surgery–Examination Questions. WV 18.2]
  RF57
  617.5'10076–dc23
                                          2014034717

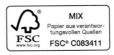

Printed in Germany   5 4 3

ISBN 978-1-60406-768-2

Also available as an e-book:
eISBN 978-1-60406-769-9

Important note: Medicine is an ever-changing science undergoing continual development. Research and clinical experience are continually expanding our knowledge, in particular our knowledge of proper treatment and drug therapy. Insofar as this book mentions any dosage or application, readers may rest assured that the authors, editors, and publishers have made every effort to ensure that such references are in accordance with **the state of knowledge at the time of production of the book.**

Nevertheless, this does not involve, imply, or express any guarantee or responsibility on the part of the publishers in respect to any dosage instructions and forms of applications stated in the book. **Every user is requested to examine carefully** the manufacturers' leaflets accompanying each drug and to check, if necessary in consultation with a physician or specialist, whether the dosage schedules mentioned therein or the contraindications stated by the manufacturers differ from the statements made in the present book. Such examination is particularly important with drugs that are either rarely used or have been newly released on the market. Every dosage schedule or every form of application used is entirely at the user's own risk and responsibility. The authors and publishers request every user to report to the publishers any discrepancies or inaccuracies noticed. If errors in this work are found after publication, errata will be posted at www.thieme.com on the product description page.

Some of the product names, patents, and registered designs referred to in this book are in fact registered trademarks or proprietary names even though specific reference to this fact is not always made in the text. Therefore, the appearance of a name without designation as proprietary is not to be construed as a representation by the publisher that it is in the public domain.

To my beautiful wife, for your endless support and encouragement; and to our baby girl and
rowdy boys who are the joy of our lives.

– MLC

To my incredible husband, whose endless patience and support never ceases to amaze me, and
to my new darling daughter whose in utero kicks and turns kept me motivated at night and entrance
into this world was delayed just long enough to allow me to finish my contribution to this important work.
I love you both more than you will ever know.

– KMVA

I dedicate this book to my mentors, who taught me anatomy and technique but also surgical judgment, mastery,
humility, and compassion. I thank our patients, who allow us the daily privilege of learning from them.

– DJA

To B, Bug, Button, and Bean, with whom I'd much rather be eating pancakes.

– DLP

Contents

Foreword

My first impression as I reviewed several excerpts of this superb review book is, "Why didn't I have this at my disposal during my residency training or during my preparation for the formidable board examination?!" As a former member of the Academy-appointed committee charged to prepare written questions for the board examination, and later as a guest examiner for the oral board section for several years, this is a must-read text.

With over nine thousand questions, *Otolaryngology—Head and Neck Surgery: Rapid Clinical and Board Review* covers fundamental surgical anatomy, applied physiology, embryology, and high-yield clinical pearls concerning patient evaluation and management. This book does an excellent job combining clinically relevant facts with "hard-to-remember" commonly tested minutia in an easy-to-follow, well organized format. This text is a must-have for otolaryngologists at all levels of training; whether a surgical intern just beginning residency or a seasoned clinician studying for board recertification. As a lifelong academician and clinical educator, I fully endorse this book.

Thomas J. McDonald, MD
Professor of Otolaryngology
Mayo Medical School
Mayo Clinic
Rochester, Minnesota

Preface

"The eyes do not see what the mind does not know." – Sir William Osler

While many fields are defined by a single organ system, otolaryngology–head and neck surgery encompasses a tremendous breadth of anatomy, physiology, and pathology unique to the head and neck region. The management principles and surgical skillset required to treat advanced stage oropharyngeal squamous cell carcinoma are substantially different than those employed for cosmetic septorhinoplasty, or during microsurgical resection of lateral skull base tumors. Furthermore, without a true medical counterpart, the otolaryngologist is often the final stop for patients seeking medical management of conditions such as chronic sinus disease, voice disorders, and vestibulopathy. As our field continues to expand, the volume of knowledge required for clinical and surgical competency will only grow.

In the United States, all otolaryngology residents take a yearly written test and a final written and oral board examination at the end of residency training. In addition, all practicing otolaryngologists who received board certification after 2002 require maintenance of certification testing every ten years. This book will provide medical students, residents, fellows, and practicing otolaryngologists with a well-organized and concise resource for rapid clinical and board review. Our intended audience maintains a very busy schedule and will use this resource between surgical cases, in the car, on the airplane, and during any other "down time." With this in mind, we have created a pocket-sized book containing succinct and high-yield facts using a short-question, short-answer format in addition to paired multiple-choice questions, covering all subspecialty topics.

This book was created "for the people, by the people" and we would like to keep an informal, open line of communication between the readers and authors. If there are any comments or suggestions for how this book could be improved we would love to hear from you at **otorapidreview@gmail.com**.

Contributors

David J. Archibald, MD
Founder, Center for Plastic Surgery at Castle Rock
Castle Rock, Colorado

Joseph T. Breen, MD
Resident Physician
Department of Otorhinolaryngology–Head and Neck
  Surgery
Mayo Clinic
Rochester, Minnesota

Matthew L. Carlson, MD
Assistant Professor
Department of Otorhinolaryngology–Head and Neck
  Surgery
Mayo Clinic
Rochester, Minnesota

Amy C. Dearking, MD
Resident Physician
Department of Otorhinolaryngology–Head and Neck
  Surgery
Mayo Clinic
Rochester, Minnesota

Colin L. W. Driscoll, MD
Department Chair and Professor
Department of Otorhinolaryngology–Head and Neck
  Surgery
Mayo Clinic
Rochester, Minnesota

Benzon M. Dy, MD
Mayo Clinic
Rochester, Minnesota

Dale C. Ekbom, MD
Assistant Professor
Department of Otorhinolaryngology–Head and Neck
  Surgery
Mayo Clinic
Rochester, Minnesota

Kyle S. Ettinger, MD, DDS
Department of Otorhinolaryngology–Head and Neck
  Surgery
Mayo Clinic
Rochester, Minnesota

W. Jonathan Fillmore, MD, DMD
Department of Otorhinolaryngology–Head and Neck
  Surgery
Mayo Clinic
Rochester, Minnesota

Brian C. Gross, MD
Department of Otorhinolaryngology–Head and Neck
  Surgery
Mayo Clinic
Rochester, Minnesota

Kathryn L. Hall, MD
Assistant Professor of Facial Plastic and Reconstructive
  Surgery
Department of Otolaryngology–Head and Neck Surgery
University of South Florida
Tampa, Florida

Cody A. Koch, MD
Instructor and Chief Resident
Department of Otorhinolaryngology–Head and Neck
  Surgery
Mayo Clinic
Rochester, Minnesota

Ian J. Lalich, MD
Resident Physician
Department of Otorhinolaryngology–Head and Neck
  Surgery
Mayo Clinic
Rochester, Minnesota

Eric J. Moore, MD
Associate Professor
Department of Otorhinolaryngology–Head and Neck
  Surgery
Mayo Clinic
Rochester, Minnesota

Ashley G. O'Reilly, MD
Resident Physician
Department of Otorhinolaryngology–Head and Neck
  Surgery
Mayo Clinic
Rochester, Minnesota

John F. Pallanch, MD
Assistant Professor
Department of Otorhinolaryngology–Head and Neck
    Surgery
Mayo Clinic
Rochester, Minnesota

Brandon W. Peck, MD
Department of Otorhinolaryngology–Head and Neck
    Surgery
Mayo Clinic
Rochester, Minnesota

Stanley Pelosi, MD
Department of Otorhinolaryngology–Head and Neck
    Surgery
Mayo Clinic
Rochester, Minnesota

Rajanya S. Petersson, MD
Assistant Professor of Otolaryngology–Head and Neck
    Surgery
Virginia Commonwealth University Medical Center
Richmond, Virginia

Daniel L. Price, MD
Assistant Professor
Department of Otorhinolaryngology–Head and Neck
    Surgery
Mayo Clinic
Rochester, Minnesota

Jonathan J. Romak, MD
Resident Physician
Department of Otorhinolaryngology–Head and Neck
    Surgery
Mayo Clinic
Rochester, Minnesota

William R. Schmitt, MD
Resident Physician
Department of Otorhinolaryngology–Head and Neck
    Surgery
Mayo Clinic
Rochester, Minnesota

David G. Stoddard Jr., MD
Resident Physician
Department of Otorhinolaryngology–Head and Neck
    Surgery
Mayo Clinic
Rochester, Minnesota

Joshua J. Thom, MD
Resident Physician
Department of Otorhinolaryngology–Head and Neck
    Surgery
Mayo Clinic
Rochester, Minnesota

Kathryn M. Van Abel, MD
Clinical Instructor
Department of Otorhinolaryngology–Head and Neck
    Surgery
Mayo Clinic
Rochester, Minnesota

1 Pediatric Otolaryngology–Head and Neck Surgery

Ashley G. O'Reilly, Kathryn M. Van Abel, and Rajanya S. Petersson

Overview

1	What primary germ layers make up the branchial arches, grooves (clefts), and pouches?	Branchial arches and grooves (clefts) are covered externally by ectoderm and composed internally by mesoderm. Each arch has a cartilaginous, muscular, neural, and arterial component. Branchial pouches are composed of endoderm.
2	What are the three most common branchial anomalies in order of frequency?	• 70 to 95%: Second branchial arch anomalies • 8 to 10%: First branchial arch anomalies • 3 to 10%: Third and fourth branchial arch anomalies
3	What branchial cleft anomaly involves the facial nerve?	First branchial cleft anomaly tracts are close to the parotid gland, particularly the superficial lobe. The tract may pass above, between, or below the branches of the facial nerve.
4	What is the second branchial arch structure that normally regresses during development but may be associated with hearing loss and pulsatile tinnitus when present in the adolescent or adult? (► Table 1.1)	The stapedial artery

Table 1.1 Branchial arch derivatives

Branchial Arch	Cranial Nerve	Muscular Contributions	Arteries	Skeletal Elements
1	V3	Muscles of mastication (temporalis, masseter, and pterygoids), mylohyoid, anterior belly digastric, tensor veli palatini, tensor tympani	Maxillary, external carotid	Meckel cartilage: mandible, malleus head and neck, incus body and short process, anterior malleal ligament
2	VII	Muscles of facial expression, posterior belly digastric, stylohyoid, stapedius	Stapedial (normally regresses)	Reichert cartilage: manubrium of malleus, long and lenticular process of incus, stapes (middle ear surface), styloid process, stylohyoid ligament, styloid process, lesser horns of hyoid
3	IX	Stylopharyngeus, superior and middle constrictors	Common and internal carotid	Greater horns and lower body of hyoid
4	X (Superior Laryngeal)	Cricothyroid, intrinsic muscles of soft palate including levator veli palatini	Aortic arch, right subclavian, brachiocephalic	Thyroid and cuneiform cartilages
6	X (Recurrent)	Intrinsic muscles of larynx (except cricothyroid)	Ductus arteriosus, roots of pulmonary	Cricoid, arytenoid, corniculate cartilages

5	Where is the proximal opening of a second branchial cleft anomaly?	Tonsillar fossa
6	What artery can persist in adulthood from the second branchial arch?	The stapedial artery

7	What is the course of a persistent stapedial artery?	The stapedial artery rises from the internal carotid artery (ICA), enters the hypotympanum via the Jacobson canal, passes through the crura of the stapes (obturator foramen of the stapes), then passes through the cochleariform process and runs with the tympanic section of the facial nerve before exiting into the extradural intracranial space just before reaching the geniculate ganglion. It replaces the middle meningeal artery, resulting in a hypoplastic or aplastic foramen spinosum.
8	What symptoms are associated with a persistent stapedial artery?	Pulsatile tinnitus, asymptomatic incidental finding, conductive hearing loss (associated stapes ankylosis), sensorineural hearing loss (SNHL), erosion of the otic capsule (rare), and may be associated with additional vascular anomalies (i.e., the ICA)
9	Describe the pathway of a third branchial arch anomaly. (▶ Fig. 1.1)	Piriform sinus of the hypopharynx → through the inferior constrictor muscle medially → greater cornu of the hyoid bone, lateral to the superior laryngeal nerve (nerve of the fourth arch) → over the hypoglossal nerve → inferior to the glossopharyngeal nerve → posterior to the ICA → fistula opens to the skin over the anterior border of the sternocleidomastoid muscle (SCM)

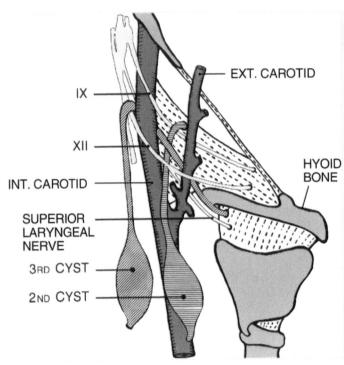

Fig. 1.1 Pathways of second and third branchial cleft anomalies. (Used with permission from Van de Water TR, Staecker H, eds. Otolaryngology: Basic Science and Clinical Review. New York, NY: Thieme; 2006.)

10	Describe the pathway of a fourth branchial arch anomaly.	Piriform sinus of the hypopharynx → medial to the superior laryngeal nerve (nerve of the fourth arch) → tracheoesophageal groove, parallel to the recurrent laryngeal nerve into the mediastinum → under the aortic arch (left) or subclavian artery (right) (both are fourth arch derivatives) → ascends along posterior surface of the common carotid artery → anterior border of the SCM; it can also follow the common carotid artery to bifurcation → between the ICA and the external carotid artery (ECA) → below the glossopharyngeal → above the hypoglossal → descends inferiorly to exit anterior to the SCM
11	What are the clinical presentations for third and fourth branchial cleft anomalies?	Both may be noted as a soft fluctuant mass, abscess, or draining tract located along the anterior border of the SCM. Acute suppurative thyroiditis can be seen. Stridor may be present in newborns with a lateral neck mass.
12	What are the typical findings in a patient with branchio-otorenal (BOR) syndrome?	Autosomal dominant syndrome: • Malformed external ears • Preauricular pits • Conductive, sensorineural, or mixed hearing loss • Renal anomalies ranging from mild hypoplasia to complete agenesis
13	At which cervical vertebral level is the cricoid cartilage of an infant located? Does this location change as the child grows?	The fourth cervical vertebra The cricoid descends to the level of the seventh cervical vertebra by adulthood.
14	Why is the thyroid notch not a palpable landmark for tracheotomy in infants?	Infants have a shortened thyrohyoid membrane, so the hyoid bone is located anterior to the thyroid notch, obscuring the thyroid notch as a landmark for tracheotomy.
15	What is the diameter of the subglottis in a full-term infant?	5 to 7 mm (< 4 mm indicates a subglottic stenosis)
16	What are the dimensions of the trachea in a full-term infant?	4 cm long × 6 mm wide.
17	What is the ratio of cartilaginous to membranous trachea?	4.5:1
18	What additional anomaly should be actively looked for in a patient who has a complete vascular ring?	Vascular sling
19	Describe how infants maintain a nasopharyngeal airway while suckling.	The more superior cervical position of the larynx allows overlap of the epiglottis and the soft palate, which allows the flow of milk or formula to be channeled around the dorsum of the tongue and laterally around the epiglottis, thus protecting the airway.
20	What is the first paranasal sinus to develop embryologically?	The maxillary sinuses begin developing at 3 weeks of fetal life and are partially pneumatized at birth. They reach full adult size by age 16 years.
21	What is the last sinus to undergo pneumatization?	Frontal sinuses Earliest pneumatization occurs at or shortly after age 2 years.
22	When do the inner ear structures reach full adult size?	The inner ear structures begin developing at 4 weeks' gestation and reach adult size by 6 months' gestation.
23	At what age would you expect to see inner ear malformations develop in a fetus?	Between 4 and 13 weeks' gestation (first trimester)
24	When does the auricle achieve the adult form?	~ 18 weeks gestation. However, it continues to grow in childhood with changes continuing into late adult life. Adult width and length are achieved at different times. Width: age 6 years in females, age 7 in males. Length: 12 in females, 13 in males); 90% of adult size achieved by age 5

25	Orbital size is what percentage of the adult size at birth?	60 to 65%. This is also the case for the length and width of the cranium. The optic nerve and eye are extensions of the brain and follow brain growth (reaches adult size by 2 or 3 years) rather than growth of the facial skeleton.

Association Syndromes and Sequences

26	What anomalies are included in the CHARGE association?	**C** Coloboma **H** Heart defect **A** Atresia, choanal **R** Retarded growth and development **G** Genital hypoplasia **E** Ear anomalies/hearing loss
27	What are poor prognostic factors in patients with CHARGE association?	Midline malformations, esophageal atresia, and bilateral choanal atresia
28	What head and neck anomalies are related to the CHARGE association?	Choanal atresia, ear abnormalities and hearing loss, facial nerve palsy, pharyngoesophageal dysmotility, laryngomalacia, vocal-cord paralysis or paresis, obstructive sleep apnea, tracheoesophageal fistula, and gastroesophageal reflux. Temporal bone abnormalities, such as hypoplasia of the semicircular canals and Mondini malformation can also occur.
29	What gene is involved in the CHARGE association?	*CHD7* gene (member of the chromodomain helicase DNA protein family), chromosome 8q12 in 75% of patients with CHARGE association
30	What is the incidence of choanal atresia in patients with CHARGE association?	>65%, >2/3 bilateral. If unilateral, left>right
31	What does VACTERL association stand for?	**V** Vertebral defects **A** Anal atresia **C** Cardiac malformations **TE** Tracheoesophageal fistula with esophageal atresia **R** Renal dysplasia **L** Limb anomalies (most commonly radial anomalies)
32	What percentage of patients with VACTERL association have a tracheoesophageal fistula?	50 to 80%
33	What are the major clinical characteristics in patients with velocardiofacial syndrome?	Clefting of the secondary palate, hypernasal speech, pharyngeal hypotonia, structural heart anomalies, dysmorphic facial appearance, slender hands and fingers, and learning disabilities
34	What chromosomal anomaly is associated with velocardiofacial syndrome?	About 80 to 100% have a hemizygous deletion of chromosome 22q11.
35	What factors lead to velopharyngeal insufficiency in patients with velocardiofacial syndrome?	Cleft palate (occult submucous cleft, overt submucous cleft or soft palate cleft), hypotonia of the pharyngeal muscles, platybasia (an obtuse angulation of the cranial base), and a small adenoid pad
36	Why do most patients with velocardiofacial syndrome have chronic otitis media and conductive hearing loss despite having a small adenoid pad?	Abnormal craniofacial anatomy, cleft palate, and associated eustachian tube dysfunction
37	What evaluation must be done when performing a pharyngeal flap on a patient with velocardiofacial syndrome? Why?	Nasopharyngoscopy (look for pulsations in the posterior or lateral pharyngeal walls), computed tomography angiography (CTA), or magnetic resonance angiography (MRA); 25 to 30% have medial displacement of their internal carotid arteries.
38	What autosomal dominant syndrome is most likely in a child with lower-lip pits, cleft lip, and/or cleft palate?	Van der Woude syndrome

39	Describe lower-lip pits in van der Woude syndrome.	Usually bilateral paramedian sinuses in the lower lips placed symmetrically on either side of midline. They can also be median, paramedian, or unilateral (usually left). A single median or paramedian lower lip pit is considered an incomplete expression of the trait.
40	Describe the embryologic formation of lower-lip pits as seen in van der Woude syndrome.	The lower lip of a 32-day embryo consists of four growth centers divided by one median and two lateral grooves. In the 38-day embryo, the lateral grooves disappear unless there is impeded mandibular growth, which results in the formation of a lower lip pit.
41	What are the clinical features of Stickler syndrome?	Typical facial characteristics (micrognathia leading to Pierre Robin sequence), hypermobility, and enlargement of joints associated with the onset of arthritis in early adulthood, myopia, retinal detachment, cataracts, and hearing loss
42	What is the genetic mutation in Stickler syndrome?	Mutations in the *COL2A1*, *COL9A1*, *COL11A1*, and *COL11A2* genes cause Stickler syndrome. These genes are involved in the production of type II, type IX, and type XI collagen, which are components of vitreous, cartilage, and other connective tissues.
43	What are the different types of Stickler syndrome, and what are the associated genetic mutations?	• Type 1 (autosomal dominant) are mutations in the *COL2A1* gene and are the most common. • Type 2 (autosomal dominant) are mutations in the *COL11A1* gene. • Type 3 (autosomal dominant) are mutations in the *COL11A2* gene. No ocular abnormalities because *COL11A2* is not present in the vitreous. • Type 4 (autosomal recessive) are mutations in *COL9A1*.
44	What are the clinical findings in Pierre Robin sequence?	Micrognathia, glossoptosis, and wide U-shaped cleft palate, leading to upper airway obstruction and feeding difficulties
45	Describe the embryology of Pierre Robin sequence.	Arrest in mandibular development at 7 to 11 weeks of gestation (micrognathia) causes the tongue to set abnormally high and posteriorly in the oral cavity (glossoptosis). This prevents fusion of the palatal shelves at week 11 and results in a U-shaped cleft palate.
46	What are the most common syndromes associated with Pierre Robin sequence?	• Stickler syndrome (most common) • Treacher Collins syndrome • Velocardiofacial syndrome • Fetal alcohol syndrome • Möbius syndrome • Nager syndrome • Beckwith-Wiedemann syndrome
47	How often is Pierre Robin sequence associated with a syndrome?	80% (20% isolated)
48	Discuss the treatment options for upper-airway obstruction in patients with Pierre Robin sequence.	• 70%: Positioning alone (i.e., prone positioning) • 20%: Nasopharyngeal airway, mandibular distraction osteogenesis (gaining popularity), tongue-lip adhesion (being performed less commonly) • 10%: Tracheostomy

Disorders of the Salivary Gland

49	Discuss the causes of acute suppurative sialadenitis in premature neonates.	• Reduction in salivary flow • Immunologic immaturity • Presence of bacteria in the oral cavity of neonates • Dehydration • Prolonged orogastric feeding • Congenital anomalies of the floor of the mouth

50	What is the treatment for acute suppurative sialadenitis in premature neonates?	Hydration and antimicrobial therapy should lead to a response within 48 to 72 hours. Gland manipulation should be avoided in a preterm child to reduce the risk of systemic septicemia. If no satisfactory improvement is seen, incision and drainage are recommended.
51	What are the causes of pediatric viral sialadenitis?	Epstein-Barr virus, parainfluenza viruses, adenovirus, human herpes virus–6, human immunodeficiency virus (HIV), Coxsackievirus, mumps virus, and influenza virus
52	What organ systems are involved in patients with mumps?	Parotid and submandibular glands (diffuse tender enlargement), gonads, pancreas, and meninges
53	What is the classic triad of symptoms seen with infectious mononucleosis?	About 80% of patients have the triad of fever, sore throat, and posterior cervical adenopathy that can involve the periparotid or perifacial (submandibular) lymph nodes with subsequent involvement of adjacent glands.
54	Discuss the clinical findings of human immunodeficiency virus (HIV)-associated benign lymphoepithelial cysts.	They occur in up to 10% of HIV-positive children, often early in the course of HIV infection with slowly progressive, asymptomatic parotid gland enlargement and often associated with cervical lymphadenopathy. Cysts are usually bilateral (up to 80%), multiple (up to 90%), and involve the superficial lobe.
55	What are the most common pathologies causing granulomatous inflammation of the major salivary glands?	Actinomycosis, tuberculosis, atypical mycobacterial infections, and sarcoidosis
56	What bacteria are associated with nontuberculous mycobacterial infections of the salivary glands?	*Mycobacterium avium-intracellulare* (70 to 90% of cases), *M. bovis*, *M. kansasii*, and *M. scrofulaceum*
57	What pathology is thought to be a form of sarcoidosis characterized by uveitis, parotid enlargement, and facial paralysis?	Heerfordt syndrome (or uveoparotid fever). Its symptoms include fever, malaise, weakness, nausea, and night sweats. Evaluation includes chest radiography looking for hilar adenopathy and an acetylcholinesterase level. A biopsy from the lip or tail of the parotid may confirm the diagnosis.
58	What pathology is characterized by recurrent episodes of nonobstructive, nonsuppurative unilateral (60%) or bilateral (40%) parotid inflammation in a 5-year-old boy?	Juvenile recurrent parotitis (JRP). The peak incidence is between the ages of 3 and 6 years, with predominance in boys. Diagnosis is made on a clinical basis and is confirmed by ultrasonography or sialography, which shows pathognomonic sialectasias (intraductal cystlike dilations).
59	What are the medical treatment options for sialorrhea?	• Oral motor training: Exercises are done to encourage swallowing, improve muscle tone and oral sensation, stabilize body and head position, promote jaw stability and lip closure, and decrease tongue thrust. • Behavioral therapy: Verbal and auditory cues can increase the frequency and efficiency of swallowing. • Anticholinergic pharmacotherapy, oral glycopyrrolate, botulinum toxin injections into major salivary glands may decrease the volume of saliva.
60	What are the surgical treatment options for sialorrhea?	• Submandibular gland excision* • Submandibular duct rerouting * • Parotid duct rerouting* • Sublingual gland excision • Ligation of parotid ducts • Transtympanic bilateral tympanic plexus neurectomy and bilateral chorda tympani nerve section • Any combination of these procedures *Highest rates of success
61	What are the most common benign pediatric tumors of the parotid gland?	Parotid gland hemangiomas constitute 50% of pediatric parotid gland tumors.

| 62 | Discuss the development and natural history of pediatric parotid gland hemangiomas. | These hemangiomas may be part of a segmental V3 hemangioma, or they may be isolated focal hemangiomas. They occur at birth or shortly thereafter and act like other hemangiomas, undergoing a rapid proliferative growth phase followed by involution. |
| 63 | What is the first-line treatment for parotid hemangiomas? (▶ Fig. 1.2) | Oral propranolol therapy |

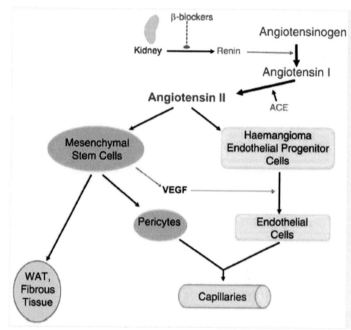

Fig. 1.2 Proposed mechanism of action of propranolol on hemangioma endothelial cell proliferation and differentiation, through blockage of renin production. (Used with permission from Itinteang T, Brasch HD, Tan ST, Day DJ. Journal of Plastic, Reconstructive 64(6):759-765.51.)

Nose and Sinus

64	What are the two most common maxillofacial fractures in children?	Nasal bone and mandibular fractures
65	If a child develops a septal hematoma after sustaining a nasal fracture and subsequently develops a septal abscess, what nasal deformity might the child develop later in life?	Saddle nose deformity, deformed columella or nasal base
66	What must be considered in the performance of a complete examination of a child who has sustained a significant nasal injury?	Sedation
67	What is the key factor that differentiates the treatment of nasal trauma in pediatric patients compared with adult patients?	Ongoing facial growth
68	Why do infants diagnosed with an obstructive septal deviation after nasal trauma require urgent evaluation?	They are obligate nasal breathers.
69	When should pediatric nasal fractures be reduced?	Reduction should be done either within 3 to 6 hours of injury, before the onset of swelling, or 3 to 10 days after the injury. If immediate reduction cannot be performed, the fractures should be evaluated 3 to 7 days after the injury, when edema has subsided.

70	What is the differential diagnosis for a congenital midline nasal mass?	• Dermoid (most common) • Glioma • Encephalocele • Epidermoid cysts • Hemangiomas • Teratomas • Neurofibromas • Lipomas • Lymphangiomas
71	Name the midline nasal epithelial-lined cyst, sinus, or tract that forms as a result of regression of the embryologic neuroectodermal tract, pulling skin elements into the prenasal space.	Nasal dermoid forms and contains keratin debris, hair follicles, sebaceous glands, and sweat glands.
72	What are the clinical findings in a patient with a nasal dermoid cyst?	• It occurs more often in male than in female patients. • Noncompressible mass. • Furstenberg sign is negative (i.e., no enlargement with compression of the jugular veins); it is firm and nontender. • It does not transilluminate. • The cyst is located in the midline, most commonly along the dorsum, resulting in a widened dorsum. • Cyst can be intranasal, extranasal, or intracranial. • It may have a sinus opening with intermittent discharge of sebaceous material. • Hair protrudes through a punctum, is pathognomonic, but not commonly seen.
73	How often do nasal dermoids extend intracranially?	In ~ 25% of cases, they most often communicate through the foramen cecum or the cribriform plate to the base of the frontal fossa with extradural adherence to the falx cerebri and are associated with an increased risk of meningitis.
74	What radiographic findings suggest a nasal dermoid with intracranial extension?	• Bifid crista galli • Enlarged foramen cecum
75	Discuss the treatment of nasal dermoids.	• Treatment involves complete surgical excision. Approaches vary depending on presence of intracranial extension, and recurrence is common. • Extracranial approach: Vertical midline incision, transverse incision, lateral rhinotomy, external rhinoplasty, inverted-U incision, and degloving procedures • Combined approach: Extracranial approach combined with a frontal craniotomy
76	What congenital nasal anomaly consists of ectopic glial tissue that lacks a patent cerebrospinal fluid (CSF) communication to the subarachnoid space but in 15 to 20% maintains a fibrous affiliation?	Nasal gliomas
77	How do nasal gliomas form?	Theories about formation: • Abnormal closure of fronticulus frontalis, isolating the brain tissue from the intracranial cavity • Nidus of ectopic neuroepithelia • An outgrowth of olfactory tissue through the cribriform plate

78	What is the clinical presentation of nasal gliomas?	*Extranasal gliomas* (60%) are smooth, firm, noncompressible masses that occur most commonly at the glabella, although they may arise along the side of the nose or the nasomaxillary suture line. *Intranasal gliomas* (30%) are polypoid pale masses that arise from the lateral nasal wall near the middle turbinate and occasionally from the nasal septum and can protrude from the nostril. *Combined* (10%) *Intracranial extension* (15%)
79	What congenital nasal anomaly consists of an extracranial herniation of the cranial contents through a defect in the skull? Meninges only? Brain matter and meninges?	Encephalocele, meningocele, and meningoencephalocele, respectively
80	How are nasal encephaloceles classified?	Location of the skull base defect: • *Sincipital* (60%): Arise between the frontal and ethmoid bones at the foramen cecum, immediately anterior to the cribriform plate. • *Basal* (40%): Arise between the cribriform plate and the superior orbital fissure or posterior clinoid fissure. *Note:* The most common congenital encephaloceles are occipital (75%).
81	What are the subtypes of sincipital encephaloceles?	• *Nasofrontal*: Defect is located at the glabella between the nasal and frontal bones. • *Nasoethmoidal*: Sac exits through the foramen cecum, passing under the nasal bones and above the upper lateral cartilages, creating a lateral nasal mass. • *Nasoorbital*: Sac transverses the foramen cecum before extending into the orbit via a defect in its medial wall.
82	What are the subtypes of basal encephaloceles?	• *Transethmoidal*: Sac extends medial to the superior turbinate via a cribriform plate defect. • *Sphenoethmoidal*: Sac protrudes into the nasopharynx via a defect between the posterior ethmoid and the *anterior sphenoid wall.* • *Transsphenoidal*: Sac also is seen in the nasopharynx, exiting intracranially through an open craniopharyngeal canal. • *Sphenoorbital*: It protrudes through the superior orbital fissure and out the inferior orbital fissure into the sphenopalatine fossa.
83	What are the common clinical findings associated with encephaloceles?	• Bluish/red mass that is soft, compressible • (Positive) Furstenburg test (expands with compression of internal jugular vein) • Pulsatile • Does transilluminate
84	What imaging is best for the diagnosis and surgical planning for an encephalocele?	CT and MRI
85	Why is surgical repair the treatment of choice for encephaloceles?	To prevent CSF leak, meningitis, and brain herniation
86	Describe the four hypotheses that have been offered to explain the development of choanal atresia.	• Buccopharyngeal membrane persistence • Abnormal neural crest cell migration • Bucconasal membrane persistence • Adhesion formation in the nasochoanal region as a result of abnormal mesoderm

87	What are the clinical features of choanal atresia?	<ul><li>1:5,000 to 8,000 live births</li><li>75% unilateral, right > left</li><li>Female-to-male ratio: 2:1</li><li>50% of patients with unilateral atresia and up to 75% of patients with bilateral atresia have other associated congenital anomalies.</li><li>Bony 30%, membranous 70%</li></ul>
88	What are the anatomic features of choanal atresia?	<ul><li>A narrow nasal cavity</li><li>Lateral bony obstruction by the pterygoid plates</li><li>Medial obstruction caused by thickening of the vomer</li><li>Membranous or bony obstruction</li></ul>
89	What syndromes are associated with choanal atresia?	<ul><li>CHARGE association</li><li>*FGFR*-related craniosynostosis syndromes (e.g., Crouzon syndrome, Pfeiffer syndrome, Apert syndrome, Jackson-Weiss syndrome, Muenke syndrome, Antley-Bixler syndrome)</li><li>Down syndrome</li><li>Treacher-Collins syndrome</li><li>Solitary medianmaxillary central incisor syndrome</li></ul>
90	At what age are most infants no longer obligate nasal breathers?	6 to 9 months
91	You are called emergently to evaluate a newborn in respiratory distress. On evaluation, you note cyanotic episodes relieved by crying. Examination is otherwise benign, and the medical history shows no complications. What is the most likely diagnosis?	Bilateral choanal atresia
92	How does unilateral choanal atresia commonly manifest?	Typically it is not seen until the patient is aged 5 to 24 months or a young adult as a result of unilateral nasal obstruction or rhinorrhea.
93	You suspect possible choanal atresia in a newborn with respiratory distress. What physical examination maneuver can be used to help determine whether choanal atresia is present?	One can attempt to pass a nasogastric tube or small catheter (< 8 French, generally a 5/6 French is used) through the nose. If it does not pass, the presence of choanal atresia is suspected and further workup is required.
94	What is the definitive diagnostic test for choanal atresia?	CT scan
95	What three surgical approaches can be considered for the treatment of choanal atresia?	<ul><li>Transpalatal</li><li>Transnasal: puncture (Fearon)</li><li>Endoscopic endonasal (transnasal, transoral, combined); puncture, drill, dilation</li></ul>
96	What symptoms might suggest congenital nasal pyriform aperture stenosis (CNPAS)?	Respiratory distress, poor feeding, failure to thrive, and recurrent cycles of cyanosis and apnea
97	What causes CNPAS?	CNPAS occurs secondary to bony overgrowth of the medial nasal process of the maxilla into the nasal aperture resulting in a pyriform aperture smaller than 11 mm.
98	What congenital anomalies are associated with CNPAS?	<ul><li>*Holoprosencephaly* (HPE): Clinical features include facial dysmorphisms such as ocular hypotelorism, midline cleft lip and/or flat nose, cerebral malformations, learning disabilities, arrhinencephaly, agenesis of the corpus callosum, hypopituitarism, single maxillary central incisor.</li><li>*Solitary median maxillary central incisor syndrome* (SMMCI): Clinical features include severe to mild intellectual disability, congenital heart disease, cleft lip and/or palate and less frequently, microcephaly, hypopituitarism, hypotelorism, convergent strabismus, esophageal and duodenal atresia, cervical hemivertebrae, cervical dermoid, hypothyroidism, scoliosis, absent kidney, micropenis, and ambiguous genitalia.</li></ul>

99	What are the treatment options for CNPAS?	• Nonoperative management: Nasal trumpets, topical steroids, and vasoconstrictive drops may be attempted until growth results in increased nasal airway size. • Operative management: A sublabial approach is done to expose the inferior and lateral pyriform aperture. A small diamond burr is then used to widen the bony lateral and inferior margins.
100	What are the features of complete agenesis of the nose (arrhinia)?	• Absence of the external nose, nasal airways, and olfactory apparatus • Hypoplasia of the maxilla • A small high-arched palate • Hypertelorism
101	What are the possible causes of congenital anosmia?	• Most commonly autosomal dominant • Defective transportation of odorants to the olfactory neuroepithelium as a result of congenital malformations in the nasal cavity • Disrupted signal transduction or signal propagation • Malformation of regions in the brain essential for olfaction
102	What syndromes are associated with congenital anosmia?	• Kallmann syndrome • Congenital insensitivity to pain • Ciliopathies including Bardet-Biedl syndrome and Leber congenital amaurosis
103	Where is the most common site of obstruction causing nasolacrimal duct cysts (dacrocystoceles)?	Inferior meatus (membrane of Hasner). *Note:* Recanalization of the nasolacrimal duct occurs from the lacrimal system inferiorly.
104	What symptoms are associated with nasolacrimal duct cysts (dacrocystoceles)?	Epiphora (tearing), nasal obstruction, respiratory distress in neonates (obligate nasal breathers), aspiration, feeding difficulty
105	What are common physical examination findings that suggest nasolacrimal duct cyst (dacrocystocele)?	Bluish swelling of the skin overlying the nasolacrimal duct, cyst in the inferior meatus, superior displacement of the medial canthal tendon, and epiphora
106	What is the first-line therapy for a nasolacrimal duct cyst?	Massage
107	When should you offer surgical intervention for a nasolacrimal duct cyst (dacrocystocele)?	Infant with significant symptoms (i.e., feeding difficulty, infection, or respiratory difficulty)
108	What is the surgical treatment of nasolacrimal duct cysts (dacrocystoceles)?	Endoscopic marsupialization (opening the cyst into the inferior meatus). Ophthalmologist may need to probe duct and possibly place stents to ensure patency.
109	During week 4 of development, a pouch forms along the dorsal stomodeum. During the week 5, the infundibular stalk and this pouch come into contact and the opening of the pouch is occluded at the buccopharyngeal junction and is separated from the oral cavity by week 6. The pituitary gland then develops from the anterior wall of the pouch (pars distalis) and a small portion of the posterior wall of the pouch (pars intermedia). Normally, the remnant pouch lumen is obliterated; if not, what is this condition called?	Rathke cleft/pouch cyst

110	Describe the characteristics of a Rathke pouch cyst.	Non-neoplastic, sellar/suprasellar epithelial lined cyst (sella turcica). Most often they are small and asymptomatic.
111	How do Rathke pouch cysts most commonly manifest?	During the fifth to sixth decade of life, female predominance. They are usually asymptomatic, but large lesions may cause visual disturbance, pituitary dysfunction, and/or headaches. They can be seen on MRI.
112	A tumor derived from a Rathke pouch is called what?	Craniopharyngioma
113	What benign cyst/bursa can form in the cleavage plane between the nasal cavity and pharynx (Rathke pouch, notochord remnant) as a result of obstruction, inflammation, or infection of the pharyngeal bursa?	Thornwaldt cyst
114	What symptoms are most commonly associated with a Thornwaldt cyst?	None. Occasionally patients complain of postnasal drip with intermittent drainage of the cyst or halitosis. If the cyst enlarges or becomes infected, nasal obstruction or eustachian ET dysfunction can result.
115	How are Thornwaldt cysts treated?	If the diagnosis is clear, observation and reassurance are recommended. If cysts are dark-colored from hemorrhage or hemosiderin, consider biopsy after obtaining an MRI to rule out intracranial communication. If symptomatic, they can be surgically removed, taking care to remove the entire cysts, which can extend to the prevertebral fascia.
116	During a routine examination, you note a smooth, mucus-covered mass within the adenoid pad. Imaging reveals a rhomboid-shaped cyst with no bony or intracranial communication. What is the likely cause?	Intra-adenoidal cyst
117	What causes are associated with pediatric sinusitis?	• Immature immune system • Small developing sinuses • Viral upper respiratory infections • Allergy/allergic rhinitis • Immunodeficiency • Gastroesophageal reflux disease • Cystic fibrosis
118	What are the diagnostic criteria for pediatric acute bacterial sinusitis?	Clinical diagnosis can be made when a child has an acute upper respiratory infection (URI) and the following (American Academy of Pediatrics [AAP] clinical guidelines, 2013) symptoms: • Persistent illness (i.e., nasal discharge of any quality or daytime cough or both lasting more than 10 days without improvement) or • Worsening course (i.e. new onset of nasal discharge, daytime cough, or fever after initial improvement) or • Severe onset (i.e., concurrent fever with temperature ≥ 39°C or 102.2°F) and purulent nasal discharge for at least 3 consecutive days (Evidence Quality: B, Recommendation)
119	What are the predominant pathogens in pediatric acute sinusitis?	*Streptococcus pneumoniae* (25 to 30%) *Haemophilus influenzae* (15 to 20%) *Moraxella catarrhalis* (15 to 20%)

120	When should imaging be obtained in the evaluation of child in whom acute bacterial sinusitis is suspected?	Only if there is concern for orbital or intracranial involvement
121	When should a clinician recommend antibiotic therapy instead of supportive care (nasal irrigation, intranasal corticosteroids, topical or oral decongestants, mucolytics, and/or topical or oral antihistamines) and close observation for a child with presumed acute bacterial sinusitis?	AAP clinical practice guidelines, 2013: • Severe onset and worsening course (signs, symptoms, or both) (Quality of Evidence B, Strong Recommendation) or • No improvement after a 3-day course of observation with persistent illness (nasal discharge of any quality or • Cough or both for at least 10 days without improvement) (Quality of Evidence: B, Recommendation)
122	What three risk factors are likely to increase the resistance of organisms to amoxicillin in both acute bacterial sinusitis and acute otitis media?	AAP clinical practice guidelines, 2013 • Day care or child care attendance • Antibiotic treatment within the previous 30 days • Age < 2 years
123	What antibiotic(s) should be considered for children with acute bacterial sinusitis?	• Amoxicillin ± clavulanate. Duration varies: continue 7 days after resolution of symptoms. • Standard-dose amoxicillin (45 mg/kg daiy divided into two doses): Mild to moderate severity illness in a child who does not attend day care, has not been treated with antibiotics in the previous 30 days, and whose age is > 2 years. • High-dose amoxicillin (80 to 90 mg/kg daily divided in two doses, maximum 2 g/day): In communities with a > 10% incidence of *S. pneumoniae* resistance • Amoxicillin-clavulanate (amoxicillin 80 to 90 mg/kg daily divided into two doses, maximum 2 g/day): Moderate to severe illness or who attend day care, have received antibiotics within 30 days, or are < 2 years of age. • Ceftriaxone (50 mg/kg dose given intramuscularly (IM) or IV) if unable to tolerate oral administration, followed by an oral antibiotic to complete therapy if improvement is noted within 24 hours. • Clindamycin = cefexime or linezolid and cefexamine or levofloxacin: If the child's condition worsens after 72 hours on high-dose augmentin • Options to consider if the child is allergic to penicillin: cefdinir, cefuroxime, cefpodoxime, clindamycin and cefexime, linezolid, or a flouroquinolone. • Inpatient IV antibiotics should be considered in pediatric patients with complicated bacterial sinusitis (AAP, 2013).
124	Describe the major complications of pediatric sinusitis.	• Orbital/periorbital inflammation from ethmoid sinuses: Preseptal cellulitis, orbital cellulitis, subperiosteal abscess, and orbital abscess • Intracranial spread from the frontal and sphenoid sinuses: Meningitis, epidural abscess, subdural empyema, intracerebral abscess, and cavernous or sagittal sinus thrombosis
125	How are orbital complications from sinusitis classified?	The Chandler Classification • Group 1: Inflammatory (preseptal) edema of eyelids without tenderness; obstruction of venous drainage; no associated visual loss or limitation of ocular movements • Group 2: Orbital cellulitis with diffuse edema of the adipose tissue in the orbital contents secondary to inflammation and bacterial infections; no abscess formation • Group 3: Subperiosteal abscess, abscess formation between the orbital periosteum and the bony orbital wall. The mass displaces the globe in the opposite direction (usually down and lateral); the proptosis may be severe with decreased ocular mobility and visual acuity. The abscess may rupture into the orbit through the orbital septum.

		• Group 4: Orbital abscess, a discrete abscess within the orbit. Proptosis is usually severe but is symmetrical and not displaced as in the subperiosteal abscess. Complete ophthalmoplegia results, and visual loss occurs in 13%. • Group 5: Cavernous sinus thrombosis; progression of the phlebitis into the cavernous sinus and to the opposite side, resulting in bilateral symptoms
126	What are the diagnostic criteria for pediatric chronic sinusitis?	American Academy of Otolaryngology (2013) • One or more symptoms of sinusitis > 12 weeks • Six or more episodes of acute sinusitis/year • Acute exacerbations without complete resolution between episodes
127	What is the role of intravenous immune serum globulin (IVIG) therapy in pediatric chronic rhinosinusitis?	IVIG may have a role in the treatment of chronic or recurrent acute sinusitis in a select group of patients whose disease is recalcitrant despite maximizing conventional medical therapy. Many believe that IVIG may not be acting as replacement therapy for a humoral immune deficiency but more so as an anti-inflammatory or immune-modulating agent that interrupts the chronic inflammatory process in patients with chronic sinusitis.
128	What conventional management options are available for chronic pediatric sinusitis?	Nasal irrigation, intranasal corticosteroids, topical/oral decongestants, mucolytics, and/or topical/oral antihistamines. Patients should also undergo a workup for allergies, reactive airway disease, headache, immunodeficiency, and cystic fibrosis as indicated.
129	Discuss the surgical options for treatment of pediatric chronic sinusitis.	• Adenoidectomy • Maxillary antral lavage • Functional endoscopic sinus surgery: middle meatal antrostomy, anterior or total ethmoidectomy
130	What are the indications for sinus surgery for pediatric sinusitis?	Absolute indications: • Complete nasal obstruction in cystic fibrosis attributable to massive polyposis or closure of the nose by medialization of the lateral nasal wall • Antrochoanal polyp • Intracranial complications • Mucoceles and mucopyoceles • Orbital abscess • Traumatic injury in the optic canal (decompression) • Dacryocystorhinitis resulting from sinusitis and resistant to appropriate medical treatment • Fungal sinusitis • Some meningoencephaloceles • Some neoplasms Relative indications: • Chronic rhinosinusitis that persists despite optimal medical management and after exclusion of any systemic disease • Optimal medical management includes 2 to 6 weeks of adequate antibiotics (IV or oral) and treatment of concomitant diseases.
131	What primary immunodeficiencies are associated with chronic sinusitis?	• Common variable immunodeficiency • Immunoglobulin (Ig)A deficiency • IgG subclass deficiencies, most commonly IgG3 deficiency (important for defense against *Moraxella catarrhalis* and *Streptococcus pyogenes*)

| 132 | Discuss the anatomical abnormalities of the sinuses in patients with cystic fibrosis. | The chronic inflammatory disease and decreased ventilation of the sinuses prevent pneumatization, resulting in diminished postnatal growth of the sinus systems already present at birth, the maxillary and ethmoid sinuses. In addition, there is a lack of development, or hypoplasia, of the frontal and sphenoid sinuses. Incidence of nasal polyposis in cystic fibrosis varies from 6 to 48% and does not usually occur before 5 years of age or after age 20. |

Neck Masses and Vascular Anomalies

133	What is the differential diagnosis for a congenital neck mass?	Lateral neck masses: • Branchial anomaly • Laryngocele • Thymic cyst • Pseudotumor of infancy Midline neck masses: • Thyroglossal duct cyst (most common midline congenital neck mass) • Dermoid cyst • Plunging ranula • Teratoma Entire neck: • Hemangioma • Lymphatic malformation
134	What congenital neck mass is most commonly seen in the first 5 years of life as a 1- to 4-cm midline cystic mass that moves cranially with tongue protrusion or swallowing and arises from the foramen cecum?	Thyroglossal duct cyst
135	Where in the neck are thyroglossal duct cysts found?	About 60% are located adjacent to the hyoid bone, 24% are between the hyoid bone and base of the tongue, 13% are between the hyoid and pyramidal lobe of the thyroid gland, and the remaining 3% are intralingual. Up to 20% of cysts are slightly off the midline, with a predilection for the left.
136	What is the cause of thyroglossal duct cysts?	Thyroglossal duct cysts form as a persistent epithelial tract during the descent of the thyroid from the foramen cecum in the base of the tongue to its final position in the anterior neck. They rarely undergo neoplastic transformation (1%).
137	Discuss the evaluation of a child in whom a thyroglossal duct cyst is suspected.	Evaluate for the presence of thyroid tissue in the cyst (45%) and whether there is functional tissue elsewhere: • Ultrasound: Median ectopic thyroid tissue would appear solid on ultrasound. • Thyroid function tests: Patients with median ectopic thyroid tissue are frequently hypothyroid, with elevated thyroid-stimulating hormone (TSH) levels and resultant hypertrophy of the ectopic thyroid tissue. • Thyroid scintiscan: This test is performed if the preceding tests indicate the presence of a median ectopic thyroid to determine whether there is functional thyroid tissue in the cyst and elsewhere.
138	What is the procedure for removal of a thyroglossal duct cyst?	Sistrunk procedure: Stresses removal of the central portion of the hyoid bone associated with the thyroglossal duct tract to decrease the risk of recurrence and removal of the tract to the level of the base of tongue.

139	What is the clinical presentation of a cervical thymic cyst?	Most occur in the first decade of life as a lateral neck mass, anterior to the SCM, most commonly to the left; 80 to 90% are asymptomatic. However, they may enlarge because of hemorrhage or infection and cause dysphagia, pain, dysphonia, and dyspnea. They are also known to expand with the Valsalva maneuver.
140	What are the possible causes of a cervical thymic cyst?	• Incomplete descent of the thymus into the chest • Sequestration of thymic tissue foci along the descent path into the chest • Failure of the thymopharyngeal duct to involute
141	What is the difference between congenital and acquired thymic cysts?	• *Congenital*: These cysts are usually unilobular and originate from persistent rudiments of the thymopharyngeal duct. They may have epithelium derived from the thyroid and parathyroid glands because of their close association during development. • *Acquired*: Cysts are multilobular and develop from degenerated Hassall corpuscles (degenerated epithelial cells); they are associated with Sjogren syndrome, apalastic anemia, and acquired immunodeficiency syndrome (AIDS).
142	What congenital neck mass is a germ cell tumor made up of ectodermal and mesodermal elements but has no endodermal elements?	A dermoid cyst, which can contain hair follicles, smooth muscle, fibroadipose tissue, and sebaceous glands
143	Where do dermoid cysts form?	Along the lines of embryonic fusion
144	How are head and neck dermoid cysts categorized?	They are categorized by location: • Periorbital region: Most common in the head and neck; develop along the naso-optic groove between the maxillary and mandibular processes • Nasal dorsum: Develop during ossification of the fronto-nasal plate • Submentum/floor of mouth: Region of fusion of the first and second branchial arches in the midline, most common location in the neck • Suprasternal, thyroidal, and suboccipital regions
145	On clinical examination, how can dermoid cysts be differentiated from thyroglossal duct cysts?	Both most commonly present as painless midline neck masses. Because of their superficial location and lack of mesodermal attachments, dermoid cysts do not move with tongue protrusion or swallowing. Infection of dermoid cysts is also rare because they have no communication with the oropharynx.
146	What is the treatment for dermoid cysts?	Surgical excision. If cervical and cannot exclude the presence of a thyroglossal duct cyst, consider a Sistrunk procedure.
147	What congenital anomaly arises from embryonic germinal epithelium of all three types: ectoderm, mesoderm, and endoderm?	Teratoma
148	What prenatal findings may indicate a cervical teratoma?	Maternal polyhydramnios: Often diagnosed during the prenatal or early neonatal period
149	Where do teratomas occur within the head and neck?	Neck (most common), nasopharynx, oropharynx, and oral cavity

150	What is the EXIT procedure?	The ex utero intrapartum treatment (EXIT) procedure is a technique used to establish an airway in neonates with airway compression from congenital anomalies diagnosed prenatally. It involves establishing an airway while the fetoplacental circulation is preserved. The fetus is partially delivered via a cesarean section, and the airway is then secured while the fetus remains attached by its umbilical cord to the placenta.
151	What abnormal dilation or herniation of the saccule of the larynx can result in an air- (most often), mucus-, or pus-filled congenital neck mass, respectively?	Laryngocele, laryngomucocele, laryngopyocele, respectively
152	What is the difference between an internal and external laryngocele?	• Internal: Dilation lies within the limits of the thyroid cartilage and is seen as cystic swelling of the aryepiglottic fold. • External: Dilation extends beyond the thyroid cartilage in a cephalad direction to protrude through the thyrohyoid membrane. • Combination: These can have internal and external components.
153	What benign congenital neck mass presents as a firm, round, nontender mass seen at the junction of the upper and middle third of the SCM that typically presents 2 to 3 weeks after birth?	Pseudotumor of infancy. Also called sternocleidomastoid tumor of infancy, fibromatosis coli, or congenital muscular torticollis.
154	What is the natural history of a pseudotumor of infancy?	It is present 2 to 3 weeks after birth, slowly increases in size for 2 to 3 months, and then slowly regresses for 4–8 months; 80 to 100% completely resolve by 12 months. Some benefit is derived from physical therapy.
155	What salivary gland is most commonly associated with a plunging ranula?	Sublingual gland
156	How do plunging ranulae most often manifest?	Intraoral component appears as a blue dome-shaped lesion in the floor of mouth, usually on either side of the midline. The extraoral portion is seen as a submental mass extending along the inferior border of one side of the mandible. It is not a true cyst.
157	What are the treatment options for plunging ranulae?	• Intraoral incision and marsupialization of cyst • Intraoral excision with removal of sublingual gland (preferred) • External cervical approach to identify the cyst, with dissection through the mylohyoid muscle. In combination, excision of the sublingual gland can be performed via an intraoral approach. • OK-432 intralesional sclerotherapy
158	How do vascular malformations differ clinically from hemangiomas?	Hemangiomas are typically absent at birth, appear during infancy, undergo rapid growth within the first year of life, and then undergo a variable period of involution. Most vascular malformations are present at birth, demonstrate growth parallel to the child's development, and do not involute over time.

159	How are vascular malformations classified?	Based on the rate of blood flow: • Low-flow lesions: Capillary malformations, venous malformations, lymphatic malformations, and a combined type that has a mixture of either two or three of the low-flow lesions • High-flow lesions: Arterial malformations and arteriovenous malformations
160	What type of malformation is located in the cutaneous superficial vascular plexus, is made up of capillary and postcapillary venules, and grows with the individual, typically becoming darker, nodular, and occasionally leading to hypertrophy of the underlying soft and hard tissues (which can lead to disfigurement)?	Capillary malformation (vascular malformation). Also known as a port-wine stain, it is commonly associated with Sturge-Weber syndrome.
161	What syndrome commonly manifests with a triad of facial dermal capillary malformation, ipsilateral central nervous system vascular malformation (leptomeningeal angiomatosis), and vascular malformation of the choroid in the eye associated with glaucoma?	Sturge-Weber syndrome
162	How are capillary malformations treated?	The superficial component can be treated with laser photocoagulation with the pulsed-dye laser (585-nm wavelength). Surgery ranging from simple excision of bleeding nodules to wide resection of hypertrophic tissues with soft tissue reconstruction may be used to treat long-standing capillary malformations.
163	Describe the manifestation of a capillary malformation.	Also termed port-wine stain, they are the most common vascular malformation, are present at birth, and grow in proportion to body development. They initially appear red and flat and over time may become more purple. They rarely involute.
164	What congenital lesion manifests as a bluish discoloration of the skin or mucosa with a soft and compressible deep component, which can swell with Valsalva maneuver or dependent positioning and has no associated thrill or pulse on examination?	Venous malformation
165	Where do venous malformations commonly occur in the head and neck?	Lips and cheeks. Intraosseous venous malformations ("soap bubble" on radiographs) can occur in the mandible, maxilla, zygoma, or calvarium.
166	What is the relationship between venous malformations and coagulopathy?	Venous malformations are commonly associated with coagulopathy resulting from the tortuous vessels, abnormal endothelium, and the low-flow characteristics. Tissue thrombosis can be detected as calcified phleboliths on plain radiographs or CT scans, as well as elevated D-dimer in the blood, and often leads to acute and chronic swelling and pain in the affected area.
167	Discuss the treatment options for venous malformations.	Surgical resection of well-circumscribed lesions, percutaneous sclerotherapy as a primary treatment modality or adjunct to surgery, and laser therapy, including pulsed-dye laser, noncontact neodymium-yttrium-aluminum (Nd:YAG) or potassium titanyl phosphate (KTP) lasers

168	How do lymphatic malformations in the head and neck manifest?	About 90% are diagnosed before age 2. They often appear as an intraoral mass or neck mass that is nontender and may cause functional concerns, such as difficulty with speech or swallowing or respiratory concerns. They can rapidly enlarge after infection or trauma caused by bleeding or swelling and may be diagnosed in utero during routine prenatal screening.
169	How are lymphatic malformations classified?	Based on the size of the cystic component: • Macrocystic: Single or multiple cysts at least 2-cm large • Microcystic: Cysts smaller than 2 cm • Mixed lesions: At least a 50% macrocystic component
170	How are cervicofacial lymphatic malformations staged?	• Stage I: Unilateral, infrahyoid • Stage II: Unilateral, suprahyoid • Stage III: Unilateral, infrahyoid and suprahyoid • Stage IV: Bilateral infrahyoid • Stage V: Bilateral infrahyoid and suprahyoid
171	What is the relationship between the type of lymphatic malformation and its anatomical location?	• Facial lymphatic malformations lateral to the lateral canthal line tend to be macrocystic, whereas medial midfacial lesions tend to be more mixed. • Midface involvement is uncommon and usually is completely microcystic. • Neck lymphatic malformations are divided into *infrahyoid* and *suprahyoid*. • *Infrahyoid disease* is generally macrocystic and suprahyoid disease is more likely to be *microcystic*.
172	Discuss the treatment modalities for lymphatic malformations.	• Surgical resection is most successful in macrocystic lesions of the posteroinferior neck and parotid regions. Microcystic and mixed suprahyoid lesions may require subtotal resection while preserving vital structures. • Percutaneous sclerotherapy (e.g., doxycycline, OK-432) may be used as primary control of macrocystic lesions and as an adjunct to subtotal resection of mixed lesions. • Carbon dioxide laser resurfacing can be used to control mucosal microcystic lesions. • Sclerotherapy with OK-432, a lyophilized, low-virulence strain of *Streptococcus pyogenes*, is best for unilateral macrocystic lesions in the infrahyoid area. • Observation: Unilocular or nearly unilocular lesions, especially if they are located in the posteroinferior neck, may spontaneously resolve.
173	What pathology results from high-flow vascular malformations that arise from a nidus of blood vessels that have abnormal precapillary communication between arteries and veins?	Arteriovenous malformations (AVMs)
174	Describe the presentation of an AVM.	It is present since birth but often expands with trauma or hormonal changes and is often warm and red or blue with an audible bruit and palpable thrill.
175	Describe the staging system for AV malformations (AVMs).	Schobinger staging system • Stage I (quiescence): Pink-bluish stain, warmth, and AV shunting on Doppler ultrasound • Stage II (expansion): Stage I plus enlargement, pulsations, thrill, bruit, and tortuous/tense veins • Stage III (destruction): Stage II plus dystrophic skin changes, ulceration, bleeding, persistent pain, or tissue necrosis. Bony lytic lesions may occur. • Stage IV (decompensation): Stage III, plus congestive heart failure with increased cardiac output and left ventricle hypertrophy

176	What are the imaging characteristics of AVMs?	• MRI: No enhancement on T2-weighted images and flow voids on both T1-weighted and T2-weighted images • Angiography: Dilatation and lengthening of arteries and early shunting of enlarged veins • CT: Skeletal involvement
177	Describe the treatment of AVMs.	The best chance at cure is a combination of endovascular embolization and surgical resection. The target for embolization is the nidus, or the abnormal network of vascular channels bridging the arterial and venous systems. Embolization can be curative in smaller lesions, palliative in complicated or unresectable lesions, or preoperative. Coil embolization is contraindicated.
178	Discuss the causes of hemangiomas of infancy.	Hemangiomas of infancy occur most commonly in the head and neck and more commonly in girls than in boys (3:1); in premature infants weighing less than 1200 g, with the risk increasing by 40% for every 500-g decrease in birth weight; and in infants born to mothers of advanced maternal age with a history of chorionic villus sampling.
179	What are the two main types of hemangiomas of infancy?	• Focal: More common; a tumor-like growth pattern • Segmental: Less common; diffuse, plaque-like lesion
180	What is the relationship between focal and segmental hemangiomas of infancy and the embryologic development of a hemangioma of the face?	*Segmental lesions* are thought to occur in embryologic prominences related to neural crest cells, which influence vascular patterning. *Focal lesions* occur in identifiable patterns associated with lines of embryonic tissue fusion, such as the central face.
181	What are the phases of hemangiomas of infancy?	• *Proliferative phase*: Rapid growth from 2 weeks to 1 year of age • *Involuting phase*: Slow regression from 1 to 7 years • *Involuted phase*: Complete regression after 8 years of age
182	What vascular tumors reach maximal size at birth and do not enter into a rapid postnatal growth phase?	Congenital hemangiomas
183	What are the two types of congenital hemangiomas?	Two major subgroups exist: • Rapidly involuting congenital hemangioma (RICH), which show accelerated regression typically by 1 year of age • Noninvoluting congenital hemangioma (NICH), which do not enter an involution stage
184	What diagnostic steps can be taken to differentiate hemangiomas of infancy from congenital hemangiomas?	Evaluation of the pattern of proliferation, the pattern of involution, and, importantly, immunostaining. Infantile hemangiomas stain positive for glucose transporter 1 (GLUT1) and Lewis Y (LeY), whereas congenital hemangiomas (RICH and NICH) do not. Placental microvasculature also stains positive for these markers.
185	What is PHACE/PHACES syndrome?	*PHACE* describes the association of facial segmental hemangiomas of infancy with one or more of the following anomalies: **P** Posterior fossa brain malformations **H** Hemangioma, covering > 5 cm of the head/neck **A** Arterial anomalies **C** Cardiovascular anomalies **E** Eye anomalies *PHACES* refers to the presence of ventral developmental defects, specifically sternal defects and/or supraumbilical raphe.

Otology and Facial Nerve Disorders

186	Discuss the embryology of the external auditory canal and middle ear structures.	• External auditory canal: First branchial groove • ET, middle ear, mastoid air cells: First branchial pouch • Malleus head, incus short process, and body: First branchial arch • Malleus manubrium, incus long process, stapes suprastructure: Second branchial arch • Stapes footplate: Otic capsule
187	What syndromes are most commonly associated with auricular deformities?	• BOR syndrome • Nager syndrome • Treacher Collins syndrome • DiGeorge syndrome • CHARGE association
188	Discuss the causes of microtia.	• Unilateral:bilateral = 4:1 • Right ear:left ear = 3:2 • Male > female • 55 to 93% are associated with external auditory canal atresia or stenosis. • 50% are associated with a congenital syndrome.
189	Describe the Marx classification system for microtia.	Marx classification • Grade I: Smaller than normal auricle with mild deformity, but all parts can be distinguished • Grade II: Abnormally small auricle with only partial helical structure preserved • Grade III: Severe deformity with mostly skin-only lobular remnant • Grade IV: Anotia
190	Describe the Weerda classification system for microtia.	Takes into account surgery required for repair. • *First-degree dysplasia*: Most structures of a normal auricle are present. Reconstruction normally does not require the use of additional skin or cartilage. • *Second-degree dysplasia*: All major structures are present to some degree, but there is enough deficiency of tissue that surgical correction requires the addition of cartilage and skin. • *Third-degree dysplasia*: Few or no recognizable landmarks, although the lobule usually is present and positioned anteriorly. Total reconstruction requires the use of skin and large amounts of cartilage.
191	What are the three types of cup ear deformities?	• *Type I*: Upper portion of the helix cupped, hypertrophic concha, reduced auricular height • *Type II*: More severe lopping of the upper pole of the ear • *Type III*: Severe cup ear deformity, malformed in all dimensions Types I and II are considered first-degree dysplasia, and type III is classified as third-degree dysplasia.
192	Describe the traditional stages of rib cartilage graft microtia repair.	Separated by 2 to 3 months, starting around 6 years of age • Stage I: Auricular reconstruction (creation of a cartilaginous framework with autogenous rib cartilage) • Stage II: Lobule transposition • Stage III: Atresia repair • Stage IV: Construction of tragus • Stage V: Auricular elevation

193	What complications have been associated with microtia repair?	• Pulmonary complications from rib harvest: atelectasis, pneumothorax, pneumomediastinum, pneumonia • Skin necrosis overlying the cartilage framework • Chondritis • Reabsorption • Malposition of auricular implant • Tissue breakdown of skin graft or of posterior aspect of ear • Keloiding of donor incision site or skin-graft areas
194	What are common otoplasty techniques?	Most common: • Mustardé technique • Furnas technique Less common: • Farrior technique • Converse technique • Pitanguay technique
195	What complication of otoplasty can be caused by too much flexion of the antihelix at a level equal to the midportion of the ear and inadequate flexion at the superior and inferior poles?	Telephone ear deformity. Can be prevented by repeatedly checking the tension on all sutures during surgery
196	Describe the Weerda classification for external auditory canal (EAC) malformations.	Weerda Classification for EAC stenosis • Type A: Marked narrowing of the EAC with an intact skin layer • Type B: Partial development of the EAC with a medial atretic plate • Type C: Complete bony EAC atresia
197	What are the minor and major malformations in congenital aural atresia?	De La Cruz classification system Minor malformations: • Normal mastoid pneumatization • Normal oval window footplate • Favorable facial nerve–footplate relationship • Normal inner ear Major malformations: • Poor mastoid pneumatization • Abnormality or absence of oval window/footplate • Abnormal course of the facial nerve • Abnormalities of the inner ear
198	What is the grading system used to predict prognosis for hearing improvement after repair of aural atresia?	Jahrsdoerfer grading system
199	What is involved in the preoperative planning for repair of congenital aural atresia?	Audiometric evidence of cochlear function: Ideally, auditory brainstem response (ABR) testing should be performed within first few days of life in patients with bilateral atresia, preferably with unilateral atresia as well. Radiographic three-dimensional evaluation of the temporal bone can be deferred until age 5 or 6 years.
200	You are reviewing the temporal bone CT scan in a 6-year-old child with bilateral aural atresia. The scan demonstrates a gray mass in the middle ear cleft on the left with associated bony erosion. What is the most likely diagnosis?	Congenital cholesteatoma (present in 15% of cases of congenital atresia)
201	What are the critical elements to review on a temporal bone CT scan that will predict hearing prognosis in congenital aural atresia repair?	• Status of the inner ear • Extent of temporal bone pneumatization • Course of the facial nerve • Presence of the oval window and stapes footplate

202	What are the two basic approaches for repair of congenital aural atresia?	• Anterior approach: Drilling area is defined by the temporomandibular joint (TMJ) anteriorly, the middle cranial fossa dura superiorly, and the mastoid air cells posteriorly. • Mastoid approach: Sinodural angle is first identified and followed to the antrum. The facial recess is opened and the incudostapedial joint separated. The atretic bone is then removed.
203	Which congenital syndrome has a wide range of clinical manifestations with the typical presentation involving epibulbar dermoids or lipodermoids, microtia, mandibular hypoplasia, coloboma, hemifacial microsomia and vertebral anomalies?	Goldenhar syndrome, also known as oculoauriculovertebral dysplasia
204	What external ear anomalies are associated with Goldenhar syndrome?	• Preauricular appendages and fistulae • Anomalies of the auricle • Atresia of the external auditory canal • Microtia or anotia
205	What are the TORCH organisms?	• Toxoplasmosis • Other infections: Syphilis, Coxsackievirus, varicella-zoster virus, HIV, and parvovirus B19, syphilis • Rubella • CMV (CMV, the most common) • Herpes
206	Discuss the type of hearing loss associated with congenital CMV infections.	Congenital CMV infections can cause SNHL in as many as 50% of children with symptomatic infections and as many as 12% of infants with asymptomatic infections. As many as 50% of cases of SNHL due to congenital CMV may have a late onset during preschool or early school years.
207	What inner ear structures are affected by CMV infection?	The exact pathophysiology of CMV-induced SNHL is not well understood: however, infants who have died of cytomegalic inclusion disease have temporal bones with characteristic cytomegalic inclusion bodies in the superficial cells of the stria vascularis, Reissner membrane, limbus spiralis, saccule, utricle, and semicircular canals.
208	What is the difference between symptomatic congenital rubella infections and asymptomatic congenital rubella infection?	• Symptomatic infection (rubella syndrome) occurs in the first trimester of pregnancy producing hearing loss in approximately 50% of patients. Other findings include cardiac malformations, visual loss (e.g., cataracts, glaucoma, retinitis, microphthalmia), osteitis, motor deficits, thrombocytopenic purpura, hepatosplenomegaly, icterus, anemia, low birth weight, and cerebral damage and mental retardation. • Asymptomatic infection results from infection during the second or third trimesters of pregnancy and is silent at birth. It is associated with hearing loss in 10 to 20% of patients. Hearing loss is most commonly seen audiometrically as a cookie-bite pattern.
209	What are the inner ear anomalies most commonly seen in congenital rubella infection?	• Cochleosaccular degeneration (Scheibe dysplasia) • Strial atrophy
210	How are early and late congenital syphilis infections defined, and how do they influence hearing loss?	• Early infection: Initial symptoms present from birth to 2 years of age. SNHL is bilateral, flat, and usually without vertigo. • Late infection: Initial symptoms can be seen anytime after 2 years of age and into the sixth decade of life. SNHL can be sudden, asymmetric, fluctuating, and progressive, accompanied often by episodic tinnitus and vertigo.

211	What are the major features of congenital syphilis infection?	<ul><li>Sensorineural hearing loss</li><li>Interstitial keratitis</li><li>Hutchinson teeth (notched incisors)</li><li>Mulberry molars</li><li>Clutton joints (bilateral painless knee effusions)</li><li>Nasal septal perforation and saddle deformity</li><li>Frontal bossing</li><li>Skeletal findings: Osteochondritis and periostitis of long bones leading to "saber shin" deformity</li></ul>
212	What are the clinical findings in congenital toxoplasmosis infection?	At birth, 90% of infants with congenital toxoplasmosis have no signs or symptoms. A subclinically infected infant may later develop progressive lesions, most commonly chorioretinitis. Other findings include progressive CNS involvement with decreased intellectual function, SNHL commonly associated with calcified scars in the stria vascularis, and precocious puberty.
213	When do the most common congenital cochlear malformations occur during development?	<ul><li>Complete labyrinthine aplasia (Michel aplasia): Arrest at week 3 of gestation</li><li>Common cavity: Arrest at week 4 or 5 of gestation</li><li>Cochlear hypoplasia: Arrest at week 5 of gestation</li><li>Cochlear aplasia: Arrest at week 6 of gestation</li><li>Incomplete partition (Mondini malformation, most common): Arrest at week 7 of gestation</li></ul>
214	What congenital anomaly results in the complete absence of differentiated inner ear structures and may be associated with stapes aplasia or malformation, anomalous facial nerve course, and vestibulocochlear nerve aplasia?	Michel aplasia
215	What is the pathophysiology of Michel aplasia?	Developmental arrest of the otic placode before gestational week 3. It has also been associated with thalidomide exposure.
216	What congenital ear anomaly results from developmental arrest of cochlear formation at week 7 of gestation, causing a failure in cochlear partitioning, an absent interscalar septum, a modiolus that is poorly formed or deficient, and a cochlea with only 1 to 1.5 turns?	Mondini malformation
217	Mondini malformation is commonly seen in what congenital syndrome?	Pendred syndrome
218	What additional inner ear anomalies are commonly seen in the evaluation of a child with Mondini malformation?	<ul><li>Enlarged vestibular aqueduct</li><li>Semicircular canal deformities</li><li>Communication with subarachnoid space (increased risk for meningitis)</li></ul>
219	Patients with a Mondini malformation are at risk of what complication during cochlear implantation?	Perilymphatic (CSF) gusher. This complication is not a contraindication to implantation, as good hearing outcomes have been demonstrated despite significant perilymphatic gusher noted intraoperatively, but patients should be counseled appropriately regarding the increased risk (although low) of a dead ear or bacterial meningitis.
220	Arrested development of the pars inferior of the otocyst causes dysplasia of the cochlea and saccule, but it does not impact the semicircular canals and utricle, which results in what congenital ear dysmorphology?	Scheibe dysplasia (cochleosaccular dysplasia)

221	What congenital anomaly results from aplasia of the cochlear duct and subsequent dysfunction of the organ of Corti, particularly the basal turn of the cochlea and adjacent ganglion cells, and how does it impact hearing?	Alexander aplasia. High-frequency hearing loss is most prominent, whereas low frequency is relatively preserved.
222	What is enlarged vestibular aqueduct syndrome?	It is a combination of SNHL, inner ear abnormalities (wide range), and enlarged vestibular aqueduct that can be associated with Pendred syndrome, distal renal tubular acidosis, Waardenburg syndrome, X-linked congenital mixed deafness, BOR syndrome, otofaciocervical deafness, and Noonan syndrome.
223	What is the radiographic definition of an enlarged vestibular aqueduct?	On CT, the vestibular aqueduct is diagnosed as enlarged when the aqueduct is greater than 1.5 mm wide at the midpoint between the common crus and its external aperture. This is roughly the diameter of the posterior semicircular canal. However, this is controversial, and diagnostic thresholds have been reported from 0.9 to 2 mm at the midpoint and 1.9 to 4 mm at the operculum.
224	What percentage of congenital SNHL is genetic?	Approximately 60% of cases of congenital SNHL can be linked to a genetic cause, with roughly 30% of these considered syndromic (most commonly Pendred) and the remaining 70% nonsyndromic.
225	Discuss the genetics of nonsyndromic hearing loss.	• 80% of cases are autosomal recessive. • 20% of cases are autosomal dominant. • <2% of cases are due to X-linked and mitochondrial mutations.
226	What disorder is characterized by hearing loss, vestibular dysfunction, and visual loss resulting from retinitis pigmentosa?	Usher syndrome. The subtypes are distinguished by the severity and progression of hearing loss and the presence or absence of vestibular dysfunction, with visual loss due to retinitis pigmentosa being common to all three subtypes.
227	What are the clinical manifestations of each type of Usher syndrome subtype?	• Type 1: Profound congenital deafness and absent vestibular function (vestibular ataxia), onset of retinitis pigmentosa before puberty (around the age of 10 years). Autosomal recessive • Type 2: Hearing loss is moderate to severe at birth. Normal vestibular function. Onset of retinitis pigmentosa is in late teens. Autosomal recessive; most common • Type 3: Progressive hearing loss. Variable vestibular function. Retinitis pigmentosa begins at puberty. Autosomal recessive • Type 4: Clinically similar to type 2 but with X-linked recessive inheritance
228	What are the pathologic temporal bone findings in patients with Usher syndrome?	Marked atrophy of the organ of Corti in the basal turn associated with spiral ganglion degeneration. These cochlear changes are similar to Scheibe inner ear dysplasia.
229	SNHL, which may be profound at birth or progressive, and abnormal iodine metabolism typically resulting in a euthyroid goiter are the classic manifestations of which congenital disorder?	Pendred syndrome
230	What inner ear abnormalities are found in patients with Pendred syndrome?	• Modiolar deficiency and vestibular enlargement (100%) • Absence of the interscalar septum between the upper and middle cochlear turns (75%) • Enlargement of the vestibular aqueduct (80%)

231	What is the most likely diagnosis for a child with congenital bilateral severe to profound SNHL, prolonged Q-T interval, and a history of syncopal events?	Jervell and Lange-Nielson syndrome (autosomal recessive)
232	What is the pathophysiology of the hearing loss in patients with Jervell and Lange-Nielson syndrome?	Two genes, *KVLQT1* and *KCNE1*, have been linked to Jervell and Lange-Nielsen syndrome. These genes encode for subunits of a potassium channel expressed in the heart and inner ear. Hearing impairment is due to changes in endolymph homeostasis caused by malfunction of this channel. Patients may suffer syncopal events, seizures, and life-threatening cardiac arrhythmias resulting in sudden death.
233	What are the criteria required for diagnosis of Waardenburg syndrome type 1?	Criteria published by the Waardenburg Consortium in 1992: Patient must have two major criteria or one major plus two minor criteria for diagnosis of Waardenburg syndrome type I: Major Criteria: • Congenital SNHL (up to 60%) • Iris pigmentary abnormality (two eyes of different colors, *heterochromia iridis*; one eye of different colors; *segmental heterochromia*; brilliant blue/sapphire iris) • *Hair hypopigmentation* (white forelock or white body hair) • *Distopia canthorum* (lateral displacement of the inner canthi, decreased visible sclera medially) • First-degree relative previously diagnosed with Waardenburg syndrome Minor Criteria: • Congenital leukodermia (several areas of hypopigmented skin) • Synophrys or medial eyebrow flare • Broad, high, nasal root • Hypoplastic alae nasi • Premature graying of hair (white scalp hair before age 30, generally occurring midline instead of at the temples) Rare: Hirschsprung disease, Sprengel anomaly, spina bifida, cleft lip and/or palate, limb defects, congenital heart anomalies, abnormal vestibular function, broad square jaw, low anterior hairline.
234	How are Waardenburg syndrome types 2, 3, and 4 classified?	All are based on type 1 requiring two major or one major and two minor criteria • Type 2: Type 1 without the dystopia canthorum • Type 3 (or Klein-Waardenburg syndrome): Type 1 with hypoplasia or contracture of the upper limbs • Type 4 (or Waardenburg-Shah syndrome): autosomal recessive or dominant; type 1 with Hirschsprung disease or other neurologic disorders
235	What gene has been implicated in Waardenburg syndrome?	*PAX3* is the only gene shown to cause Waardenburg syndrome type 1.
236	What is the pathophysiology of the SNHL in Waardenburg syndrome?	Waardenburg syndrome is due to a failure of proper melanocyte differentiation. Melanocytes are required in the stria vascularis for normal cochlear function.
237	What are the temporal bone abnormalities that can occur in Waardenburg syndrome?	• Temporal bone abnormalities occur in approximately 50% of patients • Aplasia or hypoplasia of the posterior semicircular canal (most common finding, seen in 26% of cases) • Vestibular aqueduct enlargement • Widening of the upper vestibule • Iinternal auditory canal (IAC) hypoplasia • Decreased modiolus size

238	What connective tissue disorder results in hearing loss, craniofacial anomalies (flat midface, depressed nasal bridge, short nose, micrognathia, anteverted nares, cleft palate, or Pierre Robin sequence), ophthalmologic pathology (high myopia, abnormal vitreous gel, retinal detachment), and arthropathy (joint laxity that usually progresses to osteoarthritis)?	Stickler syndrome.
239	What causes hearing loss in Stickler syndrome?	Patients with Stickler syndrome can have high-frequency SNHL, conductive hearing loss, or a mixed hearing loss. The mechanism of high-frequency SNHL is unknown. Conductive hearing loss is typically due to craniofacial abnormalities causing recurrent otitis media with effusion. Ossicular abnormalities resulting from collagen defects may also cause conductive hearing loss.
240	Do all the different types of Stickler syndrome result in similar degrees of hearing loss?	• Type 1: Normal hearing or mild impairment • Type 2: Mild to moderate hearing loss • Type 3: Moderate to severe hearing loss
241	What are the most common genetic mutations seen in the three subtypes of Stickler syndrome?	Autosomal dominant (rare autosomal recessive subtypes): • Type 1: COL2A1 → α1 chain of type II collagen (major component of cartilage, vitreous, and nucleus pulposis); type 1 vitreous subtype, most common • Type 2: COL11A1 → α1 chain of type XI collagen; also seen in Marshall syndrome, type 2 vitreous subtype • Type 3: COL11A2 → alpha α3 chain of type XI collagen, no ophthalmologic abnormality
242	What are the clinical criteria for BOR syndrome?	*BOR syndrome* is defined as the presence of • Three major criteria • Two major criteria and two minor criteria or • One major criteria and an affected first-degree relative Major criteria • Branchial anomalies (first and second branchial arches) • Deafness (90%; can be SNHL, conductive hearing loss, or mixed) • Preauricular pits/cysts • Renal anomalies (mild hypoplasia to aplasia) Minor criteria • External ear anomalies • Middle ear anomalies • Inner ear anomalies • Preauricular tags • Facial asymmetry • Palate abnormalities
243	What are the external ear anomalies seen in BOR syndrome?	• Preauricular cysts/pits (82%) • Preauricular tags • Auricular malformations (32%) • Microtia • External auditory canal stenosis or atresia
244	What are the middle ear anomalies seen in BOR syndrome?	• Ossicular malformation • Facial nerve dehiscence • Absence of the oval window • Reduction in size of the middle ear cleft • ET dilatation • Absence of the stapedius muscle

245	What are the inner ear anomalies seen in BOR syndrome?	• Cochlear hypoplasia or dysplasia • Enlargement of the cochlear or vestibular aqueducts • Hypoplasia of the lateral semicircular canal • Deviation of the labyrinthine facial nerve canal medial to the cochlea • Funnel-shaped IAC with a large porus acousticus
246	A child has malar hypoplasia, cleft zygoma, colobomas, cleft lip, choanal atresia, malocclusion, and profound hearing loss. What is the most likely diagnosis?	Treacher-Collins syndrome
247	What are the otologic manifestations of Treacher Collins syndrome?	• Microtia, aural meatal atresia, and conductive hearing loss caused by ossicular chain malformations • EAC atresia or replacement of the tympanic membrane with bony plate • SNHL and vestibular dysfunction also can be present.
248	What genetic mutation has been identified in most cases of Treacher Collins syndrome?	*TCOF-1* gene, chromosome 5q31.3–q33.3, protein: treacle. Autosomal dominant (types 1 and 2). Treacle is important in the neural crest cells of the branchial arches and may be responsible for the malformation of branchial arch 1 and 2 seen in this disorder.
249	How is Treacher Collins syndrome differentiated from Goldenhar syndrome?	Treacher Collins syndrome has symmetric facies and bilateral eyelid colobomas.
250	Mutations in which chromosomes are involved in neurofibromatosis type 1 (NF1) and type 2 (NF2)?	• NF1: 17q11.1, *NF1* gene, encodes neurofibromin, results in a loss of function mutation • NF2: 22q12.2, *NF2* gene, encodes merlin (tumor suppressor)
251	What percentage of patients with NF1 and NF2 have vestibular schwannomas?	• NF1: 5%, usually unilateral • NF2: 95%, usually bilateral
252	True or false: Vestibular schwannomas in NF2 are managed with observation, surgical intervention, or stereotactic radiosurgery only.	False. Bevacizumab, an angiogenesis inhibitor, has recently been shown to improve hearing and shrink tumors in up to 50% of NF2 patients with progressive vestibular schwannoma.
253	What are the diagnostic criteria for NF2?	• Bilateral vestibular schwannomas that usually develop by the second decade of life or a family history of NF2 in a first-degree relative, plus one of the following: • Unilateral vestibular schwannomas < 30 years of age • Any two of the following: meningioma, glioma, schwannoma, or juvenile posterior subcapsular lenticular opacities/juvenile cortical cataract
254	A patient has multiple craniofacial defects, including bicoronal synostosis and maxillary hypoplasia, hypertelorism, protruding eyes, high arched palate, hearing loss from middle ear effusion, low-set ears, and syndactyly of the hands and feet. What is the most likely diagnosis?	Apert syndrome
255	What type of hearing loss do people with Apert syndrome develop?	Conductive hearing loss, typically from persistent middle ear effusions
256	Which genetic mutation accounts for most cases of Apert syndrome?	Fibroblast growth factor receptor 2 (FGFR2), autosomal dominant, important in the growth and differentiation of mesenchymal and neuroectodermal cells
257	What are the characteristic clinical features of Crouzon syndrome?	• Craniosynostosis • Hypoplastic midface • Exophthalmos • Hypertelorism • Mandibular prognathism

258	What are the causes of the conductive hearing loss seen in patients with Crouzon syndrome?	• Chronic otitis media • Persistent middle ear effusion • Tympanic membrane perforation • Ossicular anomalies
259	What are the diagnostic criteria for Alport syndrome?	Patient must have at least three of the following four characteristics: • Positive family history of hematuria with or without chronic renal failure • Progressive high-tone sensorineural deafness • Typical eye lesion (anterior lenticonus, macular flecks, or both) • Histologic changes of the glomerular basement membrane in the kidney
260	Mutation of what structure(s) impacts the basement membranes of the eye, kidney, and cochlea resulting in Alport syndrome?	Type IV collagen
261	Discuss the hearing loss associated with Alport syndrome.	Bilateral SNHL can be detected by late childhood, is symmetric, and begins in the high-frequency ranges. Over time, it progresses to involve all frequencies over time.
262	What are the features associated with otopalatodigital syndrome?	• Hypertelorism • Frontal bossing • Flat midface • Small nose • Cleft palate • Conductive hearing loss, likely due to ossicular deformities • Abnormalities of the fingers and toes
263	List the four muscles associated with ET function.	• Tensor veli palatini • Levator veli palatini • Salpingopharyngeus • Tensor tympani
264	What are the three basic functions of the eustachian tube?	• Regulation of middle ear pressure • Clearance of middle ear secretions • Protection of the middle ear from nasopharyngeal sound and accumulation of nasopharyngeal secretions
265	What are some of the causes of eustachian tube dysfunction?	Anatomical factors (shorter eustachian tubes with a more horizontal orientation; the eustachian tube reaches adult length by 7 years of age): • Adenoid hypertrophy • Allergy • Sinonasal disease • Craniofacial anomalies (e.g., cleft palate, Down syndrome) • Neoplasm • Extraesophageal reflux • Genetic predisposition
266	What are the two general causes of negative pressure in the middle ear leading to middle ear diseases (i.e., retraction pockets, chronic otitis media, and atelectasis of the tympanic membrane)?	Negative middle ear pressure is caused by failure of the eustachian tube to open as a result of • Physical obstruction: Adenoid hypertrophy, tumor, stenosis, hypertrophy/edema of mucosa lining the eustachian tube • Physiologic obstruction: Failure of muscles involved in opening the Eustachian tube

267	What causes eustachian tube dysfunction in patients with cleft palate?	• Abnormal course and insertion of the tensor veli palatini and levator veli palatini into the posterior margin of the hard palate • Abnormal shape and development of the cartilaginous portion of the eustachian tube
268	What are the most common chronic ear diseases seen in children?	• Chronic otitis media • Chronic suppurative otitis media, with and without cholesteatoma • Chronic mastoiditis • Tympanosclerosis • Cholesterol granuloma
269	What is the definition of recurrent acute otitis media (AOM)?	Three or more documented and separate episodes of AOM in the previous 6 months, or at least four documented and separate episodes in the previous 12 months, with at least one in the prior 6 months *Note:* Persistent AOM refers to the persistence of signs/symptoms of AOM during antimicrobial therapy, signifying treatment failure, or relapse within 1 month (which may be difficult to differentiate from recurrent AOM)
270	What is the definition of chronic otitis media with effusion?	Middle ear effusion without signs or symptoms of acute ear infection for more than 3 months since the date of onset or date of diagnosis
271	What is the definition of chronic suppurative otitis media?	Chronic inflammation of the middle ear and mastoid mucosa in which the tympanic membrane is not intact (perforation or tympanostomy tube) and discharge is present
272	What are the most common pathogens causing acute otitis media?	*Streptococcus pneumoniae* (31.7%) Non-typable *Haemophilus influenzae* (28.4%) *Moraxella catarrhalis* (13.9%)
273	For infants with acute otitis media, when should antibiotics be initiated immediately and when should one offer an initial period of observation?	Immediate oral antibiotic therapy: If the child is younger than 6 months; if the child has severe signs/symptoms (e.g., moderate or severe ear pain, ear pain > 48 hours, temperature > 39°C or 102.2°F); and if the child is younger than 24 months and has bilateral AOM Observation *or* oral antibiotics: If the infant is aged 6 to 24 months and has nonsevere unilateral AOM and if the child is younger than 24 months and has nonsevere unilateral or bilateral AOM *Note:* Pain control with ibuprofen and/or acetaminophen is also important.
274	What are the antibiotics of choice for acute otitis media?	First line: Amoxicillin β-lactam resistance (i.e., patient has received a β-lactam antibiotic in the previous 30 days, has concomitant purulent conjunctivitis [commonly *Haemophilus influenza*], or has a history of resistance to amoxicillin): Amoxicillin-clavulanate. Penicillin allergy: Macrolides (e.g., azithromycin, clarithromycin, erythromycin) or clindamycin. Macrolides are not effective against *H. influenza.*
275	When should an audiogram be obtained in children with middle ear disease?	Clinical practice guideline 2013: Tympanostomy tubes in children: An age-appropriate hearing test should be obtained if otitis media with effusion (OME) is present for 3 months or longer or before surgery when the child meets the criteria for tympanostomy tube placement.

276	When should tympanostomy tubes *not* be recommended in children with middle ear disease?	Clinical practice guideline 2013: Tympanostomy tubes in children: Single episode of otitis media with effusion of less than 3 months' duration Recurrent episodes of acute otitis media without middle ear effusion in either ear at the time of evaluation for possible tube placement
277	When are tympanostomy tubes (TTs) indicated for children with middle ear disease?	Clinical practice guideline 2013: Tympanostomy tubes in children: • Bilateral TTs should be offered to children with bilateral OME for 3 months or longer (chronic OME) *and* documented hearing difficulties. • Bilateral or unilateral TTs may be offered to children with unilateral or bilateral OME for 3 months or longer (chronic OME) and symptoms that are likely related to OME, which include, but are not limited to, vestibular problems, poor school performance, behavior problems, ear discomfort, or reduced quality of life. • Bilateral or unilateral TTs should be offered to children with recurrent acute OME at evaluation. • Bilateral or unilateral TTs may be offered to at-risk children* with unilateral or bilateral OME that is unlikely to resolve quickly (flat, type B tympanogram; chronic OME) *At risk: Recurrent acute otitis media (AOM) or with OME of any duration in a child at increased risk for speech, language or learning problems, from otitis media due to baseline sensory, physical, cognitive or behavioral factors
278	How long should you recommend water precautions after placing tympanostomy tubes in a child?	Clinical practice guideline 2013: Tympanostomy tubes in children: Clinicians should *not* encourage routine, prophylactic water precautions (use of ear plugs, headbands; avoidance of swimming or water sports) for children with tympanostomy tubes.
279	What are the treatment options for chronic ear disease, which requires more aggressive intervention than tympanostomy tubes?	The least invasive approach to achieving a safe ear include the following options: • Tympanoplasty • Atticotomy • Intact canal wall tympanomastoidectomy • Canal wall down tympanomastoidectomy • Modified radical mastoidectomy • Radical mastoidectomy
280	What are the classifications of acquired cholesteatoma?	• *Primary acquired cholesteatoma*: Occurs without evidence of preexisting perforation or infection and may arise in the pars flaccida. • *Secondary acquired cholesteatoma*: Occurs as a result of traumatic or iatrogenic perforation or infection, arises in the pars tensa (most commonly in the posterior superior quadrant) or in an area of prior trauma.
281	What is a congenital cholesteatoma?	A *congenital cholesteatoma* is an epidermal inclusion cyst in the middle ear without any history of prior otorrhea, tympanic membrane perforation, or previous surgery on the ear. The examination should reveal an intact pars tensa and pars flaccida. The mass is most often located in the anterior superior quadrant of the pars tensa.

282	Discuss the "invasion theory" for congenital cholesteatoma.	Ectodermal cells within the developing external auditory canal migrate through the tympanic isthmus into the middle ear and form the substrate for the congenital cholesteatoma.
283	Discuss the "ectodermal rest theory" for congenital cholesteatoma.	Remnants of ectodermal tissue found normally in the middle ear of the developing fetus persist to form the congenital cholesteatoma.
284	What are the three most common surgical procedures for removal of cholesteatoma in the pediatric population?	Same as for the adult population: • Tympanoplasty • Canal wall-up tympanomastoidectomy • Canal wall-down tympanomastoidectomy
285	What is included in the differential diagnosis for a child with vertigo and normal hearing?	• Whiplash • Basilar artery migraine • Seizures • Posterior fossa tumor • Benign paroxysmal vertigo of childhood • Traumatic head injuries • Ocular or ophthalmological disorders • Enlarged vestibular aqueduct syndrome
286	What are the features of benign paroxysmal vertigo of childhood (BPVC)?	Spells of vertigo and disequilibrium without tinnitus or hearing loss. Children often subsequently develop migraines.
287	What is included in the differential diagnosis for a child with vertigo and hearing loss?	• Otitis media or a suppurative complication such as labyrinthitis • Perilymphatic fistula • Inner ear congenital malformation • Metabolic abnormality • Vestibular neuronitis • Congenital infection • **Ménière** disease
288	What is the treatment for Ménière disease in the pediatric patient population?	Same treatment as for adults: • Salt- and caffeine-restricted diet • Weight-dosed diuretics
289	What are the diagnostic criteria required for migraine-associated vertigo?	Episodic vestibular symptoms • Migraine according to International Headache Society criteria • At least one of the following migraine-related symptoms during at least two vertiginous attacks: migrainous headache, photophobia, phonophobia, visual or other auras • Other causes ruled out by appropriate investigations
290	How is migraine-associated vertigo differentiated from Ménière disease?	• Migraine-associated vertigo: Vertigo may last longer than 24 hours, SNHL is uncommon and rarely progressive, tinnitus is rarely obstrusive, and photophobia is often present. • Ménière disease: Vertigo can last up 24 hours but not longer, SNHL is generally progressive, tinnitus is intense, and photophobia is never present.
291	What type of migraine manifests with aura and consists of two or more of the following symptoms: vertigo, tinnitus, decreased hearing, ataxia, dysarthria, visual symptoms in both hemifields of both eyes, diplopia, bilateral paresthesias or paresis, decreased level of consciousness, followed by a throbbing headache, and occurs most commonly in female teenagers.	Basilar migraine. Also known as Bickerstaff syndrome.

292	Describe the condition of vertiginous seizures.	Dizziness may occur as an aura, followed by typical features of an epileptic seizure, or vertigo may occur as the only feature of the seizure.
293	What autosomal dominant syndrome is characterized by chronic episodic vertigo and ataxia and may include diplopia, dysarthria, tinnitus, and paresthesias?	Familial ataxia syndrome. Treated with acetazolamide.
294	How can congenital facial paralysis be classified?	• Traumatic versus developmental • Unilateral versus bilateral • Complete versus incomplete
295	What is the difference between congenital and developmental facial paralysis?	**Congenital/traumatic**: Conditions acquired at or during birth (e.g., birth trauma, etc.) **Developmental**: Abnormalities that occur during fetal development either in isolation or as a component of a named syndrome (e.g., Möbius, Goldenhar, CHARGE, etc.)
296	Why is it important to differentiate between traumatic congenital facial palsy and developmental facial palsy?	Most traumatic cases of congenital facial palsy recover spontaneously, whereas developmental causes generally carry a poor prognosis. Also important for medicolegal reasons.
297	What is the most common cause of unilateral neonatal facial paralysis?	Birth trauma
298	What are risk factors for traumatic facial nerve paralysis?	• Forceps-assisted delivery • Birth weight > 3,500 g • Primiparity • Prolonged labor
299	What clinical examination findings might suggest birth trauma as the cause of unilateral facial palsy in a newborn?	Asymmetric crying facies, hemotympanum, periauricular ecchymosis, facial swelling, other injuries
300	Describe the topographic tests available for facial nerve disorders.	• Supranuclear, nuclear, infranuclear, cerebellopontine angle facial nerve fibers: Central neurologic examination, CT scan • IAC facial nerve fibers: Electroneurography (ENG), audiologic examination, CT scan • Geniculate ganglion, greater superficial petrosal nerve: Schirmer test (tear test) • Tympanomastoid facial nerve fibers: Stapedial reflex test, salivation • Extracranial facial nerve fibers: Facial movement
301	What is the test of choice for evaluating congenital facial palsy?	Electroneuronography (ENOG) (test of choice): • Quantitative evaluation of nerve degeneration • Within 48 hours of traumatic injury, the ENOG is generally normal (can take up to 4 days for the extracranial nerve fibers to demonstrate dysfunction). • ENOG is generally absent or weak in developmental facial palsy as a result of long-standing nerve hypoplasia or aplasia. • If deterioration is greater than 90%, surgical decompression may be considered; however, most authorities recommend waiting 5 weeks with newborns. Other tests include the nerve excitability test, maximum stimulation threshold, electromyography, and topodiagnostic tests (rarely used).

302	Anomalies associated with developmental facial palsy can be placed into what four categories?	• Aplasia or hypoplasia of the cranial nerve nuclei • Nuclear agenesis • Peripheral nerve anomalies (aplasia, hypoplasia, bifurcation or anomalous course) • Primary myopathy
303	Which teratogens are associated with developmental facial palsies?	Ethanol, 13-cisretinoic acid, methotrexate, ionizing radiation, thalidomide
304	What congenital syndrome involves a range of clinical abnormalities that include bilateral or unilateral facial and/or abducens nerve palsies, as well as multiple cranial neuropathies involving the hypoglossal, vagus, and glossopharyngeal nerves? This syndrome may also be associated with lower extremity abnormalities (club foot), mental retardation, external ear deformities, and ophthalmoplegia.	Möbius syndrome
305	What is the cause of Möbius syndrome?	Studies have suggested a high incidence of vascular insults in utero. Several reports of teratogenic exposure (misoprostol, cocaine, ergotamine) resulting in vascular insults have been associated with Möbius syndrome.
306	Are facial nerve palsies a component of hemifacial microsomia?	Yes. It is also known as oculoauriculovertebral dysplasia or hemifacial microsomia and involves defects in first and second branchial arch derivatives. Patients frequently have hearing loss, and up to 50% have facial nerve dysfunction.
307	Name the autosomal recessive disorder of bone metabolism that results in osteopetrosis of the internal auditory canal and compressive neuropathies of the facial and vestibulocochlear nerves.	Albers-Schoenberg disease
308	What is the mildest form of developmental facial palsy that results from unilateral absence or hypoplasia of the depressor anguli oris muscle and is associated with cardiovascular congenital anomalies?	Congenital lower-lip palsy (asymmetric crying facies)
309	How often is developmental facial palsy a part of the CHARGE syndrome?	Around 75% of patients have at least one cranial neuropathy, and of these, up to 60% may have a developmental facial palsy.

Cleft Lip and Palate

310	What syndromes are commonly associated with facial clefts?	Apert syndrome, ectodermal dysplasia, orofacial-digital I/II, and Stickler, Treacher-Collins, Van der Woude, and Waardenberg syndromes
311	What makes up the primary palate?	• Premaxilla • Lip • Nasal tip • Columella
312	What bones form the hard palate?	• Palatine process of the maxilla • Horizontal plate of palatine bone
313	How are cleft lips classified?	*Unilateral* (right or left) or *bilateral* *Complete* (involves the entire vertical thickness of the upper lip with extension into the nasal floor, often associated with an alveolar cleft) or incomplete (extending from a slight muscular diastasis at the vermilion to a small bridge of tissue at the nasal sill called the Simonart band)

314	How are cleft palates classified?	• *Primary* (involvement anterior to the incisive foramen) or *secondary* (involvement posterior to the incisive foramen) palate • *Unilateral* (one palatal process is fused with the septum, resulting in oronasal communication on one side only) or *bilateral* (no connection between either palatal process and the septum) • *Complete* (cleft of both primary and secondary palate) or *incomplete* (involves the secondary palate only, and has varying degrees of severity)
315	Discuss the nasal deformity associated with cleft lips. (▶ Fig. 1.3)	• Lateral and inferior displacement of alar base and lateral crus, causing the dome to be flattened and rotated downward on the cleft side • Columella: Short, causing a horizontal orientation to the nostril on the cleft side • Septum: Tends to deviate toward the cleft side, with the cartilaginous base displaced off of the maxillary crest toward the cleft side. This septum malposition contributes to nasal tip tilt toward the noncleft side.

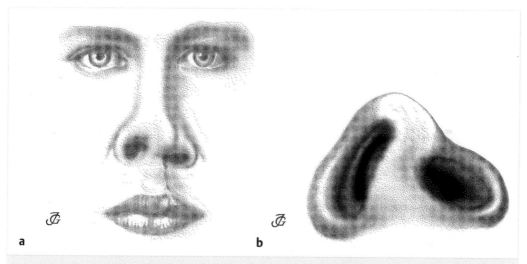

Fig. 1.3 (a,b) Nasal deformity associated with cleft lip: lateral and inferior displacement of alar base and lateral crus (dome flattened and rotated downward on cleft side), short columella (horizontal orientation of nostril on cleft side), septum deviates toward cleft side (nasal tip tilt toward non-cleft side). (Used with permission from Huizing EH, de Groot JAM. Functional Reconstructive Nasal Surgery. New York, NY: Thieme; 2003.)

316	Discuss the typical timing (i.e., age) for repair of cleft lip and palate.	6 to 12 weeks: Repair cleft lip 10 to 13 months: Repair cleft palate, consider tympanostomy tubes 2 to 5 years: Manage velopharyngeal insufficiency, consider lip/nose revision 6 to 11 years: Orthodontic evaluation and treatment, alveolar bone graft 12 to 21 years: Orthodontics and restorative dentistry, orthognathic surgery (if needed), rhinoplasty (if needed, typically the last procedure performed)

317	What criteria did surgeons historically use before proceeding with cleft lip repair?	"Rule of 10s" • At least 10 weeks old • Weighs at least 10 pounds • Hemoglobin of at least 10 g/dL In the era of modern pediatric anesthesia, these criteria are not as relevant.
318	What is a lip adhesion procedure?	A lip adhesion procedure converts a complete cleft lip into an incomplete cleft lip at between 2 and 4 weeks of age, potentially allowing the definitive lip repair to be performed with less tension.
319	What are the criteria for performing a lip adhesion?	• Wide, unilateral, complete cleft lip and palate • Symmetric, wide bilateral, complete cleft lip with a very protruding premaxilla • Introduction of symmetry to an asymmetric bilateral cleft lip
320	What are three broad classifications of techniques used to repair a unilateral cleft lip?	• Straight-line repair (Rose-Thompson repair) • Triangular flap repair (Tennison-Randall repair, Skoog repair) • Rotation/advancement repair (Millard technique, most commonly used; Mohler technique)
321	What cleft lip repair technique entails a downward and lateral rotation of the medial segment of the cleft lip combined with the medial advancement of the lateral cleft segment into the defect, which places the scar in the position of the natural philtral column? (▶ Fig. 1.4)	Millard rotation-advancement technique for cleft lip repair

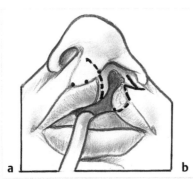 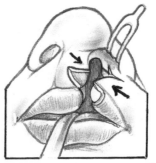 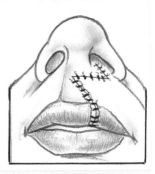

Fig. 1.4 (a,b,c) Millard rotation-advancement operation for unilateral cleft lip repair. (Used with permission from Goldenberg D, Goldstein BJ, eds. Handbook of Otolaryngology–Head and Neck Surgery. New York, NY: Thieme; 2011.)

322	What are four commonly used techniques for closure of a cleft palate?	• Wardill-Kilner technique (V-Y pushback) • von Langenbeck technique (bipedicled mucoperiosteal flaps) • Bardach two-flap palatoplasty • Furlow technique (double opposing Z-plasty)
323	What is the most common complication after palatoplasty?	Velopharyngeal insufficiency

324	What are the features of a submucous cleft palate (SMCP)?	• Bifid uvula • Zona pellucida (bluish midline region representing the muscle deficiency; abnormal insertion of levator veli palatini) • Notch in the posterior hard palate due to loss of posterior nasal spine
325	What pathologic condition, commonly seen in velocardiofacial syndrome, results when the triad of visible signs of classic SMCP palatini muscle inserts into the hard palate abnormally and there is a loss of muscularus uvulae muscle tissue in the midline?	Occult submucous cleft palate
326	What are the four velopharyngeal closure patterns? (► Fig. 1.5)	• Coronal (most common) • Circular • Circular with a Passavant ridge • Sagittal

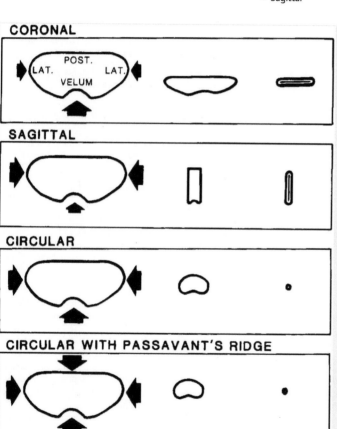

Fig. 1.5 Patterns of velopharyngeal closure. (Used with permission from Papel ID, Frodel J, Holt GR, et al, eds. Facial Plastic and Reconstructive Surgery 3rd Edition. New York, NY: Thieme; 2009.)

327	What are the surgical treatment options for velopharyngeal insufficiency?	• Nasopharyngeal augmentation • Sphincter pharyngoplasty • Pharyngeal flap • Palatoplasty

328	Name the pathologic processes that originate from remnants of the dental lamina, are located on the alveolar ridge of newborns, and occasionally become large enough to be clinically noticeable as discrete white swellings on the alveolar ridges. They are generally asymptomatic and do not produce any discomfort for the infant and typically disappear within 2 weeks to 5 months of postnatal life.	Gingival cysts of newborns (aka dental lamina cysts)
329	What is the difference between Epstein pearls and Bohn nodules?	• *Epstein pearls*: Cystic, keratin-filled nodules found along the midpalatine raphe, likely derived from entrapped epithelial remnants along the line of fusion • *Bohn nodules*: Keratin-filled cysts scattered over the palate, most numerous along the junction of hard and soft palate and apparently derived from palatal salivary gland structure

Tonsils and Adenoids

330	What is the cause of acute tonsillitis?	Viral infection often precedes bacterial infection, which can be caused by group A β-hemolytic streptococcus (most common), *Moraxella catarrhalis*, and *H. influenzae*.
331	What is the treatment of choice for culture proven acute streptococcus pharyngotonsillitis in a patient with no allergies?	Penicillin: Consider β-lactamase inhibitor. For patients who have penicillin allergies, consider clindamycin.
332	What is required for the diagnosis of recurrent/chronic tonsillitis?	• Seven or more episodes of tonsillitis in the past 12 months, or • Five or more episodes per year in the past 2 years, or • Three or more episodes per year in the past 3 years
333	What microbiology is associated with chronic tonsillitis?	Polymicrobial infection. Treatment options include long-term β-lactamase inhibitor antibiotic or tonsillectomy.
334	What are tonsilliths?	*Tonsiliths* are tonsillar concretions of retained material and bacterial growth in crypts within tonsil and adenoid tissue. They are sometimes identified in patients without a clinical history suggestive of chronic tonsil disease. Conservative therapy includes the use of water jets, manual expression, gargling, or cauterization of the crypts with silver nitrate.
335	A 5-year-old child has had 3 weeks of nasal discharge, halitosis, recurrent serous otitis media, and nightly snoring. What is the likely diagnosis?	Adenoiditis. Also associated with chronic mouth breathing, "adenoid facies" (long thin face, high arched palate, malar hypoplasia, open mouth), and hyponasal speech
336	In children with peripheral sleep disordered breathing associated with tonsillar hypertrophy, which comorbid condition(s) might improve after tonsillectomy?	Growth retardation, poor school performance, enuresis, and behavioral problems
337	What polysomnogram findings indicate sleep disordered breathing and obstructive sleep apnea in children and potentially warrant tonsillectomy?	• Abnormal study: Pulse oximetry < 92% or apnea plus hypopnea index (AHI) > 1 (more than one event in two or more consecutive breaths per hour) • AHI > 5 warrants consideration of tonsillectomy (no strict cutoff, somewhat controversial); these children should be kept in the hospital for observation after surgery.
338	How is tonsillar hypertrophy graded?	0: Not visible; tonsils do not reach tonsillar pillars 1+: Less than 25% of transverse oropharyngeal space (measured between the anterior tonsillar pillars) 2+: 25 to 49% of transverse oropharyngeal space 3+: 50 to 74% or transverse oropharyngeal space 4+: 75% or more of the transverse oropharyngeal space

339	How is adenoid hypertrophy graded?	**0:** Not visible **1+:** <25% of choanae **2+:** 25 to 49% of choanae **3+:** 50–74% of choanae **4+:** 75% of choanae
340	What are the boundaries of the peritonsillar space?	• *Medial:* Palatine tonsil • *Anterior:* Anterior tonsillar pillar • *Posterior:* Posterior tonsillar pillar • *Lateral:* Superior pharyngeal constrictor muscle (lateral to this is the parapharyngeal space) • *Superior:* Confluence of the anterior and posterior tonsillar pillars with the soft palate
341	A patient in the emergency department has drooling, stertor, muffled voice, fever, leukocytosis, odynophagia, and unilateral otalgia. She has a history of recurrent tonsillitis and on examination is noted to have uvular deviation and pharyngotonsillar asymmetry. What is the best treatment?	Treatment consists of incision and drainage of this presumed peritonsillar abscess, along with antibiotics, pain management, and consideration for steroids. Quinsy tonsillectomy should be considered in a child with recurrent tonsillitis undergoing incision and drainage of a peritonsillar abscess under anesthesia.
342	If the tonsillar bed is violated inferiorly during tonsillectomy, what nerve is at risk?	The glossopharyngeal nerve runs just lateral to the superior constrictor muscle in the floor of the tonsillar bed. Injury or postoperative edema may result in altered taste to the posterior third of the tongue and referred otalgia resulting from irritation of the tympanic nerve, a branch of cranial nerve IX.
343	What is the immunologic risk of adenotonsillectomy?	Although this tissue offers active immunologic protection via B and T cell activity, there appears to be no clinically relevant immunologic sequelae associated with performing adenotonsillectomy.
344	What are the absolute indications for tonsillectomy? (► Fig. 1.6)	• Tonsillar hypertrophy resulting in upper airway obstruction, severe dysphagia, sleep disordered breathing, cor pulmonale • Unilateral tonsillar hypertrophy, or other concern for possible malignancy • Tonsillitis resulting in febrile convulsions • Persistent or recurrent tonsillar hemorrhage

Absolute
Tonsillar hypertrophy resulting in upper airway obsruction, severe dysphagia, sleep disordered breathing, cor pulmonale
Unilateral tonsillar hypertrophy, or other concern for possible malignancy
Tonsillitis resulting in febrile convulsions
Persistent or recurrent tonsillar hemorrhage

Relative
Three or more infections per year despite adequate medical therapy
Persistent halitosis despite medical therapy
Strep carrier presenting with recurrent or chronic infection despite adequate medical therapy

Fig. 1.6 Indications for tonsillectomy.

345	What are the relative indications for tonsillectomy?	• Three or more infections per year despite adequate medical therapy • Persistent halitosis despite medical therapy • Streptococcus carrier with recurrent or chronic infection despite adequate medical therapy

		Note: Because adenoid tissue has similar bacteriology to the pharyngeal tonsils and minimal additional morbidity occurs with adenoidectomy, if tonsillectomy is already being performed, most surgeons perform adenoidectomy if adenoids are present and inflamed at the time of tonsillectomy. However, this point remains controversial.
346	Describe the relative contraindications for tonsillectomy and adenoidectomy.	• Potential for velopharyngeal insufficiency: Cleft palate, submucosal cleft palate, neuromuscular palatal dysfunction (relative contraindication for adenoidectomy, not tonsillectomy; consider superior segment adenoidectomy only) • Hematologic: Coagulopathy, hemophilia, leukemia, etc. (relative; requires hematology assistance) • Infections: Acute pharyngitis (relative)
347	What perioperative medications are recommended during routine tonsillectomy?	A single dose of intraoperative IV dexamethasone. Surgeons should *not* give routine perioperative antibiotics.
348	What should you suspect if, after adenotonsillectomy for tonsillar hypertrophy and sleep disordered breathing, your patient develops acute respiratory compromise?	Pulmonary edema
349	When does delayed hemorrhage most often occur after tonsillectomy?	7 to 10 days postoperatively as a result of sloughing of eschar
350	What are the absolute indications for adenoidectomy?	• Hypertrophy resulting in obstructive sleep apnea, obstructive daytime breathing, and chronic mouth breathing • Recurrent or persistent acute otitis media in patients > 3 to 4 years of age • Recurrent and/or chronic sinusitis
351	What are the relative indications for adenoidectomy?	• Recurrent acute adenoiditis (five to seven infections per year, five infections in 2 years, three infections in 3 years, or > 2 weeks of missed school or work in 1 year). • Chronic adenoid inflammation and infection, halitosis, or cervical lymphadenopathy • Dysphagia, not otherwise specified • Recurrent eustachian tube dysfunction requiring second set of tympanostomy tubes or recurrent sinusitis

Airway and Esophagus

352	What is the most common benign pediatric laryngeal neoplasm?	Recurrent respiratory papillomatosis (RRP)
353	What are the two most common age groups affected by recurrent respiratory papillomatosis (RRP)?	• < 5 years = juvenile-onset recurrent respiratory papillomatosis (JORRP) • > 40 years = adult onset recurrent respiratory papillomatosis (AORRP)
354	What are the three most common risk factors for development of JORRP?	Clinical triad Firstborn (longer labor) Mother is < 20 years of age (more likely a lower socioeconomic status and recent infection) Vaginal birth in a mother with genital chondylomata
355	What is the strain of human papillomavirus (HPV) most commonly responsible for JORRP, and what is the most common anatomical area infected?	HPV 6 or 11. Larynx.
356	What is the most frequent route of infection in JORRP?	Vertical transmission during vaginal birth or less commonly transplacental infection. In older children, infection can occur via accidental inoculation or sexual abuse.

357	How does the age of JORRP onset relate to disease severity?	Children < 3 years of age require more frequent operations (> four per year) and have disease involving more anatomical subsites; 19% of children with a more aggressive course will require > 40 surgical procedures in their lifetime.
358	What symptoms are associated with JORRP?	Hoarseness, dysphonia, cough, dysphagia, inspiratory stridor, and potentially respiratory distress from airway obstruction
359	The key to management of JORRP is surgical debulking procedures. Which techniques are commonly used?	Laser resection/ablation and microdebridement
360	What is the most common antiviral agent used to assist in treatment of JORRP?	Injection of cidofovir into the base of the lesion after resection. In addition, interferon-α, indol-3-carbinol, HspE7, and the mumps vaccine may be considered.
361	Why is tracheostomy reserved only for severe cases of JORRP with impending airway compromise?	There is a risk of spreading disease to the distal tracheobronchial tree.
362	Why should a biopsy be taken during surgical debulking of RRP?	Document benign disease, document human papillomavirus (HPV) infection, attain polymerase chain reaction (PCR) for HPV serotype (prognostic), rule out carcinoma.
363	What is the risk of malignant transformation in JORRP?	< 1% but increased in patients with prolonged, extensive disease and distal spread. HPV 11 is higher risk than is HPV 6.
364	The Gardasil vaccine offers immunity against which serotypes of HPV?	HPV 6, 11, 16, and 18
365	Which common pediatric pathology is considered the most common cause of acute-onset (often at night) inspiratory stridor, barky cough, hoarseness, and upper airway obstruction that can lead to respiratory compromise?	Laryngotracheobronchitis (croup)
366	What is the most common cause of laryngotracheobronchitis (croup)?	Parainfluenza virus (up to 75%). The most common subtype is parainfluenza type 1.
367	Croup is caused by viral invasion of the laryngeal mucosa that results in inflammation and edema. Which region of the airway is predominantly affected and narrowed?	Subglottis
368	How can the Westley croup scale be used to differentiate mild, moderate, and severe croup?	Westley croup scale • Level of consciousness: Normal (including sleep) = 0, altered = 5 • Cyanosis: None = 0; with agitation = 4; at rest = 5 • Stridor: None = 0; when agitated = 1; at rest = 2 • Air entry: Normal = 0; decreased = 1; markedly decreased = 2 • Intercostal retractions: None = 0; mild = 1; moderate = 2; severe = 3 Severity • Mild croup: ≤ 2 (e.g., barky cough, hoarse cry, no stridor at rest) • Moderate croup: 3 to 7 (e.g., stridor at rest, mild retractions, little to no agitation) • Severe croup: ≥ 8, (e.g., significant stridor at rest, severe retractions, anxious/agitated/lethargic)
369	Although clinical history and physical examination are generally adequate for diagnosis of croup, what imaging technique can be used when the diagnosis is in question? What is the characteristic finding?	Anterior-posterior chest radiograph; "steeple sign" or subglottic narrowing

370	Although symptoms of croup often resolve within 48 hours, children can progress to respiratory failure. Management generally rests on medical intervention; the need for intubation or tracheostomy is rare. What medical management has been shown to improve symptoms in children with mild, moderate, and severe croup?	• All children with respiratory distress may benefit from supplemental oxygen. • Mild: Single dose of oral dexamethasone • Moderate: Dexamethasone, nebulized epinephrine, and/or nebulized budesonide • Severe: Dexamethasone, nebulized epinephrine
371	If a child complains of isolated nocturnal stridor but has an otherwise normal head and neck examination with no evidence of infectious cause, what is the likely diagnosis?	Acute spasmodic laryngitis (false croup)
372	What pediatric pathology is associated with cellulitis, edema, and inflammation of the epiglottis, aryepiglottic folds, and arytenoid tissue and is limited in its inferior extent by the tightly bound epithelium of the true vocal folds?	Acute epiglottitis
373	What is the cause of epiglottitis?	Most common cause: *Haemophilus influenzae* type b (Hib) despite immunization (lack or failure of immunization). Other common causes include *Streptococcus pneumoniae*, *Staphylococcus aureus*, and β-hemolytic streptococcus. Noninfectious causes include thermal or chemical injuries, trauma, angioedema, hemophagocytic lymphohistiocytosis, and some acute leukemias.
374	Both epiglottitis and croup can manifest with fever, cough, and noisy or effortful breathing. What symptoms are more likely to be present only in epiglottitis and may help in differentiating the two?	Drooling is reliably associated with epiglottitis (3 Ds of epiglottitis are drooling, distress, and dysphagia). Less reliable hallmarks include preference for sitting or sniffing position, refusal to eat or drink, inability to swallow, odynophagia, a higher grade temperature, and vomiting.
375	True or false: Without intervention, children with epiglottitis are at higher risk for airway obstruction and death than those with croup.	True
376	How is epiglottitis diagnosed in children?	• *Mild distress* (other diagnoses are more likely): Visualize the epiglottis (using tongue depressor or flexible endoscopy). The child should be kept in a calm environment where an airway can be secured immediately. Anteroposterior/lateral radiograph: "Thumbprinting" of the epiglottis or supraglottic edema • *Moderate to severe distress*: *Do not* attempt to visualize the airway or otherwise disturb the child. IV, blood draw, rectal temperature, etc., should be performed. Remember, bag-valve-mask ventilation is feasible in almost all cases of acute epiglottitis. An experienced provider should evaluate the airway after intubation. After securing the airway, blood work and airway cultures should be obtained.
377	In a child diagnosed with epiglottitis, once the airway is secured or deemed safe for observation (in the intensive care unit, or ICU), what additional medical management is indicated?	Empiric antibiotics (third-generation cephalosporin and an antistaphylococcal agent active against methicillin-resistant *S. aureus* [MRSA]) and possibly corticosteroids (although controversial).
378	What are common criteria for extubation in the setting of acute epiglottitis?	Resolution of the inflammation, edema, and erythema of the supraglottic structures on interval airway examination (generally 2 to 3 days) and/or the presence of an air leak in addition to clinical improvement
379	What might predispose a patient to membranous laryngotracheobronchitis (bacterial tracheitis)?	Previous trauma, viral infection, or anything that alters the local immunity, thus increasing the risk of a bacterial superinfection

380	Bacterial superinfection of the larynx and tracheo-bronchial tree mucosa result in a diffuse inflammatory reaction associated with thick secretions and possible sloughing of fibrinous, mucopurulent, epithelial lining material into the airway. Why is this more problematic in the pediatric population?	The smallest diameter in the pediatric airway is at the cricoid cartilage. Any edema or narrowing of this can significantly compromise a child's respiratory status. According to Poiseuille's law, airway resistance is inversely proportional to the radius of the airway to the fourth power. So in a 4-mm infant airway, if there is 1 mm of edema, the diameter is reduced by 50%, the cross-sectional area is reduced by 75%, and resistance increases 16-fold. By contrast, in an adult airway, 1 mm of edema only causes a 25% decrease in diameter, 44% decrease in area, and 3-fold increase in resistance. More than 90% of children diagnosed with bacterial tracheitis require intubation.
381	Children with bacterial tracheitis often have fever, dyspnea, retractions, a nonpainful cough, and inspiratory stridor. What is the most common cause of mortality in these children?	Airway obstruction resulting from sloughing of fibrinous/mucopurulent debris or membrane. Mortality rates (historically high) have been decreasing as a result of early recognition, aggressive pulmonary toilet, early antibiotics, and airway protection via intubation when necessary.
382	What is the most common organism cultured from the trachea (tracheal cultures are important for diagnosis as blood cultures are often negative) during an acute episode of bacterial tracheitis?	*S. aureus*
383	True or false: Obtaining IV access in children with bacterial tracheitis is not necessary.	False. Initiation of broad-spectrum empiric antibiotics is imperative. However, IV access should not be attempted in a child demonstrating respiratory distress, as agitation may precipitate acute airway collapse. Once the airway is stable or secured, obtain IV access.
384	A 10-year-old girl has hoarseness, cough, odynophagia, general malaise, and low-grade fever. On examination, she has bilateral lymphadenopathy and coalescing pseudomembranous plaques involving her pharynx and larynx. She is a recent immigrant and has no vaccination records. What is the likely causative agent?	*Corynebacterium diphtheriae* (gram-positive bacillus). Diagnosis = culture and positive toxin assay
385	How can diphtheria lead to myocarditis, nephritis, and central nervous system (CNS) complications?	Systemic absorption of toxin
386	How is diphtheria (1) prevented, and (2) treated?	1. Vaccination: Immune individuals can be asymptomatic carriers. 2. Careful airway management (extreme caution with intubation, early consideration for tracheostomy), diphtheria antitoxin, erythromycin or penicillin, serial electrocardiograms and cardiac enzymes, serial neurologic checks, symptomatic care, consideration for prophylactic treatment of close contacts
387	What results if, during the 10th week of gestation, the epithelium that normally temporarily obliterates the laryngeal lumen fails to recanalize?	Congenital laryngeal web. Most commonly noted in the anterior commissure.
388	What is the most common chromosomal anomaly associated with laryngeal webs?	Chromosome 22q11.2 deletion
389	What congenital syndromes are related to laryngeal webs?	22q11.2 deletion syndromes (e.g., velocardiofacial syndrome, DiGeorge syndrome, conotruncal anomaly face syndrome

390	Cohen's classification of glottic webs can be helpful to describe these rare lesions. Describe this system.	Cohen's classification of glottic webs: • *Type I*: Thin anterior web, <35% glottic involvement, mild hoarseness • *Type II*: Thin to moderately thick web, 35 to 50% glottic involvement, weak cry, mild airway symptoms • *Type III*: Thick web, possible anterior cartilaginous subglottic extension, 50 to 75% glottic involvement, weak voice, moderate airway symptoms • *Type IV*: Thick web, 75 to 90% glottic involvement, cartilaginous subglottic extension, no cry, severe airway distress (tracheostomy)
391	You are performing a direct laryngoscopy on a newborn suffering from cyanosis, apnea, and stridor. Flexible fiberoptic laryngoscopy was suggestive of bilateral vocal-fold paralysis with no obvious webbing anteriorly. On palpation of the interarytenoid space, you note a thick band that is fixing the arytenoids and preventing adequate abduction. What is your diagnosis?	Posterior laryngeal web
392	You are consulted on a patient by the high-risk maternal fetal medicine team to evaluate a fetus diagnosed radiographically with congenital high airway obstruction syndrome (CHAOS) resulting from nearly complete laryngeal atresia. What procedure(s) offer a chance for survival and potential long-term survival?	EXIT (ex utero intrapartum treatment) and tracheostomy. With early detection, patients may undergo fetal bronchoscopy with attempted wire tracheoplasty as an adjunct procedure.
393	How are laryngeal webs managed?	• Mild webs: Endoscopic division can be attempted but is often unsuccessful. • Posterior webs: Tracheostomy with delayed decannulation, laryngotracheal reconstruction with posterior cricoidotomy, and grafting • Anterior webs: Laryngotracheal reconstruction or laryngofissure with Silastic keel placement, with or without tracheostomy
394	In a term infant, what measurement indicates subglottic stenosis?	Subglottic, or cricoid, diameter <3.5 mm
395	In a term infant with recurrent prolonged episodes of croup, no history of prior airway manipulation (surgical or intubation), no history of trauma, and neck films that suggest subglottic narrowing, what underlying pathology might be found in the evaluation?	Congenital subglottic stenosis
396	What are the possible causes of congenital subglottic stenosis?	Elliptical cricoid cartilage, laryngeal cleft, cricoid flattening (possibly from a trapped first tracheal ring), a large anterior lamella, generalized mucosal thickening
397	How is subglottic stenosis graded?	Cotton-Myer grading system • *Grade I*: <50% obstruction • *Grade II*: 51 to 70% obstruction • *Grade III*: >70% obstruction with a detectable lumen • *Grade IV*: No detectable lumen
398	Why is the management of congenital subglottic stenosis different from that of acquired subglottic stenosis?	Most congenital stenoses are cartilaginous and therefore do not respond to dilation or laser ablation of soft tissue.

399	How is congenital subglottic stenosis treated?	• *Grade I*: Generally conservative management • *Grade II and III*: Tracheostomy or other surgical intervention* • *Grade IV*: Tracheostomy or other surgical intervention** *Dilatation for soft stenosis, laryngotracheal reconstruction with anterior and/or posterior grafts, anterior cricoid split (rarely performed today), cricotracheal resection **Cricotracheal resecton
400	How can life-threatening subcutaneous emphysema be avoided in laryngotracheal reconstruction (LTR)?	Leave a small drain (Penrose or rubber band) to allow egress of air.
401	When creating an anterior costal cartilage graft, what is the most common shape that the cartilage is carved into, and what is done with the perichondrium?	The shape is a modified "boat" if there is no tracheostomy site to close (i.e., no tracheostomy tube in place or double-stage procedure). If performing a single-stage procedure and closing tracheostoma, a teardrop shape is used. Perichondrium is left intact facing toward the lumen.
402	In a patient with subglottic stenosis and a posterior glottic stenosis (grade II/III), what open procedure is indicated for widening the patient's airway?	Posterior cricoid split is done via laryngofissure or anterior cricoid split and placement of posterior costal cartilage graft, which may require suprastomal stenting for a period postoperatively, but often an endotracheal tube in the postoperative period will be an adequate stent.
403	When performing a laryngofissure, should the anterior commissure be divided?	No
404	What percentage of the posterior lamina of the cricoid cartilage should be divided during a posterior cricoid split?	100%. It may extend to the interarytenoid space and into the posterior tracheal wall.
405	In a single-staged laryngotracheal reconstruction (LTR), is the tracheostomy tube left in place?	No. This is the key difference between single- and double-staged LTR procedures. Patients are generally nasotracheally intubated at the end of the procedure and kept intubated for 2 to 7 days, depending on the extent of the surgical intervention.
406	True or false: Single-staged laryngotracheal reconstruction can be done only for stenosis requiring an anterior graft.	False. Single-staged LTR may include anterior grafts, posterior grafts, or both.
407	What is the relationship between the tracheostoma and the planned horizontal neck incision for open LTR?	The incision should incorporate the superior margin of the tracheostoma.
408	In patients with severe grade III or grade IV subglottic stenosis, what surgical approach may be considered instead of LTR?	Cricotracheal resection (CTR) (cricoid resection, thyrotracheal anastomosis) is the only option for grade IV subglottic stenosis. Laryngotracheal reconstruction with anterior and posterior grafts or CTR can be considered for high-grade III subglottic stenosis.
409	In a patient with a long segment of tracheal stenosis or complete tracheal rings, what procedure is often recommended?	Slide tracheoplasty
410	What are the basic steps involved in pediatric tracheostomy?	• The procedure can be done with the patient intubated with an endotracheal tube (ETT) or ventilating bronchoscope. • Horizontal incision halfway between the cricoid and sternal notch; remove the fat (lipectomy). • Dissect down to the trachea; this can be difficult to palpate because the lung apices extend further superiorly into the neck in infants and children and it can divide isthmus or retract superiorly).

		• Place right and left vertical polypropylene (e.g., 4–0 Prolene) stay sutures through the tracheal rings lateral to planned tracheal incision through the second and third rings. • You may need to mature the stoma (suture stoma skin edges to trachea), but this is usually not performed if lipectomy is adequate and the wound is not excessively deep. • Make a vertical incision through two or three rings (the ETT is placed somewhere between tracheal rings 2 and 4); no Bjork flap, no trachea removed, taking care not to injure the cricoid. • Withdraw the ETT or ventilating bronchoscope, and place the tracheostomy tube. • Using a flexible fiberoptic scope, check the tube position. • Secure the tracheostomy tube.
411	Why are stay sutures so important during pediatric tracheostomy?	Sutures allow tracheal traction into the field for emergent reinsertion of the tracheostomy tube after accidental decannulation.
412	What is the primary goal of open laryngeal surgery for pediatric patients?	Decannulation
413	In what procedure are the first and second tracheal rings, cricoid, and inferior thyroid cartilage cut in the midline to widen the diameter of the subglottis?	Anterior cricoid split. Anterior cricoid split without grafting is rarely performed today.
414	What are the most common complications of pediatric tracheostomy?	• Early: Pneumothorax. hemorrhage, accidental decannulation, tube obstruction, subcutaneous emphysema, death • Intermediate or late: Infection, accidental decannulation, subglottic stenosis, granulation tissue, suprastomal stenosis or collapse, difficult decannulation, death
415	What is the most common benign laryngeal and upper tracheal neoplasm in the newborn or infant?	Hemangioma
416	What is the natural progression of infantile subglottic hemangiomas?	Rapid growth for the first 6 months of life, relative stability for about a year, slow involution with resolution when the child is around 3 years of age
417	What congenital syndrome can be associated with subglottic hemangiomas?	**PHACE** (posterior fossa abnormalities and other brain anomalies; hemangioma(s) of the cervicofacial region; arterial cerebrovascular malformations; cardiac defects; eye abnormalities)
418	How are subglottic hemangiomas treated?	• Medical: Propranolol is first-line therapy; use steroids for propranolol failure • Surgical: Tracheostomy until resolution for obstructive lesions; external surgical approaches (e.g., submucous resection and laryngotracheal reconstruciton); can consider laser ablation
419	What disorder is caused by decreased laryngeal tone, resulting in dynamic prolapse of supraglottic tissue into the airway, inspiratory stridor, and airway obstruction?	Laryngomalacia
420	What is the most common cause of congenital stridor?	Laryngomalacia (35 to 75%)

421	Without intervention, when would you expect laryngomalacia symptoms to resolve?	18 to 20 months (at 18 months, 75% have no stridor)
422	What complications can result from severe laryngomalacia?	Difficulty feeding, failure to thrive, apnea, cyanosis, cor pulmonale, and cardiac failure
423	Whereas neurologic, genetic, and cardiac diseases are more common in infants with laryngomalacia, which comorbidity is highly associated with laryngomalacia and may need to be managed concomitantly with the airway disease?	Gastroesophageal reflux disease, or GERD
424	Why do some authorities recommend that, in addition to laryngoscopy, a full evaluation of the tracheobronchial tree be performed during the evaluation of laryngomalacia?	Up to 17.5% will have an additional, synchronous lesion.
425	What is the standard surgical treatment for laryngomalacia?	Supraglottoplasty (division of aryepiglottic folds, debulking of prolapsing arytenoid tissue, epiglottoplasty): cold steel microlaryngeal instruments, CO_2 laser, and microdebrider have been reported.
426	What are the indications for supraglottoplasty?	Laryngomalacia with failure to thrive and/or respiratory distress (apneas, cyanosis, hypoxia).
427	What complications are associated with supraglottoplasty?	Transient dysphagia and aspiration (10 to 15%), failure or partial improvement (8.8%; more common in children with additional congenital anomalies), and supraglottic stenosis (4%)
428	What condition is caused by reduction and/or atrophy of the longitudinal elastic fibers of the pars membranacea of the trachea or impaired cartilage integrity resulting in a soft and collapsible airway that is worse with increased intrathoracic pressure (Valsalva)?	Tracheomalacia
429	What is primary tracheomalacia?	Tracheomalacia is the most common congenital anomaly of the trachea; it is more often seen in premature infants and is thought to be due to tracheobronchial cartilage immaturity or irregularity. It can include true immaturity or diseases resulting in the malformation of the cartilage matrix such as polychondritis, chondromalacia, or other congenital anomalies affecting the cartilage. It can also be due to anatomical anomalies leading to insufficient cartilaginous support such as tracheoesophageal fistula.
430	What is secondary tracheomalacia?	Secondary (acquired) tracheomalacia can result from degeneration of normal cartilaginous support and is more common than primary tracheomalacia. It can be due to prolonged intubation, tracheostomy, recurrent tracheo-bronchitis, external tracheal compression (cardiovascular abnormalities, skeletal anomalies, and space-occupying lesions).
431	What is the normal ratio of cartilage to muscle within the trachea and in a child with tracheomalacia?	• Normal: Ratio of cartilage to muscle is 4.5:1. • Tracheomalacia: The amount of cartilage decreases, thus decreasing the ratio of cartilage to muscle. Some authorities recommend reserving the diagnosis of tra-cheomalacia for patients presenting with a ratio of 2:1.

432	How is tracheomalacia classified based on histologic, endoscopic, and clinical signs?	The major airway collapse (MAC) classification system (Mair and Parsons, 1992, PMID: 1562133): • *Type 1:* Congenital or intrinsic tracheal collapse without airway compression. Patients may have prematurity, esophageal atresia, or tracheoesophageal fistula, mucopolysaccharidoses, and Larsen syndrome. • *Type 2:* Extrinsic tracheal compression resulting in airway collapse. Patients may have cardiovascular anomalies, skeletal anomalies, or space-occupying lesions and may be primary or secondary. • *Type 3:* Secondary (acquired) tracheomalacia results from prolonged intubation, tracheotomy, or severe/recurrent tracheobronchitis.
433	How is tracheomalacia managed?	Although most infants outgrow the symptoms of tracheomalacia by 18 to 24 months of age, surgical intervention (correction of extrinsic compressive lesion, tracheostomy, aortopexy, stenting or possible tracheal grafts) may be required when conservative methods fail or the child develops life-threatening symptoms such as reflex apnea.
434	What normal reflex mechanism can also be amplified in children with tracheomalacia and result in "death attacks," "dying spells," or cardiorespiratory arrest when the trachea is stimulated by secretions, a bolus of food in the esophagus, or pressure from an esophagoscope or bronchoscope during examination?	Reflex apnea
435	Describe the adult vascular structure that forms from the following embryologic branchial arches: • First arch • Second arch • Third arch • Fourth arch • Fifth arch • Sixth arch • Intersegmental arteries	• None: Involutes • None: Involutes • Carotid system • Aortic arch • Atretic or never fully develops • Pulmonary artery from ventral portion; dorsal portion of right arch disappears while the left dorsal arch becomes the ductus arteriosus • Subclavian arteries
436	Any vascular anomaly that causes compression of the trachea and/or esophagus may be considered a vascular ring. How are complete and incomplete rings distinguished?	• *Complete:* Arterial derivatives of the branchial arch system that encircle the trachea and esophagus • *Incomplete:* Arterial derivatives that encircle the trachea and esophagus with and without ligaments and fibrous bands
437	What are the most common initial symptoms associated with vascular rings?	The symptoms depend on the degree of compression. Biphasic or inspiratory stridor, recurrent upper respiratory infections, cough, and dysphagia. Severe symptoms include "death spells" or acute apnea and cyanotic spells, often requiring cardiopulmonary resuscitation; these can occur with tracheal secretions, a bolus of food in the esophagus, or pressure on the trachea during esophagoscopy or bronchoscopy or they may be completely asymptomatic.
438	What are the most common findings on barium esophagram and bronchoscopy for the following vascular anomalies? • Double aortic arch • Right aortic arch anomaly • Anomalous innominate artery • Pulmonary artery sling • Aberrant right subclavian artery	Barium swallow • Posterior and bilateral compression • Right posterior and lateral compression • None • Anterior compression • Posterior compression Bronchoscopy • Anterior and bilateral compression

		• Right anterior and lateral compression • Anterior compression (left to right from inferior to superior) • Posterior compression • None Other imaging studies Chest CT angiography (or MRI/MRA) can assist in the final diagnosis and surgical planning.
439	What are the two most common forms of vascular rings?	• Double aortic arch (ascending aortic arch wraps around the trachea and esophagus, creating a complete ring; most common) • Persistent right aortic arch with a left ligamentum arteriosum and retroesophageal left subclavian artery (incomplete ring)
440	What vascular anomaly produces severe early tracheal compression, has a common site of esophageal and tracheal compression, is thought to arise from the left pulmonary artery originating from the right pulmonary artery, and is commonly associated with complete tracheal rings and distal bronchial hypoplasia?	Pulmonary artery sling
441	If the innominate artery arises from the aorta to the left of the trachea, it may result in symptomatic compression of the trachea that can be seen bronchoscopically as a triangular compression, which if compressed with an endoscope will result in dampening of the right radial pulse. What is the vascular anomaly?	Anomalous innominate artery
442	What is the likely diagnosis for a patient with solid food dysphagia and a barium esophagram that shows left to right posterior compression from inferior to superior?	Anomalous right subclavian artery
443	What term is used to describe dysphagia caused by extrinsic compression of an anomalous right subclavian artery?	Dysphagia lusoria
444	True or false: Surgical intervention in the form of pexy, reimplantation, or ligation, depending on the clinical scenario, should be recommended for all symptomatic patients with a vascular ring or anomaly.	True. Delay can increase the risk of sudden death, as well as tracheal and bronchial sequelae. Outcomes are excellent unless comorbid conditions (such as cardiac pathology) are present.
445	If a patient has no respiratory symptoms, what conservative therapy can be tried to manage dysphagia lusoria?	Dietary modification
446	A child with severe mental retardation, hypertelorism, hypotonia, microcephaly, downward slanting palpebral fissures, strabismus, low-set ears, beaklike profile, failure to thrive, and a history of a high-pitched catlike cry in infancy most likely suffers from what congenital anomaly?	Cri-du-chat syndrome (5p deletion syndrome)
447	What are the laryngeal findings in a patient with cri-du-chat syndrome?	Findings range from a normal examination (suggesting central reason to cry) to a characteristic narrow, diamond-shaped larynx during inspiration, posterior commissure air leak, and flaccid epiglottis.
448	Failed fusion of the posterior cricoid lamina and incomplete development of the tracheoesophageal septum result in what pathologies?	Posterior laryngeal clefts and laryngotracheoesophageal clefts

449	What symptoms might suggest laryngeal and laryngotracheoesophageal clefts?	Symptoms may include feeding difficulty, failure to thrive, aspiration, chronic cough, stridor, recurrent pneumonia, airway obstruction, wheezing, stridor, noisy breathing, and hoarseness. Significant defects can cause severe aspiration and respiratory distress.
450	What is the "gold standard" for diagnosis of laryngeal clefts?	Microlaryngoscopy and bronchoscopy are performed under general anesthesia with spontaneous ventilation, including palpation of the interarytenoid space and evaluation of the interarytenoid notch, which is normally about 3 mm (a deeper notch may indicate a more incompetent larynx).
451	What anatomical anomaly is frequently associated with posterior laryngeal and laryngotracheoesophageal clefts and may have a significant negative impact on surgical repair if not adequately addressed?	Tracheoesophageal fistula
452	While evaluating a patient with a type II laryngeal cleft, you perform esophagoscopy and biopsy, as well as bronchoscopy, bronchoalveolar lavage, and analysis of lipid-laden macrophages. What are you looking for?	Gastroesophageal reflux and aspiration
453	Describe the Benjamin-Inglis classification of posterior laryngeal and laryngoesophageal clefts. (▶ Fig. 1.7)	Benjamin-Inglis classification Occult cleft: Appreciated only by palpation or measurement of posterior arytenoid height. • Type 1: Limited to supraglottic interarytenoid area • Type 2: Partial clefting of the posterior cricoid cartilage

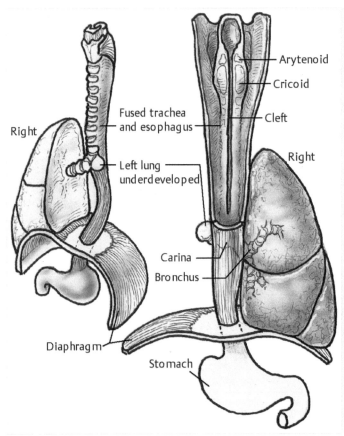

Fig. 1.7 Benjamin-Inglis type IV laryngotracheoesophageal cleft. Also shown are left-side pulmonary agenesis and microgastria. (Used with permission from Goldenberg D, Goldstein BJ, eds. Handbook of Otolaryngology–Head and Neck Surgery. New York, NY: Thieme; 2011.)

		• Type 3: Cleft of the entire cricoid cartilage and cervical portion of the tracheoesophageal membrane, stopping above the thoracic inlet • Type 4: Cleft involves a significant portion of the intrathoracic tracheoesophageal wall and may extend to the carina.
454	Describe the Meyer-Cotton classification of laryngeal and laryngoesophageal clefts.	Meyer-Cotton classification • LI: Interarytenoid cleft • LII: Partial cricoid cleft • LIII: Complete cricoid cleft • LTEI: Into cervical esophagus • LTEII: Into thoracic esophagus
455	A significant number of patients with either laryngeal or tracheoesophageal clefts have associated comorbidities. Which are the most common?	• Tracheoesophageal fistula • Esophageal atresia • Congenital heart disease • Cleft lip • Cleft palate • Micrognathia • Glossoptosis • Laryngomalacia • Opitz-Frias syndrome
456	A patient with hypospadias, hypertelorism, dysphagia, a posterior laryngeal cleft, cleft lip/palate, and bifid scrotum, uvula, and tongue is most likely to have what syndrome?	Opitz-Frias (G syndrome)
457	Patients with which congenital syndrome can develop posterior laryngotracheal cleft, polydactyly, bifid epiglottis, imperforate anus, renal abnormalities, pituitary and hypothalamic abnormalities, and hamarblastomas?	Pallister-Hall (congenital hypothalamic hamarblastomas; mutation in GLI3)
458	True or false: Patients with newly diagnosed laryngeal or laryngoesophageal clefts should undergo a trial of observation before surgical intervention is considered.	False. Early surgical intervention has been recommended to decrease the risk of irreversible pulmonary complications associated with aspiration.
459	For most clefts that involve the cricoid cartilage and all clefts that extend beyond the cricoid cartilage, would you recommend an endoscopic or open approach?	Open surgical approach. Anterior laryngofissure, two-layer approach, interposition grafting (sternocleidomastoid muscle, inferiorly based strap musculature, tibial periosteum, auricular cartilage, temporalis fascia), or tracheoesophagoplasty have all been used.
460	What comorbid condition can significantly compromise the success of surgical repair of a laryngoesophageal cleft?	Gastroesophageal reflux
461	You are evaluating an infant with inspiratory stridor and suspect a vocal-fold paralysis. What are the most common causes in newborns?	Traumatic birth, neurologic pathology, iatrogenic, or idiopathic (most common)
462	What are the most common initial clinical signs in infants and children with unilateral vocal-fold paralysis?	Breathiness, hoarseness, straining, muscle tension, and soft voice
463	In an infant diagnosed with idiopathic vocal-fold paralysis on awake flexible fiberoptic examination, what important possible cause should be investigated with a brain MRI?	Arnold-Chiari malformation (or other brainstem compressive pathologies)

464	In infants with unilateral vocal-fold paralysis, what is the likelihood of spontaneous recovery after birth trauma or after neurologic or idiopathic paralysis?	~ 70%
465	In a newborn with bilateral vocal-fold paralysis, what is the likelihood of spontaneous recovery if the cause is a neurologic disorder or idiopathic?	~ 50%
466	What is the treatment for congenital unilateral vocal-fold paralysis?	Depends on severity, age of the patient, and the cause Conservative management, tracheostomy, injection of filler material, or thyroplasty
467	Surgical intervention for congenital bilateral vocal-fold paralysis attempts to _____ the true vocal folds to improve the airway.	Lateralize
468	What diagnosis is defined as failure of the voice to drop to a normal pitch at puberty and can persist well beyond the normal age of puberty?	Mutational falsetto or puberphonia resulting from muscular incoordination, hyperfunction of the cricothyroid muscle, or psychological dysfunction
469	In patients with puberphonia or mutational falsetto, what is the first line of treatment?	Voice therapy and/or psychotherapy. For recalcitrant disease, a type 3 thyroplasty can be considered.
470	What are common nonpulmonary indications for pediatric tracheostomy?	Acquired subglottic stenosis (31.4%) Bilateral vocal-cord paralysis (22.2%) Congenital airway malformations (22.2%) Tumors (11.1%)
471	Although tracheostomy tube diameter and length must be chosen carefully on an individual basis, what helpful formula(s) can assist in predicting the correct inner and outer diameter?	Age • Inner diameter (mm) = age (years)/3 + 3.5 • Outer diameter (mm) = age (years)/3 + 5.5 Weight • Inner diameter (mm) = [weight (kg) x 0.08] + 3.1 • Outer diameter (mm) = [weight (kg) x 0.1] + 4.7
472	Describe the embryology of isolated esophageal atresia.	*Esophageal atresia* is defined as an incomplete formation of the esophagus. Isolated esophageal atresia is due to failure of the recanalization of the esophagus during the eighth week of development.
473	What percentage of patients with congenital anomalies of the aerodigestive tract has isolated esophageal atresia?	About 85% of patients with esophageal atresia have a distal tracheoesophageal fistula. Ten percent manifest with isolated esophageal atresia and about 5% with isolated tracheoesophageal fistula
474	What are the various types of esophageal atresia (EA) with or without tracheoesophageal fistula (TEF)? (► Fig. 1.8)	• EA with distal TEF (most common) • Isolated EA • Isolated TEF • EA with proximal TEF • EA with double TEF

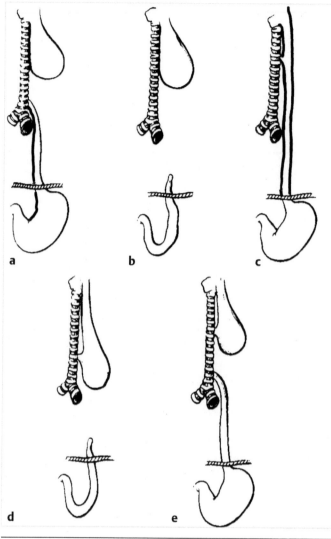

Fig. 1.8 Tracheoesophageal fistulae. (a) Esophageal atresia with distal tracheoesophageal fistula (most common); (b) isolated esophageal atresia; (c) H-type fistula (isolated tracheoesophageal fistula); (d) esophageal atresia with proximal esophagotracheal fistula; (e) esophageal atresia with double tracheoesophageal fistula. (Adapted from Morrow SE, Nakayama DK. Congenital malformations of the esophagus. In: Bluestone CD, Stool ES, Kenna MA, eds. Pediatric Otolaryngology 3rd Edition. Philadelphia: Saunders; 1996: 1122.)

475	What are prenatal signs of esophageal atresia?	• Polyhydramnios in the mother • Inability to identify the fetal stomach bubble on a prenatal ultrasonogram
476	What congenital anomalies are commonly associated with esophageal atresia?	Found in approximately 50% of patients: • Musculoskeletal: Hemivertebrae, radial dysplasia or amelia, polydactyly, syndactyly, rib malformations, scoliosis, lower limb defects • Gastrointestinal: Imperforate anus, duodenal atresia, malrotation, intestinal malformations, Meckel diverticulum, annular pancreas • Cardiac (most commonly associated): Ventricular septal defect, patent ductus arteriosus, tetralogy of Fallot, atrial septal defect, single umbilical artery, right-sided aortic arch • Genitourinary: Renal agenesis or dysplasia, horseshoe kidney, polycystic kidney, ureteral and urethral malformations, hypospadias
477	What association is commonly diagnosed with esophageal atresia with or without TEF?	VACTERL (10%): (V) vertebral defects, (A) anal atresia, (C) cardiac malformations, (TE) tracheoesophageal fistula with esophageal atresia, (R) renal dysplasia and (L) limb anomalies (most commonly radial anomalies)

2 Pediatric Malignancies

Kathryn M. Van Abel, Ashley G. O'Reilly, and Rajanya S. Petersson

Rhabdomyosarcomas

1	Second to accidents, what is the most common cause of death in children between 1 and 14 years of age?	Malignancy
2	What is the most common sarcoma of childhood?	Rhabdomyosarcoma. Up to 35% are found in the head and neck.
3	Which cell type gives rise to rhabdomyosarcoma, and what major histologic variants are described?	Primitive skeletal muscle cells (small, round blue cell tumor of childhood): embryonal, botryoid, alveolar, undifferentiated. Some include anaplastic. Embryonal and alveolar are the most common types, and embryonal type carries the best prognosis.
4	Where does pediatric head and neck rhabdomyosarcoma most commonly occur?	*Parameningeal* (50%): Paranasal sinuses, nasopharynx, nasal cavity, middle ear, mastoid, infratemporal fossa (5-year survival: 49%; considered high risk) *Orbit* (25%) (5-year survival: 84%) *Nonorbital, nonparameningeal* (25%): Scalp, parotid, oral cavity, pharynx, thyroid, parathyroid, neck (5-year survival: 70%)
5	What are the common initial symptoms associated with head and neck pediatric rhabdomyosarcoma?	Symptoms are due to progressive mass effect, local swelling, neurologic sequelae, or tissue necrosis. Bone marrow involvement can manifest as hematologic concerns.
6	What are the most important negative prognostic factors associated with pediatric rhabdomyosarcoma?	Diagnosis during infancy or adolescence; metastatic disease at diagnosis; alveolar histology; disease identified in a parameningeal location (risk for intracranial spread), in the extremities, or in the retroperitoneum or trunk; recurrence or progression during therapy
7	What diagnostic techniques are required to evaluate the primary tumor in rhabdomyosarcoma?	Biopsy: Open biopsy is done to ensure adequate tissue unless the lesion is small and difficult to access, in which case, needle biopsy may be acceptable. Imaging: CT scan and magnetic resonance imaging (MRI) to evaluate extent of disease
8	What diagnostic techniques are required to evaluate locoregional and/or distant metastases in rhabdomyosarcoma?	Laboratory work (complete blood count [CBC], electrolytes, liver function, coagulation studies, renal function tests) Technetium-99 bone scan CT chest Positron emission tomography (PET)/CT scan Aspiration/biopsy of iliac bone marrow. Distant metastases are more commonly found in the brain, lung, bone, and bone marrow.
9	Which group is credited with increasing the survival rate for patients with rhabdomyosarcoma from 30 to 70% since the 1970s?	The Intergroup Rhabdomyosarcoma Study Committee (now the Soft Tissue Sarcoma Committee of the Children's Oncology Group)
10	What is the clinical grouping or surgical pathologic staging system commonly used for staging rhabdomyosarcoma?	(▶ Table 2.1)

Table 2.1 Surgical-Histopathologic Clinical Grouping System for the Intergroup Rhabdomyosarcoma Study

Stage	Description
Group I	Localized disease, completely resected
A	Confined to organ or muscle of origin
B	Invasion outside organ/muscle of origin; regional nodes not involved
Group II	Compromised or regional resection including
A	Grossly resected tumors with microscopic residual tumor
B	Regional disease, completely resected, in which nodes may be involved and/or tumor extends into an adjacent organ
C	Regional disease with involved nodes, grossly resected, but with evidence of microscopic residual
Group III	Incomplete resection or biopsy with gross residual disease
Group IV	Distant metastases, present at onset

Data from Crist WM, Garnsey L, Beltangady MS, et al. Prognosis in children with rhabdomyosarcoma: a report of the intergroup rhabdomyosarcoma studies I and II (Intergroup Rhabdomyosarcoma Committee). J Clin Oncol. 1990 Mar;8 (3):443–52.

11	What is the tumor, node, and metastases (TNM) staging system for rhabdomyosarcoma introduced by the Intergroup Rhabdomyosarcoma Study IV?	(▶ Table 2.2)

Table 2.2 TNM staging system for rhabdomyosarcoma introduced by the Intergroup Rhabdomyosarcoma Study IV.

Stage	Description
T1	Confined to the anatomical site or origin
T2	Extension beyond site of origin A: ≤ 5 cm in diameter B: > 5 cm in diameter
N0	No clinically involved lymph nodes
N1	Clinically involved lymph nodes
NX	Clinical status unknown
M0	No distant metastasis
M1	Distant metastasis
MX	Distant metastasis unknown

Data from Neville HL, Andrassy RJ, Lobe TE, et al. Preoperative staging, prognostic factors, and outcome for extremity rhabdomyosarcoma: a preliminary report from the Intergroup Rhabdomyosarcoma Study IV (1991–1997). J Pediatr Surg. 2000 Feb;35(2):317–21.

12	Describe the staging system for rhabdomyosarcoma that combines the TNM and clinicopathologic groups to provide both prognostic and therapeutic recommendations.	Rhabdomyosarcoma prognostic stratification and standard treatment assignment (Prognosis, Event-Free Survival): Excellent (> 85%) Very good (75 to 85%) Good (50 to 70%) Poor (< 30%) This system allows for risk-directed therapy.

13	Describe the favorable and unfavorable locations for head and neck rhabdomyosarcoma.	Favorable: Orbit and eyelid Unfavorable: Parameningeal
14	True or False. In a patient with localized nonorbital, nonparameningeal head and neck embryonal rhabdomyosarcoma, if complete surgical excision can be achieved, radiation therapy may be avoided.	True. However, chemotherapy is recommended for all patients with rhabdomyosarcoma.
15	Is elective neck dissection for clinically negative necks recommended in patients with nonparameningeal rhabdomyosarcoma of the head and neck?	No
16	What are the most commonly used chemotherapeutic agents for treatment of rhabdomyosarcoma?	Vincristine, actinomycin D, cyclophosphamide
17	What are the most common late complications in patients treated for rhabdomyosarcoma of the head and neck?	Short stature, regional tissue hypoplasia, poor dentition, malformed teeth, impaired vision, decreased hearing, and learning disorders
18	What is the most common fibrous tumor of infancy?	Infantile myofibromatosis (solitary or multicentric; well-circumscribed, spindle-shaped cells, including fibroblasts and smooth muscle cells on histopathology)
19	What is the natural history of infantile myofibromatosis?	Most will involute by age 1 to 2 years. Visceral lesions causing functional impairment (e.g., pulmonary), may require surgical excision. For nonresectable, rapidly progressive, recurrent or symptomatic lesions, surgery, radiation therapy and chemotherapy should be considered.

Other Sarcomas

20	What tumor type is composed of a mixed group of mesenchymal malignancies that are generally defined as either soft tissue (80%) or bony/cartilaginous (20%) tissue?	Sarcomas. These tumors can arise from muscle, nerve, fat, vessel, fibrous tissue, bone, or cartilage.
21	What is the most common initial manifestation of head and neck sarcoma?	Painless mass. Symptoms generally are related to the structures involved and uncommonly include pain. Referred otalgia may be seen in patients with oropharyngeal or hypopharyngeal lesions. Pain can also represent bony impingement of nervous structures.
22	How are sarcomas defined in general terms?	Tissue of origin Histologic grade Anatomical subsite in the head and neck
23	List examples of high-grade and low-grade sarcomas of the head and neck.	High grade • Osteosarcoma* • Malignant fibrous histiocytoma* • Rhabdomyosarcoma* • Angiosarcoma* • Synovial sarcoma • Alveolar soft part sarcoma • Ewing sarcoma Low grade • Dermatofibrosarcoma protuberans • Desmoid tumors • Atypical lipomatous tumors • Require individual grading • Chondrosarcoma • Fibrosarcoma • Neurogenic sarcoma • Hemangiopericytoma *Most common in the head and neck (50%)

24	How does the anatomical subsite within the head and neck influence decision-making in the management of sarcomas?	The ability to resect the tumor fully, without causing undue morbidity, significantly influences surgical versus nonsurgical decision-making.
25	In the pediatric population, what percentage of sarcomas manifest in the head and neck?	Around 35% of sarcomas in children manifest in the head and neck; this rate is greater than that in adults.
26	What historical factors increase the risk of developing a sarcoma?	History of radiation of the head and neck Li-Fraumeni syndrome (*p53* mutation) Hereditary retinoblastoma (*Rb-1* mutation) Neurofibromatosis type 1 (NF-1) Gardner syndrome Nevoid basal cell carcinoma syndrome Carney triad Hereditary hemochromatosis Werner syndrome
27	How might a sarcoma differ from a squamous cell carcinoma of the same anatomical subsite during examination of the upper aerodigestive tract?	Sarcomas will appear as a submucosal mass.
28	What radiographic workup is necessary for pediatric head and neck sarcomas?	CT scan: Soft tissue extent, nodal involvement, cortical bony involvement MRI scan: Soft tissue, bone marrow, perineural extension, orbital and intracranial involvement Fludeoxyglucose (FDG)-PET/CT scan: Staging, response to therapy, surveillance
29	What is the most likely site of metastasis from head and neck sarcomas, and how does this influence diagnostic workup?	Lung. Imaging of the chest is required: chest-X-ray for low-grade lesions, CT for high-grade lesions.
30	During initial diagnosis of a soft tissue mass in the head and neck, why might core needle biopsy or excisional biopsy be preferred to FNA?	FNA may not provide enough tissue for extensive immunohistochemical analysis, and it has a higher risk of being nondiagnostic. However, FNA is minimally invasive, can be performed without conscious sedation in some children, and has a reported sensitivity of 95%.
31	What mesenchymal vascular sarcoma arises from the pericytes of Zimmerman?	Hemangiopericytoma
32	Notably, 10 to 25% of all hemangiopericytomas are in the head and neck. What is the most common subsite?	Sinonasal tract
33	True or False. All hemangiopericytomas diagnosed in the pediatric population are acquired after birth.	False. 5% of all hemangiopericytomas are congenital and are considered benign.
34	How do pediatric hemangiopericytomas most commonly present?	Most are slow-growing, soft, subcutaneous, painless masses. Compared with adult-onset hemangiopericytomas, the pediatric variant generally follows a more benign clinical course.
35	How are pediatric hemangiopericytomas managed?	*Surgical resection* to negative margins is the mainstay of treatment for malignant lesions. *Radiation and chemotherapy* may improve local and distant control, although distant metastases are less common in the head and neck. *Chemotherapy* has been used for congenital lesions.
36	What aggressive malignant sarcoma arises most commonly in the axial long bones of the lower extremities and pelvis but can arise in extraosseous soft tissue sites, such as the sinonasal tract and paranasal sinuses, orbit, scalp, and paravertebral areas of the neck?	Ewing sarcoma

37	What is the tissue of origin for Ewing sarcoma?	This topic is controversial; possible origins include totipotential mesenchymal cells and primitive neuroectodermal tumors.
38	What are the most common initial symptoms associated with Ewing sarcoma?	Pain and regional swelling
39	What proportion of patients with Ewing sarcoma manifest with metastatic disease?	Ewing sarcoma is considered metastatic at presentation in nearly all patients.
40	How is Ewing sarcoma managed?	Treatment comprises surgical excision with concurrent chemotherapy (vincristine, actinomycin-D, cyclophosphamide) and radiation therapy.
41	What tumor is a type of spindle cell sarcoma that is either associated with peripheral nerves or shows nerve sheath differentiation?	Malignant peripheral nerve sheath sarcoma is a malignant, aggressive tumor with a high rate of metastases.
42	Malignant peripheral nerve sheath tumors are masses that can be associated with pain and dysesthesia. How often is a nerve of origin identified?	~ 70%
43	What hereditary condition is a significant risk factor for the development of malignant peripheral nerve sheath tumors?	NF-1. Up to 40% of tumors develop in a preexisting neurofibroma.
44	What important prognostic factors predict poor outcome in patients with malignant peripheral nerve sheath tumors?	Tumor size > 5 cm, tumor invasiveness (T2), concomitant NF-1, head and neck location
45	What is the management strategy for malignant primary nerve sheath tumors?	Surgical resection is the mainstay of treatment and a strong predictor of survival. Adjuvant chemotherapy or radiation therapy potentially has a role.
46	Alveolar soft part sarcoma arises from which tissue type(s)?	Myogenic and neural cells (controversial)
47	Although they are extremely rare, two-thirds of head and neck alveolar soft part sarcomas arise in which anatomical subsites and manifest with what common symptom(s)?	They manifest in the orbit and tongue as a painless mass.
48	What demographic is most commonly affected by alveolar soft part sarcomas?	Females aged 10 to 30 years
49	How are alveolar soft part sarcomas treated?	Surgical resection with adjuvant radiation therapy or chemotherapy (in phase I or phase II trials)
50	What are the two most common locations for osteosarcoma within the head and neck?	Mandible and maxilla
51	What are the most common initial symptoms associated with osteosarcoma of the head and neck?	2 to 6 months of a painless mass, dental pain, or loose teeth
52	What is the mainstay of therapy for osteosarcoma of the head and neck?	Aggressive surgical resection. Postoperative radiation therapy is controversial. The addition of chemotherapy to surgery has been shown to be beneficial.
53	Despite advances in treatment, surgical resection, and reconstruction, survival for patients with osteosarcoma is poor. What prognostic factors have been identified?	Surgical margins (i.e., positive margins are associated with poor outcome), recurrence, primary tumor arising in previously radiated bone, and tumors arising in extragnathic bone (i.e., less likely to achieve wide resection). No differences have been identified between pediatric and adult populations.

Lymphomas

54	What is the most common lymphoproliferative malignancy of the head and neck in pediatric patients?	Lymphoma
55	What are common risk factors for lymphoma?	Radiation, Epstein-Barr virus, human immunodeficiency virus (HIV) or other immunosuppressive disorders, organ transplantation, common immunodeficiency syndromes (e.g., Wisckott-Aldrich syndrome, ataxia-telangiectasia, X-linked lymphoproliferative disease), organic toxins (e.g., phenols, benzene), autoimmune disorders (e.g., celiac disease, rheumatoid arthritis)
56	What cell types give rise to non-Hodgkin lymphoma?	B cells: 85% T cells: 15%
57	What is the typical age distribution of non-Hodgkin lymphoma?	Incidence increases with age.
58	According the National Cancer Institute, what are the most common types of non-Hodgkin lymphoma of childhood?	Burkitt [t(8:14)] and Burkitt-like lymphomas Lymphoblastic lymphoma Diffuse large B-cell lymphoma Other (anaplastic large cell lymphoma)
59	How do pediatric lymphomas most commonly manifest?	• Rapid enlargement of extranodal tissue (e.g., Waldeyer ring) or nodal enlargement (persisting > 4 to 6 weeks, generally > 2 cm in diameter; nodes > 1 cm should be considered suspicious) that may or may not be painful • Mass effect is dependent on location (e.g., nasal obstruction, dysphagia, airway compromise, superior vena cava syndrome). • Hepatosplenomegaly • Central nervous system (CNS) involvement (cranial nerve palsies, mental status changes, rarely with seizures)
60	What are the two symptom classes used for staging lymphomas?	Class A: Asymptomatic (better prognosis) Class B: Weight loss, fever, night sweats (poorer prognosis)
61	Most non-Hodgkin lymphomas in the pediatric population arise in the abdomen; only 5 to 10% are located in the head and neck. What are the most common subsites in the head and neck?	Salivary glands, larynx, Waldeyer ring, paranasal sinuses, orbit, and scalp
62	Non-Hodgkin lymphoma workup includes a careful history and physical examination; imaging such as CT and gallium-67 scanning; and laboratory workup including cerebrospinal fluid analysis, urinalysis, CBC, and serum chemistries. However, definitive diagnosis rests on what key step?	Biopsy or tissue specimen (excisional biopsy) for histology, cytology, immunohistochemistry and genotyping
63	What infectious agent has been shown to be associated with both endemic (85%) and sporadic (15%) cases of Burkitt lymphoma?	Epstein-Barr virus
64	What chromosomal translocation is commonly noted in Burkitt lymphoma?	t(8;14)(q24;q32)
65	The 5-year survival rate in pediatric cases of non-Hodgkin lymphoma is 80%; this rate varies depending on what important prognostic factor(s)?	Age: Worse outcome if patient is < 12 months or > 15 years of age Site of disease: Worse in mediastinum, with CNS involvement Tumor burden or lactate dehydrogenase (LDH) levels Unusual chromosomal abnormalities

| 66 | How is pediatric non-Hodgkin lymphoma clinically staged? | (▶ Table 2.3) |

Table 2.3 St. Jude's Research Hospital Staging System for NHL (the clinical staging does not take into account the cell of origin).

Stage	Description
I	Single extranodal tumor or single anatomic area (nodal) excluding the mediastinum or abdomen
II	Single extranodal site with regional lymph node involvement; two or more nodal areas on the same side of the diaphragm; two single extranodal tumors + /- regional node disease on the same side of the diaphragm; primary GI tract tumor (usually ileocecal + /- involvement of the associated mesenteric nodes)
III	Two single extranodal tumors + /- regional node disease on opposite sides of the diaphragm; two or more nodal areas on opposite sides of the diaphragm; all extensive primary intra-abdominal disease; unresectable; all primary intrathoracic tumors (mediastinal, pleural, thymic); all primary paraspinal or epidural tumors regardless of other sites
IV	Any initial CNS or bone marrow involvement (< 25%)

Data from Murphy SB, Fairclough DL, Hutchison RE, et al. Non-Hodgkin's lymphomas of childhood: an analysis of the histology, staging, and response to treatment of 338 cases at a single institution. J Clin Oncol 7 (2): 186–93, 1989.

67	What is the mainstay of management for non-Hodgkin lymphoma?	Chemotherapy: CHOP (cyclophosphamide, doxorubicin [hydroxydaunorubicin, Adriamycin], vincristine (Oncovin), prednisone (or prednisolone) Radiation can be used for localized disease or emergencies involving respiratory, nervous system, or vascular compromise.
68	What age group(s) is(are) most affected by Hodgkin lymphoma?	Bimodal distribution: Teenage adolescents and middle-age adults
69	Which sex confers a higher risk for Hodgkin lymphoma?	Male, 2:1
70	What causative agent is commonly associated with Hodgkin lymphoma?	Epstein-Barr virus
71	What tumors are most commonly associated with Epstein-Barr virus infection?	Burkitt lymphoma (non-Hodgkin lymphoma) Hodgkin lymphoma Nasopharyngeal carcinoma
72	How does Hodgkin lymphoma typically manifest?	About 80% of patients have cervical lymphadenopathy and ~ 40% with class B symptoms (night sweats, fever, weight loss). It can present with respiratory distress or superior vena cava syndrome resulting from mediastinal involvement.
73	What is the pathognomonic histopathology found in Hodgkin lymphoma?	Reed-Sternberg cells ("owl-eyes" = two or more nuclei with two or more large nucleoli) Eosinophilic inclusions Large, clonal, multinucleated cells B cell in origin, derived from germinal centers.
74	What is the histologic classification used for Hodgkin lymphoma?	The World Health Organization (WHO) 2008 Classification: 1. Nodular lymphocytic predominant 2. "Classic" Hodgkin lymphoma: Rye modification of the Lukes-Butler classification: • *Lymphocytic predominance* (< 10%): Typically manifests with localized disease; high concentration of normal-appearing lymphocytes, uncommon Reed-Sternberg cells, and no fibrosis; better prognosis

		• *Mixed cellularity* (20 to 40%): Typically manifests with extranodal involvement; mixed infiltrate; Reed-Sternberg cells more common • *Lymphocytic depletion* (< 15%): Common in HIV patients; diffuse fibrosis, few lymphocytes, bizarre Reed-Sternberg cells; poor prognosis • *Nodular sclerosis* (40 to 80%): Most common; lymphoid nodules separated by bands of collagen containing the Reed-Sternberg cells (lacunar cell variant); more commonly affects females than males
75	What is the clinical classification system used to stage Hodgkin lymphoma?	Ann Arbor Staging: • *Stage I*: Single lymph node region or single extralymphatic organ or site (IE) • *Stage II*: Two or more lymph node regions on the same side of the diaphragm or localized involvement of an extralymphatic organ or site (IIE) in addition to one or more lymph node region on the same side of the diaphragm • *Stage III*: Involvement of lymph node regions on both sides of the diaphragm, with or without involvement of an extralymphatic organ or site (IIIE), involvement of the spleen (IIIS), or both • *Stage IV*: Diffuse or disseminated involvement of one or more extralymphatic organs or sites, with or without associated lymph node involvement
76	In addition to a thorough physical examination, what radiographic studies are important for the workup of a patient with suspected Hodgkin lymphoma?	Chest X-ray Chest and abdominal CT scan PET/CT
77	What is the overall 5-year survival rate for patients with Hodgkin lymphoma?	~ 80%
78	What prognostic factors are important in Hodgkin lymphoma?	*Better:* Lymphocytic predominance types *Worse*: The presence of Reed-Sternberg cells, higher Ann Arbor stage, presence of class B symptoms
79	What is the management strategy for primary treatment of Hodgkin lymphoma?	Chemotherapy: MOPP (mechlorethamine, Oncovin [vincristine], prednisone, procarbazine); ABVD (Adriamycin [doxorubicin], bleomycin, vinblastine, dacarbazine), followed by targeted radiation therapy. Some authorities suggest single-modality radiation therapy for early disease.

Thyroid Carcinomas

80	What percentage of pediatric thyroid nodules are malignant?	About 26% (ranges have been published from < 1%, citing a referral bias in children with risk factors for thyroid cancer, to as high as 36%; most of the literature suggests an increased risk of thyroid carcinomas in pediatric thyroid nodules compared with adults) Regardless of the exact percentage, the 2009 revised American Thyroid Association (ATA) recommends the same diagnostic and therapeutic approach for children as for adults (clinical evaluation, serum thyroid-stimulating hormone [TSH], ultrasonography, FNA).
81	What are the most common benign thyroid nodules?	Multinodular goiter (sporadic) Hashimoto thyroiditis Hemorrhagic, colloid, and simple cysts Follicular adenomas Hürthle cell adenomas

82	What is the most important environmental risk factor for the development of pediatric thyroid carcinoma?	Radiation exposure
83	What genetic syndromes are associated with an increased risk of medullary thyroid cancer?	MEN 2A MEN 2B Familial medullary thyroid carcinoma
84	Name the syndrome associated with the following constellation of syndromes: • Familial adenomatous polyps, papillary thyroid carcinoma, autosomal dominant (adenomatous polyposis coli [*APC*]) gene • Primary pigmented nodular adrenocortical disease (primary adrenal hypercorticism); lentigines, ephelides, and blue nevi of the skin and mucosa; nonendocrine and endocrine tumors including papillary and follicular thyroid carcinoma • Premature aging (progeria), osteosarcoma, soft tissue sarcoma, and follicular or papillary thyroid carcinoma • Macrocephaly, autism or developmental delay, penile freckling or other benign skin lesions, vascular anomalies such as arteriovenous (AV) malformations or hemangiomas, and GI polyps	• Gardner syndrome • Carney complex type 1 • Werner syndrome • *PTEN* hamartoma syndrome (Cowden syndrome, Bannayan-Riley-Ruvalcaba syndrome)
85	What is the most common pediatric thyroid tumor (malignant or benign)?	Follicular adenoma (benign)
86	What is the most common malignant thyroid tumor in children?	Papillary thyroid carcinoma (83%): 60% papillary, 23% follicular variant papillary. Less commonly, follicular thyroid carcinoma (10%), medullary thyroid carcinoma (5%), and other rarer cancers may arise.
87	What factors increase the risk that a thyroid nodule is in fact thyroid carcinoma?	• Male • History of thyroid cancer in one or more first-degree relatives • History of previous hemithyroidectomy for thyroid cancer History of radiation exposure (external beam, ionizing radiation, etc.) • Associated genetic syndrome increasing the risk for thyroid cancer (e.g., MEN 2A, MEN 2B, Familial Medullary Thyroid Carcinoma [FMTC], Cowden, Carney, Werner, *PTEN* hamartoma syndrome, etc.) • Firm, fixed, rapidly growing nodule • New-onset hoarseness or vocal cord paralysis • Dysphagia • Odynophagia • Lymphadenopathy (up to three-fourths of patients) • FDG avidity on PET scanning
88	Does a 5-year-old diagnosed with thyroid carcinoma have a higher risk of advanced disease than an 18-year-old with the same tumor?	Yes. Prepubertal children are more likely to have advanced disease (regional metastasis, extracapsular extension, and invasion into surrounding tissue). Overall prognosis is still excellent.
89	Children diagnosed with medullary thyroid carcinoma generally have a solitary thyroid nodule or are diagnosed during workup for which three associated syndromes?	• MEN 2A (or Sipple syndrome): RET (rearranged during transfection) proto-oncogene mutation; parathyroid hyperplasia, pheochromocytoma, medullary thyroid carcinoma • MEN 2B: RET proto-oncogene; mucosal neuromas, marfanoid habitus, thickened corneal nerves, medullary thyroid carcinoma, rare parathyroid hyperplasia • Familial medullary thyroid carcinoma

90	What laboratory workup should be performed for a child in whom thyroid cancer is suspected?	• Thyroid function testing: tri-iodothyronine (T3), thyroxine (T4), TSH; generally normal in malignancy • Calcitonin: Elevated in medullary thyroid carcinoma • Thyroglobulin: If elevated, can be used for postoperative surveillance; routine preoperative measurement is not recommended by the ATA • Carcinoembryonic antigen: Elevated in medullary thyroid cancer (except in advanced disease) • 24-hour urine metanephrines: Functional pheochromocytomas or paragangliomas may result in hypertensive crises if untreated. • Genetic screening: If patient is at high risk for hereditary disorders
91	What is the first step in the imaging workup for pediatric thyroid cancer?	Ultrasonography: location, number of nodules, size, microcalcifications, infiltrative margins, hypervascularity, extracapsular spread, regional metastases, height relative to width on transverse view; can also be used to guide FNA biopsy
92	True or False. FNA biopsy is less accurate for diagnosing thyroid malignancy in pediatric patients than in the adult population.	False. There is no difference in diagnostic accuracy. FNA is first-line test for tissue diagnosis and management planning. Patient compliance may require FNA with sedation.
93	True or False. Scintigraphy does not often help to distinguish malignant from benign thyroid disease.	True. Scintigraphy is useful for identifying ectopic thyroid tissue (ectopic lingual thyroid). Hot nodules can be malignant.
94	When should a CT scan be considered in the workup of pediatric thyroid cancer?	CT of the neck and chest should be considered with extensive disease, extracapsular spread, mediastinal involvement, or regional lymphadenopathy. The risk of pulmonary metastases is as high as 20% in some series and increases with regional metastases. Pulmonary metastases can also be detected using radioactive iodine scanning.
95	How are thyroid cancers in children staged?	TNM staging *T-stage* • T1: <2 cm • T2: 2 to 4 cm • T3: >4 cm limited to the thyroid gland or with minimal extrathyroidal extension • T4a: Any size; extrathyroidal extension to involve adjacent soft tissues, larynx, trachea, esophagus, or recurrent laryngeal nerve • T4b: Any size, extrathyroidal extension to involve the prevertebral fascia or encase the carotid artery or mediastinal great vessels *N-stage* • N1a: Metastases to level VI • N1b: Metastases to any cervical or mediastinal lymph node(s) *M-stage* • M1: Distant metastases *Well-Differentiated*: • Stage I: Any T, any N, M0 • Stage II: Any T, any N, M1 *Note*: Medullary thyroid carcinoma has the same TNM system, but stages I, II, III, IVA, IVB, and IVC are delineated.
96	The American Joint Committee on Cancer (TNM) system was developed to determine the risk of death, but it does not describe the risk of recurrence. How do the 2009 ATA guidelines describe this risk?	Low-risk • No local or distant metastases • All macroscopic tumor has been resected. • No tumor invasion of locoregional tissues or structures Tumor does not have aggressive histology or vascular invasion.

		• If ^{131}I is given, there is no uptake outside the thyroid bed on the first post-treatment whole-body scan. Intermediate-risk • Microscopic invasion of tumor into the perithyroidal soft tissues at initial surgery • Cervical lymph node metastasis or ^{131}I uptake outside the thyroid bed done after thyroid remnant ablation • Tumor with aggressive histology or vascular invasion High-risk • Macroscopic tumor invasion • Incomplete tumor resection • Distant metastases • Possibly thyroglobulinemia disproportionate to what is seen on the post-treatment scan
97	In general, what is the extent of resection recommended for a solitary thyroid lesion in a child?	Hemithyroidectomy. Subtotal or completion thyroidectomy should be performed if frozen or permanent pathology confirms thyroid cancer.
98	When might thyroid lobectomy alone be sufficient as surgical therapy in the pediatric population?	Small (< 1 cm), low-risk, unifocal, intrathyroidal papillary carcinomas in the absence of prior head and neck irradiation or radiologic or clinical cervical lymphadenopathy
99	When should total thyroidectomy be considered in patients with indeterminant thyroid nodules?	Large tumors (> 4 cm), when marked atypia is seen on biopsy, when the biopsy is read as "suspicious for papillary carcinoma," in patients with a family history of thyroid carcinoma, and in patients with a history of radiation exposure
100	Discuss the pros and cons of subtotal or near-total thyroidectomy.	Pros • Potentially limit morbidity associated with recurrent laryngeal nerve injury and parathyroid devascularization • Unlikely to increase recurrence rates • May be able to maintain a euthyroid state Cons • Can interfere with postoperative radioactive iodine treatment for microscopic and distant disease • May impact postoperative surveillance
101	When should you consider elective neck dissection in pediatric patients with well-differentiated thyroid carcinoma?	Lateral neck dissection should be performed only for clinically positive nodal disease. If such disease is present, elective dissection of levels IIA, III, IV, and VB should be performed. If there is disease in level IIA, some authorities recommend dissection of level IIB. Levels I, IIB, and VA should also be included if there is clinically evident disease. Central neck dissection (level VI) should be performed therapeutically for clinically involved central or lateral neck nodes and electively (ipsilateral or bilateral) for patients with advanced primary tumors (T3 or T4).
102	When should radioactive iodine be considered in the management of pediatric thyroid carcinoma?	Indicated: • All patients with known distant metastases, gross extrathyroidal extension, and primary tumor size > 4 cm • Selected patients with 1- to 4-cm thyroid cancers confined to the thyroid with documented lymph node metastases or other high-risk features when the combination of age, tumor size, lymph node status, and individual histology predicts an intermediate to high risk of recurrence or death from thyroid cancer. Not indicated: • Solitary tumor < 1 cm in diameter without high-risk features

		• Multifocal cancer if all tumors are < 1 cm and intra-thyroidal without high-risk features
103	What are the potential side effects of radioactive iodine ablation for the management of pediatric thyroid cancer?	Short-term effects: Nausea (immediate, temporary), xerostomia, altered taste, dental carries, cytopenias, menstrual irregularities (temporary), decreased sperm counts (temporary) Long-term effects: Xerostomia, altered taste, cytopenias, nasolacrimal duct obstruction, increased lifetime risk of secondary malignancy (leukemias, salivary gland, urinary, and GI)
104	What is the extent of surgical intervention recommended for medullary thyroid carcinoma?	Total thyroidectomy (when there is high risk for multicentricity and recurrence) and elective bilateral central compartment dissection Lateral dissection is reserved for clinically evident disease or lymph node metastases in the adjacent central neck compartment. Elective lateral neck dissection should include levels IIA, III, IV, and VB. The superior level VII nodes should also be addressed in this situation.
105	A 9-month-old female infant is brought to your office for consideration of prophylactic thyroidectomy to prevent the development of thyroid carcinoma. Why might you consider this operation?	*RET* gene mutation positivity For MEN 2B (high-risk) mutations, resection may be considered in the first year of life (includes central neck dissection if patient is > 1 year). In MEN 2A or familial medullary thyroid cancer syndromes (lower risk), resection can be delayed until early childhood (age of 3 to 6 years is suggested in the literature, but no real consensus has been reached; timing of surgery depends on other risk factors; in general < 8 to 10 years of age) unless a high-risk mutation is identified.
106	True or False. Because of their young age, risk for recurrence, and aggressive disease at diagnosis, pediatric patients diagnosed with thyroid carcinoma uniformly do poorly compared with their adult counterparts.	False. The survival rate for pediatric patients is better than that for adults. Long-term survival for well-differentiated thyroid carcinoma is > 90%. Medullary thyroid carcinoma has relatively low 30-year survival rates, but the 5-year survival rate is > 90%.

Salivary Gland Malignancies

107	What are the two most common benign salivary gland tumors of childhood?	Pleomorphic adenoma and hemangioma
108	What is the risk of malignancy in pediatric epithelial salivary gland tumors compared with the risk in adults?	Pediatrics 50 to 60% vs. adults 15 to 25%
109	Name the most common and the second most common pediatric salivary gland malignancy.	Mucoepidermoid carcinoma and acinic cell carcinoma
110	What two salivary gland malignancies are seen almost exclusively in children?	Sialoblastoma (congenital, relatively high risk of local recurrence, risk of metastases) and salivary gland anlage tumor (benign, pedunculated nasopharyngeal tumor, simple surgical excision)
111	True or False. Pediatric salivary gland tumors in children are treated the same as in adults.	True

Nasopharyngeal Carcinomas

112	Although nasopharyngeal carcinoma represents only 1% of pediatric malignancies in the United States and Europe, it is more common in which geographic and international regions?	China, Southeast Asia, Alaska (Inuit population), North Africa, and some areas in the Mediterranean

113	What three subtypes of nasopharyngeal carcinoma does the WHO recognize?	WHO subtypes of nasopharyngeal carcinoma: • Type 1: Squamous cell carcinoma • Type 2: Nonkeratinizing carcinoma • Type 3: Undifferentiated carcinoma (most common in pediatric patients)
114	What virus is commonly associated with pediatric nasopharyngeal carcinoma?	Epstein-Barr virus
115	Where does nasopharyngeal carcinoma most commonly metastasize?	Bone and bone marrow, lung, liver, and mediastinum
116	What is the mainstay of treatment for pediatric nasopharyngeal carcinoma?	Biopsy for diagnosis and to assess recurrence Radiation and chemotherapy for treatment
117	With modern treatment protocols, what is the estimated 5-year survival for pediatric nasopharyngeal carcinoma?	Event-free and overall survival greater than 90%

Neurogenic Tumors

118	What solid, extracerebral pediatric tumor arises from neuroectodermal neural crest cells of the sympathetic nervous system (e.g., organ of Zuckerkandl, sympathetic chain, etc.) or adrenal medulla?	Neuroblastoma
119	What is the range of clinical outcomes associated with pediatric neuroblastoma?	Spontaneous resolution vs. rapid metastases (70% at diagnosis) and death
120	What are the common age groups affected by neuroblastoma?	50% by age 1 year, 80% by age 5 years
121	What are the common manifestations of neuroblastoma in the head and neck?	Horner syndrome, asymmetric crying facies, heterochromia irides, mass effect (airway compression, pharyngeal compression, proptosis, periorbital ecchymosis or "raccoon eyes," trismus, etc.)
122	Where are the potential sites of distant metastases in neuroblastoma?	Head and neck: skull base, periorbital bones, maxillofacial bones, paranasal sinuses Other: bone marrow, liver, skin, other organs
123	In addition to neck CT and MRI, abdominal CT and MRI, chest X-ray, bone scans (technetium radionuclide scan or I123-metaiodobenzylguanidine [MIBG] scan), and bone marrow aspirates, what additional tests are important in evaluating a patient with neuroblastoma?	Histology (core needle or open biopsy, not FNA), urinary catecholamine metabolites (vanillylmandelic acid, homovanillic acid), and possibly urinary dopamine, serum LDH, or serum ferritin
124	Although several genetic markers have been linked to neuroblastoma, which has the most significance when considering prognosis and risk stratification?	MYCN amplification
125	What is the staging system used for pediatric neuroblastoma?	International Neuroblastoma Staging System • *Stage 1*: Localized tumor with complete gross resection, with or without microscopic residual disease; ipsilateral lymph nodes; not attached to the primary specimen; microscopically negative for tumor • *Stage 2A*: Localized tumor with incomplete gross resection, ipsilateral lymph nodes, not attached to the primary specimen, microscopically negative for tumor • *Stage 2B*: Localized tumor, with or without gross resection; ipsilateral lymph nodes; not attached to the primary specimen; microscopically negative for tumor • *Stage 3*: Unresectable unilateral tumor infiltrating across the midline, with or without regional lymph node involvement; or localized unilateral tumor with contralateral regional lymph node involvement; or midline tumor with bilateral extension by infiltration (unresectable) or lymph node involvement

		• *Stage 4*: Any primary tumor with distant metastases to lymph nodes bone, bone marrow, liver, skin, or other organs (except as noted for stage 4S) • *Stage 4S*: Localized primary tumor (1A–2B) with dissemination limited to skin, liver, or bone marrow in an infant < 1 year of age
126	Why might it be reasonable to offer close observation for infants less than 12 to 18 months of age (excluding neonates < 2 months of age) diagnosed with neuroblastoma?	Most of these tumors undergo spontaneous regression (stage 4S). High-risk features such as age < 2 months, diploidy, undifferentiated pathology, and/or MYCN amplification are contraindications to observation.
127	What treatment options are available for patients with neuroblastoma based on the Children's Oncology Risk stratification schema (stage, age, histology, International Neuroblastoma pathology classification, and clinical picture)?	• Primary surgical resection or surgery combined with other treatment strategies • Upfront chemotherapy to shrink the tumor followed by resection • Multiagent chemotherapy as primary treatment • Radiation for unresectable tumors that are unresponsive to chemotherapy, high-risk disease, or life-threatening compression
128	What benign tumor contains Schwann cells, mast cells, and fibroblasts?	Neurofibromas
129	What clinical criteria are required to diagnose NF-1?	• Two or more of the following are required for a diagnosis: Six or more café-au-lait macules > 5 mm (prepubertal) or > 15 mm (postpubertal) in diameter • Two or more neurofibromas of any type or one plexiform neurofibroma • Axillary or inguinal freckling • Optic glioma • Two or more Lisch nodules (raised, pigmented hamartomas of the iris) • Distinctive bony lesion (i.e., sphenoid dysplasia, thinning of the long bone cortex with or without pseudoarthrosis) • A first-degree relative with NF-1 based on these criteria Note: 46% of children < 1 year of age with sporadic NF-1 fail to meet these criteria; 95% meet criteria by 8 years and 100% by 20 years.
130	What gene is responsible for NF-1?	NF-1 gene on chromosome 17q11.2, which results in mutation of neurofibronin, a tumor suppressor gene; autosomal dominant
131	For a child with a large, light brown-pigmented macule suggestive of a cafe-au-lait spot, what conditions must be considered?	• Neurofibromatosis • McCune-Albright syndrome • Fanconi anemia • Tuberous sclerosis
132	What are the four possible neurofibroma subtypes?	• Cutaneous • Subcutaneous • Nodular plexiform • Diffuse plexiform (has the highest risk for malignancy)
133	What is a plexiform neurofibroma?	A plexiform neurofibroma demonstrates angiogenic and invasive properties. It can be nodular (with clusters along peripheral nerve roots, with or without compressive spinal symptoms, etc.), or diffuse (congenital lesion, involves long segments of nerves.

134	What is the rate of malignant conversion in NF-1?	10% (soft tissue sarcoma: malignant nerve sheath tumors; most commonly arise from plexiform neurofibromas)
135	When should neurofibromas be resected?	When causing compressive or cosmetic symptoms, neurofibromas should be resected. Diffuse plexiform neurofibromas are often impossible to resect completely.
136	What is the most common intracranial tumor associated with NF-1?	Optic pathway glioma (less common: astrocytomas, brain stem gliomas)
137	What are the most common extracranial tumors associated with NF-1?	• Rhabdomyosarcoma • Gastrointestinal stromal tumors • Chronic myeloid leukemia • Pheochromocytoma

Teratomas and Dermoids

138	What pediatric tumor arises from all three germ cell layers and occurs most commonly in the soft tissues of the neck, face, infratemporal fossa, orbit, and upper aerodigestive tract when it occurs in the head and neck?	Teratoma
139	True or False. All congenital teratomas manifest with impressive respiratory distress and are benign.	False. Although most do present with respiratory distress requiring interventions such as tracheostomies or extracorporeal membrane oxygenation and EXIT (ex utero intrapartum treatment) procedures, a small number do metastasize and are therefore considered malignant. Malignancy does not indicate maturity of tissue on histopathology, which tends to reflect the age of the host.
140	Do all metastatic teratomas result in progressive disease and death?	No. Many actually differentiate in the metastatic location and do not result in significant harm. However, fatal disease has been reported in children, and aggressive malignant disease is more common in adults.
141	What is the treatment of choice for malignant congenital teratomas?	Surgical resection of the primary tumor is the treatment of choice, as in "benign" teratomas, with consideration of chemotherapy for metastatic disease. There are limited data to guide decision-making for malignant disease.
142	What congenital, subcutaneous lesions contain trapped epithelium and its adnexa (i.e., hair follicles, hair, sebaceous glands) and form along embryologic fusion lines?	Dermoid cysts
143	Where are the most common locations for dermoid cysts in the head and face?	Anterior fontanelle, bregma, upper lateral forehead, upper lateral eyelid, and submental region are the most common locations. *Note*: These cysts can occur in other body sites, such as the ovaries, anywhere in the face, along the skull base, or spinal axis.
144	How do dermoid cysts manifest?	These cysts are solitary, rubbery, firm, painless (unless infected) mases, nonpulsatile, noncompressible, present since birth, but often noted after minor trauma. If associated with a sinus tract, they may have a dermal pit with or without an associated tuft of hair. If the tract extends to the CNS (common in the midline or nasal dermoid cysts), the patient may have meningitis. Tumors with infratemporal extension can result in midface widening, hypertelorism, and other issues associated with mass effect and altered growth.

145	What is the most important imaging modality when evaluating a midline dermoid cyst?	MRI
146	When should you remove a dermoid cyst?	Surgical resection is recommended for all dermoids to decrease possible associated complications (e.g., infection, meningitis, bony erosion).

Cutaneous Lesions

147	You are evaluating a 14-year-old girl with a well-defined tan (or yellow orange) verrucous/papillomatous hairless plaque on her scalp. This lesion has been present since birth, but it was not particularly bothersome. However, as she has begun to go through puberty, it has become significantly more prominent. What is the likely diagnosis and explanation for this change?	Nevus sebaceous. Puberty results in hyperplasia of the sebaceous and apocrine glands within the lesion.
148	What is the potential risk of simply observing nevus sebaceous in children?	A (very low) risk of developing basal cell carcinoma. Other benign tumors may also develop from these lesions (syringocystadenoma papilliferum, trichoblastoma, nodular hydradenoma, sebaceous carcinoma, etc.). All can be removed by simple excision.
149	What is the preferred management of nevus sebaceous in children?	Observation and education are preferred over surgical excision (which is indicated for cosmetic concerns as excision may be easier in infancy or childhood or for the development of a benign or malignant neoplasm).
150	A worried mother brings her son for evaluation of several "dots" she has noted on his face that were not present at birth. On evaluation, these "lesions" are light brown, homogeneous, and round. They are flat and appear rather symmetric. What is the likely diagnosis?	Acquired melanocytic nevi (typical/acquired) (i.e., freckles)
151	What is the most likely cause of a well-demarcated lesion on an infant's neck or chest?	Congenital melanocytic nevi: an error in proliferation and migration of melanocytic progenitor cells (neuroectoderm) during embryogenesis
152	What are the size categories for congenital melanocytic nevi, and how do these categories relate to the potential for malignant conversion?	• Small: < 1.5 cm • Medium: 1.5 to 2 cm • Large: > 20 cm • Giant: > 50 cm Malignant potential (melanoma, neurocutaneous melanocytosis, rhabdomyosarcoma) increases with increasing size. An increasing number of satellite lesions also increases the risk.
153	How are congenital melanocytic nevi managed?	Treatment should be individualized based on cosmetic and emotional impact, as well as the risk for malignancy. Options range from surgical excision to dermabrasion and chemical peels to simple observation.
154	Name the pediatric skin lesion that is generally smaller than 1 cm in diameter, dome shaped, and well circumscribed; it can be purple, red, black or brown; it is composed of spindled and/or large epithelioid cells; and it can be quite difficult to differentiate from melanoma.	Spitz nevus

155	What are the three subtypes of Spitz nevi?	Conventional Spitz tumor (benign or low-grade melanocytic neoplasm) Atypical Spitz tumor (larger, irregular, more atypia, increased risk for local lymph node involvement, and often difficult to differentiate from melanoma) Malignant Spitz tumor/melanoma (histologically difficult to differentiate from melanoma, malignant lesion)
156	How are Spitz tumors managed?	Conventional Spitz nevi should be excised with surgical margins of 3 to 5 mm. Atypical Spitz nevi should be excised with wider margins (up to 1 cm), with consideration for sentinel lymph node biopsy and completion lymphadenectomy for positive nodes. (Note: Up to 50% of sentinel lymph node biopsies will be positive, with questionable impact on survival/outcome.) Malignant Spitz tumor/melanoma: Treat as malignant melanoma
157	Describe some common characteristics of a dysplastic nevus.	A skin lesion with a macular (flat, nonpalpable) component, irregularly distributed pigmentation, indistinct boundary ("fried egg"), size > 5 mm, irregular border, and a background of erythema. This lesion is commonly seen on the scalp but not in chronically sun exposed areas such as the face.
158	What is the clinical significance of dysplastic nevi or a family history of melanoma?	It carries an increased risk for melanoma, although atypical nevi generally do not represent a premalignant lesion.
159	What is required to diagnose familial dysplastic nevus syndrome?	> 100 melanocytic nevi, at least one clinically dysplastic nevus, and at least one nevus > 8 mm
160	When is biopsy indicated for a dysplastic nevus?	Biopsy is done when clinically and dermoscopically it is difficult to differentiate the lesion from melanoma.
161	What is required for the diagnosis of familial atypical mole and malignant melanoma syndrome?	> 50 common and/or atypical nevi + a history of melanoma in one or more first-degree relatives. (Autosomal dominant, genetic association: *CDKN2A* gene mutations).
162	What clinical criteria are required to diagnose nevoid basal cell carcinoma syndrome (,i.e., Gorlin syndrome, basal cell nevus syndrome)?	Two major or one major and one minor criteria: *Major criteria*: • More than two basal cell carcinomas (BCCs) or 1 basal cell carcinoma in a patient < 20 years old • Odontogenic keratocyst of the jaw (histologically proven) • Three or more palmar or plantar pits • Bilamellar calcification of the falx cerebri • Bifid, fused, or markedly splayed ribs • First-degree relative with the disease *Minor criteria*: • Macrocephaly • Congenital malformations (i.e., cleft lip/palate, frontal bossing, coarse facies, moderate/severe hypertelorism) • Skeletal anomalies (i.e., Sprengel deformity, marked pectus deformity, marked syndactyly) • Radiographic anomalies (i.e., bridging of the sella turcica, vertebral anomalies, modeling defects of the hands and feet, or flame-shaped lucencies of the hands and feet) • Ovarian fibroma or medulloblastoma
163	What is the genetic defect associated with nevoid basal cell carcinoma syndrome?	*PTCH1* (patched) gene, chromosome 9q22.3, tumor suppressor gene

164	What treatment options are available for nevoid basal cell carcinoma syndrome?	Surgical resection (wide local excision, Mohs surgery, laser ablation), topical therapy (imiquimod, tretinoin, 5-fluoro-uracil), photodynamic therapy, systemic therapy (oral retinoids, vismodegib). Radiation is largely avoided because of the risk of developing basal cell carcinomas. *Note:* Vismodegib has shown good efficacy in treating this disease.
165	You are examining a 5-year-old girl with a mobile, rock-hard mass on her lateral cheek in the deep dermis or subcutaneous layer of the skin. The mass has been present for some time and has shown slow growth. It has an irregular border and is completely asymptomatic. What is the likely diagnosis?	Pilomatricoma (mutations in the ß-catenin gene arises from the outer root sheath of hair follicles).
166	Although most pilomatricomas are isolated lesions located predominantly in the head and neck (lateral cheek, preauricular area, and periorbital area), when they occur as multiple lesions, what additional diagnoses should be investigated?	Gardner syndrome, myotonic dystrophy, Rubenstein-Taybe syndrome, Turner syndrome
167	What is the recommended management for pilomatricomas?	Surgical excision. They do not spontaneously regress.
168	Infantile hemangiomas are the most common benign neoplasm in childhood and are differentiated from other vascular malformations by the presence of what molecular marker?	Glucose transport protein 1 (GLUT-1)
169	A 12-month-old infant is undergoing inpatient medical treatment of a bright red, large, vascular growth involving her right cheek and orbit. What is the medication, and what side effects may occur with this treatment?	Propranolol: hypoglycemia and rarely hypotension and bradyarrythmias
170	You are examining an infant with a well-demarcated, dome-shaped, yellow-brown (or reddish-orange) papule (or nodule) on the neck. What is the likely diagnosis?	Juvenile xanthogranuloma: Benign, spontaneously regressing lesion with an excellent prognosis, occasionally associated with neurofibromatosis
171	Juvenile xanthogranulomas of the head and neck can be single or multiple, involve ocular structures (more common with multiple lesions in children under 2 years of age), regress within 2 years, and can be confirmed on biopsy if the diagnosis is suspect. What findings would you look for on pathology to confirm the diagnosis?	Dense infiltrate of foamy histiocytes in the dermis and cells containing a wreath of nuclei surrounded by eosinophilic nuclei (Touton giant cells)
172	What autosomal recessive genetic disorder results in extreme sensitivity to sunlight (i.e., early freckling, intense/prolonged burns), the potential for neurologic sequelae (i.e., cognitive impairment, ataxia, choreoathetosis, sensorineural hearing loss, spasticity, seizures, and peripheral neuropathy), and a greatly elevated incidence of cutaneous malignancies (i.e., basal cell carcinoma, squamous cell carcinoma, and melanoma)?	Xeroderma pigmentosum
173	What is the genetic defect associated with xeroderma pigmentosum?	A defect in the DNA repair mechanism; autosomal recessive; eight genes have been identified (XPA–XPG, excluding XPF)

174	What management options improve the prognosis for patients with xeroderma pigmentosum?	Aggressive sun protection and early detection and management of cutaneous malignancies improve prognosis. Patients without neurologic involvement may have a good prognosis with this strategy.
175	Although pediatric head and neck melanoma is quite rare, what is the prognosis compared with adult populations?	Similar survival time but shorter disease-free intervals
176	How is pediatric head and neck melanoma managed?	Wide local excision, sentinel lymph node biopsy, neck dissection for positive sentinel nodes, and consideration of interferon α-2b in high-risk individuals

3 Rhinology, Allergy, and Immunology

Cody A. Koch, Kathryn M. Van Abel, Ian J. Lalich, Matthew L. Carlson, and John F. Pallanch

Overview

1	What cells contribute to the formation of the nose during the 4th week of embryogenesis?	Neural crest cells
2	Before closure during embryogenesis, what are the following spaces called? • Between the frontal and nasal bones • Between the frontal and ethmoid bones • Between the nasal bones and nasal capsule	Fronticulus nasofrontalis Foramen cecum Prenasal space
3	What embryologic structures form within the thickened ectoderm of the nasal placodes of the frontonasal process and after dividing each placode into medial and lateral nasal processes become the early nasal cavities?	Nasal pits
4	Into what structures do the (1) medial and (2) lateral processes of the nasal pits and the (3) maxillary process of the maxilla develop?	• Medial: Nasal septum (from the globular processes of His), philtrum, premaxilla • Lateral: Nasal alae • Maxillary process: Lateral nasal wall
5	What embryologic membrane separates the nasal and oral cavities, and normally degenerates to allow open passages as the choanae are formed by the deepening olfactory pits during development?	Nasobuccal membrane
6	The nasal bones attach to what structures within the facial skeleton?	Frontal bone, nasal process of the maxilla, upper lateral cartilages, contralateral nasal bone, perpendicular plate of the ethmoid, and cartilaginous septum
7	What are the three different regions of the paired lower lateral cartilages of the nose?	• Medial crus • Intermediate crus • Lateral crus
8	What is the name of the area that connects the lower lateral cartilages with the upper lateral cartilages?	Scroll region
9	What are the boundaries of the internal nasal valve? (▶ Fig. 3.1)	• Caudal septum • Head of the inferior turbinate • Remainder of tissues around the piriform aperture • Upper lateral cartilage, distal end *Note*: Also called the valve area, nasal valve region

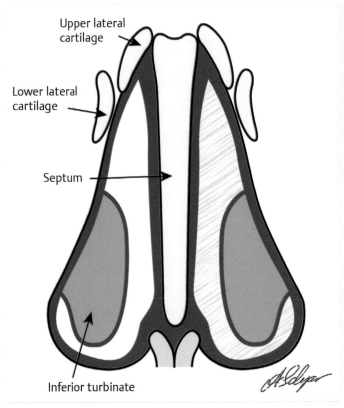

Upper lateral cartilage

Lower lateral cartilage

Septum

Inferior turbinate

Fig. 3.1 Drawing of the external and internal nasal valves. Shaded region represents the cross-sectional area of the internal valve. The boundaries of the the internal valve include the caudal septum, head of the inferior turbinate, remainder of tissues around the pririform aperture, and the distal end of the upper lateral cartilage. (Used with permission from Georgalas C, Fokkens W, eds. Rhinology and Skull Base Surgery. New York, NY: Thieme; 2013.)

10	What structure does the frontal process of the maxilla, nasal floor, and lateral fibrofatty tissue form?	Piriform aperture
11	What are the boundaries of the external nasal valve?	• Caudal septum • Lower lateral cartilage (caudal edge of the lateral crus, junction with the upper lateral cartilage) • Piriform aperture
12	Name the components of the nasal septum. (▶ Fig. 3.2)	• Perpendicular plate of the ethmoid bone • Quadrangular cartilage • Vomer • Maxillary crest • Palatine bone

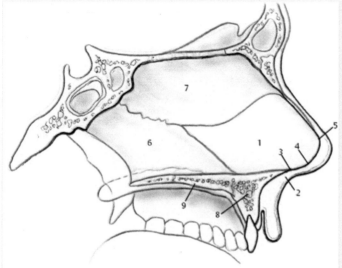

Fig. 3.2 Anatomy of the nasal septum. 1, Quadrangular cartilage; 2, nasal spine; 3, posterior septal angle; 4, middle septal angle; 5, anterior septal angle; 6, vomer; 7, perpendicular plate of ethmoid bone; 8, maxillary crest, maxillary component; 9, maxillary crest, palatine component. (Used with permission from Becker DG, Park SS, eds. Revision Rhinoplasty. New York, NY: Thieme; 2008.)

13	What is the blood supply of the nasal septum?	• Anterior and posterior ethmoid arteries (superior septum) • Sphenopalatine artery branches/posterior septal branch (posterior/inferior septum)
14	Most cases of epistaxis arise in what area?	Kiesselbach plexus (Little area), anterior septum
15	The uncinate process is an extension of what bone?	Ethmoid bone
16	What are the three most common superior attachment points for the uncinate? (▶ Fig. 3.3)	• Lamina papyracea • Skull base • Middle turbinate

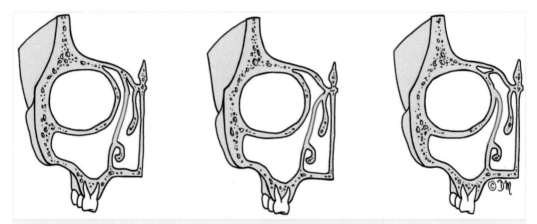

Fig. 3.3 The three most common superior attachment points of the uncinate process: (a) skull base; (b) middle turbinate; (c) lamina papyracea. (Used with permission from Levine HL, Clemente MP, eds. Sinus Surgery: Endoscopic and Microscopic Approaches. New York, NY: Thieme; 2005.)

17	How does the superior attachment of the uncinate process relate to the drainage of the frontal sinus outflow tract?	When attached to the lamina papyracea, the frontal sinus usually drains medial to the uncinate, and when it is attached to the skull base or middle turbinate, it often drains lateral to the uncinate.
18	What is the opening to the space between the uncinate process and the ethmoid bulla called?	Semilunar hiatus
19	The uncinate process covers the medial aspect of which space that provides a common drainage pathway for some of the anterior sinuses?	(Ethmoidal) Infundibulum
20	True or False. The uncinate attaches to the ethmoid crest of the maxilla, the lacrimal bone, the ethmoidal process of the inferior turbinate bone, and the palatine bone via the lamina perpendicularis.	True
21	The lamina papyracea is formed by which bone?	Ethmoid bone
22	The nasolacrimal duct empties under what structure in the nose?	Inferior turbinate (via the Hasner valve)
23	What is the name for a pneumatized middle turbinate, which is an extension of the ethmoid bone?	Concha bullosa
24	The middle turbinate attaches superiorly to the lateral aspect of the cribriform plate, laterally to the lamina papyracea/maxillary sinus, posteriorly to the lateral wall just anterior to the crista ethmoidalis of the palatine bone, and anteriorly near the agger nasi to what structure, which is a part of the frontal process of the maxilla?	Cristal ethmoidalis of the maxilla
25	What structure separates the anterior and posterior ethmoid sinuses?	Ground or basal lamella
26	What are the five ethmoturbinals, and what do they become?	First → Agger nasi (ascending portion) and uncinate process (descending portion) Second → Middle turbinate Third → Superior turbinate Fourth and fifth fuse → supreme turbinate
27	List the first four ethmoid lamellae. (▶ Fig. 3.4)	• Uncinate process • Ethmoid bulla • Basal lamella of the middle turbinate • Lamella of the superior turbinate

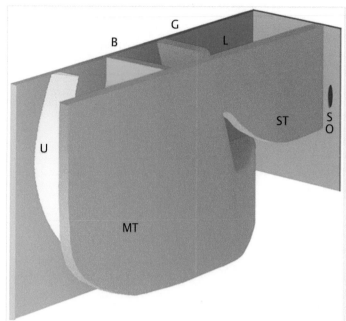

Fig. 3.4 Diagram of the ethmoid complex demonstrating the four ethmoid lamellae: (U) uncinate process, (B) ethmoid bulla, (G) ground lamella of the middle turbinate (lamella of the superior turbinate not depicted). Also shown are the (L) lamina papyracea, (MT) middle turbinate, (ST) superior turbinate, and the (SO) sphenoid sinus ostium. (Used with permission from Kennedy DW, Hwang PH, eds. Rhinology: Diseases of the Nose, Sinuses, and Skull Base. New York, NY: Thieme; 2012.)

28	What is the horizontal plate of the ethmoid bone that forms the roof of the ethmoid sinus and separates the ethmoid air cells from the anterior cranial fossa called?	Fovea ethmoidalis
29	What are the three infundibular cells that are anterior ethmoid air cells?	• Agger nasi cells • Terminal cell (recessus terminalis) • Suprainfundibular cell
30	Which cell type is the most anterior of the ethmoid cells and forms near the attachment of the middle turbinate to the lateral nasal wall?	Agger nasi cell(s)
31	After removing the uncinate process, the ethmoid bulla typically sets just anterior to the basal lamella. Where does this sinus drain?	Suprabullar or retrobullar recess (sinus lateralis)
32	What arterial structure typically runs through the roof of the ethmoid bulla?	Anterior ethmoid artery
33	The middle meatus, uncinate, infundibulum, anterior ethmoid cells, and ostia (frontal, ethmoid, maxillary) collectively are referred to as what? (▶ Fig. 3.5)	Ostiomeatal complex

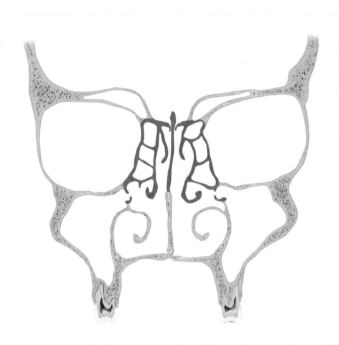

Fig. 3.5 Bony structure of the paranasal sinuses. (Used with permission from Thieme Atlas of Anatomy: Head and Neuroanatomy, © Thieme 2007, illustration by Karl Wesker.)

34	What is the name of the infraorbital ethmoid air cells that pneumatize into the maxillary sinus and can narrow the maxillary sinus ostium?	Haller cells
35	In the adult, the posterior ethmoidal complex consists of one to five cells, which typically drain into which space?	Superior or supreme meatus
36	Air cells that pneumatize lateral or posterior to the anterior wall of the sphenoid sinus are called what?	Onodi cells (sphenoethmoidal cell)
37	What is the first sinus to develop embryologically?	Maxillary sinus
38	What structure must be removed to visualize the natural ostium of the maxillary sinus?	Uncinate process
39	Where is the most common location for the maxillary ostium within the infundibulum?	Inferior third (65%)
40	Where are the anterior and posterior nasal fontanelles located?	Located anterior and posterior to the inferior aspect of the uncinate process
41	What structure runs through the roof of the maxillary sinus?	Infraorbital nerve
42	A series of three or four frontal furrows arise out of the ventral middle meatus and give rise to what?	• First frontal furrow = agger nasi cell • Second frontal furrow = frontal sinus • Third and fourth furrow = anterior ethmoid cells
43	What is the last sinus to fully develop, and at what age has it typically reached full size?	Frontal sinus. Late teens
44	The frontal sinus drains via the frontal sinus outflow tract or frontal recess into which space?	Ethmoid infundibulum (most common)

45	The frontal or frontoethmoidal cells are located superior to the agger nasi cell and can have quite variable pneumatization. Describe the four Kuhn types of pneumatization.	• Type I: Single cell superior to the agger nasi but not extending into the frontal sinus • Type II: Tier of two or more cells above the agger nasi but below the orbital roof • Type III: Single cell extending from the agger nasi into the frontal sinus • Type IV: Isolated cell within the frontal sinus
46	What type of cell can be found posterior to the frontal sinus and superior to the orbit? (▶ Fig. 3.6)	Supraorbital ethmoid cells

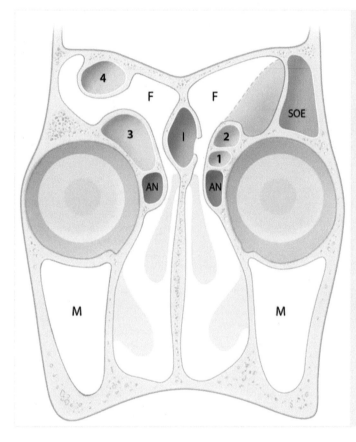

Fig. 3.6 Anatomic variations of the frontal sinus and frontal recess. M, maxillary sinus; F, frontal sinus; AN, agger nasi cell; 1–4, type 1–4 frontal cells; SOE, supraorbital ethmoid cell; I, frontal intersinus septal cell. (Used with permission from Kennedy DW, Hwang PH, eds. Rhinology: Diseases of the Nose, Sinuses, and Skull Base. New York, NY: Thieme; 2012.)

47	The spread of frontal sinus infections intracranially is commonly thought to pass through what structures?	Foramina of Breschet (small venules that drain the frontal sinus mucosa to the dural veins)
48	How is the sphenoid sinus formed during development?	Nasal mucosa invaginates into the cartilaginous nasal capsule, which forms the cupolar recess. The wall of this recess becomes ossified later in development into the ossiculum Bertini. The cartilage is resorbed in the 2nd and 3rd years of life, and the ossiculum attaches to the sphenoid bone. Pneumatization then progresses and is complete in the 9th to the 12th years.

49	What is the most posterior paranasal sinus, and where does its natural ostium drain?	Sphenoid sinus; sphenoethmoidal recess (between the superior turbinate and the anterior wall of the sphenoid sinus)
50	Describe four surgical landmarks to help safely identify the natural ostium of the sphenoid sinus.	• 6.2 to 8.0 cm from the anterior nasal spine • 30 to 40 degrees from the nasal floor • Medial to the posterior end of the superior turbinate (85%) • ~ Halfway up the anterior sphenoid wall
51	The carotid artery is reported to be dehiscent in the sphenoid sinus in what percent of patients?	~ 15%
52	What are the main types of sphenoid pneumatization in the Hamberger classification?	• Conchal type: No pneumatization • Presellar type: Pneumatization restricted anterior to a vertical plane passing through the anterior clinoid process • Sellar type: Well-pneumatized, most common (90%); can be complete or incomplete depending on whether the pneumatization extends to the clivus
53	When removing the intersinus septum within a sphenoid sinus, attachment of this septation to what critical structure must be considered? (▶ Fig. 3.7)	Internal carotid artery

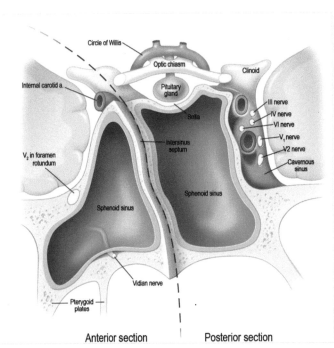

Fig. 3.7 Oblique view of the sphenoid sinus. Dashed line demonstrates the proximity of the intersinus septum to the internal carotid artery. Also note that cranial nerve 6 is the most medial cranial nerve in the cavernous sinus explaining why abducens palsy may be preferentially affected in sphenoid disease. (Used with permission from Kennedy DW, Hwang PH, eds. Rhinology: Diseases of the Nose, Sinuses, and Skull Base. New York, NY: Thieme; 2012.)

54	What is the space between the internal carotid artery and the optic nerve within the sphenoid sinus called?	Opticocarotid recess
55	What portion of the internal carotid artery can be seen within the sphenoid sinus?	(Inter)cavernous portion: • Presellar: Anterior vertical segment and anterior bend • Infrasellar: Short horizontal segment • Retrosellar: Posterior bend and posterior vertical segment

56	What neurovascular structures set within the parasellar cavernous sinus?	• Internal carotid artery • Cranial nerves III, IV, and VI • Cranial nerves V1 and V2
57	What anatomical structures pass through the optic canal?	• Optic nerve • Ophthalmic artery • Ophthalmic vein
58	The vidian nerve is formed by which two nerves before it runs through the vidian canal and exits into the pterygopalatine fossa? (▶ Fig. 3.8)	• Greater superficial petrosal nerve from the geniculate ganglion of the facial nerve (parasympathetic fibers from the superior salivary nucleus) • Deep petrosal nerve from the sympathetic plexus of the internal carotid artery (sympathetic fibers)

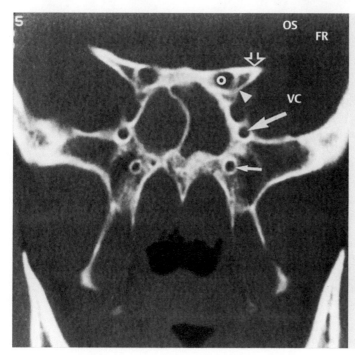

Fig. 3.8 Coronal CT scan at the sphenoid sinus and pterygoid plates. The vidian canal (VC), foramen rotundum (FR), optic strut (OS), and optic canal (O) can be seen. (Used with permission from Mafee MF, Valvassori GE, Becker M. Imaging of the Head and Neck 2nd Edition. New York, NY: Thieme; 2005.)

59	What is the lateral craniopharyngeal canal that may persist in the adult patient anad lead to encephalocele formation and cerebrospinal fluid (CSF) leak and most commonly is noted in patients with significant lateral pneumatization of the sphenoid sinus?	Sternberg canal
60	The cribriform plate lies medially within the anterior skull base, surrounded laterally by what structure?	Fovea ethmoidalis (roof of the ethmoid sinuses): Joins the cribriform plate via the lateral lamella of the cribriform plate, which is often quite thin
61	According to Keros et al (Laryngol Rhinol Otol, 1965), the anterior skull base can be described based on the depth of the cribriform plate in relation to the fovea ethmoidalis according to which three classifications? (▶ Fig. 3.9).	• Type I: 1 to 3 mm • Type II: 4 to 7 mm • Type III: 8 to 16 mm (highest risk for iatrogenic injury)

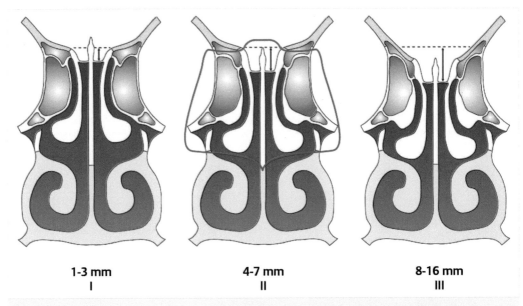

1-3 mm	**4-7 mm**	**8-16 mm**
I	**II**	**III**

Fig. 3.9 Keros classification measuring the depth of the cribriform plate (olfactory fossa) compared to the height of the fovea ethmoidalis. (Used with permission from Georgalas C, Fokkens W, eds. Rhinology and Skull Base Surgery. New York, NY: Thieme; 2013.)

62	Describe the slope of the anterior skull base from anterior to posterior.	Highest anteriorly, lowest posteriorly
63	What major branches of the internal maxillary artery provide arterial blood supply to the nose?	• Sphenopalatine artery • Descending palatine artery → greater and lesser palatine arteries
64	The sphenopalatine foramen is located posterior to the attachment of the middle turbinate to the lateral nasal wall, may have several foramina, and almost always is demarcated by what small, raised, bony crest just anterior or anteroinferior to the foramen?	Crista ethmoidalis of the palatine bone
65	The sphenopalatine artery can exit the foramen in up to 10 separate branches, what are the most common branches and their distribution?	• Lateral nasal artery: Lateral nasal wall including the turbinates • Posterior septal artery: Posterior/inferior septum
66	When ligating the anterior ethmoid artery via an external approach, the vessel can be found running in what suture line?	Frontoethmoid suture
67	What is the distance between the anterior lacrimal crest of the maxilla's frontal process to the anterior ethmoid artery?	20 to 25 mm
68	What is the average distance between the anterior and posterior ethmoid arteries?	10 to 19 mm
69	What is the average distance from the posterior ethmoid artery to the optic nerve?	3 to 7 mm
70	What intranasal vessels are branches of the internal carotid artery?	Anterior and posterior ethmoid arteries

71	What is the blood supply to the nasal septum?	• Superior labial artery (anteriorly) • Greater palatine artery (posteriorly) • Anterior and posterior ethmoid arteries (superiorly) • Posterior septal artery (posterior and inferiorly)
72	What arterial plexus is formed along the posterior lateral nasal wall just under the inferior turbinate by branches from the ascending pharyngeal, posterior ethmoid, sphenopalatine, and lateral nasal arteries?	Woodruff plexus
73	True or False. Venules within the respiratory mucosa of the nasal and paranasal cavities do not have valves.	True
74	Where do the (1) sphenopalatine, (2) ethmoid, (3) angular, and (4) anterior facial veins drain?	• Pterygoid plexus • Superior ophthalmic vein • Ophthalmic vein → cavernous sinus • Common facial vein → internal jugular vein
75	What is the primary blood supply to the external nose?	• Angular artery (facial artery) • Superior labial artery (facial artery)
76	What arterial supply contributes to the formation of the Kiesselbach plexus (the Little area)?	• Posterior septal artery (sphenopalatine artery, external carotid artery) • Anterior ethmoid artery (ophthalmic artery, internal carotid artery) • Greater palatine artery (internal maxillary artery, external carotid artery) • Septal branches of the superior labial artery (facial artery, external carotid artery)
77	What major nerve branches arise from the nasociliary nerve (V1), and what regions of the nose do they supply?	• Infratrochlear nerve → medial eyelid skin • Anterior ethmoid nerve → anterior/superior nasal cavity, lateral nasal wall, and septum, external skin of nasal tip
78	After exiting the foramen rotundum, the maxillary nerve (V2) contributes fibers to the pterygopalatine (sphenopalatine) ganglion, which then supplies innervation to the nose via which branches?	• Infraorbital nerve → anterior area of inferior meatus, anterior nasal floor, nasal vestibule • Superior nasal branches (medial/lateral posterior) → posterior superior/middle turbinates, posterior ethmoid sinuses, face of the sphenoid, nasal vault, posterior septum • Nasopalatine nerve → anterior hard palate • Greater palatine nerve → middle/inferior meatus, posterior aspect of inferior turbinate
79	Where do the parasympathetic fibers that provide vasodilation and secretomotor stimulation to mucous glands synapse?	• Pterygopalatine (sphenopalatine) ganglion • Superior salivatory nucleus → nervus intermedius → geniculate ganglion → vidian nerve → pterygopalatine ganglion → sphenopalatine nerve branches → vasodilation/secretomotor function
80	Postganglionic sympathetic fibers that ultimately control vasoconstriction in the nose arise from what ganglion?	• Superior cervical ganglion • T1–T3 → superior cervical ganglion → internal carotid artery plexus → join greater superficial petrosal nerve → vidian nerve → pterygopalatine ganglion → sphenopalatine nerve branches → vasoconstriction
81	Where do olfactory neurons synapse?	• Olfactory bulb • Olfactory receptor neurons → unmyelinated axons → myelinated fascicles → olfactory fila/cribriform plate/→ olfactory bulb → olfactory tract

| 82 | Name the bones of the orbit. (▶ Fig. 3.10) | • Lacrimal bone
• Ethmoid bone
• Frontal bone
• Maxillary bone
• Sphenoid bone
• Zygomatic bone
• Palatine bone |

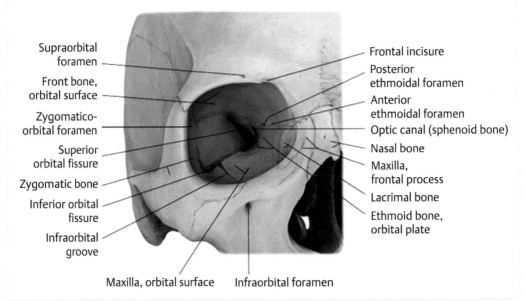

Supraorbital foramen

Front bone, orbital surface

Zygomatico-orbital foramen

Superior orbital fissure

Zygomatic bone

Inferior orbital fissure

Infraorbital groove

Frontal incisure

Posterior ethmoidal foramen

Anterior ethmoidal foramen

Optic canal (sphenoid bone)

Nasal bone

Maxilla, frontal process

Lacrimal bone

Ethmoid bone, orbital plate

Maxilla, orbital surface   Infraorbital foramen

Fig. 3.10 Bones of the orbit: lacrimal, ethmoid, frontal, maxillary, sphenoid, zygomatic, palatine. (Used with permission from Thieme Atlas of Anatomy: Head and Neuroanatomy, © Thieme 2007, illustration by Karl Wesker.)

83	What extraocular muscle is at highest risk during medial orbital decompression for Graves ophthalmopathy?	Medial rectus muscle
84	What epithelium covers the cribriform plate bilaterally, extending to the superior and middle turbinates?	Olfactory neurepithelium: Pseudostratified columnar epithelium containing bipolar spindle-shaped olfactory receptor cells (cranial nerves I and V), columnar sustentacular cells, microvillar cells, and basal cells. *Note*: This sets on a vascular lamina propria containing Bowman (olfactory) glands and no submucosa.
85	What part of the nasal cavity is composed of stratified keratinizing squamous epithelium, hair follicles, sebaceous glands, and sweat glands?	Nasal vestibule
86	What ectodermally derived epithelium lines most of the nasal and paranasal cavities?	Ciliated pseudostratified columnar (respiratory) epithelium with ciliated and nonciliated columnar cells, mucoserous (minor salivary) glands within the submucosa, goblet cells, and basal cells *Note*: Anterior third → squamous and transitional cell epithelium, posterior two-thirds → pseudostratified columnar epithelium

87	Ciliated columnar cells may contain 50 to 200 cilia per cell with each cilia arranged in a specific pattern. On electron microscopy, what do you expect to see for a normal ciliary structure?	"9 + 2" microtubules in doublets (dynein arms)
88	What is another name for the ciliated pseudostratified columnar epithelium that lines the nasal and paranasal cavities?	Schneiderian membrane (ectodermally derived)
89	In normal individuals, the mucosa of one nasal passageway will be congested compared with the contralateral side owing to cyclic engorgement of the nasal turbinates. What is this normal physiologic phenomenon, which may function to optimize humidification and warming of the air, called?	Nasal cycle
90	What is the length of the average nasal cycle? What factors can cause an increase or decrease in "congestion" on a given side?	• Average cycle: 2 to 4 hours • Decreased exercise, increased heart rate • Increased: on "down" side when lying on one's side
91	True or False. The nasal mucosal microvasculature is under parasympathetic tone.	False. Sympathetic tone → vasoconstriction → when tone decreases → increased vasodilation. Changes in tone result in the normal nasal cycle.
92	What is typically the narrowest area inside the nose, which creates the area of greatest resistance to airflow?	Internal nasal valve
93	Without changing nasal resistance, injecting lidocaine into the nose can result in the sensation of nasal obstruction, whereas inhaling menthol, camphor or eucalyptol can result in the sensation of a more "open" nasal passageway. Why?	Change in the level of activity of cold receptors, located predominantly in the nasal vestibule
94	On what is airflow through the nose dependent?	• Cross-sectional area of the nasal passageway • Pressure differential across the nose • Laminar vs. turbulent airflow
95	Describe the Bernoulli principle with respect to the nasal valve.	The speed of a fluid through a tubular structure is greatest at the point of smallest diameter. At the point of maximum velocity, the pressure reaches a nadir. The difference between intranasal pressure at the nasal valve and atmospheric pressure leads to potential for collapse.
96	As air moves from the nasal vestibule to the nasopharynx, the relative humidity increases by approximately what percent?	95%
97	What nasal structure filters out large particles (20 to 30 μm) from the air?	Nasal vibrissae • Nasal septum and turbinates filter particles 10 to 30 μm. • Bronchial tree mucosa filters out particles 2 μm in diameter. • Particles 0.2 to 0.5 μm in diameter tend to remain suspended and are exhaled.
98	The nose filters out particles from the air larger than what size? Particles smaller than this size are able to reach the alveoli of the lungs.	5 μm
99	What are the two mucous layers associated with the nasal mucociliary system? (▶ Fig. 3.11)	• Upper gel layer: Trap inhaled particle; formed by goblet cells and submucosal glands • Lower sol layer; surround cilia of epithelium; formed by microvilli

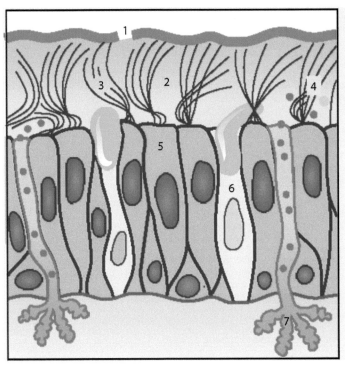

Fig. 3.11 Mucociliary apparatus. 1, Gel layer; 2, sol layer; 3, cilia (beating); 4, cilia (recovering); 5, ciliated epithelial cell; 6, goblet cell; 7, seromucous gland. (Used with permission from Behrbohm H, Kaschke O, Nawka T, Swift A. Ear, Nose, and Throat Diseases: With Head and Neck Surgery. New York, NY: Thieme; 2009.)

100	What cells are responsible for producing the airway mucus?	• Goblet cells: Secrete mucins • Submucosal Seromucous glands: secrete mucins • Epithelial cells: Hydration of the mucus via active transepithelial transport systems • Venules: Plasma proteins
101	What factors can contribute to decreased mucociliary clearance?	• Dysfunction of cilia: Trauma, environmental damage, genetic disorder (i.e., primary ciliary dyskinesia, Kartagener syndrome, cystic fibrosis, etc.) • Altered mucus production or viscosity: Cystic fibrosis
102	What test can be used to measure mucociliary transport time in the nose?	Saccharin test: A saccharin pellet is placed in the anterior nasal cavity and dissolves, passing toward the oropharynx via the mucociliary system and resulting in the sensation of a sweet taste. Time for placement to sensation: < 20 minutes.
103	What nasal reflex results in congestion/swelling of the nasal mucosa when lying in a dependent position?	Postural reflex
104	Which nerves contribute to the overall experience of an odor?	• Olfactory nerve • Trigeminal nerve • Vagus nerve • Glossopharyngeal nerve
105	What produces the nasal mucus, a key component of olfaction?	Bowman glands found within the lamina propria beneath the olfactory epithelium and goblet cells and submucous glands found within the adjacent respiratory epithelium produce mucus
106	What type of cell is responsible for olfaction?	Olfactory receptor cells are bipolar ciliated neurons.

107	What layer(s) must odorants penetrate to reach the olfactory receptor neurons?	Olfactory mucus
108	What organ is often noted in the anteroinferior nasal septum as a small pit whose function in humans is unknown but in many other mammals is thought to be related to the detection of pheromones?	Vomeronasal organ (Jacobson organ)
109	What characteristics of particles are important for their recognition by the olfactory nerves?	For particles to be recognized by the olfactory nerves, the particles must be volatile substances that are lipid soluble.
110	What terms are associated with each of the following? • Normal olfaction • Complete loss of smell • Decreased sense of smell • Altered perception of smell • Perception of odor without stimulus present • Altered perception of an odor in the presence of an odorant stimulus	• Normosmia • Anosmia • Hyposmia • Dysosmia • Phantosmia • Parosmia or troposmia
111	Describe the two main types of olfactory dysfunction.	• Conductive olfactory loss: Occurs secondary to obstruction of the nasal airflow to the olfactory cleft • Sensorineural or nonconductive olfactory loss: Occurs secondary to damage or dysfunction of the olfactory neurons anywhere along the olfactory system
112	What are common causes of conductive olfactory loss?	• Chronic rhinosinusitis (CRS), allergic rhinitis, polyps, septal deflection, tumors • Also occurs with diverted airway (tracheostomy or laryngectomy) from diminished or absent airflow through the nose
113	What are common causes of sensorineural olfactory loss?	Post-upper respiratory tract infection (UTI; viral) loss, CRS (certain patients), head trauma, toxin exposure, congenital disorders, dementia, Alzheimer disease, Parkinson disease, multiple sclerosis
114	How often does olfactory loss occur after head trauma, and when does it occur?	5% to 10% The amount of loss usually correlates with the severity of trauma. Onset is often immediate but can be delayed for months.
115	What is the mechanism thought to be associated with olfactory dysfunction resulting from head trauma?	Shearing of the olfactory nerve axons, contusion/hemorrhage within the olfactory regions of the brain, or structural alteration of the sinonasal tract The most common trauma type is impact to the frontal region, followed by trauma to the occiput.
116	How does post-traumatic olfactory dysfunction differ in the pediatric population compared with that in adults?	Olfactory dysfunction is less common: 3.2% transient dysfunction and 1.2% with permanent dysfunction.
117	What percentage of adults will recover their sense of smell after experiencing anosmia from a head trauma?	5 to 10%
118	What is the most common cause of olfactory loss?	Persistent olfactory dysfunction after URI. This type of olfactory loss is more common in women, typically women older than 50 years (70 to 80% of cases).
119	What proportion of patients will likely recover their sense of smell following a postviral URI, regardless of treatment?	~ One-third

120	Olfaction is dependent on the health of the olfactory neural elements, which are slowly lost over time, resulting in an age-dependent decline in olfaction, most noticeable after what decade(s)?	Sixth and seventh
121	Olfactory function can be lost after exposure to specific toxins, such as formalin or cigarette smoke. What factors most strongly influence the olfactory dysfunction?	• Type of toxin • Concentration and duration of exposure
122	In what two neurologic diseases is olfactory loss thought to be one of the earliest signs?	Parkinson disease and Alzheimer disease
123	What disorder is associated with anosmia and hypogonadism?	Kallmann syndrome (hypogonadotropic hypogonadism); can be X-linked (*KAL 1* gene) or autosomal dominant (*KAL 2* gene)
124	Describe Kallmann syndrome and its relation to congenital olfactory dysfunction.	Gonadotropin-releasing hormone neurons fail to migrate from the olfactory placode to the hypothalamus. Magnetic resonance imaging (MRI) may demonstrate the absence of olfactory bulbs.
125	In what familial autosomal dominant condition do patients develop anosmia, early baldness, and bilateral vascular headaches?	Familial anosmia
126	What advice is critical to relay to patients with significantly impaired olfaction?	It is critical to review the risks of inability to smell "warning" odors, such as smoke, natural gas, and spoiled foods, and to recommend the use of smoke alarms and natural gas detectors.
127	Describe the principle of olfactory threshold testing and one method of performing it.	Absolute threshold of detection is identified, which is the lowest concentration of an odorant that can be detected reliably. An odorant in one sniff bottle and water in another bottle are presented at varying concentrations from weak to strong (based on distance).
128	Describe the principle of odor identification tests.	This is a quantitative test (number of odorants identified). Odorants are presented at suprathreshold concentrations to a patient who is asked to identify the odorants.
129	Describe the University of Pennsylvania Identification Test (UPSIT).	The UPSIT is a self-administered test with four "scratch and sniff" booklets, each containing 10 odorants. Each odorant has a question with four answers. The patient is required to answer even if he or she does not recognize the odorant. Random-chance performance would be 10 of 40, so scores lower than 5 are concerning for malingering. The UPSIT has been studied extensively, and the reliability of the test is high.
130	Describe the Cross-Cultural Smell Identification Test (CC-SIT).	This test is a variant of the UPSIT. It comprises 12 items (banana, chocolate, cinnamon, gasoline, lemon, onion, paint thinner, pineapple, soap, smoke, and turpentine) and is based on odorants most consistently identified by subjects representing various countries (China, France, Germany, Italy, Japan, Russia, and Sweden).
131	What are the most common side effects of second-generation histamine type 1 (H1) blockers?	Headache, urinary retention, dry mouth, blurry vision, and GI upset
132	What is the most common side effect of intranasal steroid sprays?	Epistaxis resulting from incorrect technique
133	What are the most common side effects of pseudoephedrine?	Nervousness, hypertension, and urinary retention
134	What is the onset of action of cocaine?	5 to 10 minutes

135	What is the duration of action of cocaine?	6 hours
136	What is the maximum recommended dose of cocaine?	Varies between 1 and 3 mg/kg; 3 mg/kg is most common. Commonly comes in a 4% solution, and it is estimated that < 40% is truly absorbed.

Disorders of the Nasal Valve and Septum

137	What are the two general forms of nasal valve obstruction?	• Static = does not change with respiration (i.e. caudal septal deviation) • Dynamic = changes with respiration, causes collapse of the structures of the nasal valve (i.e. internal nasal valve collapse)
138	While examining a patient, you use lateral distraction on the cheek while asking the patient to breathe in and out and tell you whether this maneuver increases airflow. What is the name of this test, and what is it most useful for?	Cottle maneuver. Nonspecific. Almost all nasal obstruction improves with this maneuver. It can point to internal nasal valve collapse, which can also be demonstrated with Breathe Right strips.
139	How does the modified Cottle maneuver differ from the Cottle maneuver?	The modified Cottle maneuver is performed by placing an ear curette or end of a Q-tip inside the nose with gentle support of the internal and/or the external nasal valve while the patient breathes to determine whether his or her breathing improves. The modified test is a better test than the Cottle maneuver.
140	What test can be used to determine whether the inferior turbinates are a significant contributor of nasal airway obstruction?	Spray the patient's nasal cavities with phenylephrine spray to decongest the patient's inferior turbinates and determine whether nasal obstruction improves.
141	What is the point of highest resistance in the adult airway?	Internal nasal valve
142	What structure visualized on anterior rhinoscopy is responsible for two-thirds of upper airway resistance at the internal nasal valve?	Inferior turbinate
143	On anterior rhinoscopy you note a normal, but enlarged, middle turbinate. On CT scan, there is an air-filled sinus within the head of the middle turbinate. What is the most likely cause?	Concha bullosa: Pneumatized middle turbinate
144	What percentage of the population will have a concha bullosa?	25%
145	What is the approximate angle between the septum and upper lateral cartilage within the internal nasal valve?	10 to 15 degrees
146	Identify treatment options for both internal and external nasal valve collapse.	Septoplasty, batten grafts, spreader grafts, lateral crural strut grafts, lower lateral cartilage suture suspension
147	List the possible causes of nasal septal perforation.	• Iatrogenic: Prior septal surgery, prior cauterization, nasogastric tube placement, nasotracheal intubation, etc. • Trauma: Nose picking (i.e., digital trauma), septal hematoma • Inhalants: Cocaine abuse, intranasal corticosteroids, chronic vasoconstrictor use, glass dust, etc. • Autoimmune: Wegener granulomatosis, sarcoidosis, systemic lupus erythematosus, Crohn disease, etc. • Infectious: Syphilis, leishmaniasis, tuberculosis, acquired immunodeficiency syndrome (AIDS), etc. • Neoplastic: T-cell lymphomas, etc. • Miscellaneous: Lime dust, cryoglobulinemia, renal failure • Idiopathic

148	What common symptoms are associated with septal perforation?	• Asymptomatic (vast majority) • Nasal crusting • Epistaxis • Nasal obstruction • Postnasal drip • Whistling
149	Where are septal perforations most commonly found in the septum, and how large are they usually?	Anterior septum. Most commonly 1 to 2 cm
150	When should you take a biopsy of a septal perforation?	When there is concern for malignancy, a biopsy should be taken, although this is controversial and not recommended routinely; yield is low when biopsy is done for vasculitic disease, etc.
151	What size septal perforation has a high risk of failed surgical closure?	Large perforation (> 2 cm)
152	What perforations should you treat with conservative management, and what does this involve?	Asymptomatic perforations. The goal is to keep the perforation moist (i.e., nasal saline sprays, Vaseline, saline irrigations, etc.).
153	For large septal perforations not amenable to surgical closure or smaller symptomatic perforations, what nonsurgical option can be offered that can decrease epistaxis, nasal crusting, obstruction, and whistling?	Septal button placement. Prefabricated or custom buttons are available. Custom prostheses for large or irregular perforations can be optimally sized using a maxillofacial CT scan.
154	Identify complications associated with septal button placement.	• Intranasal pain (particularly if displaced) • Erosion of perforation edges (rare, usually protects) • Intranasal crusting • Bacterial colonization/biofilm *Note*: All are relatively low risk but should be discussed.
155	Describe the surgical approaches and techniques available for nasal septal perforation repair.	Approaches: Endonasal versus open techniques: • Primary closure • Interposition grafts: Bone, cartilage, periosteum, temporalis fascia, acellular dermis • Flaps: Bipedicaled mucoperichondrial flap, rotational mucoperichondrial flap • Alternative flaps (large perforations > 2 cm): Inferior turbinate pedicled flap, tunneled sublabial mucosal flap, facial artery musculomucosal flap, radial forearm free flap, pericranial/glabellar flap
156	Describe the process and potential danger of septal hematoma.	Blood collection causes elevation of the mucoperichondrium/mucoperiosteum off the septal cartilage causing devascularization of underlying cartilage and potential for avascular necrosis and reabsorption.
157	Identify complications associated with septal hematoma.	Septal perforation, subperichondrial fibrosis, septal abscess, intracranial infection (spread to cavernous sinus through emissary veins, extremely rare)
158	What factor places children at increased risk for developing nasal septal hematoma?	Loose adherence of the mucoperichondrium and mucoperiosteum to the underlying bone and cartilage
159	What is the treatment for septal hematoma?	Incision and drainage with application of nasal stent or packing to keep the potential space reduced. The patient should be receiving prophylactic antibiotics while packing is in place.

160	What is defined as a collection of purulent material between the nasal septal mucoperiosteum/mucoperichondrium and the bony and/or cartilaginous septum?	Nasal septal abscess
161	What are the risk factors for developing a nasal septal abscess?	• Septal hematoma resulting from trauma or prior surgery • Nasal vestibule furuncle • Sinusitis • Dental infection
162	What is the recommended management for nasal septal abscesses?	• Anti-staphylococal antibiotics • Incision and drainage
163	What complications are associated with nasal septal abscesses?	Intracranial complications (abscess, cavernous sinus thrombosis), orbital cellulitis, septal perforation or weakening or loss of the nasal framework resulting in saddle-nose deformity
164	A patient with pain and itching of the nasal vestibule is examined, and you note small pustular lesions with an erythematous base, pierced by a single hair follicle. What is the diagnosis?	Nasal folliculitis
165	Facial or nasal folliculitis can be superficial or deep and is often associated with what pathogen?	*S. aureus*
166	What pathologic condition generally follows folliculitis, or hair follicle infection, and develops as a small abscess with extension of purulent material from the dermis to subcutaneous tissue?	Furuncle (boil)
167	Why are incision and drainage of nasal furuncles, if necessary, deferred for at least 24 hours after initiating antistaphylococcal antibiotics?	Risk of cavernous sinus thrombosis
168	Inflammatory nasal masses can form around a foreign body, blood clot, or secretion and grow as a result of accumulation of salts (calcium, magnesium, phosphate, carbonate) over time, potentially resulting in pressure injury to adjacent structures and causing nasal obstruction, pain, headache, infection, or recurrent epistaxis. This process is referred to as what?	Rhinolith
169	A previously healthy 3-year-old patient has had 2 days of unilateral rhinorrhea associated with a foul odor, intermittent ipsilateral epistaxis, and generalized irritability. Examination reveals a mass in the right nasal cavity. What is the most likely diagnosis?	Nasal foreign body
170	What proportion of epistaxis arises from an anterior source?	Approximately 90% to 95%
171	What are the common local causes of epistaxis?	• Trauma: Digital, fracture, nasotracheal intubation, feeding tube placement, foreign body, recent surgery • Drug related: Nasal steroid sprays, cocaine inhalation • Desiccation: Nasal oxygen, continuous positive airway pressure (CPAP) • Inflammatory or infectious • Neoplastic
172	What systemic processes can result in epistaxis?	Coagulopathy: • Genetic: Hemophilia, hereditary hemorrhagic telangiectasis (HHT), von Willebrand disease • Drug related: Coumadin, heparin, aspirin • Hypertension • Neoplastic: Pancytopenia, thrombocytopenia, etc.

173	List nonsurgical methods of epistaxis management.	ABCs (airway, breathing, and circulation): Epistaxis can be life threatening! • Direct pressure • Vasoconstrictive agents • Cautery under direct visualization • Nasal packing • Absorbable packing • Nonabsorbable packing • Control hypertension and correct coagulopathy if possible • Nasal hygiene • Saline sprays, humidity, emollients (petroleum jelly, etc.)
174	What are the surgical methods available for epistaxis control if bleeding continues despite maximum nonoperative intervention?	• Surgical ligation • Sphenopalatine artery (transnasal endoscopic, identify crista ethmoidalis, may use large maxillary antrostomy) • Internal maxillary artery (transmaxillary endoscopic, either via the Caldwell-Luc procedure, mega-antrostomy, or partial medial maxillectomy) • Anterior ethmoid artery (Lynch incision, identify fronto-ethmoid suture line) • External carotid artery (transcervical) • Endovascular embolization (most commonly internal maxillary artery; risk of stroke)
175	External ligation of the anterior ethmoid artery is obtained through what approach?	Accessed via Lynch incision, located approximately 24 mm posterior to the anterior lacrimal crest, along the fronto-ethmoid suture line
176	Describe the location of the sphenopalatine artery for endoscopic ligation.	Posterior to the inferior attachment of the middle turbinate, submucosal on the lateral nasal sidewall
177	Why are antibiotics prescribed while a patient has nasal packing in place?	To prevent toxic shock syndrome
178	What autosomal dominant disorder results in punctate hemangiomas or vascular sinuses that are irregularly shaped, associated with thin epithelium, and have no muscular or elastic layers resulting in easy bleeding?	Osler-Weber-Rendu disease (HHT)
179	What are the organs most commonly associated with HHT?	Nasal cavity, oral cavity, GI tract, lungs, liver
180	Which genetic mutations are most commonly seen with HHT?	Endoglin gene (*ENG*, *HHT1*) and activin A receptor type II-like 1 gene (*ACVRL1*, *HHT2*). Mutation detection rates are as high as 75% with sequence analysis of these two genes. *SMAD4* is less common (3%) and is associated with HHT and juvenile intestinal polyposis.
181	What are the most common sign and symptom associated with HHT?	Mucocutaneous telangiectasias and recurrent epistaxis
182	What are the nonsurgical treatment options available for HHT patients with recurrent epistaxis?	• Anemia: Iron supplementation, blood transfusions • Nasal hygiene: Oil of sesame with rose-geranium, nasal saline spray; tolerated in some patients • Intranasal bevacizumab
183	What are the surgical treatment options available for HHT patients with recurrent epistaxis?	Surgical management: • Potassium-titanyl-phosphate (KTP) laser ablation of lesions • Injection of bevacizumab • Septodermoplasty • Young's procedure

| 184 | Describe Saunder's septodermoplasty. | Denuding of nasal mucosa affected by telangiectasias and coverage of denuded area with a split-thickness skin grafts |
| 185 | In what surgical procedure are the nasal cavities closed by creating two layered flaps (nasal mucosa and skin), thus eliminating airflow through the nasal cavities? | Young's procedure |

Rhinitis

186	A patient with irritation and inflammation of the nasal mucous membranes complains of rhinorrhea, nasal congestion, and postnasal drip. What is the most likely general diagnosis based on this information?	Rhinitis
187	What are the main forms of rhinitis?	• Allergic rhinitis • Nonallergic rhinitis
188	Allergic rhinitis reflects what type of Gell and Coombs hypersensitivity?	Type I (anaphylactic/immediate) hypersensitivity with both early and late-phase reactions occurring after re-exposure to the antigen (see section on *Allergy*)
189	What are the primary subtypes of allergic rhinitis?	• Seasonal allergic rhinitis • Perennial allergic rhinitis • Mixed allergic rhinitis
190	What are the classic symptoms of allergic rhinitis?	• Sneezing • Rhinorrhea • Nasal congestion • Pruritus (nasal, palatal, ocular) • Watery eyes • Postnasal drainage • Anosmia/hyposmia
191	Diagnosis of allergic rhinitis hinges most heavily on what factor?	Clinical history
192	What comorbidities are commonly associated with allergic rhinitis?	Asthma, acute rhinosinusitis, otitis media with effusion, sleep disordered breathing, and obstructive sleep apnea
193	What treatments exist for allergic rhinitis?	Intranasal/oral corticosteroids, intranasal/oral antihistamines, leukotriene inhibitors, cromolyn sodium, immune therapy (sublingual and injection) (see section on *Allergy*)

194	A patient presents with nasal congestion, rhinorrhea, and postnasal drip but has a history of negative allergy testing. What type of rhinitis does this most likely represent? What are the major subtypes associated with this condition?	• Nonallergic rhinitis:
		  ○ Infectious rhinitis
		  ○ Vasomotor rhinitis (60%)
		  ○ Nonallergic rhinitis of eosinophilia syndrome (NARES)
		  ○ Gustatory rhinitis
		  ○ Occupational
		  ○ Hormonally induced
		  ○ Medication induced
		  ○ Atrophic
		  ○ Inflammatory/immune-related disorders

195	What are the key symptoms associated with non-allergic rhinitis?	• Sneezing • Rhinorrhea • Nasal congestion • Postnasal drainage
196	True or False. Negative allergy testing is required for the diagnosis of nonallergic rhinitis.	False

197	Viral infections (rhinovirus, respiratory syncytial virus, parainfluenza virus, adenovirus, influenza virus, and enterovirus) can result in URI symptoms, including congestion, rhinorrhea, and postnasal drip, but often they do not cause pruritic symptoms. The infection typically resolves within 7 to 10 days. What diagnosis does this describe?	Infectious rhinitis
198	In what type of nonallergic rhinitis is there excess parasympathetic tone resulting in vasodilation, which can be triggered by cold temperatures and strong smells?	Vasomotor rhinitis
199	What are the characteristics of vasomotor rhinitis?	It is a diagnosis of exclusion. Patients usually manifest this condition in older age, with copious clear rhinorrhea that is triggered by alcohol, temperature, or humidity changes or exposure to odors.
200	What are the common triggers for vasomotor rhinitis?	Changes in temperature, change in relative humidity, odors (e.g., perfumes, cleaning agents), second-hand tobacco smoke, alcohol, sexual arousal, and emotional changes can be triggers.
201	What is the underlying pathophysiology associated with vasomotor rhinitis?	This condition is poorly understood. It may be related to the increased neural efferent input to mucosal vasculature.
202	Though controversial, what surgical interventions can be considered in patients with vasomotor rhinitis?	Vidian neurectomy
203	What type of nonallergic rhinitis manifests with perennial symptoms including sneezing, watery rhinorrhea, nasal pruritus, and intermittent hyposmia/anosmia; demonstrates ~10 to 20% eosinophils on nasal smear, and is associated with negative in vivo and in vitro allergy testing?	NARES
204	A 33-year-old man has profuse watery rhinorrhea whenever he eats his favorite hot and spicy meals. What is the likely diagnosis?	Gustatory rhinitis
205	What is the underlying pathophysiology of gustatory rhinitis?	Vagally (cholinergically) mediated vasodilation after eating (especially with hot or spicy foods)
206	What type of rhinitis is can be associated with (1) inhaled protein or chemical antigens that result in an IgE-mediated response (allergic rhinitis), (2) inhaled chemical respiratory sensitizers that cause an unknown immune response, or (3) exacerbation of rhinitis and is often associated with concurrent asthma?	Occupational rhinitis
207	Pregnancy, puberty, menstruation, and hypothyroidism can all be associated with what type of rhinitis?	Hormonally induced rhinitis
208	During pregnancy, hormone-induced vasodilation, vascular pooling, and increased blood volume can contribute to congestion and rhinitis. Is it more common for this to occur as a new diagnosis of rhinitis or as an exacerbation of preexisting rhinitis?	1/3 of women = exacerbation 2/3 of women = de novo = typically resolves ~2 weeks after delivery
209	What are some common medications that can cause rhinitis?	Angiotensin-converting enzyme (ACE) inhibitors, β-blockers and other antihypertensives, erectile dysfunction or pulmonary hypertension medications (i.e., sildenafil), oral contraceptives and aspirin in sensitive individuals. Ethanol in wine, beer, and other alcoholic beverages can result in vasodilation and rhinitis.

210	What condition is associated with rebound nasal congestion secondary to using topical nasal decongestants (α-adrenergic) for more than 5 to 7 days?	Rhinitis medicamentosa
211	What condition is associated with degeneration of sinonasal sensory and autonomic nerve fibers leading to mucosal gland involution, squamous metaplasia of the sinonasal epithelium, and significant alteration of mucociliary transport and can be either primary or secondary (after surgery or trauma)?	Atrophic rhinitis (also called rhinitis sicca or ozena)
212	What organism commonly colonizes the nasal mucosa in patients suffering from atrophic rhinitis?	*Klebsiella ozaenae*
213	What are the clinical examination findings associated with atrophic rhinitis?	• Foul odor • Yellow/green crusting • Atrophic/fibrotic mucosa
214	In addition to the categories of rhinitis included above, what important inflammatory-immune diseases are also associated with nonallergic rhinitis?	• Granulomatous infections (rhinoscleroma, rhinosporidiosis) • Wegener granulomatosis • Sarcoidosis • Midline granuloma • Churg-Strauss syndrome • Relapsing polychondritis • Amyloidosis (Covered in the section on inflammatory/infectious nasal masses and *Systemic Disease* sections of this chapter)
215	What management options have demonstrated utility in the management of nonallergic rhinitis?	• Intranasal glucocorticoids* • Intranasal antihistamine (azelastine [Astelin, Astepro], olapatadine [Patanase])* • Intranasal ipratropium bromide (Atrovent) • Nasal irrigation • Adjunctive oral medications (antihistamines, decongestants) *Primary management: Use full dose daily, often in combination (results are better with intranasal steroid and antihistamine than with either alone).
216	What specific feature of nonallergic rhinitis is the target of ipratropium bromide intranasal spray?	Watery rhinorrhea
217	What is the proposed reason an intranasal antihistamine nasal spray would offer a benefit to patients with nonallergic rhinitis?	Anti-inflammatory: Decreased eosinophil activation, expression of adhesion molecules, and cytokine production. Potentially decreases neurogenic excitation from olfactory stimuli.

Acute and Chronic Rhinosinusitis

218	In the past decade, the term *rhinosinusitis* has been commonly used to describe what condition?	Inflammation of the nose and paranasal sinuses. This term is preferred over *sinusitis* because sinusitis almost always involves the nasal cavity.
219	According to the European Position Paper on Rhinosinusitis and Nasal Polyposis (2007), what are the criteria for diagnosing rhinosinusitis?	Inflammation of the paranasal sinuses, with two or more of the following: • Nasal blockage, obstruction, congestion, or nasal discharge (anterior and/or posterior) • ± Facial pain or pressure • ± Hyposmia or anosmia

220	Describe the five major classifications of rhinosinusitis based on symptom time course.	• Acute: < 4 weeks with complete resolution • Recurrent Acute: Four or more episodes per year lasting ≥ 7 to 10 days; complete resolution between episodes • Subacute: 4 to 12 weeks; controversial designation (considered as a "filler term") • Chronic (± NP): > 12 weeks, without complete resolution • Acute exacerbations of CRS: Worsening from baseline chronic symptoms, followed by return to baseline
221	What is one of the tools used to assess the *severity* of rhinosinusitis symptoms?	• 10-cm visual analog scale: "How troublesome are your symptoms of rhinosinusitis?" • Range: 0 = Not troublesome, 10 = Worst thinkable • 0 to 3 = Mild • 3 to 7 = Moderate • 7 to 10 = Severe
222	Define double worsening/sickening.	Symptoms that worsen following initial improvement
223	What type of acute rhinosinusitis occurs two to five times per year in the average adult, has a symptom peak at 2 to 3 days, progressively improves after day 5, and has symptom resolution by day 10 to 14?	Acute viral rhinosinusitis
224	What are the two most common pathogens associated with acute viral rhinosinusitis?	Rhinovirus and Influenza virus
225	What percentage of viral rhinosinusitis is estimated to progress to bacterial sinusitis?	0.5 to 2%
226	What type of acute rhinosinusitis lasts for > 10 days or manifests with worsening of symptoms after day 5?	Acute bacterial rhinosinusitis (ABRS)
227	In addition to the diagnostic symptoms associated with rhinosinusitis, what secondary symptoms may suggest ABRS?	Fever, aural fullness, cough, myalgias, or headache
228	What pathogens are most commonly involved in ABRS?	• *Streptococcus pneumoniae* (30%) • *Haemophilus influenzae* (20 to 30%) • *Moraxella catarrhalis* (10 to 20%)
229	What workup is recommended for acute rhinosinusitis?	• Not recommended: CT or X-ray • CT may be considered for severe disease, immunocompromised patients, clinically suspicious complications, preoperative evaluation, or evaluation of recurrent acute rhinosinusitis. Optional • Anterior rhinoscopy • Nasal endoscopy: Consider for initial workup, if disease is refractory to empiric treatment, for unilateral disease, when symptoms are severe or disabling • Nasal culture: Treatment failure, complications
230	When should you consider a sinus puncture using a large-bore needle through the canine fossa or inferior meatus for workup of acute rhinosinusitis?	• Clinical trials: Standard for identifying bacterial pathogens in the maxillary sinuses • Potentially useful if episodes are refractory to treatment or when rapid diagnosis and identification of pathogens are required (e.g., in an immunocompromised patient)
231	According to the European Position (EPOS) Paper on Rhinosinusitis and Nasal Polyposis (2007) and supported by data in EPOS 2012, what treatment strategy should be used for mild acute rhinosinusitis with symptoms lasting < 5 days or improving after 5 days?	Symptomatic treatment • Decongestant • Saline irrigation • Analgesics

232	Why do some guidelines on acute rhinosinusitis recommend against using mucus color to dictate antibiotic use?	Mucus color is driven by neutrophils, not bacteria.
233	If a patient has moderate to severe symptoms of acute rhinosinusitis that persist or worsen after 5 days, what is the recommended treatment according to the European Position Paper on Rhinosinusitis and Nasal Polyposis (2007) and supported by data in EPOS 2012?	Initiate intranasal corticosteroids. If no improvement is seen after 14 days → reconsider diagnosis, perform nasal endoscopy, consider an intranasal culture, and consider imaging. Also consider antibiotics, if indicated, if no improvement has occurred after 14 days.
234	For a patient with acute rhinosinusitis with a temperature > 38°C or in severe pain, what treatment is recommended?	• Intranasal corticosteroids • Antibiotics • May consider an oral steroid to decrease pain • Symptomatic management (i.e., analgesia) *Note*: Improvement is expected within 48 to 72 hours.
235	When should an antihistamine be used in the treatment of patients with acute rhinosinusitis?	Use antihistamines *only* in patients with a history of allergic rhinitis or allergic disease.
236	Although decongestants can benefit patients with rhinosinusitis by decreasing mucosal swelling and potentially relieving paranasal sinus outflow obstruction, there is no conclusive published evidence for their use in this disease. What is the maximum amount of time they should be used for?	5 days
237	The Infectious Disease Society of America's (IDSA) 2012 Guidelines for ABRS in children and adults recommends initiating antibiotic therapy for what signs and symptoms?	• Persistent signs or symptoms of ABRS for ≥ 10 days • Severe signs or symptoms for ≥ 3 to 4 days (temperature ≥ 39°C, 102°F; purulent nasal discharge, facial pain at the beginning of illness, or other concerning findings suggestive of complicated ABRS) • Worsening or double sickening at ≥ 3 to 4 days
238	In the IDSA's algorithm, once a patient meets the criteria to receive an antibiotic, the risk for resistance must be assessed. What makes a patient high risk?	• Age < 2 years or > 65 years • Attends daycare • Antibiotics taken within the past month • Hospitalization within the past 5 days • Immunocompromised status • Other comorbidities such as asthma, cystic fibrosis, etc. • Geographic region with high endemic rates of penicillin-resistant *Streptococcus pneumoniae* (> 10%)
239	If a patient meets the criteria for an antibiotic and is not considered at high risk for resistance, what is the first-line antibiotic recommended by the IDSA?	Standard-dose augmentin for 5 to 7 days (adults) These guidelines recommend against the use of amoxicillin because of concern about an increasing number of patients developing ABRS from *Haemophilus influenza* since the introduction of pneumococcal conjugate vaccines as well as increasing β-lactamase production in these strains. However, previous guidelines published in the otolaryngology literature suggest amoxicillin as first line.
240	If a patient meets the criteria for an antibiotic and is considered at high risk for resistance, what is the second-line antibiotic recommended by the IDSA?	• High-dose amoxicillin-clavulanate (amoxicillin dosed at 2 g twice daily or 90 mg/kg daily given twice daily) for 7 to 10 days • Doxycycline • Levofloxacin/moxifloxacin
241	In penicillin allergic patients, what antibiotics are recommended by the IDSA for adults?	• Doxycycline • Levofloxacin • Moxifloxacin • Cefixime/cefpodoxime and Clindamycin *Not* macrolides or trimethoprim-sulfamethoxazole because of concern for resistance

242	According to the IDSA, for a patient being treated with either a first- or second-line antibiotic for acute bacterial rhinosinusitis (who does not demonstrate symptomatic improvement or presents with worsening symptoms after 3 to 5 days of treatment), is switched to a different class of antibiotic or broader coverage, and again demonstrates no improvement or worsening after 3 to 5 days, what additional steps should be considered?	• CT and/or MRI (CT preferred) to look for anatomical problems and suppurative complications • Sinus culture to help direct pathogen specific antimicrobials • Consider referral to infectious disease or allergy specialist (and ear, nose, and throat [ENT] specialist).
243	When should surgical intervention be considered for patients with acute rhinosinusitis?	Only if complications are present that would benefit from surgical intervention or for recurrent acute rhinosinusitis thought to be caused by an anatomical abnormality
244	What criteria are required for diagnosis of CRS according to the European Position Paper on Rhinosinusitis and Nasal Polyposis (2007 and 2012) and the Clinical Practice Guidelines: Adult Sinusitis (2007)?	Two or more of the following symptoms for ≥ 12 weeks: • At least one of (1) nasal blockage/obstruction/congestion or (2) nasal discharge (anterior or posterior, mucopurulent) • Facial pain/pressure or fullness (less common in patients with NP) • Decreased or loss of smell (more common in patients with NP) • Objective evidence of inflammation • Purulent mucous or edema in the middle meatus or ethmoid region • NP • CT without contrast demonstrating inflammation in the paranasal sinuses (more commonly recommended for endonasal tumors)
245	During the workup for CRS or recurrent acute rhinosinusitis, what comorbidities should be investigated that might modify management?	• Allergic rhinitis • Cystic fibrosis • Immunocompromise • Ciliary dyskinesia • Anatomical abnormality
246	What is the classic triad associated with Kartagener syndrome?	• Situs inversus • Bronchiectasis • CRS Note: Caused by a dynein arm defect; autosomal recessive
247	What percentage of patients with CRS will also have asthma?	50%
248	If patients with CRS do not improve with standard therapy, allergy testing may be considered because 60% of these patients have significant allergies. What are the most common allergens implicated?	Perennial allergens: Dust mites, cockroaches, pet dander, fungi
249	What diagnosis is given to patients who have aspirin sensitivity, NP, and asthma?	Samter triad
250	What cytokine, or proinflammatory mediator, is thought to be primarily involved in Samter triad patients?	Leukotrienes
251	What bacterial antigen is thought to be associated with nonspecific T-cell activation and cytokine release via cross linking of T-cell receptors with major histocompatibility class (MHC) II receptors on antigen presenting cells, and has been hypothesized to be involved in the pathogenesis of CRS with NP?	Staphylococcal superantigen

252	What term defines the organized, three-dimensional bacterial structures encased in an extracelluar matrix, which protects it from conventional treatment modalities and may contribute to some cases of CRS?	Bacterial biofilms
253	In patients with refractory rhinosinusitis, according to Chee et al (Laryngoscope 2001), what underlying immunodeficiencies may be identified?	• Combined variable immunodeficiency (10%) • Selective IgA deficiency (6%) • Low titers of IgG (18%), IgA (17%), or IgM (5%)
254	What is the prevalence of rhinosinusitis in the HIV population?	20 to 70%. Patients with HIV are at increased risk because of lymphocyte dysfunction and increased mucociliary transport time.
255	What laboratory tests should be considered for a patient with refractory CRS or recurrent acute rhinosinusitis to evaluate for an underlying immunodeficiency?	• Quantitative immunoglobulin assays (IgG, IgA, IgM) • Antibody response to tetanus toxoid and pneumococcal vaccines (before and after vaccination) • T-cell number and function
256	What is the genetic inheritance and cause of CRS in cystic fibrosis?	Autosomal recessive disorder causes abnormally tenacious exocrine gland secretions involving multiple organ systems. Patients with cystic fibrosis universally develop chronic sinusitis as a result of tenacious sinonasal secretions.
257	Describe the management of CRS in patients with cystic fibrosis.	Conservative management is with mucolytics, topical antibiotic irrigations, and saline irrigations. The patient may need aggressive endoscopic surgical management followed by nasal saline irrigations and antipseudomonal antibiotic irrigations (tobramycin, especially if he or she is undergoing lung transplant.
258	What findings on CT scan should be specifically evaluated for when evaluating a patient with CRS or recurrent acute rhinosinusitis?	• Mucosal inflammation • Osseous destruction, extrasinus extension, or local invasion suggestive of aggressive disease or a malignant process • Anatomical abnormalities: Septal deviation, concha bullosa, Haller cell, maxillary sinus hypoplasia, and/or obstruction of the osteomeatal complex
259	What staging system grades the amount of mucosal disease present in the left and right frontal, anterior/posterior ethmoid, maxillary and sphenoid sinuses (0 = clear, 1 = partial opacification, 2 = complete opacification) and ostiomeatal complex (0 = clear, 2 = occluded)?	Lund-Mackay system (Annals of Otology, Rhinology, and Laryngology, 1995)
260	Although bacterial infection in CRS is often related to more common pathogens such as *Staphylococcus aureus*, *Pseudomonas aeruginosa*, *Klebsiella pneumoniae*, and *Proteus mirabilis*, over time, more rare anaerobic infections can occur. Name three such pathogens.	• *Fusobacterium* spp. • *Peptostreptococcus* spp. • *Prevotella* spp.
261	What are the three primary subtypes of CRS?	• CRS with NP • CRS without NP • Allergic fungal rhinosinusitis
262	What is a key difference between the inflammation seen in CRS with and without NP?	Without NP: Neutrophils Without NP: Eosinophils; interleukin-5 (IL-5) also increased
263	What is the treatment recommended for CRS without NP (European Position Paper on RS and NP, 2007, supported 2012)?	Mild disease (visual analog scale: 0 to 3) • Topical corticosteroids • Nasal saline irrigation • If no improvement in 3 months, treat as moderate/severe Moderate/severe disease (visual analog scale: 4–10)

		• Topical corticosteroids • Nasal saline irrigation • Long-term macrolide treatment (~3 months) (if IgE is not elevated) • Culture • If no improvement: Consider CT and surgical candidacy • If improvement noted: Continue close follow-up, nasal irrigation, and topical corticosteroids. Consider continuation of long-term macrolide treatment *Note*: Evidence for the 3-month duration cutoff is lacking.
264	Name the four macrolides that can be considered for long-term antibiotic therapy in CRS without NP?	• Azithromycin • Clarithromycin • Roxithromycin • Erythromycin
265	What is the treatment recommended for CRS with NP (European Position Paper on RS and NP, 2007)?	Mild disease (visual analog scale: 0 to 3) • Topical corticosteroids for 3 months • Benefit noted → continue therapy and review every 6 months • No benefit → 1 month of oral corticosteroid • Benefit noted → continue or switch back to topical corticosteroid drops; review after 3 months • No benefit → CT, consider surgical candidacy Moderate disease (visual analog scale: 4 to 7) • Topical corticosteroid drop for 3 months • Benefit noted → continue and review every 6 months • No benefit → 1 month of oral corticosteroid • Benefit → continue or switch back to topical corticosteroid drop • No benefit → CT; consider surgical candidacy Severe disease (visual analog scale: 8 to 10) • 1-month course of oral corticosteroid + topical corticosteroid • Benefit → continue topical corticosteroid drops only and review every 3 months • No benefit → CT; consider surgical candidacy *Note*: Antibiotics are not recommended by these guidelines. Evidence for the 3-month duration cutoff, topical corticosteroid drop vs. spray, and 1 month of steroid therapy is controversial.
266	What is the only Food and Drug Administration (FDA)-approved topical corticosteroid spray for NP?	Mometasone furoate
267	What are indications for endoscopic sinus surgery in patients with CRS?	• Allergic fungal rhinosinusitis • Failed medical therapy • Anatomical abnormalities that hinder sinus drainage or medication application • Significant NP • Complications of rhinosinusitis or previous therapy (e.g., mucoceles, synechiae, etc.)
268	After surgical intervention with polypectomy for CRS with NP, what medical management is recommended?	Maintenance therapy with topical corticosteroids and nasal irrigation
269	What are the most common sites for extrasinus complications associated with rhinosinusitis (generally acute or acute-on-chronic)?	• Orbital (60 to 75%) • Intracranial (15 to 20%) • Bony (5 to 10%)

270	Name the valveless veins that allow retrograde spread of thrombophlebitis from mucosal veins to emissary veins, which pass through the diploe between the anterior and posterior tables of cranial cancellous bone to subdural veins and ultimately to cerebral veins.	Veins of Breschet (also known as *diploic veins*)
271	What term refers to the paralysis or paresis of one or more of the extraocular muscles?	Ophthalmoplegia
272	Describe the classification system used for orbital complications associated with rhinosinusitis. (▶ Fig. 3.12)	Chandler classification groups • Preseptal cellulitis • Orbital cellulitis • Subperiosteal abscess • Orbital abscess • Cavernous sinus thrombosis

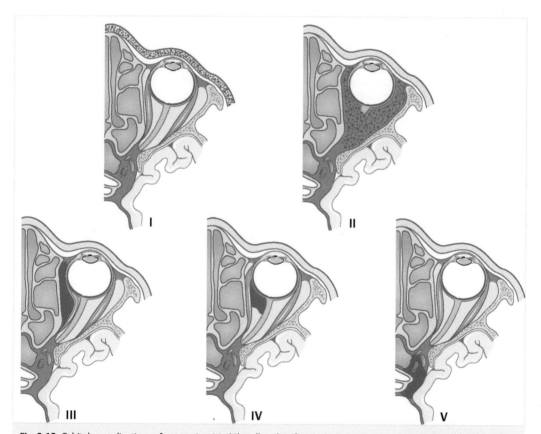

Fig. 3.12 Orbital complications of acute sinusitis (Chandler classification). Group I: preseptal cellulitis; group II: orbital cellulitis; group III subperiosteal abscess; group IV: orbital abscess; group V: cavernous sinus thrombosis. (Used with permission from Georgalas C, Fokkens W, eds. Rhinology and Skull Base Surgery. New York, NY: Thieme; 2013.)

273	You are evaluating a patient with acute rhinosinusitis who has unilateral eyelid edema, periorbital erythema, and tenderness with no evidence of proptosis, visual change, or restriction of ocular muscle movement. Imaging suggests rhinosinusitis and inflammation/infection of the periorbital soft tissues anterior to the orbital septum. What is the most likely diagnosis?	Preseptal cellulitis (Chandler group 1)
274	What is the treatment for preseptal cellulitis?	Medical therapy: IV antibiotics (may consider oral), warm compresses, elevation of the head of the bed, decongestants, mucolytics, and sinus irrigation. Close follow-up
275	You are evaluating a patient with acute rhinosinusitis who has unilateral eyelid edema and erythema, proptosis, chemosis, normal vision, decreased extraoccular motility, and pain. CT scan shows an area of low attenuation adjacent to the lamina papyracea but no discrete abscess. What is the likely diagnosis?	Orbital cellulitis (Chandler group 2)
276	Although most patients with orbital cellulitis should be treated with medical management (similar to preseptal cellulitis), what are two indications that a patient will need surgical drainage?	• Visual acuity ≤ 20/60 • Worsening or lack of improvement after 48 hours of medical therapy
277	You are evaluating a patient with acute rhinosinusitis who has unilateral proptosis, chemosis, and ophthalmoplegia with decreased visual acuity and significant orbital pain. CT scan demonstrated a rim-enhancing hypodensity with mass effect adjacent to the lamina propria. What is the likely diagnosis?	Subperiosteal abscess (Chandler group 3)
278	Although medical cure is possible in patients with subperiosteal abscesses with the use of IV antibiotics, warm compresses, and nasal decongestants/irrigation/mucolytics, surgical intervention is recommended for worsening visual acuity, increased restriction of range of motion, or lack of improvement after 48 hours. What approaches can be used?	• Endonasal endoscopic drainage: medial abscess • External ethmoidectomy via a Lynch incision • Transcaruncular transconjunctival approach
279	You are evaluating a patient with acute rhinosinusitis who has unilateral severe ophthalmoplegia, chemosis, proptosis, severe vision loss, and pain. CT scan demonstrates fluid collection within the orbital tissue. What is the likely diagnosis?	Orbital abscess (Chandler group 4)
280	What syndrome, which can result from an orbital abscess, is associated with ptosis, proptosis, ophthalmoplegia, a fixed and dilated pupil, and V1 anesthesia?	Superior orbital fissure syndrome
281	What syndrome, which can result from an orbital abscess, is associated with ptosis, proptosis, ophthalmoplegia, a fixed and dilated pupil, V1 anesthesia, and vision loss?	Orbital apex syndrome
282	True or False. Orbital abscesses associated with rhinosinusitis can be managed with outpatient antibiotics, decongestants, and an ophthalmology consultation with close follow-up.	False. Inpatient admission, IV antibiotics, decongestants, and a low threshold for surgical drainage

283	You are evaluating a patient with acute rhinosinusitis who has bilateral orbital pain, proptosis, chemosis, ophthalmoplegia, V2 sensory loss, sepsis, and meningismus. CT is suggestive of a process within the cavernous sinus, and MRI demonstrates heterogeneity and increased size of the sinus. What is the likely diagnosis?	Cavernous sinus thrombosis (Chandler group 5)
284	What imaging modality is best to diagnose a cerebral venous sinus thrombosis?	MRI (T1, T2, T2 echo, and MR venography)
285	The primary treatment for cavernous sinus thrombosis associated with rhinosinusitis includes IV antibiotics, management of increased intracranial pressure, management of predisposing factors, surgical drainage of associated abscesses, and/or sinuses. When should anticoagulation be used?	This topic is controversial! Although anticoagulation may decrease the propagation of thrombosis, it also increases the risk of intracranial bleeding.
286	Describe the symptoms of cavernous sinus thrombosis.	Orbital pain; conjunctival and lid edema; vision loss; proptosis; exophthalmos; photophobia; cranial nerves II, III, IV, V1, and VI involvement.
287	Name the five intracranial complications associated with rhinosinusitis.	• Meningitis • Epidural abscess • Subdural abscess • Intracerebral abscess • Cavernous sinus or venous sinus thrombosis
288	What symptoms are frequently seen in patients with intracranial complications associated with rhinosinusitis?	Fever, headache, nausea or vomiting, altered mental status, focal neurologic signs, seizures, visual changes, and meningismus
289	What management strategies are frequently used in patients with intracranial complications of rhinosinusitis?	IV antibiotics, often 4 to 8 weeks. Management of elevated intracranial pressure. (*Note:* Lumbar puncture is often contraindicated). Possible surgical drainage: endonasal and intracranial (bur hole vs. craniotomy, needle aspiration vs. resection)
290	Why are steroids considered controversial in the management of intracerebral abscesses?	Steroids can result in decreased encapsulation of the abscess, increased necrosis, increased risk of rupture into the ventricular system, decreased antibiotic penetration into the abscess, and possible rebound edema after discontinuation.
291	Thrombophlebitic spread of infectious material from acute bacterial rhinosinusitis into the adjacent bone with resulting osteomyelitis can occur via which vascular structures?	Diplopic veins (veins of Breschet)
292	A patient with a history of CRS has a recent exacerbation and new-onset headache, fever, nasal congestion, and rhinorrhea. On examination, you note an area of swelling, erythema, and fluctuance over the frontal bone. On CT, you note a frontocutaneous fistula through the anterior table. What is the diagnosis?	Pott puffy tumor
293	What are the cornerstones for management of Pott puffy tumor?	• Surgical drainage and removal of infected bone • IV antibiotic therapy continued for 6 weeks
294	What percentage of Pott puffy tumors can be associated with additional periorbital, pericranial, or intracranial abscesses?	60%

295	Describe the origin of a sinonasal mucocele.	Sinus ostial obstruction leading to mucus accumulation. Origins include mucus retention cyst, trauma, inflammation (chronic sinusitis, allergy), iatrogenic surgical injury, polyposis, and osteoma.
296	Which paranasal sinuses are most frequently involved by mucoceles?	The frontal sinus is most commonly involved, followed by ethmoid sinus involvement. Maxillary and sphenoid sinuses are less frequently involved.
297	Why might a patient have an enlarged sinus or dehiscent area of bone associated with a known mucocele?	Mucocele growth is expansile and can result in bony remodeling.

Fungal Disease

298	Describe the cause of allergic fungal sinusitis.	A noninvasive fungal sinusitis arising from an allergic response (type I hypersensitivity) to sinonasal fungal exposure
299	Describe the criteria presented by Bent and Kuhn (Otolaryngology HNS, 1994) for the diagnosis of allergic fungal rhinosinusitis.	Bent and Kuhn allergic fungal rhinosinusitis criteria: • Type I hypersensitivity to mold allergens (history or formal allergy testing) • Eosinophilic mucin with Charcot-Leyden crystals • Fungal hyphae without invasion into soft tissue • NP Characteristic imaging • CT: Hyperdense central mucin surrounded by a rim of hypointensity with speckled areas of increased attenuation resulting from ferromagnetic fungal elements. Unilateral > bilateral. May have bony expansion of the paranasal sinuses • MRI: T1 and T2 show central hypointensity surrounded by hyperintensity and T2 may show a central void.
300	What are the characteristics of eosinophilic mucin?	• Necrotic inflammatory cells • Eosinophils • Charcot-Leyden crystals • Fungal hyphae
301	What fungi are commonly implicated in allergic fungal rhinosinusitis?	*Alternaria, Aspergillus, Bipolaris, Curvularia, Cladosporium,* and *Dreschlera*
302	When evaluating a patient with NP, eosinophilic mucin on examination, and a history of atopy to inhaled mold allergens, what comorbid condition must also be investigated?	Asthma
303	During the workup for allergic fungal rhinosinusitis, what procedures and/or diagnostic tests are recommended?	• Allergy testing for fungi-specific IgE (skin or blood tests) • Endoscopy for assessment and procurement of mucin specimen • Pathologic analysis of eosinophilic mucin for fungal stains and possible culture • May consider total serum IgE • Strongly consider CT without contrast
304	What term was proposed by Ponikau (Mayo Clinic Proceedings, 1999) to describe patients with CRS and fungal hyphae in eosinophilic mucin but no evidence of type I hypersensitivity reactions on allergy testing?	Eosinophilic fungal rhinosinusitis
305	What is the recommended treatment for allergic fungal rhinosinusitis?	• Endoscopic surgery • Possibly systemic or topical antifungals • Consider systemic or topical steroids • Nasal saline irrigations

306	What are the two categories of fungal rhinosinusitis?	• Invasive • Noninvasive
307	Name the subtypes of noninvasive fungal rhinosinusitis.	• Fungus ball (old terms no longer recommended: *mycetoma, aspergilloma*) • Allergic fungal rhinosinusitis (see preceding) • Saprophytic fungal infestation
308	Fungus balls most frequently form in an isolated paranasal sinus as a mass of fungal hyphae with associated inflammatory debris and no evidence of mucosal invasion in immunocompetent patients and are found incidentally or manifest with associated symptoms. What is the most common fungus that is isolated?	*Aspergillus fumigatus*
309	Define the distribution of paranasal sinus fungus balls.	Maxillary > sphenoid > ethmoid > frontal sinuses
310	Paranasal fungus balls exhibit what imaging characteristics?	• Complete or subtotal opacification, usually of a single sinus • Osteal thickening or sclerosis • Noncontrast CT shows hyperattenuating lesion with punctate calcifications. The fungus ball is hypointense on T1-weighted and T2-weighted images owing to the absence of free water. • Calcifications and paramagnetic metals generate areas of signal void on T2-weighted images.
311	How are paranasal sinus fungus balls treated?	Surgical debridement and postoperative irrigations
312	What type of noninvasive fungal rhinosinusitis often has an asymptomatic or foul-smelling fungal colonization of mucous crusts after previous sinus surgery?	Saprophytic fungal colonization
313	What are the three types of invasive fungal rhinosinusitis?	• Acute invasive • Chronic invasive • Chronic granulomatous
314	An immunocompromised patient has sudden-onset and rapidly progressive periorbital or facial swelling and/or ophthalmoplegia, neutropenic fever, and a nonpainful intranasal ulcer or eschar most likely has developed what disease process?	Acute invasive fungal rhinosinusitis (old terms that are no longer recommended: *fulminant, necrotizing*)
315	True or false. *Acute invasive fungal rhinosinusitis* is defined as an invasive fungal infection that can take up to 4 weeks to develop.	True
316	What patient populations are at highest risk for development of acute invasive fungal rhinosinusitis?	Immunocompromised: • Hematologic malignancy • Hematopoietic stem cell transplant • Diabetes mellitus • Advanced HIV • Immunodeficiency • Chemotherapy induced neutropenia • Solid-organ transplant • Corticosteroids
317	What are the most common initial symptoms associated with acute invasive fungal rhinosinusitis?	Fever, facial pain,* nasal congestion, decreased sensation over malar regions,* and epistaxis, which may develop change in vision and mentation *Important complaint that warrants attention.

318	What are the most common physical examination findings suggestive of acute invasive fungal sinusitis?	*Early*: Pale, boggy mucosa, petechiae, or areas of ischemia *Late*: Black eschar, sloughing mucosa, gross hyphae, decreased sensation. Mucosa does not bleed.
319	What areas of the sinonasal cavities most commonly manifest acute invasive fungal rhinosinusitis?	The middle turbinate is reported to be the most common, followed by the septum and inferior turbinate. The palate and oral cavity must also be evaluated.
320	What findings on CT scan would be suggestive of invasive fungal sinusitis?	• Unilateral sinus involvement (more common than bilateral) • Severe soft tissue edema of the nasal cavity mucosa (turbinates, lateral nasal wall and floor, septum) • Paranasal sinus mucoperiosteal thickening • Bone erosion • Facial soft tissue swelling • Retroantral fat pad thickening (CT or MRI) • Orbital invasion • Intracranial invasion
321	When should an MRI be ordered during the workup for invasive fungal sinusitis?	If a patient is symptomatic but the CT and/or examination are equivocal or to evaluate the extent of intracranial or intraorbital invasion as suggested by CT or examination
322	What two fungal organisms are most commonly involved in acute invasive fungal rhinosinusitis?	• Mucorales • Aspergillus
323	Which fungal organisms have nonseptate (aseptate) twisted hyphae that branch at 90-degree angles, are seen in a necrotic background, and often demonstrate angioinvasion, which most commonly occurs in diabetic ketoacidosis?	Mucormycoses (order: *Mucorales*)
324	What are the most common Mucorales species associated with acute invasive fungal rhinosinusitis, and where are they found in the environment?	• *Mucor* • *Rhizopus* • *Absidia* • *Cunninghamella* • *Rhizomucor* • *Mortierella* • *Saksenaea* • *Apophysomycoses* • *Zygomycoses* Found in the soil or associated with decaying organic matter such as leaves, wood, or compost
325	What fungal organisms are known to have septate hyphae that branch at 45-degree angles and are best seen by using methenamine silver stain?	*Aspergillus* spp.
326	What are the keys to effective management of acute invasive fungal rhinosinusitis, which carries a very poor overall prognosis?	• Rapid diagnosis and intervention! • IV antifungal medications • Aggressive surgical resection • Reverse underlying immune dysfunction If a patient is cured and lifelong immunosuppression is required, then lifelong oral suppressive antifungal therapy can be used.
327	What IV antifungal medications should be considered empirically in the early management of acute invasive fungal rhinosinusitis?	IV amphotericin B (drug of choice for mucormycosis) +/- voriconazole (drug of choice for *Aspergillus*)
328	What type of rhinosinusitis results from invasion by fungal elements and tissue destruction over a period of > 12 weeks?	Chronic invasive fungal rhinosinusitis
329	What is the most common initial manifestation in patients with chronic invasive fungal rhinosinusitis?	Symptoms suggestive of CRS with few, if any, systemic complaints

330	What patient populations are most at risk for development of chronic invasive fungal rhinosinusitis?	• Mildly immunocompromised • Elderly • Diabetes mellitus • Glucocorticoid use • AIDS
331	True or False. Patients with chronic invasive fungal rhinosinusitis do not develop the severe complications associated with acute infection.	False. They can develop orbital and intracranial invasion. Prognosis is poor.
332	What are the most common CT findings associated with chronic invasive fungal rhinosinusitis?	Thickened mucosa associated with bony erosions and a mass lesion in a single paranasal sinus (most common in the sphenoid or ethmoid)
333	What are the findings on histopathology that suggest chronic invasive fungal rhinosinusitis?	• Dense accumulation of hyphae • +/- Vascular invasion • Little to no inflammatory reaction to invasion and destruction of local structures
334	What is the most common fungal species associated with chronic invasive fungal rhinosinusitis?	*Aspergillus fumigatus*
335	What is the recommended treatment for chronic invasive fungal rhinosinusitis?	Rapid diagnosis and intervention: • IV antifungal medications • Aggressive surgical resection • Reverse underlying immune dysfunction
336	What form of invasive fungal rhinosinusitis is diagnosed after 12 weeks' duration, most commonly in immunocompetent patients from Sudan, India, Pakistan, or Saudi Arabia?	Chronic granulomatous invasive fungal rhinosinusitis
337	What is the most common manifestation seen in patients with chronic granulomatous invasive fungal rhinosinusitis?	• Enlarging mass (cheek, orbit, nose, paranasal sinus) • Gradual onset of symptoms
338	What are the histopathologic findings most commonly seen in chronic granulomatous invasive fungal rhinosinusitis?	• Significant fibrosis • Noncaseating granulomas • Foreign body–type reaction • Langherhans type multinucleated giant cells • Possible vasculitis, vascular proliferation, perivascular fibrosis
339	What fungal species is most often implicated in chronic granulomatous invasive fungal rhinosinusitis?	*Aspergillus flavus*
340	What is the recommended treatment for chronic granulomatous invasive fungal rhinosinusitis?	• Surgical biopsy and debridement • Systemic antifungals

Tumors and Skull Base Disease

341	What type of papilloma arises within the nasal vestibule and nostril from stratified squamous epithelium, is more common in males, and can be treated by simple excision or cauterization?	Vestibular (keratotic) papilloma
342	What three types of papillomas arise in the nasal cavity?	• Fungiform papilloma (also called exophytic, septal, or everted papilloma) • Inverted papilloma (also called Schneiderian, epithelial, transitional cell, or Ringertz papilloma) • Oncocytic papilloma (also called cylindrical)
343	Where do everted papillomas of the nasal cavity most commonly arise?	Nasal septum (rarely: inferior turbinate, nasal vestibule, nostril)

344	Describe the gross and microscopic characteristics of everted papillomas of the nasal cavity.	• Gross: Raised, verrucous, 1 to 15 mm in diameter, single, unilateral, attached to mucosa via a broad base • Micro: Branching fronds of mucosa with a connective tissue core with stratified squamous epithelium; koilocytosis is common
345	What human papillomavirus (HPV) subtypes are commonly associated with everted nasal papillomas?	HPV 6 and 11.
346	What is the treatment for everted papillomas of the nasal cavity?	Simple excision or cauterization. Rare recurrence or transformation
347	Where do inverted papillomas most commonly arise within the nasal cavity, and from what epithelial subtype do they originate?	Lateral nasal wall. May also arise from ethmoid air cells or maxillary sinus. Unilateral >>> bilateral. Schneiderian epithelium.
348	What patient demographic most commonly has inverted papillomas?	White men (0.75F:1M) in their 60 s and 70 s
349	Describe the gross and microscopic characteristics of inverted papilloma.	• Gross: Unilateral, pale pink to reddish gray, polypoid ("mulberry") mass arising from a stalk (can be broad or narrow), irregular, friable, often firmer than inflammatory polyps, although may be difficult to differentiate • Microscopic: Hyperplastic ribbons of basement membrane and epithelium invaginating into the underlying stroma. Stroma demonstrates inflammatory changes containing fibrosis and edema. Multilayered squamous, columnar, or transitional cell epithelium (or a combination) containing mucocytes and intraepithelial mucous cysts
350	Which HPV subtypes are most commonly associated with inverted papilloma?	HPV 16 and 18 although 6 and 11 have been seen as well
351	What is the incidence of malignant degeneration of inverted papillomas to squamous cell carcinoma?	5 to 10% Note: Adenocarcinoma and small cell carcinoma have also been identified.
352	Although the risk of recurrence for inverted papilloma is high, what might increase the risk of recurrence?	Surgical approach and multicentricity of the tumor
353	What two imaging modalities are used most commonly during the workup for inverted papillomas?	• Contrast-enhanced CT: Demonstrates bony destruction, including erosion, remodeling, and sclerosis; may demonstrate areas of calcification within the lesion • Contrast-enhanced MRI: Can differentiate inspissated secretions, mucoperiosteal thickening, and inflammatory changes. T1 lesion is ~ hyperintense to muscle; T2 inspissated secretions and inflammatory polyps are hyperintense.
354	What are the treatment options available for sinonasal inverted papilloma?	• Complete surgical excision: Endoscopic or open • Radiation therapy • Observation
355	What are the surgical approaches used for endoscopic and open surgical resection of inverted papillomas?	• Endoscopic: En bloc wide local excision, medial maxillectomy, Sturman-Canfield operation (Denker operation), Draf procedure • Open: Lateral rhinotomy, midfacial degloving, osteoplastic flap, frontal sinus trephination Note: The key is subperiosteal dissection, removal of all involved mucosa, and drilling down the bone in contact or attached to the papilloma.

356	When is radiation therapy recommended for inverted papilloma?	• For aggressive, multifocal disease • For squamous cell carcinoma • If patient cannot tolerate surgery or if the functional or cosmetic results of surgical resection are not acceptable *Note*: The risks of radiation include potential for malignant conversion.
357	How long should patients be followed up for surveillance of inverted papilloma, and when should CT scans be ordered?	Minimum of 5 years. Recurrence most often occurs between 2 and 10 years. CT scans should be ordered if scarring limits full visualization of the resection cavity, if the patient is symptomatic, or there is evidence of recurrence.
358	What is the least common unilateral Schneiderian nasal papilloma?	Oncocytic (cylindrical) papilloma, 3 to 5% of all sinonasal papillomas
359	You are evaluating the pathology report on a patient with a lateral nasal papilloma; biopsy was performed at an outside hospital. The report describes endophytic invaginations of tall columnar, multilayered epithelium composed of oncocytes and containing microcysts laden with mucin and neutrophils. What is the most likely diagnosis?	Oncocytic (cylindrical) papilloma
360	What is the reported malignant potential of oncocytic papillomas, and what histologic findings have been reported?	10 to 17% (although controversial); squamous cell carcinoma (most common), mucoepidermoid carcinoma, small cell carcinoma, and undifferentiated carcinoma
361	Similar to inverted papillomas, oncocytic papillomas can be locally aggressive and have a relatively high rate of recurrence. What is the best management strategy for these tumors?	Complete surgical excision, as for inverted papillomas
362	What is the most common benign nasopharyngeal tumor that most commonly affects prepubescent males at an average age of 14 to 15 years (range: 10 to 25)?	Juvenile nasopharyngeal angiofibroma
363	Describe the major hypotheses put forth to explain the development of juvenile nasopharyngeal angiofibromas.	• Incomplete regression of the first branchial arch artery • Development from embryologic chondrocartilage of the skull base at the junction of the palatine bone, horizontal ala of the vomer, and root of the pterygoid process. • Abnormality of the pituitary androgen-estrogen axis
364	What is the most common blood supply to juvenile nasopharyngeal angiofibromas?	Internal maxillary artery *Note*: May also arise from ascending pharyngeal, external/internal/carotid artery, and occasionally from contralateral supply
365	What are the two most common symptoms described by patients with juvenile nasopharyngeal angiofibromas?	Epistaxis and unilateral nasal obstruction. More progressive symptoms can include middle ear effusion, facial deformity, headache, dacryocystitis, rhinolalia, palatal deformity, hyposmia/anosmia, cranial neuropathies, and massive hemorrhage.
366	Describe the characteristic gross appearance of a juvenile nasopharyngeal angiofibroma.	Well-circumscribed, smooth, lobulated, purple to reddish hue, compressible
367	Describe the characteristic routes of spread or patterns of growth associated with juvenile nasopharyngeal angiofibromas.	• Pterygopalatine (sphenopalatine) fossa → • Orbit → middle cranial fossa • Masticator space → intracranial cavity • Infratemporal fossa → cheek or intracranial cavity • Nasal cavity → • Paranasal sinus (i.e., sphenoid sinus → intracranial cavity) • Nasopharynx *Note*: Dural invasion is rare.

368	CT, MRI, and magnetic resonance angiography can each be used during the workup of patients with suspected juvenile nasopharyngeal angiofibromas. What characteristics are common?	• Epicenter located adjacent to the sphenopalatine foramen within the posterior nasal cavity • Hypervascularity after contrast enhancement • Distinct pattern of growth • No regional or distant metastases
369	What specific findings can be seen on CT and MRI that help distinguish a juvenile nasopharyngeal angiofibroma?	• CT: Bony remodeling without frank bony destruction • MRI: Flow voids on both T1- and T2-weighted imaging
370	Describe the Holman-Miller sign. (▶ Fig. 3.13)	Anterior bowing of the posterior maxillary sinus associated with juvenile nasopharyngeal angiofibroma

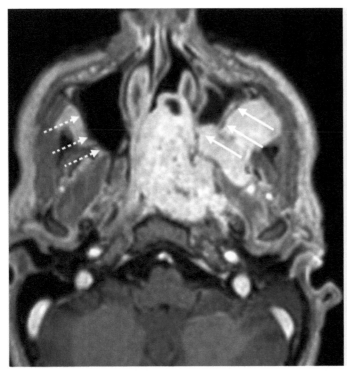

Fig. 3.13 Axial post-contrast T1-weighted MRI of a patient with a left sided juvenile nasopharyngeal angiofibroma demonstrating the Holman–Miller sign (anterior bowing of the posterior wall of the maxillary sinus). Compare the left posterior maxillary sinus wall position (solid white arrows) with the normal location of the right posterior maxillary sinus wall (dotted white arrows). (Used with permission from Duncavage JA, Becker SS, eds. The Maxillary Sinus: Medical and Surgical Management. New York, NY: Thieme; 2011.)

371	True or False. Because angiography can be used to identify a source vessel, perform carotid balloon occlusion studies if necessary, and perform preoperative embolization in patients with juvenile nasopharyngeal angiofibromas, it is considered a required step in the workup and intervention.	False. Angiography, when used 24 to 72 hours preoperatively, can provide all of this information and result in decreased intraoperative bleeding and need for transfusions and can result in shrinkage of the tumor. However, it is not required and is considered controversial.
372	What arguments have been made against the use of preoperative embolization in patients undergoing resection for a juvenile nasopharyngeal angiofibroma?	• It can potentially obscure the tumor boundaries, resulting in a higher rate of recurrence • Complications associated with embolization are not benign: cerebrovascular accident, blindness, facial paralysis, skin or soft tissue necrosis. • Some argue that tumor hypoxia can decrease the radiosensitivity of these tumors.

373	What is the most common staging system used to classify juvenile nasopharyngeal angiofibromas?	There is no universal staging system, although several have been published. The most recent is the Radkowski system (1996). • IA: Limited to nasal cavity and nasopharynx • IB: Involvement of at least one paranasal sinus • IIA: Minimal extension through the sphenopalatine foramen to involve the medial portion of the pterygopalatine fossa • IIB: Extensive involvement of the pterygopalatine fossa with a positive Holman-Miller sign and anterolateral displacement of the maxillary artery branches. Possible superior extension with orbital bone erosion • IIC: Extension through the pterygopalatine fossa to involve the cheek, infratemporal fossa, or posterior to the pterygoids • IIIA: Skull base erosion with minimal intracranial extension • IIIB: Skull base erosion with significant intracranial extension and possible cavernous sinus involvement
374	What treatment options are available for patients with juvenile nasopharyngeal angiofibromas?	• Surgical resection (gold standard; open vs. endoscopic vs. combined) • Radiation therapy (30 to 36 Gy, 20 fractions; has been shown to have similar efficacy to surgery in some situations) • Hormonal therapy (controversial and not commonly used) • Chemotherapy (potentially used for recurrences, rarely used)
375	What is the risk of recurrence for juvenile nasopharyngeal angiofibromas, and what increases this risk?	Up to 40%. Large tumors; intracranial extension; involvement of the sphenoid, base of the pterygoids, or clivus; failure to remove all the tumor; or primary radiation treatment. Most are diagnosed within the first year either based on symptoms or with MRI.
376	Sinonasal hemangiomas can arise from bone, mucosa, or submucosa within the nasal cavity and sinonasal cavities. Both cavernous and capillary subtypes can be seen. Which is more common in adults?	Cavernous hemangiomas
377	Where do sinonasal hemangiomas most commonly arise within the nasal cavity and/or paranasal sinuses?	• Cavernous hemangioma → lateral nasal wall or medial maxillary wall • Capillary hemangioma → septum
378	What are the most common symptoms associated with sinonasal hemangiomas?	Epistaxis and nasal obstruction. For patients with hemangiomas restricted to the bone, symptoms may include a firm, painless swelling associated with a pulsatile sensation.
379	Describe the imaging characteristics of sinonasal hemangiomas on CT and MRI.	• CT: Enhance on CT with contrast. It is often indistinct from turbinates and can be associated with bony destruction. • MRI: Enhance with contrast, intermediate signal intensity, ± flow voids. If intraosseous, it may have a soap-bubble, sun-ray, or honeycomb appearance.
380	What is the management of choice for sinonasal hemangiomas?	Surgical resection. Can consider preoperative embolization, especially for intraosseous lesions.
381	What pathologic lesion can be seen in the sinonasal or oral cavity as a rapidly growing mass resulting in nasal obstruction and epistaxis and is composed of proliferating capillaries separated into lobules by loose connective stroma?	Lobular capillary hemangiomas (previously known as pyogenic granulomas)

382	What theories have been presented as explanations for the formation of lobular capillary hemangiomas?	• Local trauma (e.g., nose picking, nasal packing) • Hormonal fluctuations (e.g., pregnancy) • Infection (e.g., influence of viral oncogenes) • AVM • Local production of angiogenic growth factors
383	What are the clinical examination findings associated with a sinonasal lobular capillary hemangioma?	• Purplish/red mass • Generally < 1 cm, but can be larger
384	What is the treatment of choice for lobular capillary hemangiomas?	Complete surgical excision, although recurrence has been reported in up to 40%
385	What benign neoplasm can develop from Zimmerman pericytes (contractile cells surrounding small vessels) and can be seen in the sinonasal tract, retroperitoneum, lower extremities, and pelvis?	Hemangiopericytoma
386	What is the typical clinical presentation and gross appearance of a sinonasal hemangiopericytoma?	Nasal obstruction and epistaxis. Gray/tan mass that is spongy, vascular, and polypoid in appearance and involving the sinonasal cavity and often one or more paranasal sinus
387	True or False. Sinonasal hemangiopericytomas can demonstrate malignant potential.	True. The risk is low, but regional metastases and death from disease progression have been reported.
388	What are the typical imaging characteristics associated with sinonasal hemangiopericytomas?	• CT: Homogeneous, enhancing lesions; expansile, resulting in bony remodeling • MRI: Enhance on T2-weighted imaging, intermediate enhancement on T1-weighted imaging
389	What are the management options available for sinonasal hemangiopericytomas?	Complete surgical resection. Adjuvant radiation and chemotherapy may play a role, especially in patients with positive surgical margins. Recurrence rates of up to 19% have been reported.
390	What is the most common benign tumor of the sinonasal tract that occurs as an expansile proliferation of mature bone within the membranous bones of the skull and face?	Osteoma
391	Which sinuses are most commonly involved with osteomas?	Frontal > ethmoid > > maxillary > > > sphenoid
392	What is the most likely diagnosis for a patient with multiple osteomas (often seen in the mandible), intestinal polyps, and epidermoid inclusion cysts and desmoids tumors?	Gardner syndrome (autosomal dominant)
393	What theories have been described to explain the development of osteomas?	• Embryologic theory (development from the junction of the frontal bone, which is membranous, and the ethmoid bone, which is cartilaginous) • Inflammation/infection theory • Traumatic theory • Slow growing osseous hamartomas
394	Describe the three subtypes of osteomas.	• Ivory (eburnated): Compact, dense bone, minimal fibrous tissue • Mature (spongiosum): Spongy, mature bony, trabeculum composed of fibrous tissue • Mixed: Components of both ivory and mature osteomas
395	What is the average growth rate of an osteoma?	1.6 mm/year (range: 0.44 to 6.0 mm/year)

396	Although most osteomas are asymptomatic, they can result in a mass effect such as sinus outflow obstruction and resultant pain, sinusitis, and mucocele formation or orbital symptoms, such as proptosis, diplopia, etc. Less commonly, osteomas can grow intracranially. In these situations, what complications can arise?	CSF leak, meningitis, pneumocephalus, abscess formation
397	What imaging characteristics are associated with osteomas?	• CT: Range from a high-density lesion to a less dense ground-glass appearing lesion based on the amount of mineralized bone • MRI: Necessary only to evaluate adjacent soft tissue, trapped secretions, or mucoceles.
398	How are osteomas best managed?	• Observation: For lesions that are asymptomatic and present a low risk for intracranial or orbital complications • Surgical resection: Endoscopic vs. open vs. combined
399	Name the following disorders associated with sinonasal exostoses: • Hyperostosis of the inner table of the skull, thickened cancellous bone, and intact cortex sparing the midline and frequently seen in post-menopausal women • Hyperostosis in postmenopausal women in the presence of obesity and hirsutism • Hyperostosis associated with thickened dura in adolescent males	• Hyperostosis frontalis interna • Morgagni syndrome (metabolic craniopathy) • Acromegaly
400	What characteristics can be used to differentiate an ossifying fibroma from fibrous dysplasia?	An ossifying fibroma typically has a capsule and more mature bone and is more common in black women in their 30s and 40s.
401	What are the imaging characteristics common to ossifying fibromas?	• CT: Well-defined, multiloculated lesion, surrounded by a bony capsule • MRI: Hyperintense T2-signal; T1-signal is intermediately intense centrally and hyperintense peripherally.
402	What is the treatment of choice for ossifying fibromas?	Radical surgical resection (44% recurrence rate)
403	What bony disorder is due to the replacement of normal bone with fibro-osseous tissue (woven-ossified tissue, increased bony matrix, abnormal mineralization, marrow fibrosis) that can occur in monostotic, polyostotic, or syndromic (McCune-Albright) forms?	Fibrous dysplasia
404	Describe the radiographic and histologic appearance of fibrous dysplasia.	• Radiographic pattern: Expansile lesion with relatively homogeneous smooth ground-glass appearance • Histologic pattern: Irregularly shaped, patternless woven trabecular bone within a vascularized fibrous stroma; the irregular shaped spicules can occur as (1) Chinese writing type, (2) pagetoid type, and 3) hypercellular type.
405	When should intervention, the gold standard of which is surgical resection, for fibrous dysplasia be considered?	• Aesthetic concerns • Compression of neurovasculature resulting in symptomatic or functional sequelae • Functional impairment, such as malocclusion • To rule out malignancy
406	Although rare (<4%), malignant transformation of fibrous dysplasia can occur. What is the most common cancer associated with this transformation?	Osteosarcoma

407	What is the rate of CSF production?	~ 500 mL/day or ~ 20 mL/hour
408	What is the most common cause of anterior cranial fossa CSF leaks?	Noniatrogenic trauma >> iatrogenic trauma > nontraumatic (neoplastic process, spontaneous, congenital)
409	What is the most common location for sinonasal CSF leaks to occur?	Ethmoid region (cribriform > lateral lamella) > sphenoid sinus (lateral > midline) >> frontal sinus
410	What is the name given to the congenital dehiscence seen in some patients in the lateral sphenoid roof and is thought to be due to persistence of the lateral craniopharyngeal canal?	Sternberg canal
411	Describe the *reservoir sign*.	A change in head position, generally leaning forward that results in a gush of fluid (CSF) collected in an anatomical depression or open sinus
412	How much CSF is required to test for β-2 transferrin, a protein that is highly specific to CSF?	0.4 mL
413	What imaging modality can demonstrate the site of a CSF leak in the absence of an obvious bony abnormality based on fine cut CT scanning?	CT cisternography (requires intrathecal contrast) *Note*: MRI cisternography using highly weighted T2 images does not require intrathecal contrast but does not demonstrate the bony anatomy.
414	In a patient with an anterior skull base defect resulting in CSF rhinorrhea after blunt head trauma, what is the best first course of action?	Conservative management: stool softeners, bed rest, lumbar drain, and prophylactic antibiotics
415	What are the potential side effects or complications associated with the use of low-dose intrathecal fluorescein?	In order of frequency (most to least): Malaise, headache, dizziness, nausea, vomiting, back pain, lower-extremity weakness, tinnitus, neck pain, fever At higher doses, seizures and cranial neuropathies have been reported.
416	What two grafting techniques can be used to repair skull base defects?	Overlay: Graft material is placed over the defect on the sinonasal side. Underlay: Graft material is placed over the defect on the intracranial side. The two techniques are often used in combination. Grafts may include mucosa, mucoperiosteum, bone, cartilage, synthetic material, vascularized local flaps, or free flaps.
417	Which patient demographic is at highest risk for developing idiopathic intracranial hypertension, which is thought to be due to chronically elevated intracranial pressure?	Obese women of childbearing age. Recurrent disease is associated with the number of pregnancies. *Note*: This condition was reviously referred to as *benign intracranial hypertension* and *pseudotumor cerebri*.
418	Describe the head and neck symptoms associated with idiopathic intracranial hypertension.	Headache, transient visual obscurations, papilledema, pulsatile tinnitus; no localizing signs with the exception of abducens nerve palsy
419	In patients with known idiopathic intracranial hypertension and a history of recurrent CSF leak, what additional interventions can decrease the risk of recurrence?	• Weight loss • Daily acetazolamide • Ventriculoperitoneal shunt

Systemic Diseases

420	What are the three primary granulomatous diseases that can involve the nasal airway?	• Sarcoidosis • Wegener granulomatosis (granulomatosis with polyangitis) • Churg-Strauss syndrome
421	What is the classic clinical triad seen in Wegener granulomatosis?	• Necrotizing granulomas of the respiratory tract (lung effected most commonly) • Vasculitis • Glomerulonephritis

422	Describe the otolaryngologic manifestations of Wegener disease.	• Sinonasal: Obstruction, rhinorrhea, crusting, sinusitis, epistaxis, septal perforation, saddle-nose deformity • Otologic: Conductive hearing loss with serous otitis media; less commonly, sensorineural hearing loss and vertigo • Subglottic: Stridor, dyspnea, subglottic stenosis, crusting
423	What are the nasal manifestations of Wegener granulomatosis?	Nasal inflammation, rhinorrhea, nasal crusting and purulence, CRS, septal perforation
424	The antibodies used for diagnosis of Wegener granulomatosis are directed at what protein?	PR3
425	What blood tests are highly sensitive for Wegener granulomatosis but if negative do not completely exclude the diagnosis?	c-ANCA, PR3 (most typical for Wegener, granulomatosis with polyangitis (GPA) Anti-myeloperoxidase (AMO); possibly more common with microscopic polyangiitis (MPA)
426	What pathologic findings are seen on biopsies of a patient with Wegener granulomatosis?	• Necrotizing, noncaseating multinucleated giant cell granulomas • Small and medium vessel vasculitis • Microabscesses *Note:* Biopsies are often nondiagnostic.
427	What are the three systemic medications used to treat Wegener granulomatosis?	• Cyclophosphamide (used in severe cases) • Methotrexate (used in limited Wegener granulomatosis) • Glucocorticoids
428	What is the cause of sarcoidosis?	Unknown. There is the potential for a genetic susceptibility that is triggered by exposure to an antigen (bacteria, virus, dust, etc). African Americans are 10 to 20 times more likely to be affected than are whites.
429	What is the most common nasal symptom associated with sarcoidosis?	Nasal obstruction Other symptoms include epistaxis, epiphora, nasal pain, and dyspnea. Nasal symptoms are present in < 5%.
430	Where does sarcoidosis most commonly manifest in the nose?	Septum and inferior turbinates and commonly involved with thick crusting. At later stages, yellow subcutaneous nodules can be seen.
431	What is the typical disease course of sarcoidosis?	• Spontaneous resolution within 2 years of disease onset • ~ 10% → Progressive disease and pulmonary fibrosis
432	What is the key histopathologic characteristic seen on nasal biopsy in a patient with sarcoidosis?	Noncaseating granulomas
433	What laboratory test can be used in the diagnosis of sarcoidosis?	Serum angiotensin-converting enzyme (SACE)
434	What percentage of patients with active sarcoidosis will have a positive SACE test?	~ 80%
435	How is sarcoidosis most commonly systemically managed?	Medically with one or more of the following: • Corticosteroids • Antirejection medications • Antimalarial medications • Tumor necrosis factor (TNF)-α inhibitors Rarely organ transplant can be considered.
436	What is the treatment for sinonasal sarcoidosis?	Nasal saline irrigations and topical nasal steroids. Some advocate intralesional steroid injections. In acute exacerbations of aggressive disease, systemic corticosteroids should be administered.

437	What is the clinical triad associated with Churg-Strauss syndrome?	• Asthma • Systemic vasculitis • Eosinophilia
438	What are the three phases of Churg-Strauss syndrome?	• Prodromal or allergic phase: Adult onset asthma and allergic rhinitis • Eosinophilic phase: Peripheral eosinophilia with variable organ involvement • Vasculitic phase: Systemic vasculitis
439	What are the criteria for the diagnosis for Churg-Strauss Syndrome?	Four of the following must be present in a patient with known vasculitis: • Asthma • More than 10% eosinophils in peripheral blood • Neuropathy • Pulmonary opacities on chest X-ray • Sinonasal disease • Biopsy of blood vessel showing eosinophil accumulation
440	What is the management of sinonasal Churg-Strauss disease?	Nasal saline irrigations and topical nasal steroids, antibiotics as needed
441	What are the two most common causes of midline granuloma syndrome?	• Wegener granulomatosis • T-cell lymphoma Improved diagnostic techniques have largely proven that these two are the only true diagnostic entities. Other older terms, such as *malignant midline granuloma, lethal midline granuloma*, and others, generally should not be used).
442	Describe the typical clinical presentation of T-cell lymphoma as a midline granuloma.	• Most common in Asian men • Associated with Epstein-Barr virus • Initial symptoms include nasal obstruction, drainage, pain, epistaxis, fatigue, weight loss, and potentially night sweats. May demonstrate external midface destructuring with advanced disease.
443	What criteria are needed to make a diagnosis of relapsing polychondritis?	Michet et al criteria: • Chondritis of two of three sites (auricular, nasal, or laryngotracheal) or • Chondritis of one of the above-listed sites, with two other features (ocular inflammation, seronegative inflammatory arthritis or vestibular dysfunction, hearing loss)
444	What are the nasal symptoms commonly seen in 48 to 72% of patients with relapsing polychondritis?	• Acute and painful chondritis • Sensation of fullness over the nasal bridge • Mild epistaxis • Long-standing disease → saddle-nose deformity
445	What are the treatment options available for relapsing polychondritis?	• Immune-suppressing medications: Corticosteroids, dapsone, azathioprine, cyclophosphamide, cyclosporine, penicillamine • Plasma exchange • Airway surgery: Tracheostomy, tracheal stent placement, etc. • Reconstructive surgery: Rhinoplasty for saddle nose can be considered if disease is well controlled.
446	What are the clinical manifestations of anhidrotic ectodermal dysplasia?	Abnormal development of the skin, hair, nails, teeth, and sweat glands
447	What is the method of inheritance associated with the most common form of anhidrotic ectodermal hypoplasia?	X-Linked recessive

448	What triad is associated with anhidrotic ectodermal hypoplasia?	Anhydrosis, hypotrichosis, and anodontia Patients often have hypotrichosis, hypodontia, eczema, and atrophic rhinitis.
449	What percentage of patients with primary ciliary dyskinesia will have situs inversus?	50%. May also have recurrent sinopulmonary infections and infertility
450	Nasal biopsy followed by electron microscopy looking at the ultrastructure of the cilia is a useful test when looking for what disorder?	Ciliary dyskinesia. Looking at the number of inner and outer dynein arms and evaluating ciliary orientation can assist in differentiating primary from secondary causes.
451	What nasal disorder results from hypertrophy of the sebaceous glands in both the nasal skin and fibrosis?	Rhinophyma
452	Describe two early signs of rhinophyma.	• Dilated (patulous) pores • Telangiectatic vessels on the distal nose
453	Rhinophyma may manifest as the final stage of what other skin disease?	Acne rosacea, although not all patients with rhinophyma have a history of rosacea
454	What malignant condition can be associated with rhinophyma?	Basal cell carcinoma
455	What patient populations are affected by rhinophyma?	Although acne rosacea is more common in women (3:1) compared with men, rhinophyma almost always affects men (30:1). The disease typically afflicts white males in their 50s to 70s.
456	How is rhinophyma managed?	Inflammation can be managed conservatively, similar to rosacea. For significant hypertrophy, deformity, and nasal obstruction, surgical recontouring can be performed using most commonly a carbon dioxide laser with or without dermabrasion.
457	Rosacea is a chronic skin disorder that can appear with erythematotelangiectatic, papulopustular, phymatous, or ocular characteristics and is thought to be related to what underlying cause?	• Immune disorder • Inflammatory reaction to infection (e.g., *Demodex folliculorum, Bacillus olenorium, Helicobacter pylori*) • Other: UV radiation, vascular hyperreactivity, family history
458	What is the infectious cause of rhinoscleroma, an infectious granulomatous disease that is endemic to Africa, southeast Asia, and Central America and affects the nasal cavity and occasionally the larynx, paranasal sinuses, and nasopharynx?	*Klebsiella rhinoscleromatis* (Frisch bacillus)
459	What are the clinical stages associated with rhinoscleroma?	• Catarrhal (atrophic): Purulent rhinorrhea, rhinitis, honey nasal crusting • Granulomatous (hypertrophic): Painless granulomatous nodules in the upper respiratory tract • Sclerotic: Healing with extensive scar tissue formation and nasal stenosis
460	Describe the histologic findings associated with rhinoscleroma.	Mikulicz cells (foamy histiocytes), and Russel bodies (intracellular inclusions associated with excessive immunoglobulin synthesis)
461	What is the management of choice for treating rhinoscleroma?	Long-term culture-specific antibiotics and surgical debridement
462	What granulomatous infection is endemic to Africa, Pakistan, Sri Lanka, and India and manifests with strawberry-red, friable, polypoid lesions of the nose and eye causing nasal obstruction and epistaxis?	Rhinosporidiosis

463	What is the agent responsible for rhinosporidiosis, and what is the primary means of transmission?	• *Rhinosporidium seeberi* • Contaminated water
464	What is the classic histopathologic finding(s) associated with rhinosporidiosis?	Fungal sporangia with chitinous elements in the setting of pseudoepitheliomatous hyperplasia and submucosal cystic structures
465	How is rhinosporidiosis managed?	Surgical excision with close follow-up for recurrent lesions *Note*: Long-term treatment with dapsone has been effective. Other treatments that can be tried are local steroid injection, and antifungal agents.

Allergy: General

466	What hypothesis postulates that the increase in allergic and atopic diseases in the world is secondary to reductions in infectious disease as well as cleaner environments that limit our exposure to common allergens when we are young and more likely to become tolerant to them rather than allergic?	Hygiene hypothesis
467	What are the two phases of an allergic reaction?	Early and late responses
468	What is the clinical term used to refer to patients who have a genetic predisposition toward developing an allergic response after exposure to an antigen?	Atopy
469	What are the types of hypersensitivity reactions? (▶ Fig. 3.14; ▶ Fig. 3.15; ▶ Fig. 3.16; ▶ Fig. 3.17)	• Type I: Immediate/anaphylactic or antibody mediated • Type II: Cytotoxic T-cell mediated • Type III: Immune complex mediated • Type IV: Delayed hypersensitivity

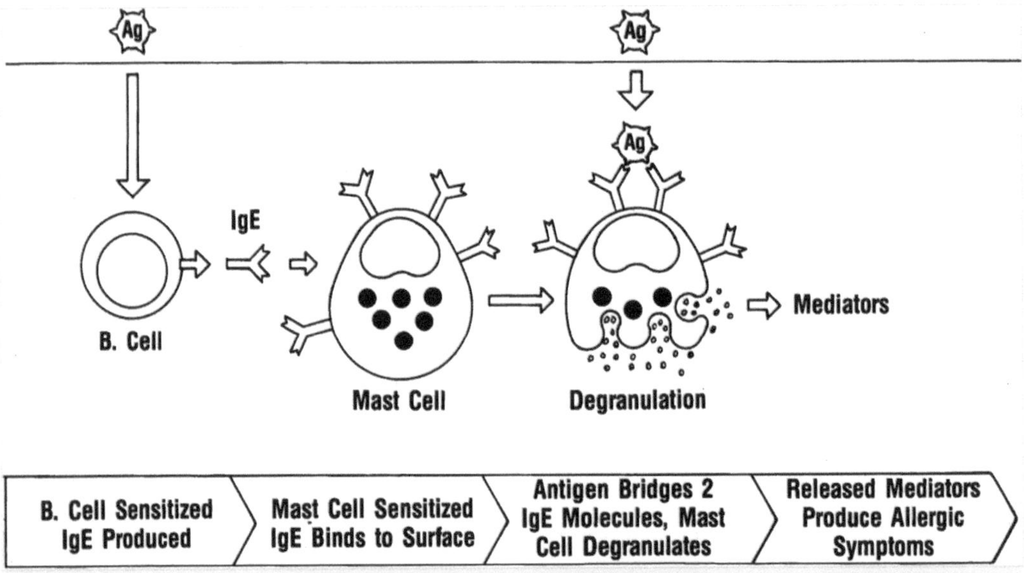

Fig. 3.14 Gell and Coombs type I hypersensitivity reaction: immediate/anaphylactic or antibody mediated. (Used with permission from King HC, Mabry RL, Gordon BR, Marple BF, Mabry CS. Allergy in ENT Practice. New York, NY: Thieme; 2005.)

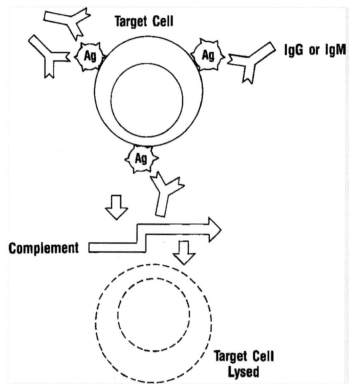

Fig. 3.15 Gell and Coombs type II hypersensitivity reaction: cytotoxic T-cell mediated. (Used with permission from King HC, Mabry RL, Gordon BR, Marple BF, Mabry CS. Allergy in ENT Practice. New York, NY: Thieme; 2005.)

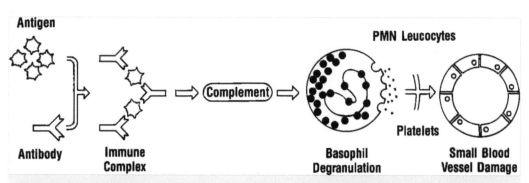

Fig. 3.16 Gell and Coombs type III hypersensitivity reaction: immune complex mediated. (Used with permission from King HC, Mabry RL, Gordon BR, Marple BF, Mabry CS. Allergy in ENT Practice. New York, NY: Thieme; 2005.)

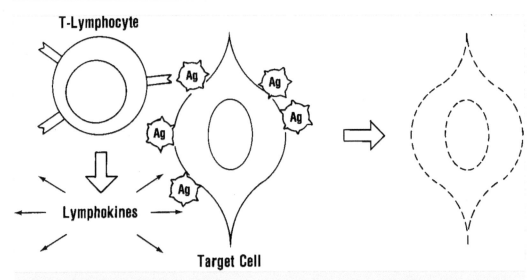

Fig. 3.17 Gell and Coombs type IV hypersensitivity reaction: delayed hypersensitivity. (Used with permission from King HC, Mabry RL, Gordon BR, Marple BF, Mabry CS. Allergy in ENT Practice. New York, NY: Thieme; 2005.)

470	What is another name for the hypersensitivity reactions?	Gell and Coombs classes
471	Anaphylaxis is a form of what type of hypersensitivity reaction?	Type I, immediate or antibody-mediated
472	What is the most important cytokine in the early or acute phase of a type I hypersensitivity reaction?	Histamine
473	What is the predominant cell type during an early or acute phase type I hypersensitivity reaction?	Mast cells
474	What is the predominant cell type during the late phase of a type I hypersensitivity reaction?	Eosinophils
475	In what type of hypersensitivity reaction might you see a systemic hypersensitivity induced by an unknown factor that results in IgG- or IgM-mediated cytotoxic action against an antigen located on the surface of a cell (or complement-mediated lysis of the cell)?	Type II (cytotoxic) hypersensitivity
476	In what hypersensitivity reaction are immune complexes formed (IgG) as a result of the presence of drugs/bacterial products, which result in complement activation and a delayed (days) acute inflammatory reaction?	Type III (immune complex mediated) hypersensitivity
477	In what hypersensitivity reaction do antigens directly stimulate T-cell activation and cell-mediated inflammation resulting in dermatitis, granulomatous disease and some fungal disease?	Type IV (delayed) hypersensitivity
478	What three cell types are required during the primary antigen exposure for the formation of antigen specific IgE antibody formation?	• Mast cells • T cells (T-helper cells type 2 [T_H2] pathway) • B Cells

479	After reexposure to an antigen, what is the result of antigen-specific IgE crosslinking on mast cell surfaces followed by release of preformed mediators (histamine, tryptase, chymase) and synthesis of newly formed mediators (leukotrienes, prostaglandins, platelet activating factor, interleukins, etc) that results in allergic symptoms within minutes?	Early phase allergic response
480	After reexposure to an antigen, what occurs after the release of newly generated inflammatory mediators that cause eosinophil, basophil, monocyte, and lymphocyte migration, infiltration, and cell-mediated inflammation, which can take hours (i.e., 3 to 12 hours) to occur and can last for up to or more than 24 hours?	Late-phase allergic response
481	What is the definition of *anaphylaxis*?	A severe life-threatening generalized or systemic hypersensitivity reaction that may involve urticaria, angioedema, bronchospasm, hypotension, and shock

482	What are the criteria for diagnosing anaphylaxis?	• Criterion 1: Acute onset (minutes) of illness with involvement of skin, mucosa, or both with either respiratory compromise or hypotension
		• Criterion 2: At least two of the following occurring within minutes of an exposure to a likely allergen:
		  ○ Involvement of skin-mucosa tissue
		  ○ Respiratory compromise
		  ○ Hypotension
		  ○ Persistent gastrointestinal symptoms
		• Criterion 3: Hypotension after exposure to a known allergen for the patient

483	What are the two most common causes of anaphylaxis?	• Foods • Drug reactions
484	What medication, not including antibiotics, most commonly causes drug-induced anaphylaxis?	ACE inhibitors
485	A patient has multiple recurrent episodes of anaphylaxis with an unidentified cause. The patient states his allergist asked him to have a laboratory test in the emergency department the next time he had an episode of angioedema in an effort to confirm the diagnosis. What test does the allergist want, and when should it be drawn?	Serum tryptase. Serum tryptase peaks in 30 minutes and should be drawn within 3 hours of the start of the episode.
486	What percentage of patients with anaphylaxis initially have cutaneous findings?	Greater than 90%
487	What is the most common condition to be mistaken for anaphylaxis?	Vasodepressor reaction, usually triggered by trauma or stress and manifesting as flushing, pallor, weakness, diaphoresis, hypotension, and at times loss of consciousness
488	What is the initial treatment of a patient with anaphylaxis?	• Advanced cardiovascular life support (ACLS) protocol, and secure the airway if necessary • Elevate lower extremities in recumbent position if possible • Supplemental O_2 (100%, 8 to 10 L by open face mask) • Gain peripheral IV access (two large-bore IVs) → fluid resuscitation

- First-line medications:
  - Vasopressors (i.e., intramuscular epinephrine) if hypotension is not responding
  - Second-line medications
  - IV H1- or H2-antihistamine (e.g., diphenhydramine 50 mg IV)
  - Nebulized ß2-adrenergic agonist
  - Administer corticosteroids (e.g., dexamethasone 8 to 10 mg IV)

Remember, death can occur in minutes!

489	What dose of epinephrine should be given during anaphylaxis to adults and children?	Intramuscular administration is preferred to subcutaneous: 1 mg/1 ml (1:1000), mid-outer thigh • Adult: 0.3 to 0.5 mg • Child: 0.01 mg/kg, maximum 0.5 mg Can repeat at 5- to 15-minute intervals *Note*: Autoinjectors generally have 0.3-mg doses for adults and 0.15-mg doses for children who weigh < 25 kg.
490	What is the primary reason for administering an antihistamine to patients with anaphylaxis?	Resolution of cutaneous manifestations of anaphylaxis
491	A patient taking what kind of class of drugs might be refractory to the treatment of anaphylaxis?	β-blockers
492	What type of anaphylaxis results in recurrence of symptoms after the initial resolution of associated symptoms without any additional allergen exposure?	Biphasic anaphylaxis (23% of adults, 11% of children; generally 8 to 10 hours after initial reaction)
493	What is the definition of *angioedema*?	Significant swelling of deep dermal or subcutaneous tissues; less often associated with pruritus and more commonly associated with burning or pain
494	What is the most common cause of angioedema presenting to emergency departments today?	ACE inhibitors
495	What is the cause of hereditary angioedema?	The condition is caused by high levels of activated C1 in the bloodstream secondary to deficiency of C1 inhibitor.
496	What is the mechanism of inheritance of hereditary angioedema?	Autosomal dominant
497	What is the treatment for hereditary angioedema?	Attacks usually spontaneously abate in 3 to 4 days. Many patients respond to androgen derivatives, such as danazol, that stimulate the production of C1 inhibitor and C4 but help even at levels that do not stimulate the production of these proteins. Purified C1 inhibitor is now starting to be used in Europe for acute attacks or monthly preventative therapy. Laryngeal involvement may not respond to subcutaneous epinephrine, and a tracheostomy may be needed.
498	Inhalant allergens include proteins such as pollens, animal dander, and molds. How is an inhalant allergy classified in the United States, and based on the World Health Organization (WHO) ARAI (allergic rhinitis and its impact on asthma) guidelines?	U.S. Classification • *Seasonal allergy* (outdoor allergen): Seasonal occurrence, winter/spring = tree, summer = grass, fall = mold • *Perennial allergy* (indoor allergen): No consistent seasonal pattern, dust mites, animal dander, etc WHO ARAI Guidelines • *Intermittent allergic rhinitis*: Present < 4 days/week, < 4 weeks/year • *Persistent allergic rhinitis*: Present > 4 days/week, > 4 weeks/year • *Mild*: Does not impact quality of life or function • *Moderate/severe*: Does impact quality of life or function

499	During which seasons would you expect to see seasonal allergic rhinitis in response to the following inhalant allergens? • Elm, birch, ash, oak, aspen, maple, box elder, hickory, sycamore, cedar, etc. • Bermuda grass, Johnson grass, sweet vernal grass, Timothy grass, Orchard grass, etc. • Ragweed, nettle, mugwort, sage, lamb's quarter, goosefoot, sorrel, etc.	• Winter/spring (February-May) • Late spring/summer (April-August) • Late summer/fall (July to first hard frost)
500	What are some measures to decrease exposure to house dust mite antigen?	• Wash bedding weekly at > 130°F • Use impermeable covers over pillows and bedding • Use hardwood flooring or laminates instead of carpet • Keep humidity levels at less than 45%
501	How long after removing a pet from a home can it take for the amount of allergen to decrease below clinically significant levels?	4 months
502	What is the definition of urticaria?	Pruritic, erythematous cutaneous elevations that blanch with pressure
503	What percentage of the general population will develop urticaria at some point in their lives?	10 to 20%
504	A patient with aspirin-sensitive asthma and urticaria. In addition to NSAIDs, what chemical, used in foods, would you recommend they avoid as well?	Tartrazine (Yellow #5); as many as 15% of affected individuals also react to this.
505	Infection with what pathogenic organism is most commonly associated with eosinophilia and urticaria?	Helminth infections such as *Ascaris lumbricoides*
506	What is cold urticaria, and what should patients be warned to avoid?	Rapid swelling, erythema, and pruritus after exposure to cold objects or weather. It affects only the areas exposed to the cold. There have been reported deaths, secondary to hypotension, of people who swam in cold water.
507	What clinical test might be used to determine whether a patient suffers from cold (temperature) urticaria?	Clinical history is most important. However, the ice cube test can be used to confirm the diagnosis. Place an ice cube on the forearm for 4 minutes, and then observe the area for 10 minutes. Symptoms should develop in 2 minutes.
508	Stroking of the skin with a fingernail or tongue blade causes a wheal and flare reaction where the skin was touched. What is the diagnosis?	Dermatographism
509	What form of allergy testing must be used in patients with dermatographism?	Radioallergosorbent test (RAST) or enzyme-linked immunosorbent assay (ELISA)-based blood assays
510	What is the treatment for dermatographism?	Patients are typically treated with diphenhydramine or hydroxyzine 25 to 50 mg daily. Use of second-generation antihistamines works for mild symptoms. Doses needed are typically two or three times the advised doses.
511	A patient has a history of developing itchy red skin on any sun-exposed skin and intense hives if he or she spends any significant time in the sun. The patient does not report a similar reaction when exposed to heat not associated with sunlight. How is this type of reaction classified?	Solar urticaria is classified by the wavelength of light that causes immediate hypersensitivity.
512	What immunoglobulin mediates most food allergies?	IgE

Allergy: Diagnostic Testing

513	Although it is no longer regularly used in the United States, what test can be used to look for eosinophils versus neutrophils in the nasal mucus in an effort to distinguish eosinophilic rhinitis from other rhinitis?	Nasal cytology
514	Allergy testing to specific allergens can be done via which two broad techniques?	• In vivo (skin testing) • In vitro (serum testing)
515	What immunoglobulin is being tested for with in vivo skin testing?	Antigen-specific IgE
516	What are the two most common locations for performing skin testing?	• Volar surface of the forearm • Back
517	What type of in vivo allergy test is performed using scratch, prick/puncture, or patch to challenge a patient by introducing allergen into the epidermis only?	Epicutaneous testing
518	What type of in vivo allergy test is performed using intradermal techniques to place antigen into the superficial dermis?	Percutaneous testing
519	What variables impact both epicutaneous and percutaneous skin testing?	• Age of the skin (very young and very old may be less sensitive) • Area of the body being tested (sensitivity: upper back > lower back > upper arm > lower arm) • Skin pigmentation (darker skin colors may be less sensitive) • Concurrent medications • Potency and biologic stability of the allergen test extract • Dermatopathology: Dermatographism, eczema → contraindications, including degree of sensitization, recent anaphylaxis, recent exposure, prior immunotherapy
520	During skin testing, what controls are commonly used?	• Negative control: Glycerin-saline, saline, allergen diluent • Positive control: Histamine (10 mg/mL)
521	During skin testing, what term is used to describe the white (blanched) raised area at the site of the allergen application? The area of erythema that extends beyond this raised region?	Wheal Flare
522	Why is scratch testing (small superficial lacerations made in the skin, a drop of concentrated antigen then applied) not recommended for skin testing?	Poor reproducibility, variable sensitivity, poor specificity, frequent false-positives, painful, and reaction may be due to trauma to skin instead of reaction to allergen
523	During an in vivo epicutaneous allergy test, a drop of antigen is placed on the patient's skin. The tester then uses a needle, lancet, or prick device (single or multiple tines) to puncture or prick the skin through the drop of antigen and deliver the antigen to the epidermis. What is this called?	Skin-prick or puncture testing. It is the most commonly used test.
524	What instrument(s) can be used to perform a skin prick or puncture test?	Hypodermic needle, solid-bore needle, lancet ± bifurcated tip, multiple-head devices (more commonly used because of OSHA concerns regarding inadvertent health care worker needle sticks) Pass through the droplet, then the skin at a 45- to 60-degree angle to the skin, lift and break the skin without causing bleeding for the prick test; or the skin device can be passed through the drop at a 90-degree angle to the skin for puncture test.

525	After performing a skin prick or puncture, how long should you wait before assessing the response?	15 to 20 minutes
526	How can you assess the allergic response to a skin test (epicutaneous or percutaneous)?	Direct measurement: Recommended scoring system • Longest diameter or longest diameter and orthogonal diameter (perpendicular) of wheal in millimeters • Presence or absence of flare and size in millimeters as in preceding • Presence or absence of pseudopods Classically based on a 0 to 4+ system: Based on wheal and flare compared with the negative control and the presence or absence of pseudopods Subjective analysis is no longer recommended by the American Academy of Allergy, Asthma and Immunology because of interphysician variability in scoring and interpretation.
527	The American Academy of Allergy, Asthma, and Immunology guidelines for skin testing recommend that wheals < 3 mm should not be considered positive. Why?	Trauma can affect wheal size.
528	What are the major disadvantages to skin-prick tests?	Semiqualitative (less objective than intradermal testing). Low degrees of sensitivity may be missed → false-negative results.
529	When should you use an intradermal/percutaneous allergy test?	When the primary goal of testing is increased sensitivity, or for evaluating drug or venom anaphylactic reactions
530	Describe the technique used for single dilutional intradermal (percutaneous) allergy testing.	1. Using a small needle (generally 26- or 27-gauge needle at 45-degree angle), inject 0.02 to 0.05 mL of antigen diluted to 1:500 to 1:1000 weight/volume intradermally (create a 2- to 3-mm bleb in dermis). 2. Positive control: Histamine (0.001 mg/mL) if needed; can be excluded if reaction was proven by prick testing. Negative control also performed. 3. Wait 10 to 15 minutes, and then assess response.
531	What is the major risk in using intradermal allergy testing, and how can this risk be decreased?	Significant systemic reaction (anaphylaxis). Patients should be screened with prick/puncture testing initially. They can also be screened with very dilute concentrations administered intradermally.
532	What part of the body is commonly used for intradermal testing and why?	Volar surface of the forearm. To allow a tourniquet to be placed in case of systemic symptoms
533	True or False. Single-dilution intradermal skin testing is more specific than it is sensitive.	False. High sensitivity, less specificity. It has a higher false-positive rate than skin prick testing.
534	What type of allergy test requires the sequential administration of fivefold-diluted antigens intradermally, beginning with dilute concentrations?	Intradermal dilutional testing, also called *skin endpoint titration*
535	What does the American Academy of Allergy, Asthma and Immunology recommend as a starting dose of intracutaneous extract solution in patients with a preceding negative prick test?	100- to 1000-fold dilutions of the concentrated extracts used for prick/puncture tests.
536	What size needle/syringe is recommended during intradermal dilutional testing?	0.5- or 1.0-mL syringe with a 26- to 30-gauge needle (can come as a single unit)
537	What volume of antigen concentrate should be injected during intradermal dilutional testing?	0.01 mL (Goal is to create a 4-mm round wheal.)

538	After injection of 0.01 mL and creation of a 4-mm wheal, you appropriately wait 10 minutes to measure the final wheal. If the injected solution was inert diluent, what diameter do you expect based on passive physical diffusion in the skin?	5 mm
539	What is required for a whealing response to be considered positive during intradermal dilutional testing?	A final wheal size of 7 mm, which is 2 mm larger than the expected size at 10 minutes from physical diffusion alone. Flare is not measured during this type of testing. This topic is somewhat controversial, as many practitioners use 3 mm.
540	During intradermal dilutional testing, you note that the no. 6 dilution produces a 5-mm wheal after 10 minutes. You then inject the no. 5 dilution and again note a 5-mm wheal after 10 minutes. You therefore inject the no. 4 dilution and note a 7-mm wheal. What should you do?	The no. 4 dilution demonstrated progressive whealing, so you must perform a confirmatory wheal by injecting the no. 3 dilution. If this is > 7 mm, it would suggest progressive whealing, and the no. 4 dilution would be considered the end point of the examination. A confirmatory wheal must grow by at least 2 mm.
541	Describe the technique used for intradermal dilutional testing.	• Dilutions created and labeled as no. 1 to no. 6, with no. 6 representing the weakest concentration and the least likely to induce a response • Inject a negative control: 4 mm wheal → 5 mm or less. • Inject a positive control (histamine: 0.0004 mg/mL): 4-mm wheal → 7 mm or more • 0.01 mL of the no. 6 dilution is injection intradermally to create a 4-mm wheal • Wait 10 minutes. • If the wheal is 5 mm, it is considered negative. If it is 7 mm or larger, it is considered positive. Continue with dilution no. 5. • If at any dilution you note growth of the wheal > 2 mm over the negative wheal (so 7 mm or more), continue with the next dilution. • It the next dilution demonstrates progressive growth (an additional 2 mm), stop the test. The first wheal to demonstrate growth is the endpoint dilution, and the second dilution to demonstrate progressive whealing is the confirmatory wheal.
542	After a positive fivefold sequential intradermal dilutional testing, what dilution should be used as a safe starting point for immunotherapy?	The endpoint dilution (the wheal that initiated progressive whealing)
543	What test uses skin-prick/puncture testing to determine the approximate degree of allergic sensitization, followed by specific sequential intradermal dilutional tests to assess further the prick/puncture results and to determine an endpoint dilution that can be used for initiating immunotherapy?	Modified quantitative testing (MQT) MQT is Frequently used by otolaryngologists practicing in the allergy field. It is used for its reproducibility, decreased cost, high sensitivity and specificity, and excellent correlation with full intradermal dilutional testing batteries.

544	Describe the technique used when performing a modified quantitative test for allergic disease?	• Use mutlitest (a device with multiple skin prick/puncture device).
		• Wait 20 minutes.
		• Wheal < 3 mm → Place no. 2 dilution in upper arm. → Wait 10 minutes → assess wheal
		  ○ ≤ 6 mm = Negative
		  ○ ≥ 7 mm = Endpoint: no. 3 dilution
		  ○ Wheal 3 to 8 mm → place no. 5 dilution in upper arm.
		• → Wait 10 minutes → assess wheal:
		  ○ ≤ 5 mm = Endpoint: no. 4 dilution
		  ○ 7 to 8 mm = Endpoint: no. 5 dilution
		  ○ ≥ 8 mm = Endpoint: no. 6 dilution
		  ○ Wheal ≥ 9 mm = Endpoint: no. 6 dilution

545	What medications can suppress the wheal and flare response for 48 to 72 hours?	First-generation antihistamines (i.e., brompheniramine, chlorpheniramine, clemastine, diphenhydramine, hydroxyzine)
546	Which medications should be avoided for 7 days because of suppression of the wheal and flair response?	Second-generation antihistamines and tricyclic antidepressants
547	What are the second-generation antihistamines that should be avoided at least 7 days before skin testing?	Cetirizine, loratidine, fexofenadine, levocetirizine. Note: Desloratidine should be avoided for > 14 days.
548	True or False. Leukotriene receptor antagonists should always be stopped at least 7 days before to skin testing.	False. They have not been shown to routinely inhibit wheal and flare response. They can be stopped in individual patients in whom the wheal and flare response is thought to be impacted by the medication.
549	What impact do intranasal or systemic corticosteroids have on the wheal and flare response during skin testing?	Little to none
550	To resuscitate a patient adequately in the unlikely event he or she develops anaphylaxis after skin testing in your office, what medication(s) should be stopped?	β-blockers (both topical and systemic)
551	What test measures serum concentrations of allergen-specific IgE antibodies?	RAST and modified RAST (has better sensitivity and more consistent scoring but is based on the original RAST immunoassay)
552	Describe the steps involved in the original RAST immunoassay?	• Allergen-bound paper disk is placed in test tube. • Patient's serum is added and antigen-specific IgE binds the antigen. • Excess serum and IgE are washed away. • Radiolabeled anti-IgE antibodies are added to the test tube and bind the antigen-specific IgE already bound to antigen on the paper disk. • Excess is washed away. • Gamma counter is used to determine the amount of bound IgE.
553	What are the benefits of immunoassay testing for allergic disease over skin testing?	Condition of skin does not matter, the results are not affected by drugs, no risk of anaphylaxis, greater patient convenience, quality control is easier, allows for quantitative assessment in preparation for immunotherapy, greater specificity. It may be less sensitive and is more expensive.
554	What are the benefits of skin testing over immunoassay for allergic disease?	Less time and expense to perform, increased sensitivity, wider variety of antigens to test, faster results
555	What level of total IgE in a patient's serum is suggestive of allergy?	> 200 IU. However, lower concentrations do not rule out allergy.
556	When should in vitro studies be recommended?	Patient is uncomfortable undergoing skin testing. Patient is not responding to medical therapy or doing poorly on immunotherapy. Patient is unable or unwilling to stop taking antihistamines, tricyclic antidepressants, or β-blockers. Patient has eczema or dermatographism. Patient has venom sensitivity Patient has possible IgE-mediated food sensitivity.
557	During a nasal provocation test, a patient is exposed to an allergen to determine whether exposure to a clinically significant allergen results in symptoms. The outcome can be measured based on symptoms and what other diagnostic tool?	Rhinomanometry

Allergy Management

558	What are the three main strategies used to manage allergy?	• Environmental modification • Pharmacotherapy • Immunotherapy
559	What drug class works on H1 receptors as antagonists, is most effective in treating early phase allergic response related symptoms and can cause sedation as a major side effect?	Antihistamines
560	Why do first-generation antihistamines result in sedation, psychomotor impairment, and central nervous system suppression?	They are highly lipophilic and cross the blood brain barrier.
561	In addition to sedation, what two side effects should be considered when prescribing first generation antihistamines?	• Anticholinergic side effects (i.e., urinary retention, dry mucous membranes, constipation, etc.) • Tachyphylaxis
562	Why are second-generation antihistamines currently preferred?	• Lipophobic → Do not cross the blood-brain barrier • Fewer or no anticholinergic side effects • Less or no tachyphylaxis
563	Provide examples of systemic first-generation antihistamines.	• Diphenhydramine • Chlorpheniramine • Azatadine • Hydroxyzine • Tiprolidine • Brompheniramine. • Clemastine (Tavist)
564	Provide examples of systemic second-generation antihistamines.	• Desloratidine* (Clarinex) • Loratidine (Claritin) • Fexofenadine* (Allegra) • Cetirizine (Zyrtec) • Levocetirizine* (Xyzal) * Can be considered third-generation antihistamines.
565	Name two second-generation topical antihistamines that have relatively rapid onset and effectiveness in treating congestion.	• Azelastine • Olopatadine
566	What drug class works primarily as α1-receptor agonists resulting in vasoconstriction?	Decongestants
567	What are the primary side effects associated with systemic decongestants such as phenylephrine and pseudoephedrine?	• α-Adrenergic side effects: Hypertension, increased appetite, tachycardia, arrhythmia • Tachyphylaxis (rebound rhinitis)
568	Name four medications that function as topical decongestants.	• Tetrahydrozoline • Naphazoline • Oxymetazoline • Phenylephrine
569	What condition can occur as a result of tachyphylaxis associated with topical decongestants when used for as little as 3 days?	Rhinitis medicamentosa
570	What are the three most commonly used oral corticosteroids for allergic rhinitis, which function to decrease the inflammatory reaction in as little as 12 to 24 hours?	• Prednisone • Methylpredisolone • Dexamethasone
571	What is the only topical corticosteroid nasal spray that is pregnancy class B?	Budesonide (Rhinocort Aqua)

572	What intranasal topical corticosteroids are commonly used?	• Budesonide (Rhinocort Aqua) • Triamcinolone acetate (Nasacort) • Fluticasone propionate/furoate (Flonase/Veramyst)* • Mometasone furoate (Nasonex)* • Ciclesonide (Omnaris) • Flunisolide (Nasarel) *Onset of action within 12 hours
573	Which intranasal corticosteroids are approved for patients as young as 2 years of age?	Mometasone furoate and fluticasone furoate
574	What side effect of intranasal corticosteroids has been related to drying and thinning of the nasal mucosa and can be related to improper intranasal application?	Epistaxis
575	What intranasal topical medication can be used prophylactically to stabilize mast cell degranulation, is well tolerated due to low systemic absorption (lipophobic), but must be redosed multiple times per day (short half-life)?	Cromolyn sodium
576	Name the leukotriene receptor antagonist that is approved for allergic rhinitis and can be used in children as young as 6 months.	Montelukast
577	What conditions have been shown to benefit from immunotherapy?	Allergic rhinitis, allergic conjunctivitis, allergic asthma, and stinging insect hypersensitivity. Potential uses include prevention of asthma in patients with allergic rhinitis and management of atopic dermatitis and aeroallergen sensitization.
578	For a patient to be considered for immunotherapy, what conditions must be met?	The allergen must cause clinically significant symptoms, and allergen-specific IgE must be demonstrated through in vivo or in vitro testing. Environmental avoidance and medical management should have been optimized.
579	What are the contraindications for immunotherapy?	• Non-IgE mediated symptoms • Symptoms controlled with maximal medical treatment and environmental avoidance • Atopic dermatitis (small studies suggest some benefit if induced by aeroallergens) • Food allergy • Allergies related to very short seasonal allergen exposure • Poorly controlled asthma • Use of β-blockers
580	Describe the major impact(s) immunotherapy has on the immune system resulting in allergic tolerance and decreased associated symptoms over time.	• Increase in the number of T_H2 cells and increased numbers of T_{reg} cells. • Increase in IL-10 and IL-12, decrease in IL-4 and IL-5 • Decreased release of early and late phase inflammatory mediators. • Decreased migration of inflammatory cells • Suppression of antigen-specific IgE over time following initial rise • Increased levels of IgG_4 (blocking antibody vs. T-helper regulatory cell)
581	What is the length of time normally required for immunotherapy to achieve good effect?	3 to 5 years
582	What technique is used to administer gradually increasing concentrations of allergy-provoking antigen over time to the patient in an effort to modulate allergen-specific immune reactions and symptoms via subcutaneous injection?	Subcutaneous immunotherapy (SCIT)

583	When choosing a starting dose for SCIT, what two goals should be achieved?	• Strong enough concentration to induce rapidly an antigen-specific response • Not strong enough to induce a significant local or systemic reaction
584	What dose is considered the maximum dose that can be delivered without inducing significant local or systemic effects?	Maintenance dose (delivers a goal cumulative amount of antigen over 3 to 5 years; should control symptoms for 1 week)
585	Describe the process of dose escalation from a starting dose (generally chosen based on modified quantitative testing) to a maintenance dose.	• Increase antigen load by 0.05 to 0.10 mL weekly (safe). • Increase antigen load by 0.05 to 0.10 mL twice weekly in healthy patients (no significant asthma or history of anaphylaxis). • Once maintenance dose is achieved, space injections from weekly or biweekly to every 2 to 3 weeks, then every 6 to 12 months (assuming symptoms are controlled) for 3 to 5 years. • Treatment can be discontinued after 3 to 5 years, with careful observation for recurrent symptoms.
586	What might result in an unexpected systemic or significant local reaction during immunotherapy?	• Wrong patient • Wrong concentration • Administering the immunotherapy during a time of year with increased environmental allergen load • Upper or lower respiratory tract infection • Asthma, poorly controlled • Drug allergy
587	True or False. Successful immunotherapy will eliminate the need for any adjuvant medical therapy and should stop any breakthrough symptoms.	False. Some breakthrough symptoms are expected, and medications may be necessary to augment the immunotherapy effect even when successful.

588	Describe the grading system used by the World Allergy Organization for systemic complications related to SCIT.	World Allergy Organization
		Grade I: One organ system
		• Cutaneous
		  ○ General pruritis, urticaria, flushing, sensation of heat or warmth
		  ○ Angioedema (not laryngeal, tongue, or uvular)
		• Upper respiratory
		  ○ Rhinitis (sneezing, rhinorrhea, nasal pruritis, and/or congestion)
		  ○ Throat clearing (itchy throat)
		  ○ Cough (not lower airway)
		• Conjunctival
		  ○ Erythema
		  ○ Pruritis
		  ○ Tearing
		• Other
		  ○ Nausea
		  ○ Metallic taste
		  ○ Headache
		Grade II: More than one organ system
		• Lower respiratory
		  ○ Asthma (cough, wheeze, shortness of breath)
		  ○ A drop of <40% in peak expiratory flow (PEF) or forced expiratory volume in 1 second (FEV$_1$)
		  ○ Responsive to bronchodilators
		• Gastrointestinal
		  ○ Abdominal cramps, vomiting, diarrhea
		• Other
		  ○ Uterine cramps
		Grade III: More than one organ system

- Lower respiratory
  - Asthma
  - A drop of 40% or more in PEF or FEV_1
  - Not responsive to bronchodilators
- Upper respiratory
  - Laryngeal, uvular, or tongue edema with or without stridor

Grade IV: More than one organ system

- Lower or upper respiratory
  - Respiratory failure with or without loss of consciousness
- Cardiovascular
  - Hypotension with or without loss of consciousness

Grade V: Death

Note: Many patients report a sense of impending doom with worsening complications.

589	What form of immunotherapy relies on fixed or escalating-dose schedules for antigen administered sublingually or orally with the goal of decreasing allergic symptoms, modulating the immune system, and providing a safe and easy method for immunotherapy?	Sublingual immunotherapy (SLIT). Used in Europe. Currently, SLIT is used off-label in the United States as a physician-prepared serum (similar to that given subcutaneously) and is not covered by third-party payers.
590	True or False. Sublingual immunotherapy has predominantly been used for single antigen therapy.	True

Immunology

591	What are the two major types of immunity? (▶ Fig. 3.18)	• *Innate* (nonspecific): First line of defense; antigen independent, immediate maximal response, no immunologic memory • *Adaptive* (specific immunity): Antigen dependent, delayed maximal response, immunologic memory, lymphocytes and lymphocyte-derived immunity

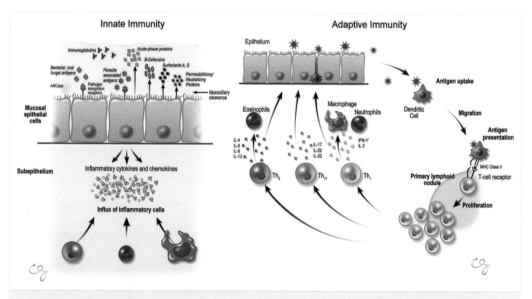

Fig. 3.18 Sinonasal immune response types. (a) Innate immunity (non-specific): first line of defense; antigen independent, immediate maximal response, no immunologic memory. (b) Adaptive immunity (specific): antigen dependent, delayed maximal response, immunologic memory, lymphocytes and lymphocyte derived immunity. (Used with permission from Kennedy DW, Hwang PH, eds. Rhinology: Diseases of the Nose, Sinuses, and Skull Base. New York, NY: Thieme; 2012.)

592	What are the three major components of innate (nonspecific) immunity?	• Anatomical boundaries: Epithelium; mechanical movement and trapping from cilia, tears, saliva, and mucus; competition from normal flora • Humoral barrier: Cytokine system, complement system, coagulation; fatty acids, lysozyme, lactoferrin, transferrin, phospholipase, defensins, surfactants, IL-1, TNF-α, interferons (IFNs) • Cellular barrier: Polymorphonuclear cells, macrophages, NK cells, and eosinophils
593	In what type of immunity do toll-like receptors coordinate the responses of cytokine-complement-phagocytic responses?	Innate (nonspecific) immunity
594	How do NK cells differ from NK T cells?	They are part of the innate immune system but can participate in the adaptive immune response. They arise from the lymphoid progenitor cell, which gives rise to T and B cells, do not have common T cell–specific markers (CD3, TCR, MHC, etc), they express CD-16, CD-56, and often CD8. They can be activated by IFN to target virally infected or tumor formation within 3 days based on the absence of "self" markers.
595	The anti-tumor effect of NK cells is thought to be due to their unique ability to recognize what?	The absence of self. Although T cells and many other immune effector cells are programmed to recognize nonself proteins produced by viruses or bacteria, NK cells have the ability to recognize when self peptides and proteins have been downregulated as a result of tumor transformation or what might be seen with viral infections. The most commonly encountered down regulated self molecule that might be "recognized" by NK cells are MHC molecules.
596	The adaptive immune system reacts specifically to individual antigens (proteins, polysaccharides, or macromolecules). What is the region of the antigen that is recognized by antigen-specifc receptors (T and B cells) and immunoglobulins within the adaptive immune system called?	Epitope (determinant)
597	What is the term that defines the ability of a host to ignore self and demonstrate immunologic unresponsiveness to self for both innate and adaptive immune responses?	Tolerance
598	Name the two subtypes of adaptive immunity.	• Humoral immunity → B cells, antibodies • Cell-mediated → T cells, cytokines
599	Describe the three basic steps of adaptive immunity.	• Recognition of antigen • Lymphocyte activation → production of cytokines, cytokine receptors, and other proteins; clonal expansion of lymphocytes; cellular differentiation (i.e., B cell into plasma cell) • Removal of the offending antigen (clearance)
600	What are the primary lymphoid organs?	• Thymus • Bone marrow
601	What are the secondary lymphoid organs, and what is their purpose?	• Systemic (spleen and lymph nodes) • Mucosal immune system (tonsils, Peyer patches, intraepithelial lymphocytes, lamina propria of mucosal tissues) • Cutaneous immune system
602	Where do myeloid (erythrocytes, neutrophils, platelets, basophils, eosinophils, monocytes/macrophages, and dendritic cells) and lymphoid cells (T cells, B cells, NK cells, plasma cells) arise from?	Bone marrow

603	Name the immature dendritic cell found in the skin and mucosa that contains Birbeck granules, is most prominent in the stratum spinosum of the skin, and is involved in antigen processing.	Langerhans cells
604	Name the specialized mucosal immune cell that is responsible for transocytosis (pinocytosis) of antigens across the follicular epithelium to germinal centers within Peyer patches within tonsillar tissue.	M (microfold) cells
605	Immune responses to hematogenous antigens and encapsulated organisms occur predominantly in the spleen, where lymphoid follicles surround small arterioles forming what structure?	Periarteriolar lymphoid sheaths
606	Lymphocytes can be identified by what specialized molecules on their surface that can help other cells (and researchers/clinicians) recognize their level of maturity, lineage, and extent of immune activation?	Cluster of differentiation (CD) markers
607	Name the cell associated with the following CD markers: • CD2 • CD3 • CD4 • CD8 • CD25	• All T cells • All T cells • T_H1 or T_H2 cells • T-suppressor cells (cytotoxic T cells) • + CD4 = T_H17 or T regulatory cells
608	What cell is required to undergo maturation in the thymus, and what are the possible outcomes of differentiation?	T cells differentiate in the thymus via both positive and negative differentiation: • Apoptosis • CD4 + helper T cell • CD8 + precytotoxic T cell
609	What percentage of CD4 + and CD8 + T cells survive selection in the thymus?	Less than 5%; most say 2% or less
610	Where does negative selection of developing T cells occur?	Thymic medulla
611	The process by which developing T cells that react too strongly with self peptides are deleted is called what?	Negative selection
612	What is the process called by which developing T cells that react appropriately with self peptides are signaled to survive and continue to develop?	Positive selection
613	What cell type is stimulated to develop from naïve CD4 cells (T_H0) by intracellular pathogens and IL12 and subsequently inhibits B cells, produces INF-γ and IL2, and stimulates cell-mediated immunity (activates cytotoxic CD8 cells, etc)?	T_H1 cells
614	What cell type is stimulated to develop from naïve CD4 cells (T_H0) by allergens and IL-4 and subsequently recruits/activates eosinophils, activates B cells; produces IL-4, IL-5, IL-6, IL-10, and IL-13; and is involved in both allergic disease and humoral immunity?	T_H2 cells
615	How does the immunologic T-cell response to oral antigens differ compared with more systemic responses?	Oral antigens are more likely to induce T-cell anergy or T-cell tolerance than T-cell activation.

616	What are the two types of MHC molecules?	• MHC Class I: Display self and nonself antigens (8–10 amino acids), membrane associated glycoprotein. • MHC Class II: Display extracellular proteins (various length, generally longer, 18 to 20 amino acids) that are phagocytosed and processed intracellularly before presentation
617	What type of MHC molecules are expressed by almost all nucleated cells and when downregulated can result in targeted destruction by NK cells and present endogenous antigen?	MHC class I
618	What type of MHC molecules are expressed primarily on antigen-presenting cells and lymphocytes (B cells, macrophages, endothelial cells, or dendritic cells primarily) and present processed exogenous antigen?	MHC class II
619	What type of T cell recognizes antigen presented by MHC class II molecules?	T_H cells (CD4+)
620	What type of T cell recognizes antigen presented by MHC class I molecules and kills cells presenting that antigen?	Cytotoxic T cells (CD8+)
621	What are the components of MHC molecules?	• Extracellular peptide binding region • Pair of Ig-like domains (bind CD4 and CD8) • Transmembrane region • Cytoplasmic tail
622	To activate T_H cells, antigen-presenting cells must present antigen via an MHC class II molecule, as well as secrete which important cell signal?	IL-1
623	Which cells secrete antibodies, and how are they activated?	B cells phagocytose antigen and present it to T_H cells via MHC class II molecules. T-cell then stimulates the B cell via IL-2 and IL-4 to mature into an Ig-producing plasma cell. Alternatively, large antigens can crosslink enough B-cell receptors to lead to direct activation of the cells and antibody production.
624	What cell type can be identified by the CD markers 19 and 21?	B cells
625	How is antibody isotype switching induced in B cells?	B cells encounter antigen and migrate out of follicles to a B cell-T cell interface, where they encounter activated T_H cells. The B cells present their processed antigen in the context of MHC class II recognized by the T-cell receptors. The costimulatory molecule CD40L interacts with the CD40 receptor, providing survival signals and isotype switching. The type of cytokine environment encountered at the time this is happening helps determine which isotype is then secreted.
626	What glycoprotein molecules are produced by plasma cells in response to humoral immune stimulation?	Immunoglobulins
627	What are the basic functions of immunoglobulins?	• Antigen binding • Effector functions: complement fixation, neutralization, or antibody-dependent cellular cytotoxicity via opsonization ("tagging" an antigen for ingestion and destruction by a phagocyte), stimulation of phagocytosis, etc.
628	What is the basic structure of an immunoglobulin?	Four chains (two heavy, two light), variable regions (bind antigen), constant regions, and hinge regions

629	What component of an immunoglobulin molecule is responsible for most of the effector functions of an antibody?	Fc domain of the antibody
630	What component of an immunoglobulin molecule is responsible for the specificity of antibodies?	Variable region of the antibody
631	Cleavage at the hinge region of an immunoglobulin results in production of what three fragments?	• 1–2. Fab fragments: Two identical fragments that contain the light chain and the variable and first constant domain of the heavy chains; binds antigen • 3. Fc fragments: One fragment containing the remaining heavy chains and their constant regions; may stimulate complement
632	What are the five classes of immunoglobulins produced in the body, which vary based on the amino acid sequences in the constant region of the heavy chain?	• IgA (serum, monomer; secretions, dimer) • IgD (monomer) • IgE (monomer) • IgG (monomer) • IgM (pentamer)
633	Which immunoglobulin makes up more than 70% of the total body immunoglobulin (only 15% of serum immunoglobulin), is found in mucosal secretions (nasal, pulmonary, lacrimal, salivary, colostrum, sweat, GI tract, and genitourinary), and is important in preventing microrganisms from invading the body?	IgA
634	How do IgA molecules primarily mediate mucosal immunity?	They are weak activators of complement and mediate their affects primarily via neutralization of antigen and prevention of systemic access.
635	What are the two subclasses of IgA?	• IgA1 (~85% serum): Strong immune response to protein antigens. Some response to polysaccharide and lipopolysaccharides • IgA2 (~15% serum): Key player in defense against mucosal invasion via immune response to polysaccharide and lipopolysaccharide antigens
636	What are the two forms of IgA found in the body?	• Monomeric serum IgA: Fc portion binds phagocytic cells, stimulating ingestion and destruction. • Dimeric secretory IgA: Two IgA molecules + J (joining) chain and a secretory piece; secreted by plasma cells located below the basement membrane of the basement epithelial surfaces
637	How does IgA gain access to extravascular secretions and tissues?	IgA is produced in a monomeric form and is joined with a J chain to form a dimer that is too large to diffuse across cellular membranes. The IgA dimer binds to polymeric IgA receptors on cells, which results in endocytosis and passes through the cell. The immunoglobulin is secreted on the luminal side of the cell still attached to the receptor. The receptor is then degraded, and the IgA molecule is free to diffuse throughout the lumen.
638	Which immunoglobulin deficiency is largely asymptomatic, correlating with the poorly understood function of its associated monomeric glycoprotein?	IgD
639	What is the structure of IgM?	IgM is a pentamer made up of five immunoglobulin subunits linked by a J chain.

640	What immunoglobulin is produced first in a humoral immune response and is excellent at binding complement?	IgM
641	What monomeric immunoglobulin is implicated in allergic responses to environmental allergens?	IgE
642	What conditions can lead to high levels of IgE antibodies?	Allergic diseases, lymphoma, IgE myeloma, systemic parasitosis, tuberculosis, HIV infection, Churg-Strauss, among others
643	Which monomeric immunoglobulin class is the most prevalent both in the serum and in extravascular spaces, is the only immunoglobulin to cross the placenta; play an important role in immunologic memory; and function to fix complement and activate macrophages, monocytes, polymorphonuclear cells, and some lymphocytes via opsonization?	IgG
644	Describe the function of the four IgG subclasses, which are divided based on structural variation of the Fc and hinge region, as well as the difference in number of disulfide bonds.	• IgG1 (60 to 70%): Opsonization, strong C1q binding, and classic complement cascade activation, response to protein and viral antigens • IgG2 (20 to 30%): Opsonization, weak C1q binding and classic complement cascade activation, response to bacterial polysaccharide antigens (i.e., *Pneumococcus*) • IgG3 (5 to 8%): Opsonization, strong C1q binding and classic complement cascade activation, response to protein and viral antigens • IgG4 (1 to 4%): Minimal opsonization, no complement activation, may be involved in immune response to parasites (*Schistosoma* and *Filaria* spp.)
645	What component of the nonspecific immune system functions to opsonize bacteria, recruit and activate polymorphonuclear cells and macrophages, participate in antibody regulation, clear immune complexes, clear apoptotic cells, and can result in inflammation and anaphylaxis?	Complement system
646	What are the four pathways involved in complement activation?	• Classic pathway (C1qrs, C2, C3, C4; C1-INH, C4-BP); antibody dependent • Lectin pathway (mannan binding protein, mannan-associated serine protease); antibody independent • Alternative pathway (C3, Factors B and D, properdin; decay accelerating factor, CR1, etc); antibody independent • Lytic (membrane attack) pathway (C5–9; protein S) *Note*: The classic, lectin, and alternative pathways can all result in the cleavage of C3 and activation of C5 convertase. C5 convertase is required for activation of C5 and the lytic (membrane attack) pathway.
647	How is the mannose-binding lectin pathway of complement activated?	Microbes containing mannan are recognized by mannan binding lectins, which in turn activate serine proteases (MASPs) which mediate cleavage of C1, C4, and C2, leading to the C3 convertase
648	How is the alternative pathway of the complement system activated?	Microbial structures neutralize inhibitors of spontaneous complement activation leading to unimpeded complement activation.
649	What are considered the anaphylatoxins produced by the complement cascade?	C3a, C4a, and C5a

650	What nonantibody proteins act as mediators between cells, result in signaling cascades, and can be produced both by immune (innate and cell mediated) and nonimmune system cells?	Cytokines
651	Name the general cytokine subtype associated with the following: • Results in an antiviral response • Produced by lymphocyte • Produced by leukocytes and effect the function of other leukocytes • Result in an acute inflammatory response to Gram-negative bacteria • Influence maturation and release of bone marrow cell populations	• INF • Lymphokine • Interleukin • TNF • Colony stimulating factor
652	Name the cytokine associated with adaptive immunity system described by the following: • Produced by T_H cells, major growth factor for T cells, B cells, and NK cells • Stimulated bone marrow immune cells to expand, especially mast cells and eosinophils • Produced by macrophages, mast cells, and T cells; stimulates development of T_H cells, stimulates B-cell immunoglobulin class switch to IgE • Produces by T_H cells, promotes maturation of B cells, and eosinophils • Produced by T cells, among others, and inhibits proliferation of T cells and macrophages and inhibits the effect of proinflammatory cytokines on polymorphonuclear cells and endothelial cells	• IL-2 • IL-3 • IL-4 • IL-5 • Transforming growth factor (TGF)-β
653	Which cytokine functions to regulate both the innate and adaptive immune system by inhibiting macrophages, cytokine synthesis, and antigen-presenting cells and is produced by macrophages and CD4 + T cells?	IL-10
654	Name the cytokine associated with the innate immunity described by the following: • Produced by activated macrophages (response to lipopolysaccharide of Gram-negative bacteria), mediates acute inflammation, stimulates thalamus to produce a fever • Produced by activated macrophages, mediates acute inflammation, stimulates T cells • Produced by many different cells (i.e., lymphocytes, macrophages, endothelium, and keratinocytes) to inhibit viral replication, increase MHC class I expression in cells making them more susceptible to cytotoxic T cells, activate NK cells • Produced by T_H1 cells, produces a myriad of direct cytotoxic effects	• TNF-α • IL-1 • Type I interferons (INF-α and INF-β) • INF-γ
655	What is the clinical impact of IgG1 deficiency?	Generalized hypogammaglobulinemia. Often associated with IgG3 deficiency.
656	When patients have significant IgG1 deficiency in combination with IgA and/or IgM deficiency. What is the diagnosis?	Common variable immunodeficiency

657	Although rare, selective IgG1 deficiencies (i.e., no other detectable immunoglobulin abnormality) can occur and can result in frequent and/or repeated infections of what two organs?	Upper (i.e., sinuses) and lower respiratory tracts.
658	You are evaluating a child with recurrent sinusitis, otitis media, and bronchitis. Immunologic workup suggests deficiency in the IgG subclass, which is important in the defense against polysaccharide capsular antigens. What is the likely diagnosis and to which bacteria is this child most susceptible?	IgG2 deficiency. *Streptococcus pneumoniae, Haemophilus influenza* type b, *Neisseria meningitidis*
659	IgG3 deficiency can result in increased susceptibility to viral infections, as well as *Moraxella catarrhalis* and *Streptococcus pyogenes*, resulting in recurrent sinopulmonary and GI infections, as well as recurrent lymphocytic meningitis. What additional IgG subtype is often deficient in these patients?	IgG1
660	You are evaluating a patient with sialadenitis and salivary gland enlargement. Biopsy reveals lymphoplasmacytic infiltrate IgG+ plasma cells and fibrosis. The condition seems to respond to glucocorticoids. Which IgG subclass is likely involved?	IgG4 (IgG4-related systemic disease). May also result in autoimmune pancreatitis
661	What is the clinical impact of IgA deficiency?	Patients are often asymptomatic, although the deficiency may be one of the most common primary immunodeficiency syndromes. May have recurrent sinopulmonary or GI infections, skin infections, anaphylaxis with transfusions, or autoimmune disorders
662	A patient has eczema, thrombocytopenia, and recurrent otitis media, pneumonia, and sinusitis. What immunodeficiency syndrome do you suspect, and how is it inherited?	Wiskott-Aldrich syndrome (X-linked)
663	A 6-month-old patient has severe and recurrent otitis media, sinopulmonary infections, pneumonia, and associated autoimmune disorders and is found to have an underlying immunodeficiency affecting B cells, but not T cells. What are the most likely diagnosis, inheritance pattern, and genetic defect?	Bruton agammaglobulinemia: X-linked, defect in tyrosine kinase (Bruton tyrosine kinase), resulting in inability of pro-B cells to mature
664	Patients with Bruton agammaglobulinemia develop masses in what organ?	Thymus (thymoma)
665	Patients with X-linked agammaglobulinemia have recurrent infections secondary to a low level of which antibody isotype(s)?	All antibody isotypes
666	Abnormality of the third and fourth branchial arches leading to thymic hypoplasia or agenesis, hypoplastic parathyroids with resultant hypocalcemia, and abnormalities of the face and aortic arch results in what syndrome?	DeGeorge syndrome (22q11.2 deletion)
667	What form of immune responses are impaired in DeGeorge syndrome?	T-cell–mediated immune responses are impaired or absent secondary to thymic agenesis.

668	Severe combined immunodeficiency (SCID) results from deficient or malfunctioning T and B cells. It presents early in life with severe infections (viral, bacterial, and fungal) involving the sinopulmonary system and other organ systems. Often these children present with severe oral candidiasis as well. If diagnosed early, this disease can be effectively managed with what treatment?	Bone marrow transplantation
669	What virus invades T cells via the CD4 + marker and synthesizes proviral DNA from reverse transcriptase, which is then integrated into the host DNA, and what is the result?	HIV Decreased T-cells, macrophages, and dendritic cells as a result of direct cytotoxic effects, which causes progressive immunodeficiency in the host
670	How are HIV infections diagnosed?	• ELISA anti-HIV antibody (screening test) • Western blot (confirmation test) • PCR for viral DNA • CD4 + count • Viral load • Viral susceptibility testing
671	What are the diagnostic criteria for AIDS?	An AIDS-defining illness (e.g., Kaposi sarcoma) or a CD4 + T cell count less than 200 cells/μL or a CD4% less than 14%
672	What disorder results in the inability of phagocytes to kill catalase-positive organisms as a result of dysfunction of intracellular hydrogen peroxide production via the nicotinamide adenine dinucleotide phosphate oxidase enzyme complex?	Chronic granulomatous disease (most commonly X-linked)
673	At what age do patients with clinically significant deficiencies in antibodies typically begin to have recurrent infections and why?	7 to 9 months. As maternal antibodies begin to clear from the patient's system, his or her own immune system must take over.
674	What is the most common cell lineage to be defective in immunodeficiency?	B cells
675	What are the recommended screening tests for T-cell immunodeficiency if one is suspected based on clinical history?	• Absolute lymphocyte count • Chest X-ray looking for the presence of thymic shadow in children • Delayed hypersensitivity skin testing to antigen • Flow cytometry to quantitate T-cell subsets
676	What are the recommended screening tests for B-cell immunodeficiency if one is suspected based on clinical history?	• Quantification of serum immunoglobulins and subclasses • Antibody (IgG) responses to a vaccine challenge after a minimum of 1 month. • Protein antigen: Tetanus, diphtheria, *Haemophilus influenzae* type B • Polysaccharide antigen: Pneumovax, meningococcal vaccine • Flow cytometry to quantify B cells

4 General Otolaryngology

Kathryn M. Van Abel, Matthew L. Carlson, and David J. Archibald

Statistics

1	Define *sensitivity*. (▶ Fig. 4.1)	The ability of the test to identify correctly those patients with the disease

	Affected (+)	Non-affected (-)
(+) Test	True Positives (TP)	False Positives (FP)
(-) Test	False Negatives (FN)	True Negatives (TN)
	All Affected (TP + FN)	All Non - affected (FP + TN)

Prevalence	(TP+FN)/ TP+FN+FP+TN
Sensitivity	TP/(TP+FN)
Specificity	TN/(TN+FP)
Positive Predictive Value	TP/(TP+FP)
Negative Predictive Value	TN/(TN+FN)

Fig. 4.1 Biostatistics calculations.

2	Define *specificity*.	The ability of the test to identify correctly those patients without the disease
3	Is high sensitivity or high specificity most important for a screening test?	Sensitivity
4	Define a *type 1 error*.	The chance of testing positive among those without the condition; false-positive rate = 1 specificity.
5	Define a *type 2 error*.	The chance of testing negative among those with the condition; false negative rate = 1-sensitivity.

6	Define positive *predictive value*.	The chance of having the condition among those that test positive
7	Define negative *predictive value*.	The chance of not having the condition among those that test negative

Imaging

8	A cervical spine X-ray revealing a greater than 5-mm widening of the predentate space (between the anterior surface of the dens and the posterior surface of the C1 tubercle) is worrisome for what traumatic injury?	Atlantoaxial dissociation
9	Conventional radiography of the facial bones and neck has been largely replaced by computed tomography (CT). What traditional views were used to view the following: • Frontal, maxillary, and sphenoid sinus • Frontal sinuses, posterior ethmoid air cells, orbital floors • Maxillary sinuses, anterior ethmoid air cells, orbital floors • Sphenoid sinuses, anterior and posterior walls of the frontal sinuses • Soft tissue of the neck	• Lateral view (5 degrees off true lateral) • Caldwell view (15 degrees off caudal angulation) • Waters view (neck in 33 degrees of extension) • Submentovertex view (anteroposterior [AP] projection, head in 90 degrees of extension) • AP and lateral views
10	In a stable pediatric patient with stridor, what radiography is appropriate?	AP and lateral neck films to evaluate for retropharyngeal abscess, croup, epiglottitis, and radiopaque foreign body
11	What are the most common findings on chest radiography in a patient with a witnessed foreign-body aspiration and clinical signs suggestive of aspiration?	Mediastinal shift, unilateral hyperinflation, atelectasis, and a foreign object if radiopaque
12	Although they have been largely replaced by CT scan, radiographs of the temporal bone are occasionally necessary. Name the following views: • Lateral view of the mastoid with 30 degrees of cephalocaudad angulation • View of the petrous apex with patient facing the film, head slightly flexed and turned 45 degrees opposite the film • Comparison of both mastoid bones and petrous pyramids via AP view with a 30-degree tilt	• Schüller view • Stenvers view • Towne view
13	Why is a CT scan typically a more appropriate imaging study in evaluating patients with a potential deep neck space infection instead of magnetic resonance imaging (MRI)?	Although MRI provides better soft tissue definition, it is expensive and requires a lengthy scan time compared with CT and therefore may necessitate sedation of a child or a distressed patient and increase the likelihood of airway compromise.
14	On T1-weighted MRI, contrast-enhancing tumors may be hidden by surrounding fat. What technique can be used to achieve better visualization of the tumor?	Fat suppression
15	Describe the T1-weighted appearance of water and fat on MRI.	Low intensity and high intensity, respectively
16	What are some of the contraindications to MRI use?	Electromagnetic force can cause serious malfunction to cardiac pacemakers and cochlear implants (although new techniques have been developed that allow cochlear implant recipients the ability to have MRI studies). Some older vascular clips and ossicular prostheses contain paramagnetic components, and unless these are known to be MRI compatible, another modality should be used.

17	What does *SUV* stand for in regard to positron emission tomography (PET) imaging?	*Standardized uptake value*, which provides a semiquantitative index of radio tracer uptake
18	What does the presence of an echogenic (fatty) hilum typically indicate during ultrasound examination of the neck?	Benign disease. Normal lymph nodes have an echogenic hilum, whereas it is reported that there is an absent hilum in 96 of metastatic lymph nodes.
19	Can the location of normal parathyroid glands be identified on ultrasound examination of the thyroid and neck?	Normal parathyroid glands are not usually visible because of their small size and similar echo texture to adjacent thyroid tissue.
20	What is *acoustic shadowing* in ultrasound imaging?	Diminished sound or loss of sound posterior to a strongly reflecting or attenuating structure

Pharmacology

21	Review the differences between first-generation and second-generation antihistamines.	Compared with first-generation antihistamines, second-generation medications generally have a longer duration of action, have less central nervous system (CNS) penetration, and are less sedating.
22	Review contraindications to glucocorticoid steroid use.	Psychosis, severe diabetes, peptic ulcer disease, congestive heart failure, severe hypertension, systemic tuberculosis, osteoporosis
23	Describe the features of ototoxicity associated with salicylate use.	Reversible sensorineural hearing loss and tinnitus, hypothesized to result from disruption of oxidative phosphorylation. Its use does not produce histologic changes.
24	What severe neurologic side effect is associated with intramuscular administration of prochlorperazine?	Extrapyramidal side effects including focal dystonia
25	List the different amide and ester local anesthetics.	Amides have two "i's," whereas esters only have one "i" in their generic name. Examples of esters include benzocaine, cocaine, and tetracaine. Examples of amides include bupivacaine, lidocaine, and mepivacaine. Esters are more likely to cause an allergic reaction
26	What topical anesthetic reversibly binds to and inactivates sodium channels, thus inhibiting excitation of nerve endings and causing vasoconstriction?	Cocaine
27	What is the maximum dose of lidocaine hydrochloride?	4 to 5 mg/kg, maximum total dose of 300 mg
28	What medication can be given to reverse the effects of local injectable epinephrine?	Local infusion of 1.5 to 5 mg of phentolamine
29	What is the mechanism of action for β-lactam antibiotics?	Binds to DD-transpeptidase (also called *penicillin-binding protein*) and inhibits the formation of peptidoglycan cross-links in the bacterial cell wall
30	What is the mechanism for acquiring penicillin resistance?	Enzymatic deactivation of penicillin G through β-lactamases and altered penicillin binding proteins
31	What is the mechanism of action of aminoglycosides?	They irreversibly bind to the 30S ribosome and freeze the 30S initiation complex. Additionally, they cause misreading of the mRNA code (bactericidal).
32	A mutation in which a gene may lead to increased aminoglycoside toxicity even at low doses?	Mitochondrial 12S ribosomal RNA gene
33	What are the earliest signs of aminoglycoside ototoxicity?	Tinnitus, high-frequency hearing loss, and dizziness
34	What is the mechanism of action of macrolides?	They inhibit translocation of the peptidyl tRNA from the A to the P site on the ribosome by binding to the 50S ribosomal RNA (bacteriostatic).

35	What is the treatment of *Clostridium difficile* colitis?	IV or oral (PO) metronidazole or PO vancomycin
36	What are the most common antibiotics that have been implicated in the development of *C. difficile* colitis?	Second- and third-generation cephalosporins, ampicillin/amoxicillin, and clindamycin
37	A child develops gray staining of the teeth with a prominent horizontal line across the upper and lower teeth after being prescribed an antibiotic. Which antibiotic was most likely prescribed?	Tetracycline
38	What is the mechanism of action of aspirin?	Irreversible acetylation of serine 529 of cyclooxygenase (COX) 1. Rapid onset of action if dose is 160 mg or greater. The effects of use last for the lifetime of the platelet, which is 7 to 10 days.
39	What is the mechanism of action of thienopyradines (e.g., clopidogrel bisulfate)?	Irreversible inhibition of the cysteine residue of the P2Y12 platelet receptor. Onset of action is rapid if patient is given a loading dose, and the effects last for the lifetime of the platelet (7 to 10 days).
40	What drug can be given to reverse the antiplatelet effects of nonsteroidal anti-inflammatory drugs (NSAIDs)?	Desmopressin acetate (DDAVP)
41	In the event of significant bleeding following administration of heparin, what medication should be considered?	Protamine. Give 1 mg for every 100 units of heparin, and closely monitor activated partial thromboplastin time (aPTT).
42	What is the mechanism of action of warfarin?	It is a vitamin K antagonist that inhibits the production of vitamin K-dependent clotting factors.

Critical Care

43	Describe the mechanism of malignant hyperthermia.	It is caused by a combination of a volatile inhalational anesthetic (commonly halothane) and the short-acting paralytic succinylcholine. An abnormal ryanodine receptor causes overwhelming amounts of calcium to be released from the sarcoplasmic reticulum of skeletal muscle, thereby initiating prolonged and intense muscle contraction.
44	What is the initial treatment for malignant hyperthermia?	Stop the anesthetic, give dantrolene (which prevents the release of calcium from endoplasmic reticulum), increase oxygen, and initiate cooling measures including ice packs.
45	What are the physical examination findings of cardiac tamponade?	Tachycardia, paradoxical pulse with respirations, hypotension, jugular vein distension, muffled cardiac sounds, decreased QRS amplitude on electrocardiogram (ECG)
46	What are the four basic classifications of shock?	• Hypovolemic shock: Loss of blood volume • Obstructive shock: Decreased circulation resulting from external or intrinsic compression • Septic shock: Related to vascular dilation • Cardiogenic shock: Impaired perfusion from lack of sufficient cardiac output
47	What is the formula describing the rate of fluid maintenance for the pediatric patient?	The 4:2:1 rule = 4 mL/kg hourly for the first 10 kg, adding 2 mL/kg per hour for the second 10 kg, and adding 1 mL/kg per hour for each kilogram over 20 kg
48	What is the formula used to calculate the rate of fluid resuscitation of a burn victim?	The Parkland formula: Fluid for the first 24 hours (milliliter) = 4 x patient weight (kg) x % body surface area involved; the first half is given over 8 hours, the second half over the remaining 16 hours. Rule of 9's for determining percentage of burned: 9% = head, each arm; 18% = chest, back, each leg

49	What preoperative condition is associated with immunosuppression, poor wound healing, decreased basal metabolic rate, longer hospitalization, and an increased mortality rate?	Preoperative malnutrition
50	Why should gastric residuals be checked every 4 hours in a patient receiving enteral nutrition via tube feeds?	Regurgitation and aspiration are risks of tube feeding
51	What is involved in the refeeding syndrome that is observed in severely malnourished patients following initiation of feeds?	Malnourishment leads to hypoinsulinemia and electrolyte abnormalities including intracellular hypophosphatemia. Within 4 to 5 days of reinitiation of carbohydrate metabolism and subsequently increased insulin production, patients can develop severe hypophosphatemia.
52	You are rounding on a patient who underwent major surgery for polytrauma and required 20 units of packed red blood cells. The patient is complaining of perioral numbness and tingling. What is the likely diagnosis and treatment?	Citrate toxicity with subsequent hypocalcemia. Treat with calcium gluconate. This should be given for symptomatic patients only.
53	What medications can be given as pretreatment to prevent mild hypersensitivity and nonhemolytic febrile reactions in a patient receiving blood transfusion with a history of mild reactions?	Acetaminophen and antihistamines such as diphenhydramine
54	What complications may be encountered in a patient who has received massive intraoperative transfusions?	Volume overload, hyperplasia or hypokalemia, hyperammonemia, acidosis, thrombocytopenia, coagulation factor depletion, coagulopathy, hypothermia, transfusion related acute lung injury, and citrate toxicity
55	What is transfusion-related acute lung injury?	Acute respiratory distress and noncardiogenic pulmonary edema that develops during or within 6 hours of blood transfusion. Treatment includes supportive measures, often including mechanical ventilation, high-inspired oxygen, and positive end expiratory pressures.
56	Mechanical ventilation is most commonly delivered via positive-pressure ventilation (PPV). What are the two most common subtypes of PPV that focus on the transition from inspiration to expiration?	• Volume control: A set volume is delivered per breath • Pressure control: A set pressure is delivered per breath
57	What common rule can be used to select the tidal volume and rate for a patient on assist control mechanical ventilation?	12–12 rule: 12 mL/kg of lean body mass delivered 12 times a minute. It is useful for patients without preexisting lung disease. It must be adjusted for patients with known chronic obstructive pulmonary disease (COPD), etc.
58	What technique can be used in mechanical ventilation to maintain a patient's airway pressure above atmospheric pressure at the end of expiration?	Positive end expiratory pressure (PEEP)
59	What is the difference in the 1-second forced expiratory volume FEV1 to vital capacity (FVC) ratio in COPD compared with that in restricted lung disease?	In COPD, the FEV_1/FVC ratio decreases, whereas the ratio is preserved or increased in restrictive lung disease.
60	Describe the difference between the two types of postobstructive pulmonary edema.	• Type 1. Follows an acute severe cause of upper airway obstruction (epiglottitis, laryngospasm, strangulation) and usually manifests within 1 hour of the event • Type 2. Follows relief from a chronic obstruction (obstructive sleep apnea (OSA), choanal stenosis, subglottic stenosis) and usually manifests within 6 hours of reversing the obstruction

61	What is the treatment of postobstructive pulmonary edema?	Oxygen and supportive care in mild cases and PEEP in more severe cases. Diuretic therapy can be instituted, although the benefit is not clear.
62	What is the most common cause of fever in the immediate postoperative period?	Within the first 48 hours of surgery, fever is likely due to an inflammatory reaction to surgical insult or reaction to medication or blood product given intraoperatively. It is unlikely to be infectious. Evaluate for possible source of infection, but prophylactic antibiotics are not indicated. Patient may be treated with antipyretic and monitor for change in clinical status.
63	In the acute postoperative setting, how can the mnemonic "Wind, Water, Walk, Wound, Wonder Drugs, What did you do?" help in the evaluation of a febrile patient?	• Wind: Pneumonia? Aspiration? Atelectasis? • Water: Urinary tract infection? • Walk: Thrombophlebitis? Deep venous thrombosis? Pulmonary embolus? • Wound: Surgical-site infection? • Wonder drugs: Drug reaction (β-lactam antibiotic? Sulfa antibiotic?) • What did we do? Catheter-related infection? IV site infection?

Otolaryngologic Manifestations of Systemic Disease

64	What is *eosinophilic granuloma*?	*Eosinophilic granuloma* is the most common form of Langerhans cell histiocytosis and is characterized by the formation of solitary or multiple discrete nodules within bones.
65	What is Hand-Schüller-Christian disease?	It is multifocal Langerhans cell histiocytosis with bone "granulomas," associated with the triad of exophthalmos, lytic skull lesions, and diabetes inspidus.
66	True or false. Most patients with Langerhans cell histiocytosis have multisystem disease.	False. Approximately two-thirds of patients have disease involving one site.
67	What is Letterer-Siwe disease?	Systemic Langerhans cell histiocytosis is the rarest (~ 10% of cases) and the most severe form of disease. Initial symptoms often include generalized skin eruption, anemia, and hepatosplenomegaly.
68	Extranodal natural killer cell (NK)/T-cell lymphoma, nasal type, is commonly associated with which virus?	Epstein-Barr virus
69	How is extranodal NK/T-cell lymphoma, nasal-type, commonly treated?	Chemotherapy (CHOP: cyclophosphamide, doxorubicin, vincristine, prednisone) in conjunction with radiotherapy
70	Compared with other types of lymphoma involving the head and neck, what is the prognosis for extranodal NK/T-cell lymphoma, nasal type?	Much poorer
71	What is the most common laryngeal manifestation of Wegener granulomatosis?	Subglottic stenosis
72	What is the most common otologic manifestation of Wegener granulomatosis?	Serous otitis media
73	What histopathologic findings are seen in Wegener disease?	Necrotizing granulomas and arteritis involving small vessels
74	What laboratory test is used to diagnose and follow Wegener disease?	Antineutrophil cytoplasmic antibody (C-ANCA). Test will be positive in more than 90% of cases.
75	What histopathological findings are seen in sarcoidosis?	Noncaseating granulomas
76	What condition is characterized by uveitis, parotid swelling, fever, and facial nerve palsy?	Heerfordt syndrome (uveoparotid fever), a manifestation of sarcoidosis

77	What is the most common site of laryngeal involvement of sarcoidosis?	Supraglottis
78	What is the most common head and neck manifestation of sarcoidosis?	Cervical lymphadenopathy
79	Describe a common presentation for pyogenic granuloma.	Less than 1-cm lobular red or purple lesion that develops on the gingiva or nasal mucosa that is friable and prone to bleeding. It occurs more commonly in women and is associated with trauma and pregnancy.
80	Describe the treatment of pyogenic granuloma.	Lesions frequently resolve spontaneously when associated with pregnancy. If frequent bleeding or cosmesis is a concern, conservative cauterization or excision can be pursued.
81	Describe the natural history of untreated necrotizing sialometaplasia.	Spontaneous resolution over weeks to months
82	How does blastomycosis typically manifest?	A common triad includes cutaneous disease, pulmonary involvement, and constitutional symptoms. Skin lesions may involve the face with verrucous growth and scarring. Oropharyngeal and laryngeal involvement are rare.
83	Describe the clinical manifestations of coccidiomycosis.	It is the cause of "valley fever." Most patients have an influenza-like illness that includes malaise, fever, myalgia, arthralgia, and cough. Initial symptoms are pulmonary, mucocutaneous involvement with maculopapular rash, cervical lymphadenopathy, and/or meningeal involvement.
84	Where is *Coccidioides immitis* endemic?	Desert Southwest including New Mexico, Nevada, California, Texas, Utah, and northern Mexico
85	Histoplasmosis most commonly occurs in which geographic location?	The Ohio, Missouri, and Mississippi River valleys
86	Describe the head and neck manifestations of disseminated histoplasmosis.	Granulomatous lesions involving the lips, gingiva, tongue, larynx, and pharynx manifesting with painful ulcers containing heaped edges
87	What is the most common site of laryngeal involvement of histoplasmosis?	Supraglottis
88	How is histoplasmosis diagnosed?	Histoplasma antibody latex agglutination test, fungal stains, blood or urine antigens using enzyme-linked immunosorbent assay or polymerase chain reaction (PCR), or histoplasma skin test
89	What pathogen is responsible for the development of rhinosporidiosis?	The parasite *Rhinosporidium seeberi*
90	What are the common head and neck clinical manifestations of rhinosporidiosis?	Fleshy, friable strawberry-like lesions most commonly involving the inferior turbinate, oropharynx, conjunctiva, and perineum
91	What is the treatment for rhinosporidiosis?	Wide local excision or prolonged dapsone therapy
92	What is the causative organism in syphilis?	The spirochete *Treponema pallidum*
93	What is the treatment of syphilis?	Penicillin G benzathine
94	Describe the presentation of primary syphilis.	A painless ulcer (chancre) at the site of transmission demonstrating a rolled edge and punched-out base is present after 3 to 6 weeks at the site of exposure.
95	Describe the presentation of secondary syphilis.	Secondary syphilis is characterized by systemic spread of disease with manifestations including fever, myalgias, arthralgias, and lymphadenopathy. A mucocutaneous rash often develops including the oral mucosa and the palms and soles. Finally, condyloma lata and patchy alopecia may develop.

96	What are the three categories of tertiary syphilis?	The three categories are gummatous syphilis, cardiovascular syphilis, and neurosyphilis.
97	Describe the findings of congenital syphilis.	"Snuffles" with sinonasal drainage, saddle nose, saber shins, Hutchinson teeth, and mulberry molars
98	Describe the Argyll-Robertson pupil.	A pupil that does not react to light but does constrict during accommodation. Associated with syphilis
99	Describe the manifestation of otosyphillis.	Otosyphilis is associated with either congenital or tertiary acquired syphilis and manifests with sensorineural hearing loss beginning in the high frequencies, fluctuating tinnitus, and vertigo.
100	What is the Hennebert sign?	Rotary nystagmus when positive or negative pressure is applied to the tympanic membrane
101	Describe the Jarisch-Herxheimer reaction.	After treatment of syphilis, dying spirochetes may trigger a cytokine cascade that manifests with myalgias, fever, headache, and tachycardia.
102	What tests are commonly used for syphilis screening?	Venereal Disease Research Laboratory (VDRL), rapid plasma reagin (RPR) test
103	What confirmatory test should be ordered after a positive or equivocal screening test for syphilis?	FTA-ABS
104	What is the most common cause of subacute pediatric cervical lymphadenopathy?	Atypical *Mycobacterium*, most commonly *M. avium-intracellulare*, *M. haemophilum*, and *M. scrofulaceum*
105	How is brucellosis transmitted?	It is transmitted from contaminated meat or dairy products or via direct contact through broken skin.
106	What are the clinical manifestations of cat-scratch disease?	The primary lesion develops as an erythematous, non-pruritic pustule 1 week affter inoculation. Lymphadenitis of the axilla, neck, and inguinal region commonly develops 2 to 4 weeks after exposure. Suppuration with acute tenderness and fever frequently occurs. Lymphadenopathy usually resolves over 2 weeks but may persist for up to 2 years.
107	What are the pathogens associated with leprosy (Hansen disease)?	*Mycobacterium leprae* and *Mycobacterium lepromatosis*
108	What is the treatment for Hansen disease?	Dapsone
109	What pathogen is responsible for the development of rhinoscleroma?	*Klebsiella rhinoscleromatis*
110	What histologic findings are strongly suggestive of the diagnosis of rhinoscleroma?	Russell bodies (immunoglobulin containing inclusions in plasma cells), pseudoepitheliomatous hyperplasia, Mikulicz cells (foamy histiocytes containing *Klebsiella*)
111	What is the treatment for rhinoscleroma?	Tetracycline or ciprofloxacin
112	What tests are helpful in diagnosing systemic lupus erythematosus?	Antinuclear antibody (ANA), anti-Sm, anti-DNA, anti-ribonuclear protein (anti-RNP), and anticardiolipin antibody
113	What are the typical clinical manifestations of a patient with mixed connective tissue disease?	Raynaud phenomenon, arthralgias, inflammatory myopathy, lymphadenitis, skin or mucosal lesions, and serositis
114	What is the definition of *mixed connective tissue disease*?	Mixed connective tissue disease is characterized by a combination of overlapping features of systemic lupus erythematous, scleroderma, and polymyositis. Patients may manifest Raynaud phenomenon, arthralgias, inflammatory myopathy, lymphadenitis, skin or mucosal lesions, and serositis.
115	Which joints in the head and neck are most commonly affected by rheumatoid arthritis (RA)?	RA can affect any diarthrodial joint, including the temporomandibular, cricoarytenoid, and ossicular joints.

116	What does the acronym *CREST* stand for?	Calcinosis, Raynaud phenomenon, esophageal dysmotility, sclerodactyly, and telangiectasias. CREST syndrome is a limited cutaneous form of systemic scleroderma.
117	What are the histologic findings in a minor salivary gland lip biopsy performed in a patient with Sjogren disease?	Focal lymphocytic infiltrate with atrophic acini
118	What head and neck sites are commonly affected by relapsing polychondritis?	Ear, nasal septum, and larynx
119	What is the most common head and neck manifestation of relapsing polychondritis?	Episodic auricular chondritis, presenting with erythema and pain of the pinna with sparing of the fatty lobule. Eventually presents in ~ 90% of patients
120	What are common symptoms of giant cell arteritis?	Headache (predominantly temporal region), jaw claudication (~ 50% patients), vision loss or visual disturbance, fatigue, general malaise, fever, anorexia, weight loss, night sweats, and tongue pain
121	What histologic finding on temporal artery biopsy is suspicious for giant cell arteritis?	Inflammatory infiltrates in at least the adventitia and media, with elastic lamina fragmentation
122	What imaging study may be useful in the diagnosis of giant cell arteritis?	Duplex ultrasound. High-resolution MRI has been reported to have very similar diagnostic power, but more data are needed before it can be recommended as a diagnostic tool.
123	What is the classic triad of Wegener granulomatosis?	Granulomas of the respiratory tract, progressive glomerulonephritis, and necrotizing vasculitis of small to medium-sized arteries and veins
124	What condition is characterized by uveitis, oral aphthous ulcers, and genital ulcers?	Behçet disease

Neck Space Anatomy

125	What are the two primary fascia networks of the neck? (▶ Fig. 4.2)	Superficial cervical fascia and the deep cervical fascia

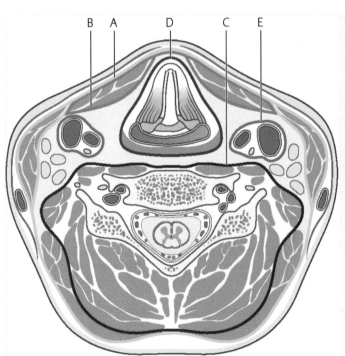

Fig. 4.2 Layers of the cervical fascia at level of C5 vertebra: (A) superficial cervical fascia; (B) muscular layer of the middle cervical fascia, (C) prevertebral fascia, (D) visceral layer of the middle cervical fascia, and (E) carotid sheath. (Used with permission from Behrbohm H, Kaschke O, Nawka T, Swift A. Ear, Nose, and Throat Diseases: With Head and Neck Surgery. New York, NY: Thieme; 2009.)

126	Describe the anatomy of the superficial cervical fascia.	It lies just deep to the dermis and superficial to the deep cervical fascia. It extends from the zygoma to the clavicle and envelops the platysma and muscles of facial expression.
127	Describe the anatomy of the deep cervical fascia.	It is composed of the superficial (investing), middle (visceral and muscular), and deep (prevertebral and alar) layer. The carotid sheath fascia is created by all three layers of the deep cervical fascia.
128	Describe the anatomy of the superficial (investing) layer of the deep cervical fascia.	It surrounds the neck and inserts superiorly at the nuchal ridge, mastoid, zygoma, and mandible and inferiorly at the clavicles, sternum, scapula, and acromion. It envelops the sternocleidomastoid muscle, trapezius, muscles of mastication, submandibular glands, and parotid gland. Inferiorly, its manubrial insertion splits to form the suprasternal space of Burns.
129	Describe the anatomy of the middle (visceral and muscular) layer of the deep cervical fascia.	It extends superior to the cranial base and inferiorly to the upper mediastinum. It is subdivided into the muscular and visceral layers. The *muscular division* surrounds the infrahyoid strap muscles; the *visceral portion* surrounds the pharyngeal constrictors, esophagus, trachea, and thyroid and creates the buccopharyngeal fascia. Both divisions contribute to the carotid sheath.
130	Describe the anatomy of the deep (prevertebral and alar) layer of the deep cervical fascia.	It is subdivided into the alar and prevertebral fascia. Both extend superiorly from the cranial base, but the alar fascia fuses with the middle cervical fascia and extends into the upper mediastinum, and the prevertebral fascia extends to the level of the coccyx. The alar fascia and prevertebral fascia fuse at the vertebral transverse processes and after joining, envelop the paraspinous muscles.
131	Describe the anatomy of the suprasternal space (space of Burns).	The inferior insertion of the superficial (investing) fascia splits just above the manubrium attaching anterior to the manubrium and posteriorly to the interclavicular ligament. This small potential space contains a portion of the anterior jugular veins, and the sternal heads of the sternocleidomastoid muscle.
132	Define the boundaries of the buccal space.	The buccal space is created by the buccinator muscle medially; the superficial layer of the deep cervical fascia and the muscles of facial expression laterally and anteriorly; and the muscles of mastication, mandible, and parotid gland posteriorly. It primarily contains adipose tissue (buccal fat pad), minor salivary glands, accessory parotid tissue, and facial/buccal arteries, veins, and lymphatics. The buccal fat pad is pierced by the parotid duct as it courses to the buccinator and eventually enters the mouth opposite the second upper molar.
133	Define the mechanism of spread of infection (or tumor) to and from the buccal space.	It permits spread between the mouth, parotid space, and masticator space from deficient fascial compartmentalization along the superior, inferior, and posterior limits.
134	Define the boundaries of the carotid space.	The carotid sheath contains the carotid artery, internal jugular vein, vagus nerve, and jugular lymphatic chain. All three divisions of the deep cervical fascia form the carotid sheath. It extends from the skull base to the mediastinum; anteriorly lies the sternocleidomastoid muscle, posteriorly the prevertebral space, and medially the visceral compartment.
135	Review the risk factors for carotid blowout.	Radiation, salivary fistula, malnutrition, hypothyroidism, T-incision over the great vessels, radical neck dissection

136	Define the boundaries of the *danger space*.	The *danger space* is a potential space that rests between the alar fascia and the prevertebral fascia. Infections in this area can communicate with the thorax (mediastinum) to the level of the diaphragm.
137	Define the boundaries of the masticator space.	The masticator space is created from the superficial layer of the deep cervical fascia surrounding the masseter laterally and the pterygoid muscles medially. It contains masseter muscle, pterygoid muscles, inferior tendon of the temporalis muscle, ramus, and posterior body of the mandible, internal maxillary artery, and the inferior alveolar neurovascular bundle.
138	Define the boundaries of the parapharyngeal space. (▶ Fig. 4.3)	It is shaped as an inverted pyramid with the base at the cranial base and the apex at the hyoid bone. Anteriorly, it is bound by the pterygomandibular raphe, posteriorly be the prevertebral fascia, medially by the superior pharyngeal constrictor, and laterally by the parotid, mandible, and lateral pterygoid.

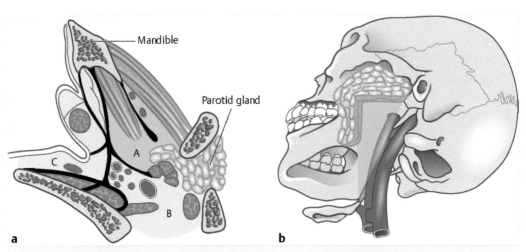

Fig. 4.3 Axial cross section of the left parapharyngeal space. (a) The prestyloid (A) and post-styloid (B) compartments of the (C) parapharyngeal space. (b) The inverted pyramid of the parapharyngeal space, with the base of the pyramid at the cranial base (superiorly) and the apex at the greater cornu of the hyoid bone (inferiorly). (Used with permission from Bradley PJ, Guntinas-Lichius O, eds. Salivary Gland Disorders and Diseases: Diagnosis and Management. New York, NY: Thieme; 2011.)

139	How is the parapharyngeal space commonly divided?	Prestyloid and poststyloid compartments are divided by the tensor-vascular-styloid fascia connecting the tensor veli palatini and the styloid process.
140	What structures are contained within the prestyloid space?	Fat, lymph nodes, minor salivary gland tissue, internal maxillary artery, and the inferior alveolar, auriculotemporal and lingual nerves
141	What structures are contained within the poststyloid space?	Carotid artery, internal jugular vein, cranial nerves 9 through 12, and the superior sympathetic chain
142	What is the syndrome that follows the parapharyngeal space or parotid surgery that causes pain with the onset of eating?	First-bite syndrome

143	Define the boundaries of the parotid space.	It is created by the superficial layer of deep cervical fascia as it surrounds the mandible and parotid gland and contains the parotid gland and parotid lymph nodes, the facial nerve, posterior facial vein, and facial artery.
144	Describe the mechanism of infection or tumor spread from the parotid space to the parapharyngeal space.	The superomedial parotid space fascia is deficient, allowing for direct spread into the parapharyngeal space via the stylomandibular tunnel.
145	Define the boundaries of the peritonsillar space.	It is bound by the palatine tonsil medially and the superior pharyngeal constrictor, palatoglossus, and palatopharyngeus medially, superiorly, inferiorly, anteriorly, and posteriorly. It contains loose areolar tissue and minor salivary glands.
146	Define the boundaries of the prevertebral space.	It extends from the skull base to the coccyx and is bordered anteriorly by the prevertebral fascia, posteriorly by vertebral bodies, and laterally by the transverse processes of vertebrae.
147	Describe the sequential layers and spaces (superficial to deep) of the posterior pharyngeal wall.	Mucosa, pharyngeal constrictor, buccopharyngeal fascia, retropharyngeal space, alar fascia, danger space, prevertebral fascia, prevertebral space
148	Define the boundaries of the sublingual space.	It contains the sublingual gland, Wharton duct, and lingual and hypoglossal nerves and is bound superiorly by the mucosa of the floor of mouth, laterally by the mandible, inferiorly by the mylohyoid, medially by the genioglossus, and anteriorly by the mandible.
149	What are the two divisions of the submandibular space?	It is subdivided into the *sublingual* and *submaxillary* spaces, which are separated by the mylohyoid. These two spaces communicate at approximately the second molar.
150	Define the boundaries of the submaxillary (submylohyoid) space.	It contains the submandibular gland and is bound superiorly and medially by the mylohyoid muscle, inferiorly and posteriorly by the digastric muscle, and laterally and anteriorly by the superficial layer of the deep cervical fascia and mandible.
151	Define the boundaries of the infratemporal fossa. (▶ Fig. 4.4)	• Located inferior and medial to the zygomatic arch • Anterior: Posterolateral portion of maxillary sinus • Lateral: Ramus of the mandible • Medial: Lateral pterygoid plate • Superior: Greater wing of the sphenoid bone • Inferior: Medial pterygoid muscle • Posterior: Articular tubercle of the temporal bone, glenoid fossa

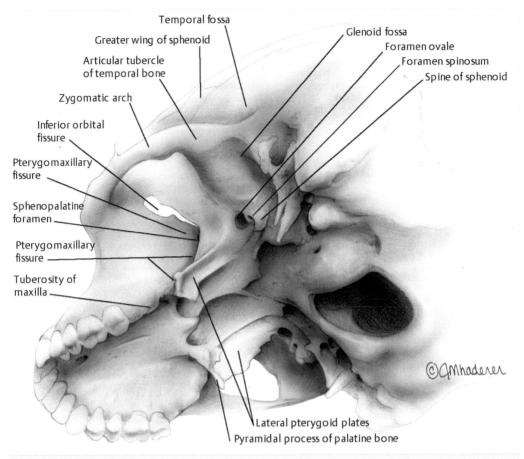

Temporal fossa

Greater wing of sphenoid

Articular tubercle
of temporal bone

Zygomatic arch

Inferior orbital
fissure

Pterygomaxillary
fissure

Sphenopalatine
foramen

Pterygomaxillary
fissure

Tuberosity of
maxilla

Glenoid fossa

Foramen ovale

Foramen spinosum

Spine of sphenoid

Lateral pterygoid plates

Pyramidal process of palatine bone

Fig. 4.4 Oblique view of the left infratemporal fossa and its boundaries: Anterior: posterolateral portion of maxillary sinus; Lateral: ramus of the mandible (removed); Medial: lateral pterygoid plate; Superior: greater wing of the sphenoid bone; Inferior: medial pterygoid muscle (not shown); Posterior: articular tubercle of the temporal bone, glenoid fossa. (Used with permission from Levine HL, Clemente MP, eds. Sinus Surgery: Endoscopic and Microscopic Approaches. New York, NY: Thieme; 2005.)

152	Describe the branches of the three segments of the internal maxillary artery. (▶ Fig. 4.5)

- First (lateral) portion: Deep auricular artery, anterior tympanic artery, middle meningeal artery, inferior alveolar artery, accessory meningeal artery
- Second (middle) portion: Masseteric artery, pterygoid branches, anterior and posterior deep temporal arteries, buccal artery
- Third (medial) portion: Sphenopalatine artery (terminal branch), descending palatine artery, infraorbital artery, artery of the vidian canal, anterior, middle, and posterior superior alveolar artery

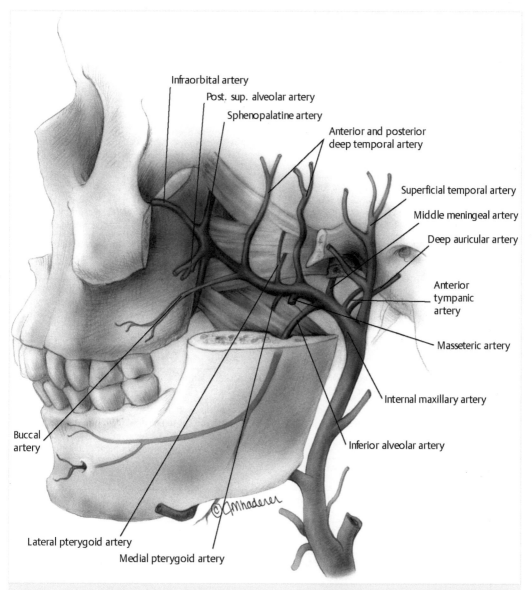

Fig. 4.5 Left lateral view of the internal maxillary artery and its primary divisions. First (lateral) portion: deep auricular artery, anterior tympanic artery, middle meningeal artery, inferior alveolar artery, accessory meningeal artery (not shown); Second (middle) portion: masseteric artery, pterygoid branches, anterior and posterior deep temporal arteries, buccal artery; Third (medial) portion: sphenopalatine artery (terminal branch), descending palatine artery (not shown), infraorbital artery, artery of the vidian canal (not shown), anterior, middle, and posterior superior alveolar artery. (Used with permission from Levine HL, Clemente MP, eds. Sinus Surgery: Endoscopic and Microscopic Approaches. New York, NY: Thieme; 2005.)

153 Define the boundaries of the pterygopalatine fossa.	• Located medial to the infratemporal fossa • Anterior: Posteromedial portion of maxillary sinus • Lateral: Pterygomaxillary fissure and infratemporal fossa • Medial: Perpendicular plate of the palatine bone • Superior: Body of the sphenoid bone • Inferior: Pterygopalatine canal • Posterior: Root of the pterygoid plates

154	Name the foramina communicating with the pterygopalatine fossa.	• Anterior: Inferior orbital fissure • Lateral: Pterygomaxillary fissure • Medial: Sphenopalatine foramen • Interior: Greater palatine canal • Posterior: Vidian canal, foramen rotundum
155	What important structure may be encountered if the vidian canal is followed posteriorly?	The second genu of the internal carotid artery
156	Define the boundaries of the temporal fossa.	It is located between the superficial layer of the temporalis fascia and the periosteum of the squamosal portion of the temporal bone and is subdivided into the superficial and deep layer by the temporalis muscle. It contains the internal maxillary artery and inferior alveolar nerve.
157	During submandibular gland excision, the marginal mandibular nerve cannot be readily identified. What strategy can be used to decrease the risk of marginal mandibular nerve injury?	The common facial vein can be identified low, ligated, and divided and then reflected superiorly because the marginal mandibular nerve rests superficial to the common facial vein and facial artery in the region of the mandibular notch.
158	Describe the location and course of the hypoglossal and lingual nerves in the region of the submandibular gland.	It is located deep to the digastric muscle and mylohyoid and superficial to the hypoglossus muscle. The lingual nerve is located cephalad to the hypoglossal nerve.
159	What landmarks can be used for identification of the accessory nerve during level 2 neck dissection?	Transverse process of C1, anterolateral to the internal jugular vein, two fingerbreadths below the mastoid tip, or just as it runs posterior to the sternocleidomastoid 1 to 2 cm above the Erb point
160	Describe the location of the phrenic nerve and superior sympathetic chain.	It is located anterior to the anterior scalene muscle. The phrenic nerve runs lateral to the sympathetic chain.
161	The hypoglossal nerve is "pinned" by what artery as it descends behind the digastric muscle?	The occipital artery
162	Describe five methods or landmarks for identifying the facial nerve during parotidectomy.	The tragal pointer, tympanomastoid suture line, level of the digastric groove (posterior digastric muscle), retrograde from marginal mandibular nerve at mandibular notch, anterograde from the vertical segment of the mastoid
163	During deep-lobe parotidectomy, what arteries must be divided for en bloc removal?	External carotid artery, superficial temporal artery, internal maxillary artery
164	Which cervical rootlets contribute to the ansa cervicalis?	C1, C2, and C3
165	Which deep neck spaces involve the entire length of the neck?	Four: the retropharyngeal, danger, prevertebral, and carotid spaces
166	Describe the parasympathetic innervation to the parotid gland.	Inferior salivatory nucleus → cranial nerve IX (Jacobson nerve) → lesser superficial petrosal nerve → otic ganglion → auriculotemporal nerve (V3) → parotid gland
167	Describe the parasympathetic innervation to the submandibular gland and sublingual glands.	Superior salivatory nucleus → nervus intermedius → cranial nerve VII → chorda tympani → lingual nerve → submandibular ganglion → submandibular gland
168	Describe the parasympathetic innervation to the lacrimal gland.	Superior salivatory nucleus → greater superficial petrosal nerve → vidian nerve → sphenopalatine ganglion → lacrimal branch V1 → lacrimal gland

Benign Neck Masses

169	Describe the condition of benign symmetric lipomatosis.	This condition involves diffuse lipomatosis of the head, neck, shoulders, and proximal upper extremities. It is more common in men than in women. Patients often have a history of alcoholism and diabetes.
170	True or False. Most liposarcomas develop from a preexisting benign lipoma.	False. Most liposarcomas develop de novo.

171	What is the most common type of monomorphic adenoma?	Basal cell adenoma
172	What is the most common paraganglioma of the head and neck? (▶ Fig. 4.6)	Carotid body tumor, which develops within the adventitia of the carotid bifurcation and are of neural crest origin

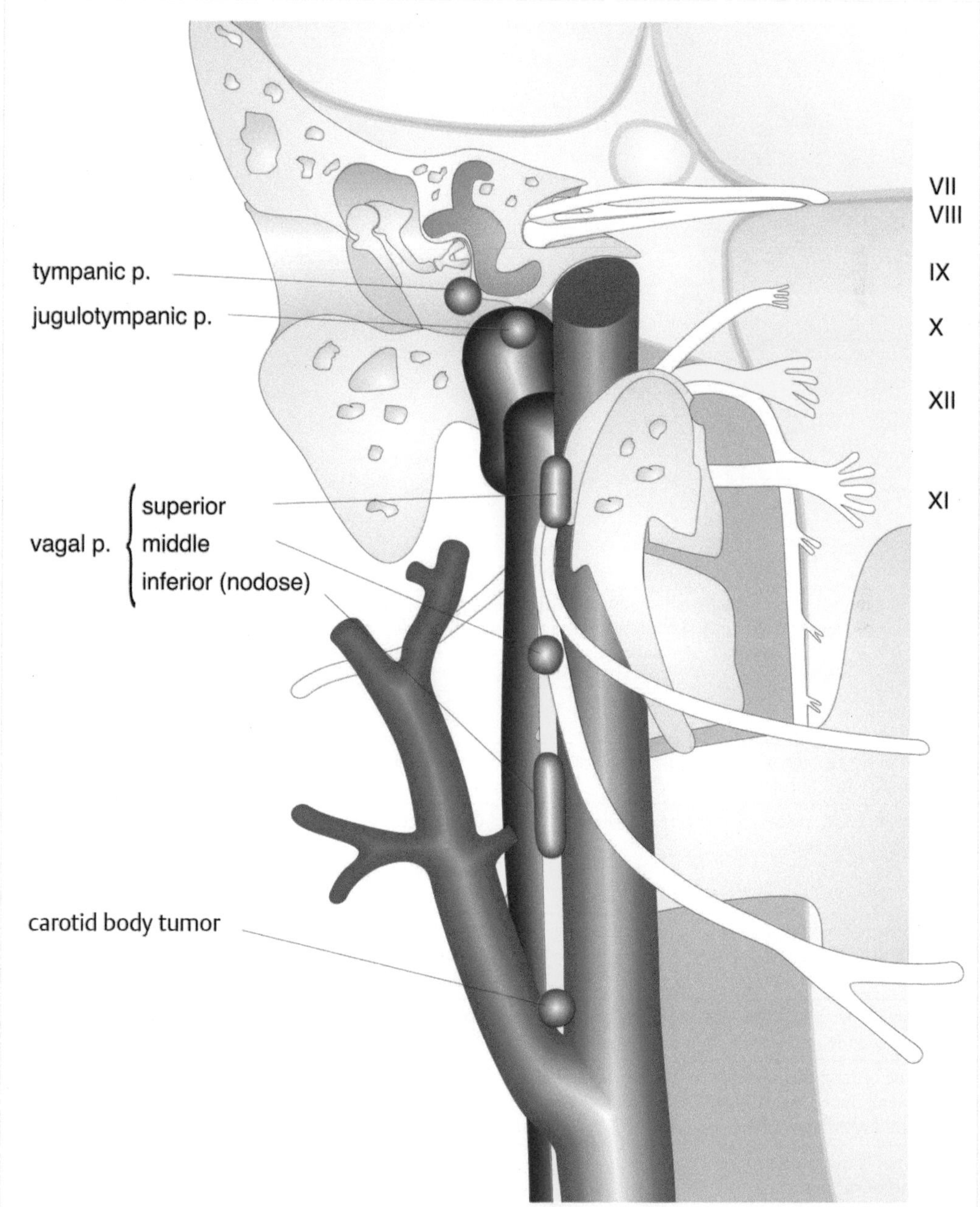

Fig. 4.6 Paragangliomas of the head and neck: tympanic paraganglioma (glomus tympanicum), jugulotympanic paraganglioma (glomus jugulare), vagal paraganglioma (glomus vagale) and carotid body tumor (most common). (Used with permission from Sanna M, Piazza P, Shin SH, Flanagan S, Mancini F, eds. Microsurgery of Skull Base Paragangliomas. New York, NY: Thieme; 2013.)

173 Describe the Lyre sign. (▶ Fig. 4.7)

- Splaying of the internal carotid artery and the external carotid artery at the carotid bifurcation
- Seen with carotid body tumors
- Glomus vagale and sympathetic chain paragangliomas on the other hand displace the carotid system anteriorly.

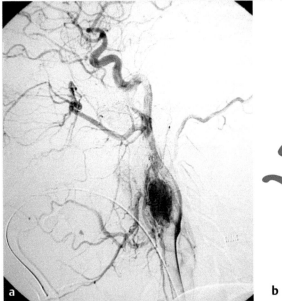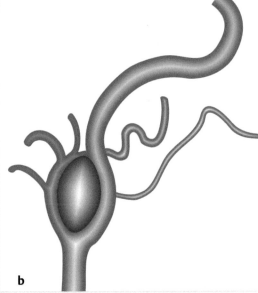

Fig. 4.7 Angiography (a) and schematic drawing (b) demonstrating splaying of the internal carotid artery and the external carotid artery at the carotid bifurcation by a carotid body tumor (Lyre sign). (Used with permission from Sanna M, Piazza P, Shin SH, Flanagan S, Mancini F, eds. Microsurgery of Skull Base Paragangliomas. New York, NY: Thieme; 2013.)

174	What percentage of head and neck paraganglio-mas are functional?	Less than 3%
175	What cellular pattern is characteristically seen in paragangliomas?	Cells of Zellballen. Alveolar-like clumps of tumor cells are surrounded by a network of thin-walled capillaries. Thick bands of collagenous tissue divide the tumor. Five to 20 epithelial cells compose a nest or group of cells.
176	What percentage of head and neck paraganglio-mas are malignant?	Less than 10%. Paragangliomas are determined by the presence of lymph node metastasis, not by cellular atypia or local invasion.
177	Familial paraganglioma syndromes are caused by a mutation in genes that encode for what enzyme?	Succinate dehydrogenase
178	True or false. Neural fascicles can be more easily spared during resection of a schwannoma com-pared with a neurofibroma.	True
179	What is the most common poststyloid parapha-ryngeal space tumor?	Schwannoma of the vagus or sympathetic chain
180	Which benign salivary gland tumors have pro-nounced fluorodeoxyglucose (FDG) uptake on PET imaging?	Oncocytoma, and Warthin tumor. Both tumors are com-posed of large eosinophilic granular cells containing high mitochondrial concentrations.
181	What is the most common type of tumor to arise within the prestyloid parapharyngeal space?	Benign salivary gland tumors

182	Describe the MRI findings of pleomorphic adenoma.	Well-circumscribed mass with low intensity on T1- and hyperintensity on T2-weighted sequences. Frequently demonstrates homogeneous gadolinium uptake
183	What is the most common prestyloid parapharyngeal space tumor?	Pleomorphic adenoma is the most common overall. Mucoepidermoid carcinoma is the most common malignancy.
184	What are the main access routes to the parapharyngeal space?	Cervical, submandibular/cervical, cervical parotid, cervical parotid with mandibular osteotomy, transoral (not recommended)
185	When should a mandibulotomy be considered for parapharyngeal space tumors?	• Tumors > 5 cm • Tumors with extensive skull base disease • Extensive invasion
186	What are laryngoceles?	Air-filled dilations of the laryngeal ventricle that may be congenital or acquired
187	Describe the three types of laryngoceles.	• Internal: Connects the ventricle with the paraglottic space, false cord, and aryepiglottic fold • External: Ventricular dilation extends through the thyrohyoid membrane to the lateral neck. • Combined: Both internal and external extension
188	What are plunging ranulas, and how do they differ from nonplunging ranulas?	Plunging ranulas form from obstructed sublingual gland ducts leading to the formation of an epithelial-lined retention cyst. A plunging ranula requires that the cyst extend through the mylohyoid, most commonly to the submandibular space.
189	Review the characteristic signs and symptoms of Kawasaki (lymphomucocutaneous) disease.	Fever for more than 5 days with at least four of the following five findings: • Bilateral nonsuppurative conjunctivitis • One or more changes of the mucous membranes of the upper respiratory tract, including pharyngeal injection, fissured or erythematous lips, and "strawberry" tongue • One or more changes of the extremities, including peripheral erythema or edema and periungual and generalized desquamation • Polymorphous rash • Cervical lymphadenopathy > 1.5 cm in diameter (usually unilateral)
190	Describe the cardiac complications associated with Kawasaki disease.	Coronary artery aneurysms occur in up to 25% of untreated patients. Death may occur secondary to coronary artery thrombosis or aneurysm rupture. An ECG and echocardiogram should be obtained in all patients suspected of having Kawasaki disease.
191	Describe the clinical manifestation of Kikuchi-Fujimoto disease.	A benign, self-limiting necrotizing lymphadenitis that most commonly affects young Japanese women. Initial symptoms may include malaise, fever, fatigue, arthralgias, weight loss, and hepatosplenomegaly.
192	Describe Castleman disease.	Castleman disease is a rare lymphoproliferative disorder that can manifest with localized or multicentric disease. It is commonly associated with human immunodeficiency virus (HIV) and human herpes virus (HSV) 8.

Infectious Diseases of the Neck

193	What is the most common cause of deep neck space infections in the adult population?	Odontogenic infection
194	What is the most common cause of deep neck space infections within the pediatric population?	Tonsillitis

195	Describe the head and neck manifestations of *Actinomyces israelii* infection?	Development of a "lumpy jaw" and multiple painless, red or bluish raised, firm lesions containing multiple draining sinus tracts
196	Describe the histologic appearance of *Actinomyces israelii*?	Gram-positive, non–acid-fast, anaerobic bacilli demonstrating a filamentous fungal-like growth pattern and "sulfur granule" formation
197	What are the most common sites of the head and neck to develop *Mycobacterium* infections?	Anterior superior cervical region near the submandibular space, followed by the posterior cervical, middle cervical, and supraclavicular regions. Atypical mycobacterial infection is sometimes found in the preauricular region
198	What is the most common manifestation for atypical *Mycobacterium* infections involving the neck?	Persistent firm painless cervical adenopathy with overlying violaceous skin discoloration
199	What is the current recommended management of atypical *Mycobacterium* infections involving the neck?	Persistent lesions are best managed by surgical excision or incision and curettage. Common antibiotic choices include clarithromycin, ethambutol, isoniazid, and rifampin, depending on the species.
200	What tests should be ordered for patients with suspected mycobacterial infections involving the head and neck?	PPD, chest plain film, cultures (Ziehl-Neelson stain, Lowenstein-Jensen medium), nucleic acid probes, and PCR
201	Are PPD tests usually positive in patients with atypical mycobacterial infections of the head and neck?	No. PPD tests are generally negative or weakly reactive.
202	Why are mycobacteria called *acid-fast bacteria*?	Once they are colorized with a red dye, they cannot be decolorized with acid solutions.
203	What is the most common head and neck manifestation of tuberculosis?	Cervical lymphadenopathy
204	What is the treatment of cervical lymphadenopathy associated with tuberculosis?	Isoniazid, rifampin, ethambutol, and pyrazinamide
205	What pathogen is associated with cat-scratch disease?	*Bartonella henselae*
206	Name the three types of Langerhans cell histiocytosis.	• Eosinophilic granuloma • Hand-Schüller-Christian (disseminated chronic) • Letterer-Siwe (disseminated acute)
207	What condition manifests with the triad of osteolytic skull lesions, exophthalmos, and diabetes insipidus?	Hand-Schüller-Christian disease (disseminated chronic)
208	Which type of Langerhans cell histiocytosis is associated with early in life onset and a rapidly progressive course?	Letterer-Siwe (disseminated acute)
209	What is Lemierre syndrome?	Septic thrombophlebitis of the neck that most commonly results from *Fusobacterium necrophorum*. It often begins with pharyngitis progressing to lymphadenopathy, fevers, chills, and rigors. Septic emboli may involve the lung, brain, spleen, and liver, among other sites.
210	What is the most common cause of pediatric cervical lymphadenopathy?	Reactive lymphadenopathy from viral infection
211	What is the most common cause(s) of pediatric suppurative lymphadenopathy?	Group A *Streptococcus* and *Staphylococcus aureus*
212	What is the test of choice for primary syphilis?	The FTA-ABS test evaluates for the presence of treponemal antibodies. The test is positive in 90% of patients who seek therapy for primary syphilis and remains positive for life.

213	What are the symptoms of meningeal neuro-syphilis?	Headache, nuchal rigidity, nausea, and vomiting. Cranial nerve involvement is seen in 40% of patients resulting in hearing loss, facial paralysis, and visual disturbances.
214	What constitutes the Hutchinson triad of congenital syphilis?	Small notched teeth, deafness, and interstitial keratitis
215	What test is most useful in establishing the diagnosis of neurosyphilis?	Reactive cerebrospinal fluid (CSF) VDRL and a CSF white blood cell count of 20 cells/μL or greater
216	What is the definition of otosyphilis?	The presence of a positive FTA-ABS in the setting of unexplained sensorineural hearing loss
217	What are the causes of syphilis-associated hoarseness?	Laryngeal chancres, mucous membrane manifestations of secondary syphilis involving the upper aerodigestive tract, and gummata of the larynx may directly cause hoarseness. Long-term syphilis may result in infraglottic stenosis, adhesions between vocal folds or arytenoid fixation. Neurosyphilis may result in recurrent laryngeal nerve paresis.
218	Describe the common initial symptoms of toxoplasmosis.	Fever, malaise, pharyngitis, and myalgias, with cervical lymphadenopathy occurring in the most patients
219	What are the pathogen, vector, and carrier responsible for the development of tularemia?	*Francisella tularensis, Amblyomma americanum* (lone star tick), rabbits, and wild rodents, respectively
220	What are the early symptoms of tularemia infection?	Fever, headache, chills, myalgia, photophobia, diminished visual acuity, and lymphadenopathy
221	What are the possible side effects of amphotericin B?	Nephrotoxicity, anemia, fever, chills, nausea, and vomiting
222	What is the mechanism of action of the "azole" antifungal medications?	Fungistatic. All azoles work by inhibiting a cytochrome P-450–dependent enzyme that is required to convert lanosterol to ergosterol.
223	What are the five recognized forms of fungal sinusitis?	• Acute fulminant invasive fungal sinusitis • Chronic invasive fungal sinusitis • Granulomatous invasive fungal sinusitis • Fungus ball • Allergic fungal rhinosinusitis
224	What is the most common causative organism in chronic invasive fungal sinusitis?	*Aspergillus fumigatus*
225	Describe the condition of HIV lymphadenopathy.	Diffuse lymphadenopathy (> 2 cm) involving two or more extrainguinal sites for longer than 3 months. Two thirds of patients infected with HIV will develop this syndrome shortly after seroconversion.
226	What are the anatomical boundaries of the deep neck space involved in Ludwig angina?	The submandibular space is bound superiorly by the mucosa of the floor of mouth, laterally and anteriorly by the mandible, and inferiorly by the superficial layer of the deep cervical fascia. It contains two divisions (sublingual and submaxillary), separated by the mylohyoid muscle.
227	How do submandibular infections spread to other deep neck space compartments?	Communication between potential spaces exists at the buccopharyngeal gap, which connects the submandibular and lateral pharyngeal spaces.
228	Why is there a lack of trismus in patients suffering from Ludwig angina?	Trismus develops from irritation of the masticatory muscles (masseter and pterygoids), which insert into the mandibular ramus. The submandibular space is not contiguous with these muscles.
229	What is the mechanism of airway compromise in patients with Ludwig angina?	Increased swelling in the bilateral submandibular space pushes the tongue superiorly and posteriorly, thereby causing progressive airway obstruction.

230	What is the best management of the airway in a patient with a progressive infection of the submandibular space with increasing airway compromise?	Awake intubation or tracheostomy
231	What is the most common causative organism in necrotizing soft tissue infections?	Group A streptococcus
232	What are the clinical characteristics of necrotizing fasciitis?	Tense edema, pain disproportionate to examination, skin discoloration, bullae, necrosis, and crepitus
233	What is the treatment of necrotizing fasciitis?	Incision and drainage are inadequate. Necrotic tissue must be debrided and the wound left open with packing. Broad-spectrum antibiotics should be administered, and the patient should be monitored in an intensive care unit setting. Hyperbaric oxygen may provide additional benefit.
234	Describe the clinical presentation of infectious mononucleosis.	Fever, fatigue, generalized lymphadenopathy, splenomegaly, and exudative pharyngitis with adenotonsillar hypertrophy

Oral Cavity Overview

235	Define the following terms: • Ageusia • Hypogeusia • Dysgeusia	• Ageusia: Inability to taste • Hypogeusia: Diminished ability to taste • Dysgeusia: Distorted sense of taste
236	Describe the taste innervation of each of the following upper aerodigestive locations: • Anterior two-thirds of the tongue • The posterior two-thirds of the tongue • The circumvallate papillae • Pharynx • Epiglottis	• Chordae tympani of facial nerve • Glossopharyngeal nerve • Glossopharyngeal nerve • Glossopharyngeal and vagus • Superior laryngeal branch of vagus
237	What is the most common cause of perceived taste dysfunction?	Olfactory dysfunction
238	What tastes and odors are detected by the trigeminal nerve?	Spice and ammonia
239	What is a Burton line?	A dark blue stippled line across the upper gingiva indicative of lead poisoning
240	Oral cavity nevi most commonly occur where?	On the palate and gingiva
241	Describe Peutz-Jeghers syndrome.	Autosomal dominant disorder characterized by intestinal hamartomatous polyps and mucocutaneous melanocytic macules involving the lips and buccal mucosa. It is associated with an increased risk of developing GI, pulmonary, and reproductive track malignancies.
242	What is the most common intraoral pigmented lesion?	Amalgam tattoo resulting from amalgam implantation from prior dental work
243	Review the risk factors for mucosal melanoma.	There are no known environmental risk factors. Smoking, chemical exposure, and sun exposure do not appear to be linked with an increased risk. A small subset may arise from junctional nevi.
244	Which common medications are associated with gingival hyperplasia?	Phenytoin, calcium channel blockers, and cyclosporine
245	Name several conditions associated with pseudoepitheliomatous hyperplasia.	Rhinoscleroma, granular cell tumor, blastomycosis, syphilis, necrotizing sialometaplasia
246	What benign process is often clinically and histologically mistaken for squamous cell carcinoma of the hard palate?	Necrotizing sialometaplasia

247	Describe the important features of granular cell tumors of the head and neck.	Most commonly involve the tongue, palate and less commonly the larynx. They are sessile gray colored lesions that are of probable neurogenic origin; they stain strongly with s100 and histologically may be mistaken for squamous cell carcinoma since they exhibit pseudoepitheliomatous hyperplasia.
248	Describe the common oral manifestations of Crohn disease.	Generalized mucosal swelling, cobblestoning of the buccal mucosa and gingiva, aphthous stomatitis, and angular cheilitis
249	Describe the common oral manifestations of Sjogren disease.	Changes largely result from xerostomia, including difficulty in swallowing and eating, disturbances in taste and speech, dental caries, cobblestoning of the tongue, and increased risk of oral candidiasis.
250	What is the most common oral manifestation of amyloidosis?	Macroglossia, occurring in 20% of patients
251	What are the histologic findings with amyloidosis?	Apple-green birefringence, Congo red stain
252	What is the most common intraoral malignancy associated with HIV?	Kaposi sarcoma
253	Review the conditions associated with the development of hairy leukoplakia.	Immunocompromised states such as HIV/AIDS and prior organ transplantation. Hairy leukoplakia is associated with Epstein-Barr virus.

Oral Infectious Disease

254	What is the natural history of primary herpetic gingivostomatitis?	Mean duration of: • Fever: 4.4 ± 2.4 days • Oral lesions: 12 ± 3.4 days • Extraoral lesions: 12 ± 3.9 days • Dysphagia to food: 9.1 ± 3 days • Dysphagia to liquid: 7.1 ± 2.5 days • Viral shedding: 7.1 ± 2.5 days
255	What is the most common presentation of a primary HSV infection in the pediatric population?	Herpetic gingivostomatitis
256	General prodromal symptoms associated with primary herpetic gingivostomatitis include what?	General malaise, fever, anorexia, irritability, and headache
257	What are primary and secondary clinical findings associated with primary herpetic gingivostomatitis?	• Primary: Painful pinhead vesicles that rupture to form ulcerative lesions, which are irregular and covered by a yellow gray membrane • Secondary: Submandibular lymphadenitis, halitosis, and dehydration from refusal to take in adequate oral hydration
258	What tests can be used to definitively diagnose an HSV-1 viral infection?	PCR, viral culture, serology, immunofluorescence. Note: Tzanck smear is not helpful for delineating HSV-1 from HSV-2.
259	What are potential complications of herpetic gingivostomatitis?	Dehydration, herpetic whitlow, herpetic keratitis, secondary bacterial infection, esophagitis, epiglottitis, pneumonitis, encephalitis, eczema herpeticum
260	What are the three most common antiviral agents used to treat herpetic gingivostomatitis, and what is their mechanism of action?	Acyclovir, valacyclovir, famciclovir. Metabolized by viral enzymes to form metabolites that interfere with DNA synthesis and cause cell death. It works best if initiated within 72 hours.
261	What benefit does valacylcovir offer compared with acyclovir for the treatment of herpetic gingivostomatitis?	The dosing is twice a day compared with three to five times per day; however, it is more expensive.

262	What is the generally accepted window of opportunity for prescribing oral acyclovir for effective treatment of primary herpetic gingivostomatitis?	Three days. This therapy has been shown to decrease the duration of the lesions (intraoral and extraoral), fever, dysphagia/odynophagia, and viral shedding.
263	Recurrent oral HSV-1 infections can be associated with what important complications?	• Disfiguring lesions • Erythema multiforme • Aseptic meningitis • Eczema herpeticum
264	What noncontagious acute gingivitis is caused by an overgrowth of common bacterial species, including *Prevotella intermedia*, α-hemolytic streptococci, *Actinomyces*, or spirochetes, among others?	Acute necrotizing ulcerative gingivitis (*trench mouth*)
265	In a patient with acute necrotizing gingivostomatitis, if the disease progresses beyond the gingiva to include other mucosal surfaces, what is this condition called?	*Noma* (cancrum oris)
266	What are common risk factors for development of acute necrotizing ulcerative gingivitis?	Stress, immune incompetence (i.e., HIV infection), poor nutrition, poor oral hygiene, alcohol or tobacco use. This is not a contagious disease.
267	What are common examination findings seen in acute necrotizing ulcerative gingivitis ("trench mouth")?	Lymphadenopathy, halitosis, mucosal edema/ulceration/inflammation, with or without a pseudomembrane
268	What is the treatment for acute necrotizing ulcerative gingivitis?	• Analgesia (NSAID, narcotics, viscous lidocaine, etc.) • Antibacterial (clindamycin, penicillin, or erythromycin) • Oral hygiene (chlorhexidine 0.12% mouth rinse, brushing, flossing, etc.) • Dental consultation for debridement and definitive periodontal therapy • Management of underlying immunocompromised status is important if present
269	What is the most common oral manifestation of HIV infection?	Oral candidiasis
270	What are the common forms of oral candidiasis?	• Pseudomembranous candidiasis (thrush) • Erythematous (atrophic) candidiasis • Angular cheilitis (perlèche) • Hyperplastic candidiasis
271	What in-office diagnostic test can you perform to confirm the diagnosis of oral candidiasis?	Scraping of erosive lesion followed by potassium hydroxide (KOH) preparation and looking for budding yeast with or without pseudohyphae
272	Review the initial treatment options for oral candidiasis.	Topical antifungal lozenges or solutions for 7–14 days: Clotrimazole troches, nystatin suspension, or nystatin pastilles
273	What can you offer as treatment for moderate to severe oral candidiasis or for patients who do not respond to topical therapy for oral candidiasis?	Oral fluconazole for 7 to 14 days
274	When is daily suppressive management with antifungals indicated for oral candidiasis?	Suppressive management is usually unnecessary (even for HIV-positive patients). Treating active infections and managing the underlying immunocompromised status are recommended. When indicated (usually assisted by Infectious Disease Physicians), management usually includes fluconazole, three times a week.

Esophagus Overview

275	The esophagus, an embryologic foregut derivative, undergoes what important process during week 8 to 10 of life?	Recanalization of the esophageal lumen

276	Describe the muscular arrangement of the esophagus.	• Outer longitudinal fibers, inner circular fibers • Inferior third smooth muscle, middle third mixed, superior third skeletal
277	What are three physiologic areas of narrowing within the esophagus?	• Upper esophageal sphincter (cricopharyngeus muscle, C6, narrowest segment) • Crossed by aorta and left main bronchus in mid chest • Lower esophageal sphincter (passes through diaphragm)
278	What is the blood supply to the esophagus?	Arterial • Segmental blood supply, extensive submucosal anastomosis • Upper esophageal sphincter and cervical esophagus: Inferior thyroid artery • Thoracic esophagus: Paired esophageal arteries (terminal branches of bronchial arteries • Lower esophageal sphincter: Left gastric artery and left phrenic artery Venous • Neck: Inferior thyroid veins • Mediastinum: Azygous and hemiazygous veins • Abdomen: Left gastric vein
279	What is the innervation of the esophagus?	• Sympathetic innervation from T6-T10 bilaterally • Greater and often lesser splanchnic nerves • Branches from the celiac plexus Note: The vagal nerves form a plexus along the distal esophagus and then reform two distinct nerves on passage through the diaphragm.
280	The upper, mid, and lower third of the esophagus drain into which nodal basin(s)?	• Upper third = Paratracheal and internal jugular lymph nodes • Middle third = Mediastinal nodes • Lower third = Gastrohepatic and celiac axis lymph nodes
281	What is the normal epithelial lining of the esophagus?	Nonkeratinizing stratified squamous epithelium
282	What are the four layers of the esophageal wall?	Mucosa Submucosa Muscularis propria Adventitia
283	What key surgical landmarks must be kept in mind when operating on the esophagus in the neck?	• It lies slightly left of midline. • Anterior: Trachea, thyroid lobe, and anterolaterally the recurrent laryngeal nerves bilaterally in the tracheoesophageal groove • Posterior: Vertebral column and longus colli muscles • Lateral: Thoracic duct on the left
284	What key surgical landmarks are relevant when dilating an esophageal stricture in the mediastinum?	• Superior mediastinum: Slightly left of midline • Posterior: Vertebral column, thoracic duct (not in direct contact, to left) • Anterior: Trachea, left mainstem bronchus, aortic arch • Left lateral: Descending aorta, left parietal pleura (direct contact) • Right lateral: Vena azygos • Inferior mediastinum: Returns to midline • Posterior: Vertebral column; inferiorly, the aorta moves posterior to the esophagus and esophagus. • Anterior: Pericardium • Left lateral: Parietal pleura (direct contact) • Right lateral: Parietal pleura (direct contact)
285	At what thoracic level is the esophageal hiatus?	T10

286	How many centimeters are the incisor teeth from the cricopharyngeus, aortic arch, left mainstem bronchus, and lower esophageal sphincter and diaphragm in an average adult?	• 15 cm • 25 cm • 40 cm
287	What two types of peristalsis propel food through the esophagus?	• Primary peristalsis: Triggered by swallowing • Secondary peristalsis: Triggered by esophageal dilation
288	What are the functional muscular components of the upper esophageal sphincter?	The cricopharyngeus muscle, thyropharyngeus, and the proximal cervical esophagus *Note*: Many muscles contribute to the function of the upper esophageal sphincter (e.g., movement of the larynx, infrahyoid musculature, etc.).
289	What is the innervation of the upper esophageal sphincter?	At rest, the upper esophageal sphincter is contracted, and during oropharyngoesophageal events (swallowing, belching, emesis), the sphincter relaxes. The major tone effect stems from contraction of the cricopharyngeus, which is modulated by cranial nerve X. Afferent information is primarily transmitted via cranial nerve IX.
290	What is the innervation of the lower esophageal sphincter?	At rest, the lower esophageal sphincter is contracting as a result of neurotransmitter and hormonal influences. Swallow-induced relaxation occurs about 1 to 2 seconds after the bolus is swallowed. The vagal efferent motor neurons inhibit neurons within the myenteric plexus, which results in a decrease in the of the baseline tone.
291	What anatomical relationship augments the function of the lower esophageal sphincter?	Diaphragmatic crura
292	What are the four main protective mechanisms against esophageal reflux?	• Upper esophageal sphincter: Tonically closed • Lower esophageal sphincter: Tonically closed • Esophageal acid clearance: Peristalsis, gravity • Epithelial resistance: Mucous layer, aqueous layer, cell membrane, and intracellular junctions
293	When should esophagoscopy be considered after caustic ingestion?	Within the first 24 hours because the risk for perforation and complications may be greater at 2 to 3 days after injury
294	What endoscopic findings suggest an increased risk of stricture formation after caustic ingestion?	Circumferential erythema with exudate and perforation
295	Most esophageal foreign-body impactions occur at what level in the esophagus?	Cervical esophagus, just below the cricopharyngeus muscle
296	Describe Boerhaave syndrome.	Elevated intraabdominal pressure results in a transmural tear within the distal esophageal wall after vomiting. This commonly occurs in the posterolateral wall of the distal esophagus.
297	Describe Mallory-Weiss syndrome.	Incomplete tear of the esophageal wall involving the esophageal mucosa and submucosal arteries, often associated with retching
298	What does the Hamman sign indicate?	• Pneumomediastinum or pneumopericardium, often from tracheobronchial injury or Boerhaave syndrome • Demonstrated by a crunching sound that is synchronous with heartbeat
299	What type of imaging study should be used In a patient with a suspected esophageal perforation?	Gastrografin swallow study

Esophageal Evaluation and Testing

300	Why should patients with findings concerning for esophageal diverticulum, complex stricture, or achalasia undergo esophageal barium swallow instead of initial endoscopy?	Barium swallow is sensitive for these findings, and these conditions are associated with a higher risk for esophageal perforation with endoscopy use.

301	Is the barium swallow examination always performed using liquid barium?	No. It can be performed with barium tablets or barium-coated food objects, such as a marshmallow or bread, to identify more subtle lesions.
302	What is esophageal impedance testing?	This test is performed by a catheter measuring multi-channel intraluminal impedance, which measures the difference in resistance when a bolus (mucosa, gas, liquid, solid) passes the detecting channels on the device. It can be used in combination with manometry or pH monitoring and can identify directionality of bolus movement.
303	What are the indications for esophageal impedance testing?	• Esophageal dysphasia • Noncardiac chest pain • Heartburn or regurgitation • Preoperative evaluation for antireflux surgery • Identification of the lower esophageal sphincter before pH catheter placement
304	In a patient for whom twice-daily proton pump inhibitor (PPI) therapy has failed and who has a normal EGD, what test can be performed to confirm GERD?	Ambulatory esophageal pH monitoring, which may also be performed to assess adequacy of treatment
305	What are the two available methods of ambulatory pH monitoring?	Ambulatory pH monitoring entails 24- to 48-hour monitoring of reflux events and clinical symptoms while eating an unrestricted diet with the patient off antacid medication for at least 7 days. It can be performed via a transnasal catheter positioned 5 cm above the lower esophageal sphincter or a capsule attached to mucosa 6 cm proximal to the Z-line
306	What main outcome measure is used when evaluating the results of ambulatory pH monitoring?	Percentage of time the intraesophageal pH is < 4, to distinguish physiologic from pathologic reflux
307	What endoscopic test allows for evaluation of the oropharynx, esophagus, stomach, and upper duodenum?	EGD
308	What test is often recommended as the initial test for GERD because it provides diagnostic (both visual and histologic via biopsy) and possibly therapeutic options to allow stratification of disease?	EGD
309	Describe three methods for esophageal endoscopy.	• Rigid transoral esophagoscopy performed with the patient under general anesthesia • Flexible transoral esophagoscopy performed with the patient under conscious sedation • Flexible transnasal esophagoscopy (TNE) performed with the patient under local and/or conscious sedation
310	What benefit does endoscopy offer as the first step in evaluating a patient with esophageal dysphagia?	Endoscopy can provide visual evaluation and pathologic tissue samples and can also intervene and provide therapeutic benefit.
311	What diagnostic test evaluates both the intraluminal pressures and coordination of the upper esophageal sphincter, esophageal body, and lower esophageal sphincter?	Esophageal manometry
312	In a patient with dysphagia, noncardiac chest pain, or a possible esophageal motility disorder, what diagnostic test should be considered?	Esophageal manometry

Esophageal Dyphagia

313	In a patient with dysphagia, how can you differentiate oropharyngeal from esophageal dysphagia based on symptoms?	• Esophageal dysphagia: Food gets stuck after the swallow is completed because of structural or neuromuscular pathology; the problem is in the esophageal body or lower esophageal sphincter. • Oropharyngeal dysphagia: Difficult to complete swallow; disorders involve the oropharynx, hypopharynx, and upper esophageal sphincter.
314	How does the differential diagnosis change if a patient with esophageal dysphagia complains of symptoms with solids only versus both solids and liquids?	Mechanical obstruction usually causes difficulty with solids (but it may progress to involve liquids later on). Motility disorders commonly result in concurrent solid and liquid dysphagia.
315	What are the most common diagnoses in a patient with solid-food esophageal dysphagia?	• Esophageal ring (intermittent) • Peptic stricture (progressive) • Malignancy (progressive)
316	What is the most common cause of acute esophageal dysphagia?	Food impaction (meat); results in saliva expectoration
317	What disease process is characterized by decreased or absent lower esophageal sphincter relaxation and decreased or absent esophageal peristalsis?	Achalasia (Greek: "does not relax")
318	Eagle syndrome is associated with what anatomical abnormality?	Elongated styloid process (about > 3 cm) and/or ossification or calcification of part or all the stylohyoid ligament. This syndrome was described in 1937 by Dr. Wyatt Eagle.
319	Dysphagia lusoria is associated with what anatomical anomaly?	Aberrant right subclavian artery
320	What histopathologic findings support the diagnosis of achalasia?	Decrease in total ganglion cells within the myenteric plexus, the presence of T cell, eosinophil, and mast cell infiltration, and increased neural fibrosis
321	What is the general age group most commonly affected by achalasia?	20 to 60 years
322	What are the primary complaints associated with loss of lower esophageal sphincter relaxation and esophageal aperistalsis (achalasia)?	Solid and liquid dysphagia, weight loss, chronic cough, chest pain, hiccups, regurgitation, heartburn, and globus
323	What three associations are often included in triple A syndrome (Allgrove syndrome), which is most commonly found in children?	• Achalasia • Adrenal insufficiency • Alacrima
324	What infectious disease can lead to clinical manifestations of achalasia?	Chagas disease
325	What management strategy can be used to reverse or stop the progression of achalasia?	None. The goal of management is to decrease lower esophageal sphincter tone and manage reflux.
326	What is first-line therapy for patients with severe achalasia?	Surgical dilation or myotomy unless the patient is a poor operative candidate
327	What medical options are available for patients with achalasia?	Nitrates and calcium channel blockers with the goal of decreasing lower esophageal sphincter tone
328	What surgical interventions are available for achalasia?	Good operative candidates may undergo pneumatic dilation or myotomy. Poor operative candidates may undergo dilation with a bougie or botulinum toxin injection.
329	What pathogen is associated with Chagas disease?	Parasite *Trypanosoma cruzi*
330	What is the vector for *Trypanosoma cruzi*?	Reduviid bugs
331	Describe the esophageal manifestations of Chagas disease?	• Megaesophagus with dilation and muscular hypertrophy • Reduction in the number of neurons in the myenteric plexus

332	What is the most common condition associated with chronic Chagas disease?	• Cardiomyopathy • Arrhythmias • Conduction blocks
333	What are the clinical manifestations of scleroderma?	Skin tightening, hyperpigmentation, and hypopigmentation of skin, sclerodactyly, Raynaud phenomenon, GERD, arthralgias, myalgias, Sicca syndrome, and dysphagia
334	How common is esophageal involvement in patients with scleroderma?	90%; 50% experience significant symptoms
335	The progressive fibrosis and atrophy within the smooth muscle of the esophagus associated with scleroderma manifest with what classic finding on esophageal manometry and barium esophagram?	• Manometry: Progressive loss of esophageal body peristalsis in distal two-thirds and decreased lower esophageal sphincter pressure • Barium esophagram: Dilated esophagus, patulous gastroesophageal (GE) junction, and uninhibited reflux events into the distal esophagus
336	What are common complications noted in patients with scleroderma and GERD?	Barrett esophagus, esophagitis, and strictures
337	What laboratory test is most sensitive and specific for dermatomyositis?	Creatine kinase
338	How is dermatomyositis commonly treated?	Systemic steroid therapy and potentially immunosuppressive and cytotoxic therapy, including methotrexate, azathioprine, and cyclophosphamide
339	Describe the potential head and neck manifestations of dermatomyositis.	Heliotrope discoloration of upper eyelids, malar rash, dysphonia, dysphagia, scaly scalp, and hair loss
340	What part of the aerodigestive tract is affected by polymyositis?	Hypopharynx and upper third of the esophagus
341	What is the cause of diffuse esophageal spasm?	Neural and muscular defects triggered by reflux events, stress, extreme temperature variability in food or drink, carbonation, or particular smells
342	What symptoms are associated with diffuse esophageal spasm?	Intermittent esophageal dysphagia, noncardiac chest pain, reflux/heartburn
343	What are the classic esophageal manometric findings in patients with diffuse esophageal spasms?	Two or more uncoordinated contractions during 10 consecutive swallows, aperistalsis in more than 30% of wet swallows, and a fifth of contractions being simultaneous

Esophageal Bars, Pouches, Rings, and Webs

344	What is the test(s) of choice to evaluate for cricopharyngeal dysfunction?	Videofluoroscopic swallow with esophagram
345	What are the theories behind the relationship between cricopharyngeal dysfunction and dysphagia?	The cricopharyngeus is normally under tonic contraction but fails to relax with swallow. There is a lack of coordination between cricopharyngeus relaxation and the propulsion of food.
346	Describe the relative contraindications to cricopharyngeal myotomy.	Advanced GERD, progressive neurologic conditions such as bulbar palsy in patients with a known proximal esophageal cancer or in patients with a history of radiation to the neck
347	What is the proposed cause of epiphrenic esophageal diverticula?	Pulsion effect created superior to the cardioesophageal junction
348	What is the proposed cause of traction esophageal diverticula?	Traction effect caused by inflammation associated with cervical adenopathy or adjacent fibrotic tissue
349	Between what muscles does a Zenker diverticulum herniate? (▶ Fig. 4.8)	Between the inferior pharyngeal constrictors and the cricopharyngeus (Killian triangle)

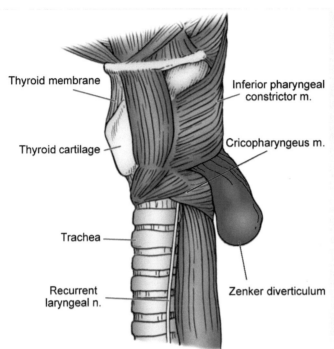

Thyroid membrane

Inferior pharyngeal constrictor m.

Thyroid cartilage

Cricopharyngeus m.

Trachea

Recurrent laryngeal n.

Zenker diverticulum

Fig. 4.8 Drawing of a Zenker diverticulum herniating between the inferior pharyngeal constrictors and the cricopharyngeus (Killian triangle). (Used with permission from Stewart MG, Selesnick SH, eds. Differential Diagnosis in Otolaryngology–Head and Neck Surgery. New York, NY: Thieme; 2011.)

350	Which side does a Zenker diverticulum most commonly involve and why?	It involves the left neck ~ 90% of the time and results from the convexity of the cervical esophagus to the left side and a more laterally positioned carotid artery on the left side, creating a space for the sac to protrude.
351	Define the *Killian-Jamieson* area.	Dehiscence between the oblique and transverse fibers of the cricopharyngeus muscle
352	Define the *Laimer triangle*.	Dehiscence between the cricopharyngeus muscles and the proximal esophageal muscles
353	What nonmalignant complication of GERD can manifest with progressive esophageal dysphagia starting with solid-food dysphagia and progressing to both solid and liquid dysphagia?	Peptic stricture
354	Describe the risk factors for developing a peptic stricture.	Older age, male gender, long history of reflux symptoms, GERD, scleroderma, Zollinger-Ellison syndrome, nasogastric tube placement, history of surgical management for achalasia (Heller myotomy)
355	What is a *Schatzki ring*?	Smooth, thin (<4 mm) web of mucosa and submucosa at the squamocolumnar junction, marking the proximal margin of a hiatal hernia
356	Describe the characteristics of a muscular esophageal ring.	Hypertrophic musculature within the esophageal body typically located within 2 cm of the GE junction
357	What disease processes increase the likelihood of developing an esophageal ring?	GERD and eosinophilic esophagitis
358	What is an esophageal web?	Thin mucosal fold covered in squamous epithelium that extends into the esophageal lumen, most commonly in the anterior cervical esophagus
359	What is the most common cause of an esophageal web?	Most often, it is idiopathic and asymptomatic.

360	What are common risk factors for the formation of an esophageal web?	Chronic GERD or iron deficiency associated with Plummer-Vinson syndrome.
361	Describe the clinical features of Plummer-Vinson syndrome.	Triad of dysphagia, iron-deficiency anemia, and esophageal webs. Additionally associated with atrophic glossitis and squamous cell carcinoma of the oral cavity, esophagus, and hypopharynx

Gastroesophageal Reflux Disease

362	What are common initial symptoms of GERD?	Heartburn 30 minutes to 2 hours after eating and regurgitation. Symptoms worsen with lying down or bending over. Less common symptoms include chest pain, chronic cough, laryngitis, asthma, and dental caries. Patients may complain of odynophagia and dysphagia in addition to belching.
363	What symptoms are worrisome for a more sinister diagnosis than isolated GERD?	Dysphagia, odynophagia, choking, weight loss, chest pain, upper GI bleed, and no or poor response to an empiric trial of antacids. If these symptoms are present, or if a patient does not improve on empiric therapy, endoscopy should be considered.
364	Why is an initial empiric trial of antacid therapy a reasonable first step in a patient with symptoms suggestive of GERD?	It is noninvasive, cost-effective, and in most cases diagnostic and therapeutic.
365	What technique offers the best evaluation of a patient's esophageal mucosa?	Endoscopic esophagoscopy
366	What is commonly seen on esophagoscopy in a patient with reflux esophagitis?	Erosions or ulcerations at the squamocolumnar junction (Z-line)
367	To determine the severity of acid reflux, demonstrate reflux in a patient with normal endoscopic findings, or to evaluate response to therapy, a 24-hour pH probe test may be performed. What is the primary limitation of this test?	A fourth of patients with erosive esophagitis and a third of patients with nonerosive esophagitis will have normal results.
368	When discussing lifestyle modifications for the management of GERD, what foods should be avoided?	Fatty foods, chocolate, coffee, excess alcohol, colas, red wine, orange juice, large meals, peppermint, basically anything that increases pH or decreases sphincter tone
369	Beyond dietary considerations, what lifestyle modifications should be considered to improve mild GERD?	Elevate the head of bed while sleeping, avoid eating right before sleep, exercise regularly, and lose weight.
370	Which histamine 2 (H2) blocker is the most effective for treating GERD, and what is the dose-dependent relationship between symptoms and therapy?	When adjusted for potency, no H2 blocker has been shown to be stronger or more effective than another. There is not a dose-dependent relationship. If a patient is treated with 6 weeks of standard therapy and does not respond, it is time to look to additional intervention.
371	In a patient diagnosed with erosive reflux disease, what medical management is indicated?	PPI therapy
372	Is there any difference in treatment outcome for GERD when comparing once-daily proton pump inhibitor therapy with more frequent dosing regimens?	Yes. More frequent dosing schedules (twice a day) have been shown to result in a significant improvement in gastric pH and provide a longer duration of effect.
373	After discontinuing a PPI for GERD, in what time frame do most patients who have recurrence begin to experience relapsing symptoms?	Three months
374	What risks are associated with chronic suppressive PPI therapy for reflux disease?	Potentially decreased bone density, infections, and electrolyte abnormalities

375	In a patient with long-standing esophageal reflux disease, the endoscopist identified specialized intestinal metaplasia or metaplastic cuboidal epithelium extending proximally to the natural squamocolumnar junction. What disease process is most likely associated with this finding?	Barrett esophagus
376	To classify peptic esophagitis on endoscopy and decrease interobserver variability, several classification systems have been devised. The Los Angeles classification system is most commonly used. Describe the different grades involved in this system.	Los Angeles Classification • Grade A: One or more mucosal break, each ≤ 5 mm long • Grade B: One or more mucosal break > 5 mm long, without continuity between the tops of adjacent mucosal folds • Grade C: One or more mucosa breaks continuous between the tops of adjacent mucosal folds; not circumferential • Grade D: Circumferential mucosal break *Note*: Historically the Savory-Miller grading system was the most prevalent; however, because of variable definitions, it is not as commonly used today.
377	During endoscopy for erosive esophagitis, what is the strongest predictor of Barrett esophagitis on examination?	The length of the columnar appearing epithelium segment extending from the GE junction (long segment > 3 cm, short segment < 3 cm). Specialized intestinal metaplasia is required on pathology to confirm the diagnosis.
378	What is the most feared complication of Barrett esophagus?	Esophageal adenocarcinoma. Annual incidence ranges between 0.12 and 0.5% in patients with Barrett esophagus.
379	With Barrett esophagus, how often should a patient with (1) no evidence of dysplasia, (2) low-grade dysplasia, and (3) high-grade dysplasia without eradication therapy be examined endoscopically?	1. Every 3 to 5 years 2. Every 6 to 12 months 3. Every 3 months
380	What three management strategies are available for patients with Barrett esophagus?	Controversy regarding optimal management is ongoing. Options include the following: • Management of GERD • Surveillance via serial endoscopy • Attempt to eradicate dysplasia
381	What endoscopic options are available for dysplasia eradication in patients with Barrett esophagus?	• Radiofrequency ablation • Photodynamic therapy • Endoscopic mucosal resection (recommended for patients with dysplasia and a visible mucosal irregularity to evaluate for T stage)
382	Provide several reasons why the prognosis for esophageal cancer is poor.	It often manifests late in the disease, and the esophagus is without an outer serosal layer, which may lead to early spread.

Obstructive Sleep Apnea

383	Describe the Müller maneuver.	Endoscopic evaluation during maximal inspiration, against a closed nose and mouth, at various levels in an attempt to identify anatomical regions of obstruction
384	What is the Epworth sleepiness scale?	A commonly used, statistically validated questionnaire for daytime sleepiness. A score of 0 to 5 is supernormal, 5 to 10 is normal, 10 to 15 is sleepy, 15 to 20 is very sleepy, > 20 is dangerously sleepy.

385	What is upper airway resistance syndrome (UARS)?	UARS is characterized by excessive daytime somnolence but normal sleep studies. Esophageal pressure monitoring shows abnormally increased negative intrathoracic pressures leading to increased work of breathing and sleep arousals. UARS is associated with crescendo snoring. In contrast to OSA, UARS is seen as frequently in women as in men, occurs in nonobese patients, and is more common in young adults than in elderly adults.
386	What cephalometric findings are associated with OSA?	The skull base appears to be shorter. The sagittal dimension of both jaws is smaller and in a more retrognathic position. The height of the lower face is increased, as the mandible tends to be rotated posteriorly. The chin and tongue are retruded, the soft palate is elongated, and the upper airway space is narrowed.
387	What is the definition of OSA?	OSA is a sleep disorder characterized by periodic complete or partial upper airway obstruction during sleep, causing intermittent apneas, hypopnea, or both despite ongoing respiratory effort. There is no universally accepted definition, but it is usually defined as a respiratory disturbance index (RDI) of 5 or greater. Measurements of the severity of OSA are based on the RDI, the severity of oxygen desaturation, and the level of daytime sleepiness.
388	What medical therapies exist for treatment of OSA?	• Weight control, CPAP (continuous positive airway pressure), and oral appliances • Medical conditions such as acromegaly and hypothyroidism should be ruled out. • Medications or substances such as alcohol, sedative hypnotics, narcotics, anesthetics, and sedating antihistamines should be avoided.
389	What are potential complications or sequelae of Uvulopalatopharyngoplasty (UPPP)?	Persistent snoring or OSA, bleeding, nasopharyngeal regurgitation of liquids, oropharyngeal dryness, oropharyngeal dysphagia, and pharyngeal stenosis
390	What does the Friedman staging system assess?	This staging system is used as a clinical predictor of which patients may have successful improvement of their OSA after UPPP surgery.
391	What is the most common surgical treatment of children with OSA?	Adenotonsillectomy. Less commonly, lingual tonsillectomy may be performed.
392	What craniofacial syndromes are closely associated with snoring and sleep apnea?	Achondroplasia, Pierre Robin syndrome, Treacher-Collins syndrome, Crouzon disease, Down syndrome, Prader-Willi syndrome, and Apert syndrome
393	What is the mechanism of radiofrequency tissue volume reduction used for the treatment of snoring?	Inserting electrodes and applying thermal energy will create a definable "thermal lesion" that over time will be replaced by stiff fibrotic tissue with reduced vibratory capacity.
394	Describe tongue base and hyoid bone suspension procedures for treatment of OSA.	A screw, with two sutures attached, is drilled into the lingual cortex of the mandibular symphysis. The two sutures are then submucosally secured to the tongue base or wrapped around the hyoid and tied under tension.

5 Laryngology

Jonathan J. Romak, Kathryn M. Van Abel, Daniel L. Price, and Dale C. Ekbom

Overview

1	What embryologic structures give rise to the larynx?	The endodermal lining and splanchnic mesenchyme of the foregut formed by branchial arches IV through VI.
2	Match the branchial arch with its laryngeal derivative: A. Corniculate, arytenoid, and cricoid cartilages; some laryngeal muscles; recurrent laryngeal nerve B. Upper body of the hyoid bone and its lesser cornu C. Epiglottis, thyroid cartilage, cuneiform cartilages, pharyngeal constrictors, some laryngeal musculature, superior laryngeal nerve D. Lower body of the hyoid bone and its greater cornu	A. V/VI B. II C. IV D. III
3	The anlagen of the larynx, trachea, bronchia, and lungs arise from what embryologic structure?	The tracheobronchial groove, a ventromedial diverticulum of the foregut
4	What structure obliterates the ventral primitive laryngopharynx during embryologic development?	Epithelial lamina
5	In the postnatal period, the larynx undergoes changes in axis, shape, length, and position. Describe the position of the larynx related to the cervical vertebra in an infant versus an adult.	• Infant: C1–C4 • Adult (by age 6 years): C4–C7
6	What are the nine laryngeal cartilages?	*Unpaired* 1: Cricoid cartilage 2: Thyroid cartilage 3: Epiglottis *Paired* 4,5: Arytenoid cartilages 6,7: Corniculate cartilages 8,9: Cuneiform cartilages
7	Name the six intrinsic muscles of the larynx, and describe both their function and innervation. (► Fig. 5.1; ► Fig. 5.2)	• *Cricothyroid*: Lengthens the vocal cord; external branch of the superior laryngeal nerve (cranial nerve [CN] X) • *Posterior cricoarytenoid*: Abducts the vocal cords; recurrent laryngeal nerve (CN X) • *Lateral cricoarytenoid*: Adducts the vocal cords; recurrent laryngeal nerve (CN X) • *Oblique arytenoid*: Adducts the vocal cords, recurrent laryngeal nerve (CN X) • *Transverse arytenoid*: Adducts the vocal cords; recurrent laryngeal nerve (CN X) • *Thyroarytenoid*: Relaxes, shortens, and adducts the vocal cords; recurrent laryngeal nerve (RLN; CN X)

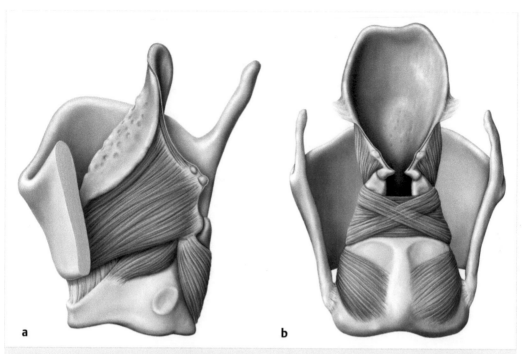

Fig. 5.1 Intrinsic muscles of the larynx: cricothyroid, posterior cricoarytenoid, lateral cricoarytenoid, transverse arytenoid, thyroarytenoid. (a) Left lateral view with left half of thyroid cartilage removed; (b) posterior view. (Used with permission from Thieme Atlas of Anatomy: Head and Neuroanatomy, © Thieme 2007, illustration by Markus Voll.)

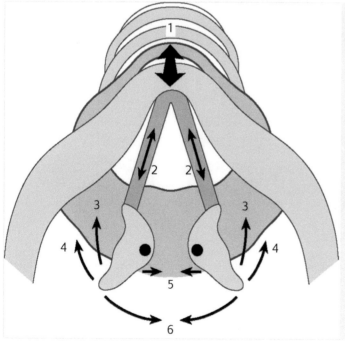

Fig. 5.2 Intrinsic muscles of the larynx and their directions of pull. (1) Cricothyroid muscle; (2) medial portion of the thyroarytenoid muscle; (3) lateral part of the thyroarytenoid muscle; (4) lateral cricoarytenoid muscle; (5) interarytenoid muscle; (6) posterior cricoarytenoid muscle. (Used with permission from Behrbohm H, Kaschke O, Nawka T, Swift A. Ear, Nose, and Throat Diseases: With Head and Neck Surgery. New York, NY: Thieme; 2009.)

8	What nerve provides sensation to the larynx?	CN X via the internal branch of the superior laryngeal nerve above the glottis and the recurrent laryngeal nerve below the glottis Glottic sensation is mainly from the superior laryngeal nerve with some sensory innervation from the RLN as well.
9	What are the extrinsic muscles of the larynx, and what is their function and innervation? (▶ Fig. 5.3)	• *Sternohyoid:* Caudal traction on the larynx; ansa cervicalis nerve • *Sternothyroid:* Caudal traction on the larynx; ansa cervicalis nerve • *Omohyoid:* Caudal traction on the larynx; ansa cervicalis nerve • *Geniohyoid:* Cephalad traction on the larynx; C1 via the hypoglossal nerve (CN XII) • *Anterior belly of the digastric:* Cephalad traction on larynx; nerve to the mylohyoid (V3) • *Mylohyoid:* Cephalad traction on the larynx; nerve to the mylohyoid (V3) • *Stylohyoid:* Cephalad traction on the larynx; facial nerve (CN VII) • *Thyrohyoid:* Caudal traction on larynx; ansa cervicalis nerve

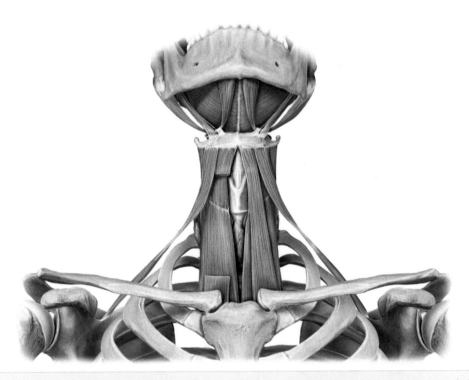

Fig. 5.3 Extrinsic muscles of the larynx: sternohyoid, sternothyroid, omohyoid, geniohyoid (not shown), anterior belly of the digastric, mylohyoid, stylohyoid, thyrohyoid. (Used with permission from Thieme Atlas of Anatomy: Head and Neuroanatomy, © Thieme 2007, illustration by Karl Wesker.)

10	Describe the subtypes of the laryngeal epithelium.	• *Supraglottis*: Pseudostratified columnar epithelium (respiratory epithelium) • *Glottis*: Stratified squamous epithelium • *Subglottis:* pseudostratified columnar epithelium (respiratory epithelium) • *Lingual surface of the epiglottis*: Stratified squamous epithelium • *Laryngeal surface of the epiglottis*: Stratified squamous merging into pseudostratified columnar epithelium
11	What are the layers of the true vocal folds, from superficial to deep? (▶ Fig. 5.4)	• Epithelium • Superficial lamina propria (SLP) • Intermediate lamina propria • Deep lamina propria • Thyroarytenoid muscle complex

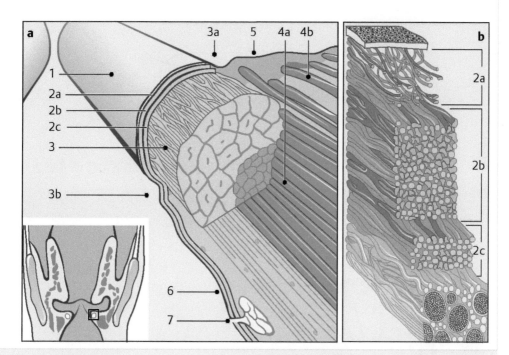

Fig. 5.4 Cross section through the membranous portion of the vocal fold. 1, Stratified squamous epithelium; 2a, superficial layer of the lamina propria; 2b, intermediate layer of the lamina propria; 2c, deep layer of the lamina propria, 2b and 2c forming the vocal ligament; 3, vocal ligament enveloping the vocalis muscle; 3a, superior arcuate line; 3b, inferior arcuate line; 4a, medial part of the thyroarytenoid muscle; 4b, lateral part of the thyroarytenoid muscle; 5, epithelium of the laryngeal ventricle (Morgagni ventricle); 6, subglottic respiratory cylindrical ciliated epithelial zone; 7, mucous gland. (Used with permission from Behrbohm H, Kaschke O, Nawka T, Swift A. Ear, Nose, and Throat Diseases: With Head and Neck Surgery. New York, NY: Thieme; 2009.)

12	What layers form the vocal fold cover, ligament, and body, respectively, involved in the cover-body theory of voice production?	• Cover = epithelium + SLP • Ligament = intermediate lamina propria + deep layers of the lamina propria • Body = thyroarytenoid muscle

Physiology of Speech and Voice

13	True/False. A unilateral cortical stroke will always result in vocal-fold paralysis.	False. True vocal-fold motion is controlled by the brainstem via both pyramidal and extrapyramidal neural systems. The cell bodies of motor nerves reside within the nucleus ambiguus, whereas sensory nerves reside within the nodose ganglion. Therefore, cortical strokes rarely result in cord paralysis.
14	Vascular insult to what structure(s) may result in loss of pain/temperature sensation in the ipsilateral face and contralateral body, ipsilateral facial pain, ataxia, nystagmus, vertigo, nausea, vomiting, dysphonia, dysphagia, and Horner syndrome? (▶ Fig. 5.5)	Vertebral artery or posterior inferior cerebellar artery (Wallenburg syndrome)

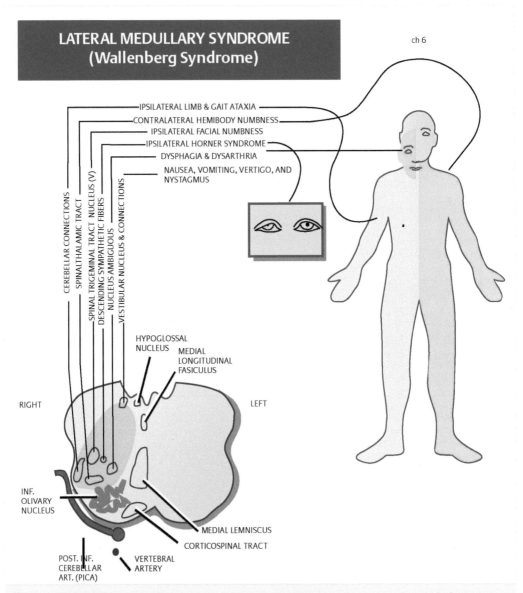

Fig. 5.5 Lateral medullary syndrome (Wallenburg syndrome) caused by a vascular insult to the vertebral artery or posterior inferior cerebellar artery. (Used with permission from Albertstone CD, Benzel EC, Najm IM, Steinmetz MP. Anatomic Basis of Neurologic Diagnosis. New York, NY: Thieme; 2009.)

15	The superior laryngeal nerve branches off the vagus nerve just caudal to what important neural structure?	The nodose ganglion
16	What are the three levels of laryngeal airway protection?	Epiglottis False vocal folds True vocal folds
17	On physical examination, you note that a patient demonstrates a protective cough reflex with palpation of the tip of epiglottis but has no response to palpation of the lower laryngeal surface of the epiglottis or arytenoid mucosa. Which nerve is most likely injured?	Superior laryngeal nerve The tip of the epiglottis receives sensory innervation from the glossopharyngeal nerve (IX), and the lower epiglottis and arytenoid regions are innervated by the internal branch of the superior laryngeal nerve.
18	The laryngeal closure reflex can be driven by several different stimuli. Name four.	• Thermal • Mechanical • Chemical • Taste
19	During intubation, what hemodynamic response may occur due to laryngeal irritation?	Bradycardia and hypotension; cardiovascular collapse Circulatory laryngeal reflex (superior laryngeal nerve [SLN], perhaps RLN as well) →central neurons →vagus →heart)
20	What are the three types of laryngeal respiratory receptors?	• *Negative pressure receptors*: Maintain airway patency during inspiration • *Airflow receptors*: Cold receptors, which are stimulated by air movement • *Respiratory drive receptors*: Provide laryngeal proprioception
21	What are three fundamental components of speech?	• *Phonation*: Vocal-fold vibration resulting in sound generation • *Resonance*: Modulation of laryngeal phonation by induction of vibration within the vocal tract • *Articulation*: Manipulation of the sound into words
22	What is required for voice production?	• Power: Adequate breath support (lungs) • Source of vibration: Larynx • Resonator: Supraglottic vocal tract and pharynx *Note*: Normal phonation requires a good vibratory medium; normal vocal-fold shape; and the ability to modify the tension, length, and shape of the true vocal folds.
23	How does injury to the superior laryngeal nerve impact voice production?	Loss of upper pitch register due to the loss of the motor innervation to the cricothyroid muscle via the external branch of the SLN, resulting in the inability to increase vocal tension
24	The intensity or loudness of sound production is directly related to air pressure in what location?	Subglottis
25	Describe the cover-body theory of voice production.	The cover (SLP) and body (thyroarytenoid muscle) move at different rates as air moves through the glottis because of their distinct masses and composition. This variation causes vibration, which results in a buzzing sound. The supraglottic vocal tract then modulates this sound to produce voice.
26	Pitch (or frequency) can be altered by adjusting the length and tension of the vocal fold. If this is done by contraction of the thyroarytenoid or cricothyroid muscle, what nerves are involved?	• Thyroarytenoid: RLN • Cricothyroid: External branch of the SLN

27	Given a constant volume of airflow through the vocal tract, the airflow velocity will increase at the level of the true vocal folds. Increased velocity results in decreased pressure and an inward movement of the vocal folds. What name is given to this effect?	Bernoulli effect
28	Describe the *myoelastic-aerodynamic theory of voice production*.	This was an early model of voice oscillation, which postulated that the Bernoulli effect would function to close the vocal folds, whereas increasing pressure in the subglottis from the lungs would function to open the vocal folds. This would occur over short bursts, resulting in a single puff of air being released. Sound production was thought to be a compilation of these puffs, dependent on the intensity of the sound source, the frequency of the source signal, and the supraglottic laryngeal tract.
29	What component of speech describes rhythm, repeated or prolonged syllables, rushes of speech, stress, and intonation?	Prosody

Evaluation

30	One of the first patient-based, voice-specific outcome measures was the Voice Handicap Index. This is a 30-question assessment that focuses on which three domains?	Functional, physical, and emotional aspects of voice disorders
31	Which voice-specific patient-reported outcome measure uses 10 questions to assess the physical functioning and social–emotional status of a patient with voice disturbance, and how is it measured?	The V-RQOL. Each question is given 1 to 5 points, with 5 representing a severe problem, and 1 representing no problem. An equation is then used to generate a score out of a total of 100, with a higher score representing better quality of life.
32	Name three important voice parameters.	• Frequency (pitch) • Intensity (loudness) • Quality (i.e., timbre)
33	What term refers to the number of repeating cycles per second (Hz) in the acoustic waveform?	Frequency
34	Define the fundamental frequency of the voice and the ranges for adult men and women.	The predominant pitch component of speech • Normal adult men into their 70s: 100 to 125 Hz • Normal adult women: 190 to 225 Hz
35	What describes the quality of a sound determined by its frequency (or fundamental frequency)?	Pitch
36	What acoustic term defines the loudness, or sound pressure level, of speech?	Intensity (normally 70 dB for both male and female conversational speech)
37	What factors most often influence loudness, or intensity?	Subglottic pressure, frequency, speech sample, glottal resistance, and airflow rate Type of equipment used, distance from the sound source, and ambient noise can also influence loudness measurements.
38	In acoustic analysis of voice, what are the most common parameters used to assess frequency?	• Average speaking fundamental frequency • Maximum phonational frequency range
39	What describes the quality or character of voice, separate from pitch, intensity, and prosody?	Quality (timbre): Roughness, breathiness, and strain
40	What is the perceptual correlate of the frequency of a sound wave?	Pitch (perceptual correlate of frequency)
41	What is the perceptual correlate of the amplitude of a sound wave?	Volume is the perceptual correlate of amplitude.

42	In acoustic analysis of voice, *jitter* is defined as cycle-to-cycle variation in what parameter?	Frequency of a wave (normal = 0.40%)
43	In acoustic analysis of voice, *shimmer* is defined as cycle-to-cycle variation in what parameter?	Amplitude of a wave (normal = 0.50 dB).
44	What are the most common measurements used to assess voice quality in acoustic analysis of voice?	Short-term perturbation measures (only reliable for nearly periodic signals): • Jitter: Cycle-to-cycle variation in frequency • Shimmer: Cycle-to-cycle variation in amplitude *Note*: No single test has been identified to reliably assess voice quality.
45	The GRBAS scale is an assessment tool, which attempts to standardize the auditory perceptual evaluation of voice quality. What does GRBAS represent, and how is this assessment scored?	**G** Grade: Overall severity **R** Roughness: Psychoacoustic impression of irregular vocal-fold vibration **B** Breathiness: Psychoacoustic impression of air leakage through the glottis **A** Asthenia: Weakness or lack of power in the voice **S** Strain: Psychoacoustic impression of hyperfunctional state of phonation 0: No deficit in parameter 1: Mild deficit 2: Moderate deficit 3: Severe deficit
46	What is the major weakness of the GRBAS scale?	It does not offer a specific protocol for administration or guidelines for analysis.
47	Which auditory-perceptual evaluation tool uses a visual analog scale (100-mm line; increasing distance from the left indicates increasing severity) to assess six parameters of voice: overall severity, roughness, breathiness, strain, pitch and loudness, and how is it scored?	Consensus Auditory-Perceptual Evaluation-Voice (CAPE-V): The score is based on two sustained vowels, six standard sentences, and 20 or more seconds of natural running speech. The six parameters are evaluated for resonance differences and whether the parameter is constant or intermittent.
48	Define the following terms: 1. Aphonia 2. Breathy voice 3. Diplophonia 4. Dysphonic 5. Flutter 6. Hoarse voice 7. Hypernasal (honky, nasal) 8. Hyponasal 9. Resonant 10. Strained (harsh, strangled) 11. Tremor	1. The inability to set the vocal folds into vibration either consistently or intermittently. *Note*: Arrest of phonation describes sudden stops. 2. Containing the sound of breathing (expiration) during phonation 3. Phonation with two independent pitches 4. Abnormal phonation 5. Phonation with amplitude or frequency modulations in the 8- to 12-Hz range 6. The combination of a rough and breathy voice 7. Voice quality when excessive acoustic energy is coupled to the nasal tract through opening of the velar port 8. Voice quality when inadequate acoustic energy is coupled to the nasal tract 9. A voice quality that rings on or "carries" well 10. A voice quality that appears effortful 11. A 1- to 15-Hz modulation of a cyclic parameter (e.g., amplitude or fundamental frequency), either neurologic in origin or interaction between neurologic and biomechanical properties
49	An important adjunct to the auditory-perceptual evaluation of the dysphonic patient is the visual-perceptual evaluation, which evaluates visible and physical facets of voice production related to cause, maintenance, or effect of dysphonia. What five categories are evaluated?	• General appearance • Posture, breathing, musculoskeletal tension • Neurologic dysfunction • Physical dysmorphology • Clinical manifestations of disease

50	When assessing a patient who has dysphonia suspicious of muscle tension or muscle misuse dysphonia, what tactile-perceptual tests can be completed in the office to provide a clinical assessment of dysfunction?	• Palpation of the suprahyoid, thyrohyoid, cricothyroid, and pharyngolaryngeal muscles both at rest and during phonation • Assessment of the thyrohyoid space for anterosuperior supraglottic compression • The clinician should assess for tension, muscle "knots," decreased space between thyroid cartilage and hyoid, or discomfort on mobilization.
51	What is the aerodynamic assessment that measures the length of time a patient can sustain a vowel after having taken a maximum inspiration?	Maximum phonatory time (indicates breath support and phonatory efficiency The longest of three trials should be reported. Typically, adult women range between 15 and 25 seconds, adult men between 25 and 35 seconds.
52	The subglottic air pressure (force/unit area) can be evaluated clinically by measuring the intraoral air pressure during a voiceless consonant. What influences the magnitude of normal pressure peak variation, and what are normative values for men and women?	Loudness, age, gender, consonant, and speech context • Men: 7.52 cm H_2O • Women: 6.43 cm H_2O
53	What term describes the minimal subglottic pressure needed for vocal fold vibration?	Phonation threshold pressure
54	Define *transglottic airflow* and its gender-specific ranges.	*Transglottic airflow* is the volume of air that passes through the glottis during a specific period. It can be traced during sustained phonation or connected speech and is associated with breathiness. • Men: 100 to 183 mL/second • Women: 91 to 156 mL/second
55	What is the term given to the ratio of translaryngeal air pressure to translaryngeal airflow? What are the normative values in each gender, and what is the perceptual correlate?	Laryngeal airway resistance • Men: 25 to 45 cm H_2O/L/second • Women: 27 to 51 cm H_2O/L/second Phonatory effort, vocal strength, strain
56	What test measures the conductance of low-frequency electrode signals between two surface electrodes on the neck to assess vocal fold vibration?	Electroglottography
57	What is the maximum number of images the retina can distinguish per second, and how does this compare with the rate of vocal fold vibration?	• Retina: Five images per second (Talbot's law) • Vocal cords: 75 to 1,000 cycles per second Therefore, vocal-fold vibration cannot be seen by the naked eye.
58	Videostroboscopy uses a xenon light with rapid on-and-off bursts to view the larynx in brief snapshots, fusing images, and "slowing" the motion of the vibration. This allows for visualization by the human retina. Why does videostroboscopy require a microphone?	The microphone is placed on the patient's neck to sense laryngeal vibration, which in turn controls the rate of xenon light firing. Light activation must be out of phase with laryngeal vibration to identify movement.
59	What five important criteria are used to grade videostroboscopy?	• Symmetry • Periodicity • Amplitude • Mucosal wave • Closure
60	Define the following terms: • Symmetry • Periodicity • Amplitude • Mucosal wave	• Symmetry: Mirrored appearance of the two vocal folds • Periodicity: Regularity of successive glottal cycles • Amplitude: Lateral excursion of the midmembranous cord • Mucosal wave: Vertical and horizontal movement of the cover (SLP) over the body (thyroarytenoid muscle)

	• Closure	• Closure: Closure of the cartilaginous and membranous portions of the glottis
61	During videostroboscopy on a normal patient, the mucosal wave will be seen traveling over what fraction of the superior portion of the true vocal fold?	From the inferior lip of the true vocal fold up the medial edge and across approximately one-half of the superior surface
62	True or False. Videostroboscopy is an excellent tool in the evaluation of all voice pathologies, including those without periodic vibration of the true vocal folds.	False. Videostroboscopy can analyze only periodic vocal-fold vibration.
63	What is the main advantage of videokymography over videostroboscopy?	*Videokymography* captures multiple images of a single glottic cycle, allowing for analysis of aperiodic vocal-fold vibration. *Videostroboscopy* is effective only in the setting of periodic vocal-fold vibration and provides an averaging of images.
64	What describes altered vocal quality, pitch, loudness, communication, or voice-related quality of life?	Dysphonia
65	What are common risk factors for dysphonia (hoarseness)?	• Upper respiratory tract infection • Recent or current infection • Significant voice use, misuse, or abuse • Recent neck trauma • Recent surgery (e.g., airway, neck or thoracic surgery) • Recent intubation • Tobacco and alcohol use • Reflux • Neurologic disorders • Psychiatric illness or stress • Hypothyroidism • Recent choking or foreign-body aspiration/ingestion
66	What type of stridor would be seen in (1) supraglottic, (2) glottic, (3) subglottic, or (4) tracheobronchial airway obstruction?	1. Inspiratory 2. Inspiratory or biphasic 3. Biphasic 4. Expiratory
67	When a suspected aspiration event has occurred, describe the most important aspects of the history and evaluation in a stable patient.	SPECS-R* S: Severity of obstruction on clinical exam P: Progression of obstruction E: Eating difficulty, failure to thrive C: Cyanotic episodes S: Sleep disturbance - R - Radiographic abnormalities (only obtain if information will change management and patient is not in acute distress) *Clinical suspicion: Witnessed aspiration, etc.

Nonoperative Therapy

68	When is voice therapy alone an appropriate treatment option for patients with dysphonia?	When medically and surgically treatable causes have been ruled out and a patient continues to have decreased voice related quality of life
69	When should antireflux medications be prescribed for hoarseness (dysphonia)?	Only when there are signs or symptoms of reflux disease or chronic laryngitis
70	True or False. Proton Pump Inhibitors (PPIs) may cause dysphonia in some patients.	True. PPI use can cause laryngeal dryness and candidiasis leading to dysphonia.

71	Why should the histamine 2 (H2) receptor antagonists cimetadine and ranitidine be pre-scribed with caution in patients taking either tricyclic antidepressants or benzodiazepines?	Cimetadine and, to a lesser extent, ranitidine inhibit the cytochrome p450 enzymes that metabolize these medi-cations and can lead to increased blood levels.
72	What are the most common side effects of PPI therapy?	Abdominal pain, diarrhea, nausea, vomiting, elevated liver function tests, candidiasis, headache, osteoporosis
73	Which asthma medications are associated with voice changes?	Inhaled and systemic steroids, β-agonists, and anticholi-nergics
74	Why should thyroid hormone levels be monitored in professional voice users?	Hypothyroidism may cause voice changes.
75	Describe the voice changes associated with hormonal therapy (androgens, estrogen, proges-terone).	Lower fundamental frequency and increased roughness
76	Describe the difference between *indirect* and *direct* voice therapy.	*Indirect voice therapy* focuses on improving vocal hygiene and decreasing phonotrauma. *Direct voice therapy* focuses on improving voice production.
77	What voice therapy technique has been proven to improve speech and speech-related activities in patients with Parkinson disease?	Lee Silverman voice therapy (LSVT)

Benign Disorders

78	Damage to the vocal folds resulting from voice abuse, misuse, and overuse can give rise to various vocal-fold lesions. This type of damage is called _____?	Phonotrauma
79	What is the most common location of true vocal fold lesions resulting from voice abuse?	Mid-membranous vocal fold
80	What is the term for benign growths in the superficial layer of the anterior and middle third of the true vocal fold, which can be either acute (edematous, erythematous, more vascular) or chronic (firm, nonvascular, thickened due to scar deposition and fibrosis)?	Vocal-fold nodules
81	What is the most common cause of vocal fold nodules?	Phonotrauma (ex: singing, screaming)
82	Before any surgical intervention for vocal-fold nodules, what is the first line of management?	Voice therapy
83	In addition to voice therapy, what two contribu-ting medical conditions should be optimized when treating a patient with vocal fold nodules?	• Laryngopharyngeal reflux • Allergies
84	Describe the pathophysiologic sequence that gives rise to vocal fold nodules.	Excessive vibration causes trauma leading to vascular congestion and submucosal edema at the midmembranous cord. If the vocal trauma continues, hyalinization of the superficial lamina propria and epithelial thickening may occur.
85	When is it appropriate to consider surgical removal of vocal-fold nodules?	When vocal impairment persists after an appropriate trial of voice therapy
86	Describe the difference between a vocal-fold nodule and a vocal fold polyp.	*Nodules* are always bilateral, are composed of inflammatory tissue, and respond to voice rest. They have a broad range of appearances (hemorrhagic/edematous, pedunculated/sessile, gelatinous/hyalinized). Polyps may be unilateral or bilateral, are full of either gelatinous material or blood, and typically do not respond to voice rest.

87	What are the two most common etiologies for vocal fold polyps?	Phonotrauma and hemorrhage
88	What is the treatment of choice for a symptomatic unilateral true vocal-fold polyp?	Voice therapy may be offered initially as a means of optimizing voice use. However, polyps only rarely respond to therapy alone, and microsurgical excision is usually necessary. Dissection should be subepithelial and just deep to the lesion within the involved SLP.
89	After a patient undergoes microsurgical excision of a vocal-fold polyp, what amount of voice use is typically recommended in the immediate post-operative period?	Complete voice rest
90	Sudden voice loss during maximal voice effort is most likely associated with what type of vocal-fold lesion?	Vocal-fold hemorrhage or unilateral hemorrhagic polyp
91	What is the treatment of choice for vocal-fold hemorrhage?	This is a laryngologic emergency, and the treatment of choice is 7 to 14 days of total voice rest with follow-up to ensure resorption of blood and to identify a varix that could be treated. If the blood has not resorbed, cordotomy and evacuation of the blood are indicated.
92	Describe the difference between *vocal-fold scar* and *sulcus vocalis*.	In *vocal-fold scar*, the lamina propria is replaced with abnormally fibrous and disorganized tissue. In *sulcus vocalis*, the lamina propria has degenerated or disappeared, leaving an epithelial-lined depression down to the vocal ligament or deeper.
93	Describe the different types of sulcus vocalis.	• Type I (physiologic sulcus): Longitudinal depression of the epithelium into the superficial lamina propria but not to the vocal ligament • Type II: Longitudinal depression of the epithelium down to the level of the vocal ligament or farther • Type III: Focal depression of the epithelium to or through the vocal ligament
94	Describe the common surgical procedures used in the management of sulcus vocalis.	• Cold instrument undermining and release of the base of the sulcus with redraping of the epithelium and superficial lamina propria • Laser undermining and redraping • Cold instrument excision • Coronal slicing to release the scar band • Fat, fascia, or alloderm implant • KTP (potassium-titanyl-phosphate) or PDL (pulsed dye laser) treatment Note: Surgical excision may improve symptoms, but techniques and results are highly variable.
95	What is the cause of dysphonia secondary to vocal-fold scar or sulcus vocalis?	Stiffening of the superficial lamina propria of the true vocal fold
96	What benign lesion often occurs on the posterior vocal fold, near the vocal process, as either an ulcerative or nodular polypoid process?	Vocal-fold granuloma
97	Vocal-fold granuloma/contact ulcer results from chronic irritation and inflammation of what structure?	Arytenoid perichondrium
98	Describe the difference between vocal-fold granuloma related to intubation and vocal-fold granuloma *not* related to intubation.	• Intubation-related granuloma tends to resolve spontaneously within a few months of extubation. • Vocal-fold granulomata not related to intubation are typically difficult to treat, requiring thorough evaluation to identify and eliminate causative factors such as reflux, voice abuse, chronic cough, or allergies.

99	What is the treatment of choice for vocal-fold granuloma?	• Intubation-related granulomas will likely resolve spontaneously. • Non–intubation-related granulomas should be treated conservatively with primary voice therapy in addition to elimination of contributing factors (e.g., antireflux medication, possibly steroids to limit inflammatory response). • Surgery is a last resort in both cases (e.g., large, pedunculated lesion).
100	You are performing an interval airway examination on a 21-year-old man who survived a motor-vehicle accident 10 days earlier. He suffered a tracheal laceration and polytrauma and has required ongoing sedation because of the extent of his neurologic injuries. He has an 8-0 endotracheal tube in place, and although his tracheal repair has healed nicely, you note the growth of a pedunculated lesion on his posterior true vocal fold and vocal process. What immediate intervention should you recommend?	Downsize his endotracheal tube (ETT).
101	A patient has dysphonia. Laryngoscopy reveals bilateral pale, watery, sessile, mobile collections of fluid on the superior surface and margins of the true vocal folds. What is the most likely diagnosis?	Reinke edema (also called bilateral diffuse polyposis or smoker's polyps)
102	What is the mechanism leading to the voice changes observed in bilateral diffuse polyposis (Reinke edema) of the true vocal folds?	Accumulation of gelatinous material in the superficial lamina propria leading to increased vocal-fold mass
103	What risk factors have been associated with the severity of Reinke edema?	Age, laryngopharyngeal reflux, vocal abuse, vocal hyperfunction, smoking, and hypothyroidism
104	True or False. The polypoid changes associated with Reinke edema are permanent.	True. However, the degree of edema and turgidity may fluctuate with voice use and exacerbating factors.
105	What is the initial treatment of choice for a patient with bilateral diffuse polyposis (Reinke edema) of the true vocal folds?	Smoking cessation, management of reflux, and reduction of phonotrauma
106	If conservative therapy for a patient with Reinke edema fails, what is the primary surgical intervention?	Mucosal sparing microflap polyp reduction, which results in decreased postoperative voice dysfunction compared with vocal cord stripping
107	What are the two mechanisms by which upper airway angioedema may occur?	Mast cell mediated and bradykinin induced
108	What laboratory test should be ordered if you suspect a diagnosis of hereditary angioedema?	C1 esterase inhibitor level
109	Describe three types of laryngeal cysts.	• Saccular cysts • Ductal cysts • Intracordal vocal fold cysts
110	Intracordal vocal-fold cysts generally arise within the superficial lamina propria (although they may arise from the vocal ligament or epithelium). They may be open to the epithelium of the vocal fold and can be associated with a sulcus, and they are also commonly associated with a contralateral nodule. What are the two most common subtypes?	• Mucus-retention cysts (wax and wane) • Epidermoid/keratin cysts (fairly stable, more white)
111	What is the preferred management for intracordal cysts?	For lesions that persist after conservative therapy, including a trial of voice therapy, microflap resection with preservation of the epithelium and superficial lamina propria, possibly followed by infusion of saline (or other substance, such as collagen) into the SLP

112	A cyst arising from which branchial cleft may involve the larynx?	Third branchial cleft
113	A large cyst is noted along the laryngeal surface of the epiglottis, resulting in partial obstruction. The cyst is covered in smooth mucosa and is round and slightly translucent. What is the best treatment?	Endoscopic incision and drainage followed by marsupialization (mucus-retention cyst)
114	A patient with a history of having been intubated for less than 24 hours develops stridor and respiratory difficulty. A subglottic cyst is identified. What is the most likely cause for development of this lesion?	Acquired subglottic (ductal) cysts develop as a result of mucosal damage, which obstructs the duct of a mucous gland
115	What structure consists of a blind sac between the false vocal fold and the thyroid cartilage, which opens into the anterior third of the laryngeal ventricle, is lined with ciliated respiratory epithelium and mucous glands, and is responsible for lubricating the vibrating vocal folds?	Laryngeal saccule (laryngeal appendix)
116	When the saccular opening becomes blocked resulting in a mucous filled dilation within the false vocal fold, what pathologic condition results?	Saccular cyst
117	What are the most common reasons for saccular cyst formation (obstruction of the saccular opening)?	Infection, recent intubation, cancer, or mass effect
118	What type of saccular cyst extends posteriorly and superiorly to involve the aryepiglottic fold?	Lateral saccular cyst
119	What type of saccular cyst extends medially into the laryngeal lumen between the true and false vocal folds?	Anterior saccular cyst
120	What is the difference between an *anterior* and a *lateral* saccular cyst?	An *anterior* saccular cyst lies between the true and false vocal folds. A *lateral* saccular cyst lies between the false vocal fold and the aryepiglottic fold.
121	What are the most common initial signs and symptoms associated with saccular cysts?	• Infants: Respiratory distress, cyanosis, stridor, difficulty feeding • Adults: Dysphonia, dyspnea, dysphagia, pain, neck mass
122	What is the treatment of choice for saccular cysts?	Marsupialization or complete excision Biopsy should be performed in adults to rule out cancer.
123	What are the medial and lateral boundaries of the laryngeal saccule?	The saccule is bordered medially by the false vocal cord and laterally by the thyroid cartilage.
124	What results when the saccule becomes dilated or herniated, is filled with air, and maintains a patent orifice?	Laryngocele
125	Describe the similarities and differences between a *laryngocele* and a *saccular cyst*.	Both laryngoceles and saccular cysts are dilations of the saccule. A *laryngocele* is an air-filled dilation that communicates with the laryngeal lumen. A *saccular cyst* is a fluid-filled dilation that does not communicate with the laryngeal lumen.
126	What type of laryngocele is confined to the larynx?	Internal laryngocele
127	What type of laryngocele extends through the thyrohyoid membrane, laterally into the neck?	External or combined laryngocele
128	Describe the difference between an *internal* laryngocele and an *external* or *combined* laryngocele.	• Internal laryngocele: Contained within the thyroid cartilage • Combined (external) laryngocele: Extends through the thyrohyoid membrane

129	What are the most common symptoms associated with a laryngocele?	Most are asymptomatic. However, symptoms can include dysphonia, dyspnea, weak cry, and aphonia. External laryngoceles may manifest with an intermittent lump in the neck.
130	How are internal laryngoceles treated?	Complete excision, either via endoscopic or external approaches. Marsupialization is not recommended.
131	How should a large combined or external laryngocele be treated?	Generally, external approaches are recommended with complete excision through the thyrohyoid membrane and transection close to the orifice of the saccule. However, complete endoscopic excision has been successfully reported even for large lesions.
132	What is the greatest risk associated with surgical repair of bilateral combined laryngoceles?	Aspiration secondary to bilateral injury to the internal branch of the superior laryngeal nerve
133	When a saccular cyst is filled with purulent debris, what is it called?	Laryngopyocele
134	How are laryngopyoceles managed?	A laryngopyocele can be a surgical emergency. Secure an airway, drain endoscopically, and culture. Either at the time of drainage or after resolution of the acute infection, complete excision either endoscopically or externally is indicated. Medical management of the acute episode includes IV antibiotics, antipyretics, and steroids.
135	Describe the normal effect of advancing age on the fundamental frequency of the speaking voice.	In both men and women, the speaking pitch decreases with age to a point and then begins to increase.
136	Describe the changes that occur in the larynx with age.	Muscle atrophy, thinning of the vocal ligament, mucous glad degeneration, cartilage ossification and epithelial thickening.
137	Name three physiologic changes that contribute to the perception of a voice as sounding "elderly."	• Air escape • Laryngeal tension • Tremor
138	In a patient with paresis of the external branch of the left superior laryngeal nerve, which direction will the petiole of the epiglottis deviate during high-pitched phonation?	Left. Toward the side of the weak cricothyroid muscle
139	True or False. Presbylaryngis is likely to be the sole cause of a voice complaint in an elderly patient.	False. Voice disorders in elderly patients are much more likely to be caused or confounded by diseases of aging and associated medications than by presbylaryngis alone. Presbylaryngis is a diagnosis of exclusion after all possible causes have been ruled out.
140	How does *chronic* laryngitis differ from *acute* laryngitis?	Chronic laryngitis results in chronic dysfunction.
141	What three habits should be limited or eliminated to improve laryngeal hygiene?	• Tobacco use • Alcohol use • Caffeine consumption
142	What are the most common symptoms associated with reflux laryngitis?	• Hoarseness • Cough • Globus • Throat clearing Notably, fewer than 50% have gastrointestinal symptoms of reflux.
143	Describe the key difference between *laryngopharyngeal reflux* (LPR) and *gastroesophageal reflux*.	Patients with LPR are less likely to have esophagitis (25%) or heartburn (< 40%) and are less likely to have prolonged periods of esophageal acid exposure or dysmotility. Patients are more often "daytime" refluxers, and the cause is thought to be upper esophageal sphincter dysfunction.

144	How is LPR diagnosed?	There is significant controversy regarding the best diagnostic criteria and tests to use. However, diagnosis is commonly made based on the following: • Clinical history: Reflux symptoms while upright, dysphonia/hoarseness, cough, globus pharyngeus, throat clearing, and dysphagia • Symptomatic improvement with empiric treatment with PPIs as indicated by a patient's reflux findings score • Laryngoscopy: Mucosal edema, injury, inflammation • Reflux events identified by use of a dual pH probe, oropharyngeal probe or impedence probe.
145	What is the treatment for LPR?	A combination of diet and behavior modifications is recommended. The use of PPIs and H2 blockers, although recommended by the American Academy of Otolaryngology–Head and Neck Surgery (AAO-HNS) consensus statement, is still somewhat controversial for isolated LPR.
146	What are the most common risk factors for developing laryngeal chondronecrosis (radionecrosis)?	Radiation dose/timing, infection, poor vascular health (i.e., smoker, diabetic, and such conditions)
147	Describe the Chandler classification system for laryngeal radionecrosis and the corresponding treatment recommendations.	• Grade I: Slight hoarseness/dryness; slight edema, telangiectasias; symptomatic care: humidification, antireflux medication, smoking cessation • Grade II: Moderate hoarseness/dryness; similar signs and treatment • Grade III: Severe hoarseness with dyspnea, moderate odynophagia, and dysphagia; Severe impairment of vocal-cord mobility or fixation of one cord, marked edema, skin changes; symptomatic care, steroid, antibiotics, tracheostomy or laryngectomy, if necessary • Grade IV: Respiratory distress, severe odynophagia, weight loss, dehydration; fistula, fetor oris, fixation of the skin to the larynx, airway obstruction, fever; tracheostomy, laryngectomy
148	In addition to symptomatic care, antibiotics, and steroids, what additional conservative measure can be tried before laryngectomy for laryngeal chondronecrosis and radionecrosis?	Hyperbaric oxygen therapy

Benign Neoplasms

149	Laryngeal chondromas arise most commonly from what anatomical site?	Posterior cricoid plate
150	According to the Myers-Cotton grading system, what grade is a subglottic stenosis with 90% obstruction of the tracheal lumen? (▶ Table 5.1)	Grade III

Table 5.1 Myers-Cotton Classification: Subglottic Stenosis

Grade	Degree of Lumen Obstruction
I	0–50%
II	51–70%
III	71–99%
IV	100%

Data from Myer CM, O'Connor DM, Cotton RT. Proposed Grading System for Subglottic Stenosis Based on Endotracheal Tube Sizes. Ann Otol Rhinol Laryngol. 1994;103:19–3.

151	What is the mechanism of injury for laryngotracheal stenosis caused by endotracheal intubation?	Ischemic necrosis of the mucosa secondary to pressure of the cuff or the tube itself Healing by secondary intention leads to fibrosis and scar contraction.
152	True or False. Approximately 80% of cartilaginous tumors of the larynx are chondromas.	False. Chondroma was initially thought to represent approximately 80% of cartilaginous laryngeal tumors, but this was later determined to be an overestimation resulting from misdiagnosed low-grade chondrosarcoma. The true number of cartilaginous tumors that are chondromas is much less than 80%.
153	What is the treatment for laryngeal chondromas?	When possible, complete excision to negative margins alone
154	Approximately what percentage of all benign laryngeal lesions are neurogenic in origin?	0.1 to 1.5%.
155	What are the most common benign neurogenic laryngeal neoplasms?	Laryngeal schwannoma (most common), neurofibroma, and granular cell neoplasms. Schwannomas and neurofibromas most commonly arise from the internal branch of the superior laryngeal nerve.
156	Where are endolaryngeal neurofibromas most commonly found?	Arytenoid complex and aryepiglottic fold Although they can occur in patients with neurofibromatosis type I (von Recklinhausen disease), isolated laryngeal neurofibromas are more common.
157	Which neurogenic laryngeal neoplasm is often associated with pseudoepitheliomatous hyperplasia of the overlying mucosa, which can often be misdiagnosed as squamous cell carcinoma?	Granular cell neoplasm
158	Because granular cell tumors present a risk for malignant conversion (2 to 3%), they should be resected. What confirmatory findings for benign tumor should be looked for on pathology?	• Large polyhedral cells that may contain significant collagen, granular eosinophilic cytoplasm, and centrally located vesicular nuclei • (+) periodic acid-Schiff (PAS), (+) S-100, (+) neuron specific enolase, (+) NK1-C3
159	What is the likely cell of origin for granular cell tumors?	Schwann cell
160	How should benign neurogenic laryngeal neoplasms be managed?	Endoscopic evaluation and biopsy • Small lesion: complete endoscopic resection • Large lesion: complete resection via an external approach These are benign lesions; therefore, conservative complete excision with voice preservation should be the goal.
161	What is the most common benign neoplasm of the larynx?	Recurrent respiratory papillomatosis (RRP)
162	Of the most common human papillomavirus (HPV) subtypes causing RRP, which has a more aggressive clinical course?	HPV 11: More frequent surgical intervention and a higher incidence of airway obstruction. HPV subtypes 6 and 11 are the most common in RRP.
163	Does juvenile- or adult-onset RRP tend to have a more aggressive course?	Juvenile RRP tends to be more diffuse, exophytic, and often recurs rapidly after intervention.
164	What is the standard of care for treatment of symptomatic RRP?	Surgical excision without damaging normal structures
165	Describe the type and structure of the virus responsible for RRP.	HPV is a papillomovirus of the Papovavirus family, with a nonenveloped icosahedral capsid and a double-stranded circular DNA genome.
166	What is a laryngeal lymphatic malformation?	• A collection of lymph vessels filled with serous fluid centered in the larynx • Rarely confined solely to the larynx

167	How do laryngeal lymphatic malformations present?	• Asymptomatic versus stridor, dyspnea on exertion, and respiratory distress • Worse during infections
168	Laryngoscopy shows a soft, smooth, painless, compressible mass in the larynx. Imaging shows fluid filled areas enveloped by connective tissue. What is the likely diagnosis?	Lymphatic malformation
169	What treatment options are available for laryngeal lymphatic malformations?	For symptomatic or disfiguring lesions, surgical debulking is the treatment of choice. Sclerotherapy may be considered for macrocystic lesions. Up to 50% of patients with extensive disease of the head and neck will require tracheostomy.
170	True or False. Both cystic hygromas and cavernous/microcystic lymphangiomas respond well to surgical excision.	False. *Cystic hygromas* are composed of large cysts that are amenable to surgical excision. *Cavernous/microcystic lymphangiomas*, however, are composed of very small cysts that are difficult to resect and tend to recur after surgery.
171	Although laryngeal hemangiomas in adults are rare, how do they manifest?	Airway symptoms including bleeding, stridor, dysphonia, mild dyspnea, dysphagia, and snoring
172	True or False. Laryngeal hemangiomas are more common on the left side of the larynx than on the right.	True
173	How are laryngeal hemangiomas diagnosed, and what is their natural history?	They are seen on examination covered by thin, friable mucosa overlying a vascular stroma. T2-weighted MRI can be helpful to delineate extent. These are most commonly seen in the supraglottis in adults and generally do not spontaneously regress.
174	What is the treatment of choice for an asymptomatic laryngeal hemangioma in an otherwise healthy adult patient?	Hemangiomas in adults should not be actively treated unless they are symptomatic. Corticosteroids or radiotherapy may be considered if necessary.
175	At what age do infantile hemangiomas typically begin to involute, and at what age is involution likely to be complete?	Infantile hemangiomas begin to involute between 12 and 24 months of age; 50% will have involuted by age 5 and 70% by age 7.

Infectious Disorders

176	What viruses have been associated with acute viral laryngitis?	Rhinovirus, parainfluenza, influenza, adenovirus, respiratory syncytial virus (RSV), herpes simplex virus (HSV), coronavirus
177	What medication has been shown to significantly improve discomfort associated with acute viral laryngitis?	Nonsteroidal anti-inflammatory drugs (NSAIDs) In a prospective, double-blinded study, flurbiprofen lozenges were shown to significantly improve sore throat associated with acute viral laryngitis compared with placebo.
178	Should steroids be given for acute viral laryngitis?	Treatment is primarily supportive (hydration and voice rest) with escalation for evidence of airway compromise (steroids, PPI, antibiotics for secondary infection, humidification). However, a single dose of dexamethasone (0.16 mg/kg) has been shown to decrease overall severity of moderate to severe laryngotracheitis in pediatric patients during the first 24 hours after injection.
179	Describe the clinical manifestations of parainfluenza virus infection in adults.	• Immunocompetent: Mild upper respiratory tract infection • Immunocompromised: Pneumonia (can be fatal)

180	What infectious agents are potential causes of epiglottitis in adults?	• A broad range of bacterial (*H. influenzae* type b[Hib]), other *Haemophilus* strains, *Streptococcus pneumonia*, *Staphylococcus aureus*, β-hemolytic streptococci, etc.), viral (HSV type 1, varicella zoster virus, parainfluenza virus type 3, influenza B virus, Epstein-Barr virus), and fungal (candida) infections • Noninfectious causes are also possible (thermal, mechanical, or chemical injury).
181	How does *adult supraglottitis* (*epiglottitis*) differ from *pediatric epiglottitis*?	Manifestation is often less dramatic, with the most common initial symptoms and signs including sore throat, dysphagia, fever, and dyspnea. Airway intervention is required in less than 20% of cases.
182	In an adult with epiglottitis demonstrating mild respiratory distress, <50% obstruction of the laryngeal inlet, without stridor, drooling, or cyanosis, what is the management strategy of choice?	Close monitoring in the intensive care unit (ICU) with an emergency airway cart available is preferred, as well as empiric antibiotics including a third-generation cephalosporin and an anti-staphylococcal antibiotic with activity against MRSA (methicillin-resistant *Staphylococcus aureus*). Glucocorticoids can be considered but are not routinely recommended.
183	Primary infection of the laryngeal cartilage can occur after trauma, radiation, intubation, tracheostomy, or foreign body aspiration. Cancer and relapsing polychondritis are also risk factors. Such an infection is called what?	Chondritis (primarily impacting the cartilage) or perichondritis (impacting the perichondrium +/- underlying cartilage)
184	What organism is the most common cause of acute fungal laryngitis?	*Candida albicans*
185	How do you confirm the diagnosis of candidal laryngitis?	Tissue biopsy is generally done to rule out carcinoma or swab and fungal stains (not routinely performed).
186	What fungal strains are responsible for chronic fungal laryngitis?	*Blastomycoces* (Southern United States), *Histoplasma* (Ohio and Mississippi River valleys), *Coccidioides* (southwestern United States and Mexico), *Paracoccidioides*, and *Cryptococcus* spp. Candidal laryngitis is more commonly acute, but it can be chronic as well.
187	What are risk factors for fungal laryngitis?	Laryngopharyngeal reflux, immunosuppression, systemic or inhaled steroid use, broad-spectrum antibiotic therapy, and smoking
188	How is fungal laryngitis treated?	Systemic antifungals (i.e., amphotericin B, ketoconazole, itraconazole, fluconazole, nystatin). Topical therapy can also be used in the form of troches or lozenges (i.e., miconazole, clotrimazole, nystatin); however, this therapy is not recommended for invasive or systemic infections and often does not lead to long-term control.
189	What risk factors predispose a person to developing chronic bacterial laryngitis?	Previous prolonged intubation, relapsing polychondritis, history of recent viral laryngitis, compromised immune status, reflux

Systemic Diseases

190	What is the most common subsite affected by laryngeal sarcoidosis? (▶ Fig. 5.6)	Epiglottis

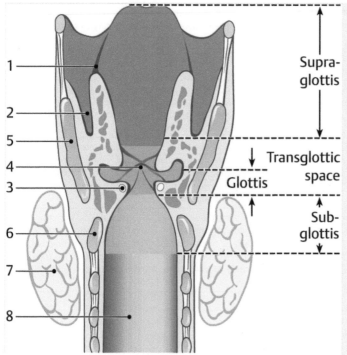

Fig. 5.6 Subsites and structures of the larynx: (1) The aryepiglottic fold; (2) piriform sinus; (3) vocal ligament; (4) anterior commissure; (5) thyroid cartilage; (6) cricoid cartilage; (7) thyroid gland; and (8) trachea. (Used with permission from Behrbohm H, Kaschke O, Nawka T, Swift A. Ear, Nose, and Throat Diseases: With Head and Neck Surgery. New York, NY: Thieme; 2009.)

Supra-glottis

Transglottic space

Glottis

Sub-glottis

191	True or False. Laryngeal sarcoidosis can occur in isolation without evidence of disease elsewhere in the body.	True (1 to 5%)
192	What is the pathognomonic finding of laryngeal sarcoidosis during laryngoscopy?	Diffuse pale, edematous enlargement of the supraglottis
193	True or False: An ACE (angiotensin-converting enzyme) level is the test of choice for diagnosing sarcoidosis.	False. An ACE level is useful for monitoring disease in patients with sarcoidosis but is not recommended as a diagnostic test due to low sensitivity (60%).
194	What percentage of patients with granulomatosis and polyangitis (Wegener) will develop subglottic stenosis?	10 to 20%
195	What are the expected biopsy findings in a patient with granulomatosis with polyangiitis (Wegener)?	Necrotizing granulomas and necrotizing vasculitis of small arteries, arterioles, capillaries, and venules
196	In a patient with symptomatic subglottic stenosis secondary to granulomatosis with polyangiitis (Wegener), what will be found on flow-volume loops during pulmonary function testing?	Flattening of both inspiratory and expiratory phases, indicating a fixed airway obstruction
197	What site within the larynx is most commonly affected by amyloidosis?	The true and false cords and the ventricles
198	What is the most common type of amyloid protein deposit found in the larynx?	Amyloid light chain
199	What autoimmune disorder results in episodic, severe, and progressive inflammation of cartilage most commonly within the ears, nose, and laryngotracheobronchial tree?	Relapsing polychondritis

200	What is the mechanism of respiratory distress in relapsing polychondritis?	Two mechanisms are possible: airway narrowing secondary to fibrosis or airway collapse secondary to cartilage destruction and fibrosis.
201	What is the most common manifestation of airway involvement in relapsing polychondritis?	Tracheobronchomalacia
202	What percentage of patients with rheumatoid arthritis develop cricoarytenoid joint involvement (i.e., arthritis, ankylosis, etc)?	25 to 30%. May also see cricothyroid joint dysfunction or rheumatoid nodules on the true vocal folds, but these are less common in the literature. May see tenderness on palpation of the larynx.
203	What percentage of patients with rheumatoid arthritis have radiologic evidence of cricoarytenoid joint involvement?	54 to 72%. The most common findings on CT are cricoarytenoid prominence, density and volume change, subluxation, decreased joint space, and pyriform sinus narrowing. However, radiologic involvement does not always correlate with symptoms.
204	How is cricoarytenoid joint dysfunction associated with rheumatoid arthritis treated?	Mild symptoms: High-dose corticosteroids or immune modulating medications used for rheumatoid arthritis. If this fails, corticosteroid injection of the cricoarytenoid joint can be considered. For acute airway obstruction (rare), consider tracheostomy, arytenoidectomy, or arytenoido-pexy.

Vocal-Fold Paralysis

205	The motor neurons of the recurrent laryngeal nerve originate in what brainstem nucleus?	Nucleus ambiguous
206	How can neuronal injuries be classified?	Sunderland and Seddon injury table with neurosensory impairment and recovery potential
207	What accounts for the small amount of continued vocal fold adduction that may exist after trans-ection of the ipsilateral recurrent laryngeal nerve?	Bilateral innervation of the interarytenoid muscle
208	What is the most common cause of unilateral true vocal-fold paralysis	Surgical iatrogenic injury
209	What is the most common malignant cause of unilateral true vocal-fold paralysis?	Lung carcinoma
210	Imaging of what region(s) should be obtained to evaluate unilateral true vocal-fold immobility of unknown cause?	Skull base to the upper chest to examine the full course of the recurrent laryngeal nerve. CT or MRI is most commonly used.
211	What is the most common swallowing problem associated with unilateral true vocal-fold immo-bility?	Aspiration of liquids
212	Unilateral true vocal-fold immobility may cause dyspnea by what mechanism?	Incomplete glottic closure leading to air escape during speech
213	What medications are known to have neurotoxic effects that can lead to true vocal-fold paralysis?	Vinca alkaloids (vincristine, vinblastine) and cisplatinum
214	After a high vagal nerve injury, will the palate elevate toward or away from the injured side?	The palate will elevate away from the injured side.
215	What mucosal wave finding on videostrobosopy is associated with unilateral vocal-fold paralysis?	Increased amplitude on the paralyzed side
216	A patient is evaluated for hoarseness and aspira-tion after suffering a known stroke involving the posterior inferior cerebellar artery. What is likely to be seen on flexible laryngoscopy?	Paralysis of the ipsilateral true vocal fold Wallenberg syndrome, or lateral medullary syndrome, results in hoarseness secondary to true vocal-fold paralysis, dysphagia, loss of pain and temperature sensation on the ipsilateral face and contralateral body, and ipsilateral Horner syndrome.

217	What is the role of laryngeal electromyography (EMG) in management of vocal-fold immobility?	EMG can differentiate paralysis from fixation and may provide prognostic information regarding the potential for recovery of mobility.
218	What is the primary goal of surgical intervention for bilateral true vocal-fold paralysis?	Improving the airway while preserving voice and swallowing
219	What options, other than tracheotomy, exist for management of airway compromise secondary to bilateral true vocal-fold paralysis in the early postinjury period?	• Endotracheal intubation • Suture lateralization • Botox injection
220	For a patient who is tracheostomy dependent as a result of bilateral true vocal-fold paralysis, what is the chance of decannulation after transverse cordotomy and medial arytenoidectomy?	59 to 100%

Neurogenic Disorders

221	Intermittent strangled or strained voice breaks during speech, particularly during words starting with vowels, is suggestive of which diagnosis?	Adductor spasmodic dysphonia
222	Describe the difference between *adductor spasmodic dysphonia* (ADSD) and *muscle-tension dysphonia* (MTD) during auditory – perceptual evaluation?	ASD is task dependent, whereas MTD is not. Patients with both disorders may have a strangled or strained voice quality, but in MTD this will be constant across all vocal tasks. In ADSD, symptoms will be worse during sentences rich in voiced consonants and during connected speech and will improve during sustained vowels and sentences with predominantly voiceless consonants.
223	Which laryngeal muscles are selectively injected during botulinum toxin treatment of adductor spasmodic dysphonia?	Thyroarytenoid muscles
224	What are the most common adverse effects of botulinum toxin injection for ADSD?	Breathy voice and aspiration of fluids, which are usually self-limiting
225	True or False. Breathy voice and aspiration of liquids after botulinum toxin injection for adductor spasmodic dysphonia are likely to last up to 2 weeks and then resolve spontaneously.	True
226	Describe the voice and speech characteristics associated with abductor spasmodic dysphonia.	Intermittent breathy voice breaks during speech, particularly following voiceless consonants
227	Which laryngeal muscles are selectively injected during botulinum toxin treatment of abductor spasmodic dysphonia?	Posterior cricoarytenoid muscles
228	Describe paradoxical vocal-cord motion.	Inappropriate adduction of the true vocal folds during inspiration
229	What spirometry finding is associated with paradoxical vocal-fold motion?	Flat inspiratory portion of the flow-volume loop
230	How can you test for suspected exercise-induced paradoxical vocal-fold motion in the office?	Provocation testing. Ask the patient to exercise until he or she becomes symptomatic, and then immediately perform flexible fiberoptic laryngoscopy. The diagnosis will be confirmed with observation of adduction of the vocal folds during inspiration.
231	What is the treatment of choice for paradoxical vocal-fold motion?	• Voice therapy • Relaxation and breathing exercises, such as laryngeal control therapy
232	What percentage of patients with essential tremor will develop vocal tremor?	10 to 20%

233	What muscles are selectively injected with botulinum toxin in the treatment of vocal tremor?	The strap muscles and/or intrinsic laryngeal muscles may be injected, based on which muscles appear most tremulous on examination.
234	What diagnosis must be considered in a patient with Parkinson disease and vocal-fold motion abnormalities?	Shy-Drager syndrome, a form of multiple-system atrophy, is a Parkinson-plus syndrome that may lead to life-threatening sleep apnea. Tracheotomy may be required.
235	What are the voice and speech characteristics observed in amyotrophic lateral sclerosis?	Monotonous hoarse voice with hypernasal and dysarthric speech
236	Describe the distinctive vocal features of spastic dysarthria.	Harsh quality, low fundamental frequency, strained/strangled sound, and pitch breaks resulting from injury of the pyramidal and extrapyramidal tracts
237	Injury to what structure(s) results in flaccid dysarthria?	Damage to any of the cranial nerves involved in speech (V, VII, X, XII) results in flaccid dysarthria.
238	Describe the speech pattern associated with ataxic dysarthria.	Ataxic dysarthria is associated with disorders of the cerebellum and is characterized by a harsh, breathy voice with a strained tremulous quality and fluctuating pitch and volume. Tremulous laryngeal muscle contractions are noted during speech but not at rest.
239	Describe the characteristic features of dysarthria associated with Parkinson disease.	Hypokinetic dysarthria: Low volume, reduced pitch variation, rushed speech, and reduction of articulation-associated movements
240	Describe the key features of muscle tension dysphonia.	Posterior glottic chink, high larynx, suprahyoid muscle tension, breathiness, and glottal fry
241	True or False. Muscle tension dysphonia is often the result of an unconscious attempt to compensate for glottic insufficiency.	True. Therefore, treatment focuses initially on voice therapy.
242	What physical examination findings are associated with excessive laryngeal muscle tension?	Pain on palpation of the larynx and extrinsic laryngeal muscles, small thyrohyoid space, high hyoid bone and larynx, difficulty rotating the larynx
243	Describe the voice characteristics associated with *dysphonia plica ventricularis*.	*Ventricular dysphonia*, or *dysphonia plica ventricularis*, refers to phonation resulting from false vocal-fold vibration as opposed to true vocal-fold vibration. The resulting voice is characteristically low pitched and hoarse, with intermittent voice breaks and diplophonia.

Surgical Airway

244	What are the indications for a surgical airway?	<ul><li>More than three failed attempts at intubation by an experienced laryngoscopist</li><li>> 10 minutes since initiation of induction</li><li>O_2 saturations < 65% during the first or second intubation attempt</li><li>Difficulty or inability to mask ventilate</li><li>Experienced airway staff decides that additional intubation attempts would be unsuccessful</li></ul>
245	In an emergent "can't intubate, can't ventilate" situation, what is traditionally the preferred surgical airway approach?	Cricothyrotomy (Some studies report that in practice tracheotomy may be used more often than cricothyrotomy.)
246	Describe the relative contraindications to cricothyrotomy.	<ul><li>Child younger than 10 to 12 years</li><li>Inability to palpate landmarks (neck trauma)</li><li>Expanding cervical hematoma</li><li>Subglottic extension of known laryngeal disease</li></ul>
247	Describe the surgical steps involved in cricothyrotomy.	<ul><li>Palpate landmarks (correctly identify cricothyroid space) and stabilize the larynx in your nondominant hand, maintaining the position of the cricothyroid membrane with your pointer finger.</li></ul>

		• Make a vertical incision through skin to, but not through, the laryngeal cartilaginous framework. • Horizontal incision through the cricothyroid membrane • Spread open the space using a clamp, back end of the scalpel, or other available instrument. • Carefully place cuffed breathing tube (tracheostomy or ETT).
248	When is needle cricothyrotomy or transtracheal needle ventilation indicated?	• It is indicated only in unique emergency settings in which intubation and surgical airway are not possible or in pediatric patients in whom a surgical airway is considered unsafe because of compressibility of the laryngeal cartilage framework. • It is used as a temporizing measure until a secure airway is possible. In adults, this is seen more in the prehospital setting. However, staff must be comfortable putting the equipment together and ventilating through this approach, which can be challenging.
249	How long can a patient be ventilated via transtracheal needle ventilation?	Reports range from 30 minutes to 2 hours.
250	Describe the technique of needle cricothyrotomy and subsequent ventilation.	• Connect a 12- or 14-gauge angiocatheter to a 3-mL syringe filled partially with saline or a commercially available needle cricothyrotomy device such as the Ravussin catheter. • After identifying the cricothyroid space, the needle is advanced at a 0- to 30-degree (caudal) angle while pulling back on the plunger. Once air is aspirated, the catheter is inserted over the needle at a 30- to 45-degree angle. • The angiocatheter is then connected to 100% oxygen at 50 psi using a Luer-Lok connector or oxygen tubing containing a y-connection attached to a jet insufflator and oxygen source (preferred). If this is not available, the angiocatheter can be connected to a bag-valve system via a 3.5-mm ETT connector, a 3-mL syringe without the plunger, and a 7.0 ETT connector, a 10-mL syringe without the plunger, and a 7.0 ETT inserted into the syringe with the cuff inflated or via cut IV infusion tubing connected to a 2.5 ETT connector. • Ventilation is most effective with a jet ventilation system: however, the airway may be temporized with a bag-valve system.
251	Describe the primary indications for tracheotomy	• Prolonged endotracheal intubation • Upper airway obstruction • Management of tracheobronchial secretions (pulmonary toilet) • Airway management associated with head and neck surgery • Management of major head and neck trauma
252	What are the nonemergent indications for surgical tracheotomy?	P Pulmonary toilet: Aspiration, inability to clear secretions (e.g., stroke, neurologic impairment, etc.) O Obstruction: Malignancy, obstructive sleep apnea (not amenable to noninvasive treatment) P Prevent complications associated with prolonged intubation (e.g., subglottic stenosis, tracheal erosion, etc.)
253	Tracheotomy should be performed after how many days of endotracheal intubation?	Although tracheotomy is generally performed after 14 days, there is no specific rule regarding optimal timing and should be individualized based on risk of continued intubation (i.e., subglottic stenosis) versus the likelihood of extubation.

254	At what level should the tracheal incision be made during open tracheostomy?	Between the second and third tracheal rings (or third and fourth if necessary)
255	What are the basic steps in open surgical tracheotomy?	<ul><li>A horizontal incision is placed between the sternal notch and cricoid cartilage at approximately the level of the second tracheal ring.</li><li>Dissection through the subcutaneous tissue to the strap musculature</li><li>Division of the midline raphe between the sternohyoid and sternothyroid muscles</li><li>Division (electrocautery or clamp and tie) or displacement of the thyroid isthmus</li><li>Identification of the cricoid cartilage and tracheal rings</li><li>Horizontal incision between rings 2–3 or 3–4</li><li>Creation of a Bjork flap using scalpel or heavy scissors and fixation of flap to subcutaneous tissue and or skin</li><li>Withdrawal of the ETT, suctioning, if needed, and placement of the desired tracheostomy tube</li><li>Inflate the cuff and secure tracheostomy with sutures to skin and tracheostomy tie.</li></ul>*Note*: Minimal lateral dissection around the trachea will limit disruption of the vascular supply to the trachea and resultant stenosis as well as injury to the recurrent laryngeal nerves.
256	What pressure is the maximum pressure acceptable for any endotracheal or tracheostomy tube cuff and why?	30 cm H_2O; must not exceed mucosal capillary pressure
257	When should a tracheostomy tube cuff be deflated?	When the patient no longer needs mechanical ventilation and is not aspirating
258	What are early and late complications of tracheostomy?	<ul><li>*Early*: Tracheostomy tube occlusion, granulation tissue formation, false passage, tube dislodgement, hemorrhage, wound infection, subcutaneous emphysema (possible pneumothorax or pneumomediastinum), postoperative pulmonary edema</li><li>*Late*: Hemorrhage (e.g., tracheoinnominate fistula), tracheoesophageal fistula, tracheal stenosis, persistent tracheocutaneous fistula (after decannulation)</li></ul>
259	When should a tracheostomy tube be removed?	<ul><li>Resolution of original indication for tracheostomy</li><li>Successfully corked/capped for 24 to 72 hours.</li><li>No anticipated need for general anesthetic or tracheostomy ventilation in the near future</li><li>Patient has adequate pulmonary toilet</li><li>No evidence for tracheal granulation tissue or other potentially compromising lesions</li></ul>
260	Your patient has met the criteria for tracheostomy decannulation. After removing the tube, cleaning the wound, and removing any stitch (i.e., from the Bjork flap), what type of dressing should be placed?	Occlusive dressing (changed once a day, when saturated, or when no longer sticking)

Laryngeal Surgery

261	What size ETT should be used during laryngeal surgery?	The smallest ETT that will allow adequate ventilation and is long enough to extend from the lips to the subglottis
262	What are the four most common ventilation techniques used during laryngeal surgery?	<ul><li>Endotracheal intubation</li><li>Jet ventilation</li><li>Spontaneous breathing</li><li>Apneic technique</li></ul>

263	What are the three types of jet ventilation?	• Supraglottic • Subglottic • Transtracheal
264	What is the most common major complication of subglottic jet ventilation?	Air trapping leading to pneumothorax/pneumomediastinum
265	What physical examination findings may be associated with difficult endotracheal intubation?	Long incisors, retrognathia, poor mandibular protrusion, small interincisor distance, Mallampati grade 3 or 4, high arched palate, short neck, thick neck, thyromental distance less than three finger breaths, limited neck range of motion
266	Describe the 4 modified Mallampati classes.	With the mouth fully open and the tongue protruded: • Class 1: Tonsillar pillars, tonsils, and uvula visible • Class 2: Uvula partially obscured by tongue base, upper tonsils visible • Class 3: Soft palate and base of uvula visible • Class 4: Only hard palate visible
267	What is the average duration of effect for deep true vocal-fold injection using the following materials: Gelfoam, bovine collagen, micronized Alloderm (Cymetra), fat, Teflon, calcium hydroxylapatite (Radiesse)?	• Gelfoam: 4 to 6 weeks • Bovine collagen: 3 to 4 months • Micronized Alloderm: 3 to 4 months • Fat: Several years • Teflon: Indefinite • Calcium hydroxylapatite: 2 years, some longer
268	The use of Teflon in true vocal-fold injection augmentation has been limited by what complication?	Teflon granuloma
269	Patients with what finding on videostroboscopy are less likely to benefit from true vocal-fold injection augmentation?	Posterior glottic gap. Laryngeal framework surgery has a higher chance of success.
270	What test must be obtained before performing true vocal-fold injection augmentation with bovine collagen?	Allergy skin testing is required due to the risk of allergic reaction to the material.
271	What are the two different types of vocal fold injection augmentation?	• Superficial (intracordal) • Deep injection augmentation
272	What are the preferred needle-placement locations for deep true vocal-fold injection augmentation?	The ideal location is at the intersection where a line drawn laterally from the vocal process tip intersects the superior arcuate line (transition from the superior surface of the vocal fold to the ventricle). A second injection, if needed, is often done along the superior arcuate line at the level of the mid-membranous vocal fold.
273	Define the *superior arcuate line of the true vocal fold*.	The *superior arcuate line* is the transition point from the superior surface of the true vocal fold to the ventricle.
274	What is the desired depth of injection for deep true vocal-fold injection augmentation?	3 to 5 mm into the thyroarytenoid muscle
275	What are the three approaches used for trans-cervical true vocal fold injection augmentation?	• Thyrohyoid • Cricothyroid • Translaryngeal
276	Define the desired effect on the true vocal folds in each of the four types of thyroplasty.	• Type I: Medial displacement • Type II: Lateral displacement • Type III: Shortening/relaxing • Type IV: Lengthening/tightening
277	To avoid airway compromise after medialization laryngoplasty, what should be true regarding the contralateral true vocal fold?	It should be able to abduct completely during inspiration.

278	What materials are commonly used for Implantation in medialization laryngoplasty?	Silastic, hydroxyapatite, and Gore Tex strips
279	To avoid fracture of the thyroid cartilage after type I thyroplasty, what is the minimum width of cartilage strut that must be left below the thyroplasty window?	3 mm
280	To externally determine the horizontal plane of the true vocal fold within the thyroid cartilage, what anatomical landmark must be completely exposed along the inferior border of the thyroid cartilage?	The inferior muscular tubercle of the thyroid cartilage must be completely exposed to define the plane of the inferior border of the thyroid cartilage, which parallels the long axis of the true vocal fold.
281	Why is the window for placing a Silastic implant during type I thyroplasty placed more posteriorly in men than in women?	The thyroid cartilage in men tends to have a more acute anterior angle. The window is therefore placed more posteriorly to avoid overmedialization of the anterior true vocal fold.
282	What are the indications for performing arytenoid adduction in addition to type I thyroplasty?	Large posterior glottic gap or vocal-fold level mismatch
283	What landmarks can be used to help identify the muscular process of the arytenoid during arytenoid adduction?	After a window has been created in the posterior thyroid lamina and the pyriform sinus mucosa has been retracted, the muscular process of the arytenoid must be identified. This can be done by palpation, by following the fibers of the posterior cricoarytenoid muscle superiorly to their attachment to the muscular process, or by looking approximately 1 cm superior to the cricoarytenoid joint.
284	During microflap excision of submucosal pathology of the true vocal fold, where should the incision be located?	Directly over or just lateral to the pathology
285	During microflap excision of submucosal pathology of the true vocal fold, what is the desired plane of elevation?	In the most superficial plane possible
286	Describe the available techniques for laryngeal reinnervation after injury to the RLN.	Primary RLN anastomosis, ansa cervicalis-to-RLN neurorrhaphy, ansa cervicalis-to-thyroarytenoid neuromuscular pedicle, ansa cervicalis-to-thyroarytenoid neural implantation, hypoglossal nerve-to-RLN neurorrhaphy and cricothyroid muscle-nerve-muscle neurotization
287	True or False: Laryngeal reinnervation procedures restore normal movement of the true vocal fold in unilateral true vocal-fold paralysis.	False. Laryngeal reinnervation procedures improve voice and other symptoms of unilateral vocal-fold paralysis by maintaining tone and bulk of the laryngeal adductor muscles, not by restoring normal movement.
288	What are the advantages of laryngeal reinnervation techniques relative to other procedures in the treatment of unilateral true vocal-fold paralysis?	<ul><li>Avoiding thyroarytenoid muscle bulk loss</li><li>Preservation of laryngeal anatomy to allow for additional procedures if needed</li><li>No alteration of vocal-fold vibratory potential</li><li>The ability to perform the procedure under general anesthesia</li></ul>
289	What is the key principle in surgical repair of upper airway stenosis?	Providing sufficient skeletal support
290	What systemic diseases have been shown to increase the risk of laryngotracheal stenosis after endotracheal intubation?	<ul><li>Laryngopharyngeal reflux</li><li>Congestive heart failure</li><li>Diabetes mellitus</li><li>Stroke</li></ul>

291	What are the indications for using an endolaryngeal stent in the repair of upper airway stenosis?	• Holding cartilage, bone grafts, or fragments in position • Stabilizing epidermal grafts, separating denuded surfaces • Maintaining a patent lumen when scar tissue is required
292	What is the mechanism of action of mitomycin C?	Mitomycin is both an antibiotic and an antineoplastic agent. It acts as an alkylating agent, causing DNA cross-linking and inhibition of DNA and RNA synthesis. This may lead to decreased cell division, decreasing fibroblast activity and protein production.
293	What is the preferred surgical technique for repair of complete tracheal stenosis?	Resection and primary anastomosis
294	What percentage of the adult trachea can be resected and still allow for primary anastomosis?	50% (5–7 cm)
295	What is the best surgical treatment for circumferential fibrous stenosis of the trachea with intact cartilage?	Staged partial excisions of the fibrous tissue, spaced 2 to 4 weeks apart to prevent recurrence.

6 Otology, Neurotology, and Lateral Skull Base Surgery

Matthew L. Carlson, Joseph T. Breen, Stanley Pelosi, and Colin L.W. Driscoll

Overview

1	Describe the sensory innervation of the pinna and external auditory canal (EAC).	Sensation of the auricle is provided by the greater auricular and lesser occipital nerve (from the cervical plexus), as well as small sensory branches of the facial nerve and auriculotemporal nerve. The EAC is supplied by overlapping contributions from cranial nerves (CN) V, VII, IX, and X.
2	What is the foramen of Huschke?	The foramen of Huschke is a developmental defect resulting from incomplete fusion of the greater and lesser tympanic spines. When present, it creates a connection between the EAC and the parotid gland, glenoid fossa or infratemporal fossa.
3	What are the fissures of Santorini?	The fissures of Santorini are anatomical communications that allow lymphatic movement between the anterior cartilaginous EAC and the parotid gland and glenoid fossa.
4	What is the notch of Rivinus?	The notch of Rivinus is the deficient portion of the tympanic annulus where the pars flaccida attaches to the squamous portion of the temporal bone.
5	How are the *pars flaccida* and *pars tensa* of the tympanic membrane structurally different?	The *pars flaccida* is, as its name implies, more compliant than the pars tensa. The *pars tensa* is slightly thicker and contains a middle fibrous layer in addition to an outer skin layer and inner mucosal layer.
6	The tympanic membrane is formed by what embryonic layer(s)?	The outer epidermal layer from the first branchial cleft (ectodermal origin); middle fibrous layer from neural crest mesenchyme (mesodermal origin); inner mucosal layer from the first pharyngeal pouch (endodermal origin)
7	Where does the carotid artery lie in relation to the eustachian tube?	The carotid artery courses just medial to the more anterior cartilaginous portion of the eustachian tube.
8	In patients with cleft palate, dysfunction of which muscle is most strongly implicated in causing recurrent otitis media?	Tensor veli palatini
9	What is the most common intratemporal location of facial nerve dehiscence?	It occurs most commonly near the oval window, second most commonly at the second genu.
10	Describe the origin, insertion, and action of the tensor tympani muscle.	The tensor tympani originates from the greater wing of the sphenoid, cartilage of the eustachian tube, and the walls of the semicanal of the tensor tympani. Its tendon then wraps around the cochleariform process to insert onto the medial aspect of the neck and manubrium of the malleus. It functions to medialize the tympanic membrane and increase the impedance of the ossicular chain.
11	What landmarks may be used to help identify the facial nerve during middle ear surgery?	The Jacobson nerve, located on the cochlear promontory, can be followed superiorly to the cochleariform process. The facial nerve is immediately medial and superior to the cochleariform process and tensor tympani. The facial nerve can also be identified immediately superior to the oval window.

12	Aside from the muscles of facial expression, what muscles does the facial nerve innervate?	In addition to the muscles of facial expression, the facial nerve innervates all the other muscles of the second branchial arch, specifically, the stapedius muscle, the stylohyoid, and the posterior belly of the digastric.
13	What is the *cog*?	The cog is a coronally oriented bony septum located just anterior to the head of the malleus that seperates the anterior epitympanic recess (supratubal recess) from the attic.
14	When looking at the external surface of the mastoid cortex, what landmark can be used to approximate the level of the middle cranial fossa?	The temporal line, which represents the inferior insertion point of the temporalis muscle, can be used as a landmark.
15	Describe the boundaries of the Macewen triangle (suprameatal).	The suprameatal crest, posterior margin of the external auditory canal, and the tangential line from the posterior ear canal bisecting the suprameatal crest are the boundaries of the Macewen triangle, which approximates the antrum.
16	What is the Körner septum?	The Körner septum is a bony plate dividing the mastoid air cells superficial to the antrum. Embryologically, it is the junction between the petrous and squamous portions of the temporal bone and creates a "false bottom" during mastoidectomy.
17	Which cells are primarily responsible for transducing acoustic energy into neural signals?	Inner hair cells are the primary cells onto which afferent auditory neurons (spiral ganglion cells) synapse. The outer hair cells also contribute to transformation of acoustic energy into neural signal; however, they primarily play a role in "tuning" the cochlea to improve frequency selectivity and sensitivity.
18	What are the boundaries of the scala media? (▶ Fig. 6.1)	In the cross-section of the cochlea, the scala media is separated from the scala vestibuli by the Reissner membrane. The basilar membrane and osseous spiral lamina separate the scala media and scala tympani. The boundaries of the outer periphery of the scala media are the stria vascularis and the spiral ligament.

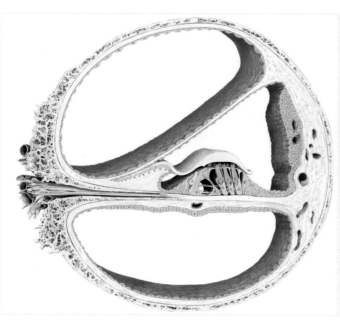

Fig. 6.1 Cross section of the cochlea and organ of Corti. (Used with permission from Thieme Atlas of Anatomy: Head and Neuroanatomy, © Thieme 2007, illustration by Karl Wesker.)

19	What two structures are connected by the perilymphatic (periotic) duct?	The perilymphatic duct, which runs in the bony canal of the cochlear aqueduct, connects the scala tympani of the cochlea and the subarachnoid space of the posterior cranial fossa.
20	Which structures are innervated by the superior and inferior vestibular nerves, respectively?	Superior vestibular nerve innervates the superior and lateral semicircular canals and the utricle. Inferior vestibular nerve innervates the posterior semicircular canal, and the saccule.
21	Where is the primary auditory cortex located?	Brodmann areas 41 and 42 of the upper temporal lobe
22	Describe the geometric anatomy of the semicircular canals and the physiologic significance of this arrangement.	The three semicircular canals are located in three mutually perpendicular planes. This orientation provides the vestibular system with independent resolution of rotational movements in three different axes (pitch, roll, and yaw).
23	Describe the course and functions provided by the nervus intermedius.	The taste, secretory, and sensory fibers of the facial nerve are carried by the nervus intermedius. It exists as a distinct nerve in the cerebellopontine angle (CPA) and internal auditory canal (IAC), but on entering the meatal foramen, these fibers exist within the body of the facial nerve.
24	What cell bodies are located in the geniculate ganglion?	Cell bodies of the special sensory taste neurons carried by the chorda tympani nerve
25	What nerve fibers are carried by the greater superficial petrosal nerve?	Preganglionic parasympathetic fibers that synapse in the pterygopalatine ganglion, as well as afferent special sensory taste fibers that supply the soft palate
26	What percentage of temporal bone specimens demonstrate dehiscence of the geniculate ganglion on the floor of the middle fossa?	16%
27	What is the prevalence of internal carotid artery dehiscence at the floor of the middle cranial fossa?	Approximately 20%
28	Describe the boundaries of the Glasscock triangle (posterolateral).	Greater superficial petrosal nerve, V3, line connecting foramen spinosum and arcuate eminence
29	Describe the boundaries of Kawase triangle (posteromedial).	V3, greater superficial petrosal nerve, arcuate eminence, superior petrosal sinus. It marks the boundaries of anterior petrosectomy for gaining access to the posterior fossa.
30	What extratemporal branches of the facial nerve arborize proximal to the pes anserinus?	The postauricular nerve, nerve to the stylohyoid, and nerve to the posterior belly of the digastric muscle

31	The external ear is formed by what mesodermal structures? (▶ Fig. 6.2)	The six hillocks of His:
		• First Arch
		  1: Tragus
		  2: Helical crus
		  3: Helix
		• Second Arch
		  4: Antihelix
		  5: Antitragus
		  6: Lobule

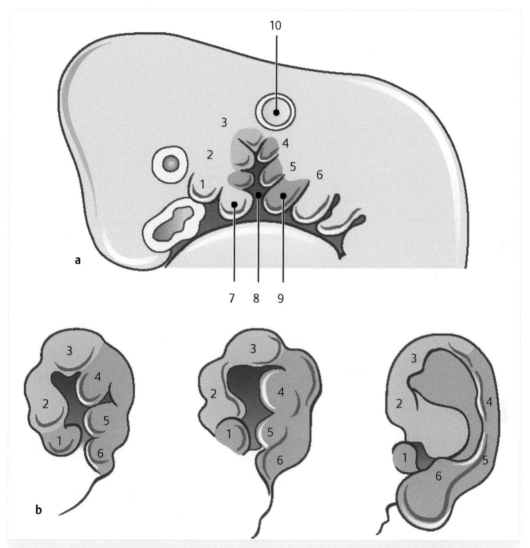

Fig. 6.2 Embryologic development of the external ear. (a) Embryo, lateral view; (b) external ear develops from six hillocks (1–3 are derived from the first branchial arch and 4–6 from the second branchial arch). 1, Tragus; 2, crus helicis; 3, helix; 4, crus anthelicis; 5, antihelix; 6, antitragus; 7, first branchial arch; 8, branchial cleft; 9, second branchial arch; 10, auricular plate. (Used with permission from Behrbohm H, Kaschke O, Nawka T, Swift A. Ear, Nose, and Throat Diseases: With Head and Neck Surgery. New York, NY: Thieme; 2009.)

32	Incomplete fusion or supernumerary development of the hillocks of His may lead to what conditions?	Preauricular cysts, pits, or tags
33	Describe the embryologic basis of a persistent stapedial artery.	The stapedial artery is derived from the second branchial arch. This is normally a transient structure, but in rare instances, it can persist into adulthood.
34	What skull base abnormality is classically seen with a persistent stapedial artery?	Lack of an ipsilateral foramen spinosum

35	Describe the embryologic origin(s) of the ossicles.	The head and neck of the malleus, as well as the incus body and short process, are derived from the first branchial arch (Meckel cartilage). The manubrium of the malleus, long process and lenticular process of the incus, and the stapes superstructure are derived from the second branchial arch (Reichert cartilage). The vestibular half of the stapes footplate and annular ligmanent are thought by many authorities to be derived from the otic capsule.
36	From which germ cell layers and branchial arch(es) does the otocyst arise?	First seen at the end of the 3rd week of development, the otic placode is a thickening of the ecdodermal surface of the first branchial groove. This invaginates into the underlying mesoderm, which it eventually becomes surrounded by to form the otocyst. This structure goes on to develop into the otic labyrinth.
37	List the primary acoustic functions of the external ear.	• Filter to reduce low-frequency background noise • Resonator to amplify mid frequency sounds (up to 20 dB) • Direction-dependent filter to augment spatial perception at high frequencies
38	Compared with adults, what anatomical characteristics of the eustachian tube in young children predisposes toward development of acute otitis media?	The eustachian tube is narrower, shorter, and oriented more in a horizontal plane in children, putting the middle ear at a higher risk for exposure to nasopharyngeal secretions and poor aeration.
39	Describe the acoustic transformer mechanism of the middle ear.	The three "levers" provide an average gain of 20 to 30 dB: • *Catenary lever*: Elastic properties of stretched tympanic membrane fibers directing sound to the centralized malleus • *Ossicular lever*: The length of the manubrium of the malleus divided by the length of the long process of the incus (1:3 ratio) • *Hydraulic lever*: A 22:1 ratio of the tympanic membrane to the oval window
40	Describe the electrolyte composition of the cochlear fluids.	Perilymph located in scala vestibul and scala tympani is similar to serum and cerebrospinal fluid (CSF) in electrolyte composition (high Na and low K concentration). Endolymph is located within the scala media and is similar to intracellular fluid in electrolyte composition (low Na and high K concentration).
41	How are movements of the oval window (stapes footplate) and the round window membrane related?	They are out of phase by 180 degrees. In other words, motion at the oval window into the vestibule leads to an outward movement of the round window membrane into the middle ear. If pressure is exerted on both the round window and oval window simultaneously and equally, phase cancellation occurs resulting in significant hearing loss.
42	Describe the tonotopic organization of the cochlea.	The cochlea (specifically the basilar membrane) is tonotopically "tuned," such that the high frequency sounds are most effectively transduced at the basal cochlea, whereas low-frequency sounds are best transduced in the apical segments.
43	What effects do ampullopedal and ampullofugal displacement of the semicircular canal kinocilia have on the firing rates of the vestibular nerves?	Ampullopetal (toward the vestibule) displacement of the kinocilia of the horizontal canal and ampullofugal (away from the vestibule) displacement of the kinocilia of the superior and posterior canals increase vestibular nerve firing rates.

Vestibular Evaluation

44	Define *first-degree*, *second-degree*, and *third-degree nystagmus*.	• *First degree*: Occurring when gazing in the direction of the fast component

		• *Second degree*: Occurring when gazing in the direction of the fast component or at midline • *Third degree*: Occurring when gazing in all directions
45	Describe Alexander's law?	The amplitude of the nystagmus will intensify when the patient looks in the direction of the fast phase. Alexander's law describes the pattern of nystagmus in a patient with a unilateral peripheral vestibular deficit.
46	Describe Ewald's three laws?	1. The axis of nystagmus parallels the anatomic axis of the semicircular canal that generated it. 2. In the lateral semicircular canals, ampullopetal endolymph movement causes greater stimulation than ampullofugal movement. 3. In the superior and posterior semicircular canals, the reverse is true.
47	Describe examination findings that help distinguish between *central* and *peripheral vestibular deficits*.	• *Central deficits* may occur in any direction (vertical, horizontal, or torsional), may alternate direction, do not suppress with visual fixation, do not fatigue, rarely are associated with hearing loss, often have other abnormal neurologic examination findings, have minimal latency with positional change, and often less severe. • *Peripheral deficits* are unidirectional; horizontal only (no vertical component), suppresses with visual fixation, often with concurrent hearing loss, otherwise normal neurological examination, positional nystagmus that often has a 2 + second latency, generally more severe.
48	Describe the direction of nystagmus with *irritative* and *destructive* vestibulopathy?	*Irritative vestibulopathy* is associated with a fast phase beating toward the affected ear, whereas *destructive vestibulopathy* is associated with a fast-phase beating away from the affected ear.
49	What is the purpose of *Frenzel goggles*?	• Frenzel goggles assist in evaluating for nystagmus. • Frenzel goggles magnify and illuminate the patient's eyes and prevent gaze fixation.
50	What inner ear structure and nerve do thermal calorics testing interrogate?	Thermal calorics measure the responsiveness of the horizontal semicircular canal (and superior vestibular nerve) to thermal stimuli and is one of the few quantitative evaluations that can test the two ears independently.
51	Describe the effects of cold and warm irrigation during caloric testing.	Cold causes the fast phase of nystagmus to beat toward the opposite ear, whereas warm causes the fast phase to beat toward the ipsilateral ear.
52	How is electronystagmography (ENG) or videonystagmography (VNG) useful in the evaluation of the dizzy patient?	Nystagmography comes in several forms (ENG or VNG) and serves to quantitatively measure eye movements while performing positional testing or calorics.
53	What is computerized dynamic posturography?	This technique, used to quantify postural control in an upright (standing) position in either static or dynamic conditions, requires coordination of sensory input, motor output, and central integration.
54	What inner ear structure and cranial nerve does VEMP testing interrogate?	Saccule and inferior vestibular nerve
55	How is computerized dynamic posturography performed?	The patient is placed on a platform that is capable of performing various movements and sensing patient sway (oscillations). Additionally, a visual backdrop is placed in front of the patient and can be held stationary or can move. The patient is then subjected to six increasingly difficult tests.

56	What pattern of results may be seen in a malingering patient during computerized dynamic posturography?	The patient has poor scores with easier tasks, but as the task difficulty increases, the patient may do disproportionately better.
57	What does the dynamic visual acuity test evaluater?	It tests for impaired ability to preceive objects accurately during head movement. Normally, the vestibular ocular reflex maintains the direction of gaze on a fixed target by moving the eyes in the opposite direction of head movement.
58	Dysdiadochokinesia is a sign of dysfunction involving what structure?	*Dysdiadochokinesia*, the difficulty with performing rapid alternating movements, is considered a sign of cerebellar pathology.
59	How is the Fukuda test performed, and what does it evaluate?	The patient is asked to march in place with eyes closed for 50 steps. Rotation (> 30 degrees) may indicate asymmetrical labyrinthine function. Rotation generally occurs toward the side of the lesion.
60	What is purpose of the vestibulo-ocular reflex?	This reflex generates eye movements in response to head motions perceived by the peripheral vestibular system, permitting visual fixation on an object while the head is moving.
61	How do you perform a head-thrust test?	The patient is asked to fixate on the examiner's nose while the head is passively and rapidly rotated in the excitatory direction of a semicircular canal. Normally, the patient will be able to maintain fixation on the examiner.
62	What constitutes a positive head-thrust test?	In the case of a left hypoactive labyrinth, the vestibulo-ocular-reflex will be impaired, and the head-thrust test toward the patient's left side will be positive; the examiner will note the patient's eyes to rotate with the head, and after a brief delay, a "catch-up saccade" toward the right will bring the gaze back toward the examiner.
63	Describe the Hennebert sign?	Induction of nystagmus or vertigo with changes in external auditory canal pressure (tragal pressure, pneumatic otoscopy)
64	What conditions are associated with a positive Hennebert sign?	Superior semicircular canal dehiscence, perilymphatic fistula, lateral semicircular canal fistula from chronic ear disease, or otosyphilis
65	Describe a positive Tullio phenomenon.	Tullio phenomenon is noise-induced activation of the vestibular system resulting in dizziness and/or nystagmus. Historically, it is associated with syphilis but may occur with inner ear fistula and/or dehiscence syndromes.
66	How is a Romberg test performed?	The patient stands with feet close together and arms at the sides. The clinician evaluates the relative amount of body sway with the patient's eyes closed compared with when they are open.
67	What is a Romberg test evaluating?	Somatosensation and proprioception carried out by the cerebellum and dorsal column-medial lemniscus
68	In what clinical situations would rotary chair testing be useful?	Because rotatory chair testing evaluates bilateral semicircular canal function simultaneously (unlike caloric testing), it may be used for evaluating suspected bilateral vestibular loss (after meningitis, vestibulotoxic medications, etc.).
69	What symptom is classically associated with severe bilateral peripheral vestibular hypofunction?	Oscillopsia

Vestibular and Balance Disorders

70	Review the differential diagnosis of Ménière disease.	Perilymphatic fistula, vestibular migraine, Cogan syndrome, autoimmune hearing loss, syphilis, mumps, Mondini malformation
71	What percentage of patients with Ménière disease will develop bilateral involvement?	Approximately 30%
72	What medical treatments are most commonly used for symptomatic treatment of active Ménière disease?	• Vestibular suppressants (e.g., benzodiazepines promethazine) • Rest • Potentially corticosteroids
73	What are the two most commonly used surgical approaches for vestibular neurectomy?	• Middle fossa or the retrosigmoid approach • Retrolabyrinthine and transmeatal approaches have also been used.
74	How does the efficacy of endolymphatic shunt placement compare with endolymphatic sac decompression for treatment of Ménière disease?	No trials have clearly demonstrated superior results in one treatment over the other.
75	Review the clinical presentation of Ménière disease.	Low-frequency sensorineural hearing loss (SNHL, fluctuating and progressive), roaring tinnitus, aural fullness, and episodic vertigo generally lasting for hours
76	Describe Lermoyez syndrome.	Tinnitus and hearing loss that remit after an attack of vertigo
77	Define *possible*, *probable*, *definite* and *certain* Ménière disease.	• Possible: Episodic vertigo without documented hearing loss or SNHL (fluctuating or fixed) with dysequilibrium but without definitive vertigo episodes; other causes excluded • Probable: One definitive episode of vertigo, audiometrically documented hearing loss on at least one occasion, tinnitus or aural fullness in the treated ear; other causes excluded • Definite: Two or more definitive spontaneous episodes of vertigo lasting 20 minutes or longer, audiometrically documented hearing loss on at least one occasion, tinnitus or aural fullness in the treated ear, other causes excluded • Certain: Definite Ménière disease plus histopathologic confirmation
78	Describe diet modifications for treatment of Ménière disease.	• Avoidance of alcohol, caffeine, tobacco and monosodium glutamate • Adherence to a low-sodium diet (less than 1 to 2 g/day)
79	How is electrocochleography used in the diagnosis of Ménière disease?	If the ratio of the *summating potential*, generated by the organ of Corti, and the *action potential*, generated by the auditory nerve, is elevated, diagnosis is indicated. A value of 0.5 or greater is considered suggestive of Ménière disease.
80	How is electrocochleography performed?	Neural responses to presented sounds are recorded through an electrode in the middle ear (transtympanic needle electrode), on the tympanic membrane, or on a gold foil-wrapped earplug.
81	What is the role of intratympanic injections of gentamicin in the treatment of Ménière disease?	• Selectively vestibulotoxic ablative treatment for unilateral Ménière disease, often pursued after failure of more conservative measures such as low-salt diet, caffeine avoidance, diuretic therapy, and intratympanic steroid injection • Carries a 5 to 20% chance of significant SNHL

82	What is the role of intratympanic injections of corticosteroids in the treatment of Ménière disease?	These injections are considered a nonablative adjunct to medical therapy that carries little risk of inducing hearing loss. Subjects may experience a brief episode of vertigo with injection if the steroid is not body temperature and a low risk for persistent tympanic membrane perforation.
83	When is a patient considered a candidate for endolymphatic sac surgery?	Frequent vertiginous spells despite conservative treatment in patients who are not candidates for ablative procedures (bilateral disease, good residual hearing, contralateral vestibular hypofunction)
84	What is the Donaldson line?	The Donaldson line is an imaginary line running parallel to the plane of the lateral semicircular canal, extending posteriorly and inferiorly through the center of the posterior semicircular canal. The endolymphatic sac lies just inferior to this line on the posterior fossa dura.
85	What pure tone audiometric findings can be seen in patients with superior semicircular canal dehiscence?	Conductive hyperacusis is sometimes seen, with bone conductive thresholds occasionally less than 0-dB hearing loss. This can lead to an air-bone gap even when air conductive thresholds are within the normal range.
86	Describe the *third window phenomenon*.	The *third window* refers to a third opening in the inner ear, in addition to the round and oval windows, that permits pathological movement of perilymph within the labyrinth, which may induce vertigo.
87	Describe the clinical presentation of superior semicircular canal dehiscence syndrome.	Aural fullness, autophony, hearing loss (generally with an air-bone gap and often supranormal bone conduction), and dizziness often associated with loud sounds, exertion or straining
88	How can one differentiate *otosclerosis* from *superior semicircular canal dehiscence syndrome*?	Patients with otosclerosis often have type A_S tympanograms, diphasic or absent stapedial reflexes, and elevated to absent cervical vestibular evoked myogenic potentials. Patients with superior semicircular canal dehiscence will usually have normal stapedial reflexes, type A tympanograms, and diminished vestibular evoked myogenic potential thresholds (often < 70 dB).
89	How do you perform and interpret the Dix-Hallpike test?	With the patient sitting, rotate the patient's head by approximately 45 degrees to the left or the right. The patient then lies flat with the head slightly extended (~ 20 degrees). The eyes are then observed for ~ 45 seconds looking for rotary nystagmus. If rotatory nystagmus occurs, the test is positive. The direction of the fast phase reveals the side that is affected.
90	Describe the clinical manifestation of benign paroxysmal positional vertigo?	Short-lived (less than 60 seconds), room-spinning vertigo provoked by head turn
91	Which semicircular canal is most commonly involved in benign paroxysmal positional vertigo?	Posterior canal. Five percent involve the horizontal canal and the superior canal is the least common.
92	What anatomical structure is the source of otoconia in benign paroxysmal positional vertigo?	The utricle
93	What are risk factors for the development of benign paroxysmal positional vertigo?	• Advanced age, head trauma, surgery, migraine • Most patients do not have an identifiable cause (idiopathic).
94	Describe the mechanism of singular neurectomy in the treatment of benign paroxysmal positional vertigo.	The singular nerve innervates the posterior semicircular canal, which is the most commonly affected canal in benign paroxysmal positional vertigo. Division of this nerve may lead to symptom relief in refractory disease.

95	What conservative treatment options are available for benign paroxysmal positional vertigo?	• Reassurance and education about the nature of the condition • No effective pharmacologic therapy is available • Canalith repositioning maneuvers involve taking a patient through a series of positions that are designed to return dislodged otoconia to the vestibule and are the most effective nonsurgical treatment.
96	What test(s) should be ordered when vertebro-basilar insufficiency is suspected?	• MRI and magnetic resonance angiography (MRA) provide the best information regarding acute and chronic infarcts, as well as the location and severity of vascular occlusions in the head and neck. • Patients who cannot undergo MRI should be evaluated with CT and CT angiography (CTA). • Duplex ultrasound can also provide information regarding proximal vertebral arteries.
97	What symptoms may accompany episodic vertigo associated with vertebrobasilar insufficiency?	Diplopia, decrease in visual acuity, ataxia, dysarthria, dysphagia, and other focal neurologic symptoms
98	Describe the symptoms of Wallenberg syndrome.	• Loss of pain and temperature sensation on the ipsilateral face and contralateral body, dysphagia, dysarthria, ataxia, vertigo, Horner syndrome, diplopia • Caused by a lateral medullary infarct supplied by the posterior inferior cerebellar artery
99	What are typical initial symptoms of vestibular neuronitis?	• Sudden onset of severe vertigo, nausea, and vomiting lasting days to weeks, often preceded by a viral upper respiratory tract infection • Unlike labyrinthitis, hearing should remain stable.
100	What are the mainstays of treatment for vestibular neuronitis?	High-dose corticosteroids, vestibular suppressants in the acute period, antiemetics, and bed rest as needed
101	What are the diagnostic criteria for chronic subjective dizziness?	• Subjective unsteadiness or nonvertiginous dizziness that is present for 3 + months and is present most days • Hypersensitivity to one's own motion and to the movement of objects in the environment • Visual dizziness marked by exacerbation of symptoms in settings with complex visual stimuli (grocery stores) or when performing precision visual tasks (reading or working on the computer)
102	What are the treatment options for chronic subjective dizziness?	First-line pharmacologic therapy includes selective serotonin reuptake inhibitors. For patients with concurrent migraine, selective serotonin norepinephrine reuptake inhibitors or tricyclic antidepressants may be used. Behavioral intervention and psychoeducation serve as complementing therapies.
103	Describe the typical presentation of mal de débarquement syndrome.	The sensation of rocking or swaying back and forth without vertigo, difficulty concentrating, and fatigue. It most commonly occurs in middle-aged women after a week-long cruise. The mean duration of symptoms is 3.5 years.
104	What is the mechanism of motion sickness?	Disagreement between vestibular cues and visual and somatosensory input
105	Excluding benign paroxysmal positional vertigo, what is the most common cause of vertigo in the general population?	Vestibular migraine, or migraine-associated vertigo, is estimated to have a prevalence of ~ 1% in the general population.
106	What are the diagnostic criteria for vestibular migraine?	*Definite* vestibular migraine • Recurrent episodic vestibular symptoms of at least moderate severity • Current or previous history of migraine

		• Migrainous symptoms during ≥ 2 vertiginous attacks
		• Other causes ruled out by appropriate investigations
		Probable vestibular migraine
		• Recurrent episodic vestibular symptoms of at least moderate severity
		• One of the following:
		  ○ Current or previous history of migraine
		  ○ Migrainous symptoms during ≥ 2 attacks of vertigo
		  ○ Migraine precipitants before vertigo in more than 50% of attacks
		  ○ Response to migraine medications in more than 50% of attacks
		  ○ Other causes are ruled out by appropriate investigations.

107	Describe the relationship between *vestibular migraine* and *Ménière disease*.	There is substantial overlap between groups. Approximately one-fourth of patients with Ménière disease also fulfill diagnostic criteria for vestibular migraine.
108	Describe the clinical features of basilar migraine.	• Similar symptoms to vertebrobasilar insufficiency with headache • Most patients experience dizziness but may also experience ataxia, hearing loss, tinnitus, dysarthria, diplopia, and syncope. • It most commonly involves young females.
109	Describe the common neurotologic examination findings in patients with multiple sclerosis.	Abnormalities of smooth pursuit (96%), saccadic eye movements (76%), optokinetic nystagmus (53%), and defective visual suppression of nystagmus (43%)
110	What is the Charcot triad?	Nystagmus, scanning speech, and intention tremor; associated symptoms of multiple sclerosis
111	Define *balance retraining therapy*.	Specialized form of physical therapy focusing on the improvement of static and dynamic balance and gait, and promoting central vestibular compensation by taking advantage of the inherent plasticity of central balance pathways
112	What are the two phases of vestibular recovery after an acute vestibular insult?	• *Static recovery* (initial phase) occurs through a central adaptive process that rebalances tonic neural activity between vestibular nuclei • *Dynamic recovery* (second phase) involves recalibrating brain and cerebellar reflex pathways in response to sensory conflicts occurring with head and eye movements.
113	Describe the clinical findings during static compensation and dynamic compensation.	During static compensation, patients will often have marked spontaneous nystagmus and vertigo lasting from days to weeks. During dynamic compensation, patients may experience general imbalance and unsteadiness with quick head turn.
114	With regard to vestibular rehabilitation, describe the strategy of adaptation.	Exercises aimed at improving vestibule-ocular response (VOR) gain. Initially, the patient is asked to view a stationary object while moving the head back and forth. The same exercise can be repeated but with the object moving in the opposite direction of head turn. This will strengthen gaze stability through improvement of the VOR response.
115	With regard to vestibular rehabilitation, describe the strategy of *habituation*.	Patients may be exposed to repetitive visual, vestibular, or motor exercises that are designed to provoke episodes of imbalance. With repetitive exposure, there is an attenuation or modification of the response.

116	With regard to vestibular rehabilitation, describe the strategy of *substitution*.	Exercises designed to take advantage of alternate intact balance mechanisms (remaining vestibular function, visual input, somatosensory input) to compensate for specific balance system deficits
117	Describe the ideal candidate for vestibular rehabilitation.	Patient with stable unilateral vestibular hypofunction who continues to feel general imbalance that is worsened by quick head movements
118	What patients are not good candidates for vestibular rehabilitation?	Central compensation requires consistent and predictable peripheral vestibular input; therefore, patients with unstable vestibular deficits (e.g., active Ménière disease, acute viral labyrinthitis) should not enter vestibular rehabilitation until their condition has stabilized.
119	Name several conditions that negatively influence the outcome of vestibular rehabilitation.	Coexisting conditions that affect balance may result in less optimal outcomes than in patients with isolated stable vestibular hypofunction. Examples include central nervous system disorders (stroke, multiple sclerosis, Parkinson disease), sensory neuropathy (diabetes, peripheral vascular disease), motor dysfunction, and patients with vestibular migraine, to name a few.
120	Which medications potentially retard progress during vestibular rehabilitation?	Anticonvulsants and sedating medications may prolong vestibular rehabilitation. Additionally, vestibular suppressive medications hinder initial static compensation.
121	To what does *presbystasis* refer?	*Presbystasis* refers to the general balance difficulties of elderly patients that is related to cumulative age-related decline in vestibular response, visual acuity, proprioception, and motor control.

Hearing Loss Evaluation

122	Name the four different subclasses of presbycusis.	• Sensory: Loss of sensory hair cells of the basal turn, resulting in a precipitous high-frequency SNHL and preserved speech discrimination • Neural: Loss of VIII nerve fibers where speech discrimination may be disproportionately affected • Metabolic: Caused by atrophy of the stria vascularis affecting all frequencies (flat audiogram); speech discrimination is frequently preserved • Mechanical: Caused by stiffening of the basilar membrane, resulting in a gradual down sloping SNHL with proportional loss of speech discrimination
123	Define *mild*, *moderate*, *severe*, and *profound* hearing loss.	• Mild = 26 to 40 dB • Moderate = 41 to 55 dB • Moderately severe = 56 to 70 dB • Severe = 71 to 90 dB • Profound > 90 dB
124	At what air-bone gap range is Rinne testing (512-Hz tuning fork) most reliable at detecting a conductive hearing loss?	Between 17 and 30 dB; any value lower or higher is more likely to produce a false negative result.
125	What is the usual air-bone gap seen with a maximal conductive hearing loss?	Roughly 60 dB
126	What is the interaural decibel difference required for a Weber examination to lateralize?	Sound should lateralize to the ear with the largest conductive loss or the side with the "better nerve"; a minimum of a 5 dB difference is needed.
127	Describe the reliability of bedside hearing screening. (▶ Fig. 6.3; ▶ Fig. 6.4)	Finger rub, watch-tick, whispered speech, Rinne test, and Weber test all carry a relatively good specificity (60 to 100%), but they have low sensitivity (< 50%).

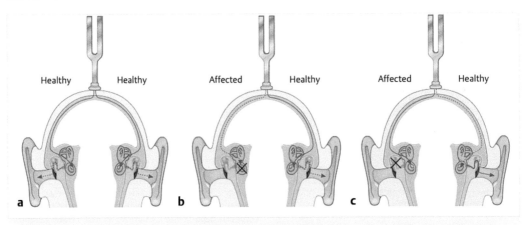

Fig. 6.3 The Weber test. A vibrating tuning fork is placed on the midline of the skull. (a) With normal hearing or symmetric hearing loss, sound is perceived with equal loudness in both ears. (b) With pure unilateral sensorineural hearing loss, sound lateralizes to the better hearing ear. (c) With pure unilateral conductive hearing loss, sound lateralizes to the poorer hearing ear. (Used with permission from Probst R, Grevers G, Iro H. Basic Otorhinolaryngology: A Step-by-Step Learning Guide. New York, NY: Thieme; 2006.)

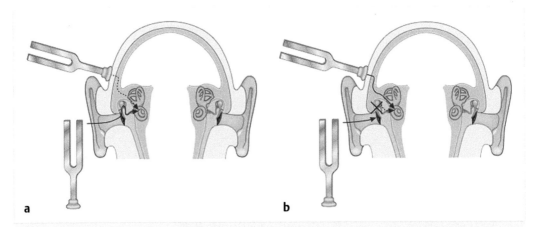

Fig. 6.4 The Rinne test. Using a vibrating tuning fork, air and bone conduction thresholds are compared in the same ear. (a) Without conductive hearing loss, air conduction is perceived louder than bone conduction. (b) With conductive hearing loss (usually greater than a 20 dB air-bone gap), bone conduction is perceived louder than air conduction. (Used with permission from Probst R, Grevers G, Iro H. Basic Otorhinolaryngology: A Step-by-Step Learning Guide. New York, NY: Thieme; 2006.)

128	Define *hearing level* as it relates to measurement of sound intensity.	*Hearing level* is a measurement (in decibels) relative to reference data from normal-hearing ears. Normal sensitivitiy is defined as decibels of hearing level, which varies in absolute intensity at different frequencies because of different frequency sensitivities of the average healthy human ear.
129	Describe the anticipated test-retest variability seen with pure tone audiometry.	Test-retest variability should be 10 dB or less.

130	Define *asymmetric hearing loss*.	Interaural differences of greater than 15 dB in two or more pure-tone thresholds or a difference of greater than 15% on speech discrimination testing
131	What are the advantages of binaural hearing?	Horizontal plane sound localization and improved speech understanding in noise from summation, squelch, and head shadow effect
132	Describe two mechanisms that permit sound localization from an "off-center" source in the horizontal plane (left- or right-sided).	• *Interaural time difference*: Sound will reach the closest ear first (low-frequency dominated). • *Interaural intensity difference*: The intensity of sound in the ear farthest from the source will be attenuated by the head shadow effect (high-frequency dominated).
133	Why is masking used during audiometric testing?	If sounds presented to the test ear are sufficiently loud, they can cross over to the non-test ear. *Interaural attenuation* is the loss of intensity that occurs before arriving at the non-test ear. If sounds are loud enough to be perceived after interaural attenuation, masking is necessary to obtain an accurate test. Interaural attenuation for air conduction and bone conduction is roughly 40 dB and 0 dB, respectively.
134	In audiometric testing, what is meant by the term *masking dilemma*?	A *masking dilemma* occurs when the required masking level is loud enough to cross over to the test ear. This most commonly occurs in patients with significant bilateral conductive hearing loss.
135	Describe the phenomenon of *recruitment*.	*Recruitment* is characterized by minimal difficulty with quiet sounds but having a disproportionately severe noise sensitivity at higher sound levels.
136	Describe the phenomenon of *rollover*.	*Rollover* is characterized by a paradoxical decrease in speech recognition with increasing sound presentation levels and is associated with retrocochlear lesions.
137	What are appropriate ages to administer the different methods of behavioral audiometric testing in children?	• 0 to 5 months: Behavioral observation audiometry • 5 months to 2 years: Visual reinforcement audiometry • 2 to 5 years: Conditioned play audiometry • 5 + years: Conventional audiometry
138	Describe how *behavioral observation audiometry* is performed.	The tester evaluates for changes in patient behavior (e.g., quieting, eye widening, startle) after presentation of unconditioned sound.
139	Describe how *visual reinforcement audiometry* is performed.	The participant is conditioned to provide a specific response when he or she is able to hear a sound. For example, a child turns the head toward the sound source and a toy lights up to reward the behavior.
140	Describe how conditioned play audiometry is performed.	The participant is conditioned to perform a play activity (e.g., throw a ball, drop a block) when he or she is able to hear a sound. After the child has demonstrated that he or she understands the "game," sound is presented at varying levels to determine frequency specific hearing thresholds and speech reponse threshold.
141	What physiologic process generates the auditory brainstem response?	Synchronized responses of specific neuron populations within the auditory pathway, with later waves corresponding to neuron groups farther down the transmission pathway: • Wave 1: Distal (lateral) auditory nerve • Wave 2: Proximal (medial) auditory nerve • Wave 3: Cochlear nucleus • Wave 4: Superior olivary complex • Wave 5: Lateral lemniscus/inferior colliculus

142	Why Is ABR testing useful in evaluating for retrocochlear pathology?	Abnormally long delays between waves (interpeak latency of Wave 1–5) suggest pathology, such as vestibular schwannoma, that is affecting the conductivity of the neurons that connect structures in the auditory pathway.
143	What types of audiometry can be used for evaluation of congenital hearing loss in a 2-month-old infant?	Behavioral observation audiometry, ABR, and otoacoustic emissions
144	What are *otoacoustic emissions*?	*Otoacoustic emissions* are sound generated by outer hair cells, either spontaneously or evoked by an auditory stimulus, that can be detected by a microphone. They are considered a form of objective audiometry because they do not rely on patient participation. Generally, this type of testing is capable of detecting losses greater than 30 to 40 dB.
145	What is the advantage of distortion product otoacoustic emissions over transient evoked otoacoustic emissions?	They are capable of providing frequency specific information.
146	What ABR pattern is expected in children with auditory neuropathy?	Severely abnormal or absent ABR with a present cochlear microphonic and otoacoustic emission response
147	Describe the following tympanometry patterns (modified Jerger classification) : As, A, Ad, B, and C. (▶ Fig. 6.5)	Tympanometry tests tympanic membrane (TM) compliance (admittance vs middle ear pressure). • Type A: Normal • Type As (shallow): Stiffened or hypomobile TM, ossicular fixation (e.g., otosclerosis, tympanosclerosis, malleus fixation), or "glue ear" • Type Ad (deep): Flaccid or hypermobile TM, ossicular discontinuity, or flaccid TM • Type B: Flat tracing with no compliance peak. Must combine with canal volume (normal child-adult 0.5 to 1.5 ml) • Type B (large volume): TM perforation or patent tympanostomy tube • Type B (normal volume): Middle ear fluid • Type B (small volume): Cerumen occlusion or probe against side wall of EAC • Type C: Left shift in peak (negative middle ear pressure) associated with eustachian tube dysfunction

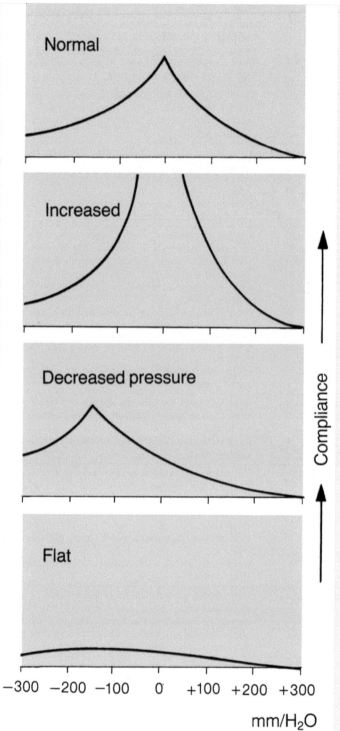

Fig. 6.5 Tympanograms (from top to bottom): Type A: normal; Type Ad (deep): Flaccid or hypermobile tympanic membrane (TM). Ossicular discontinuity or flaccid TM; Type C: Left shift in peak (negative middle ear pressure) associated with Eustachian tube dysfunction; Type B: Flat tracing with no compliance peak. In this case small volume may indicate cerumen occlusion or probe against side wall of EAC, while large volume may indicate TM perforation. (Used with permission from Becker W, Naumann HH, Pfaltz CR. Ear, Nose, and Throat Diseases. New York, NY: Thieme; 1994.)

148	Describe how *stapedial reflex testing* is performed.	Tympanometry of the ipsilateral and contralateral tympanic membrane is measured when sound, typically between 80 to 110 dB hearing level, is applied to the ear at different frequencies (500, 1,000, 2,000, and 4,000 Hz). A stapedial reflex is measured as a decrease in compliance, resulting from stapedial muscle contraction.
149	Describe conditions that may result in an absent or abnormal stapedial reflex.	Conductive hearing loss (e.g., otosclerosis, middle ear disease), severe SNHL, eighth nerve pathology (e.g., vestibular schwannoma), ipsilateral seventh nerve pathology (e.g., Bell palsy)
150	Describe the pattern of stapedial reflex testing seen with right-sided retrocochlear pathology.	• The reflexes are always absent when stimulated in the ipsilateral ear. • Left-sided stimulus: Left response present, right response present • Right-sided stimulus: Left response absent/elevated, right response absent/elevated
151	Describe the stapedial reflex pattern seen with a thick mucoid effusion in the right ear (type B tympanogram) causing a large conductive hearing loss.	• Middle ear effusion can result in dampening of the incoming auditory signal. Also, stapedial reflex detection can be impaired from decreased tympanic membrane compliance. • Left-sided stimulus: Left response present, right response absent/elevated • Right-sided stimulus: Left response absent/elevated, right response absent/elevated
152	Describe the stapedial reflex pattern seen with bilateral thick middle ear mucoid effusions (type B tympanogram) causing significant conductive hearing loss.	• Left-sided stimulus: Left response absent, right response absent • Right-sided stimulus: Left response absent, right response absent
153	Describe the stapedial reflex pattern seen with proximal right-sided facial nerve pathology.	• The reflexes on the ipsilateral side will be affected. • Left-sided stimulus: Left response present, right response absent • Right-sided stimulus: lLft response present, right response absent
154	Describe the stapedial reflex pattern seen with a large intra-axial brainstem lesion.	• In practice, the response depends largely on the location of the lesion. However, if the intra-axial lesion is large and affects the bilateral cochlear nuclei and/or the bilateral seventh nerve motor nuclei, then the following pattern may result. • Left-sided stimulus: Left response absent, right response absent • Right-sided stimulus: Left response absent, right response absent
155	Describe the phenomenon of *acoustic decay*.	A stimulus is presented in the ear of concern and a contralateral probe is placed. A continuous pure-tone stimulus is presented 10 dB above the stapedial reflex threshold and held for 10 seconds. The test is positive if the magnitude of the reflex drops by more than 50% in 10 seconds.
156	What is the difference between the *speech awareness (detection) threshold* and the *speech reception threshold*?	• *Speech awareness threshold* is the minimum volume level (in dB hearing level) at which the subject is able to detect the presence of speech stimuli 50% of the time (although the subject does not need to recognize the word). • *Speech reception threshold* is the minimum volume level at which the subject is able to correctly identify a presented word (usually a spondee) 50% of the time.

157	If a patient is found to have a PTA of 40-dB hearing level, what can be predicted regarding this patient's speech detection threshold and speech reception threshold?	Both should correspond with the PTA (average of pure-tone thresholds at 500, 1,000, and 2,000 Hz) within approximately 5 to 10 dB.
158	If there is significant discordance between the pure tone average and the speech detection threshold, what diagnosis should be strongly considered?	Exaggerated hearing loss or pseudohypacusis (factitious hearing loss)
159	Described the methods that can be used to evaluate for factitious hearing loss.	• Objective audiometry: OAE and ABR • Behavioral audiometry: Discrepancy between speech reception test (SRT) and PTA; significant difference in test-retest scores (> 15 dB) • Acoustic reflex testing • Lombard test, Stenger test
160	Describe the *Stenger test*.	Based on the principle that if tones of the same frequency are presented simultaneously to both ears, only the loudest is perceived. Two simultaneous tones with matched frequency are introduced, but the alleged poor ear receives a tone at a greater intensity (usually > 20 dB). The truthful patient with normal hearing will report the sound in the ear with the loudest sound level; the truthful patient with asymmetric hearing loss will report the sound in the better hearing ear; and the untruthful subject will deny hearing any sound.
161	Describe the *Lombard test*.	Noise is introduced into the ear with supposed hearing loss while the patient is asked to read. The noise level is gradually increased until the patient raises his or her voice or stops reading. If there is no change in the loudness of voice, this would support a true hearing loss.

Pediatric Hearing Loss

162	Which intrauterine infections are associated with the development of congenital hearing loss?	**T** Toxoplasmosis **O** Other, including syphilis, varicella, and parvovirus B19 **R** Rubella **C** Cytomegalovirus **H** Herpes simplex virus
163	What factors place a pediatric patient at particularly high risk for early SNHL?	• History of intrauterine infection • Family history of congenital hearing loss • Low birth weight (< 1,500 g) • Hyperbilirubinemia • Prolonged neonatal intensive care unit stay or prolonged mechanical ventilation • Concurrent craniofacial anomalies • Exposure to ototoxic medications • < 5 Apgar score at 1 minute, < 7 Apgar score at 5 minutes • Bacterial meningitis
164	What percentage of congenital hearing loss is genetic?	Approximately 50%
165	What percentage of patients with genetic hearing loss will have associated syndromes?	About 70% of genetic hearing loss is nonsyndromic, and 30% is syndromic.
166	What percentage of genetic hearing loss is inherited in an autosomal dominant pattern?	80% autosomal recessive, 20% autosomal dominant
167	What is the most common form of autosomal dominant hearing loss?	Waardenburg syndrome

168	Describe the four subtypes of Waardenburg syndrome.	• WS1: Autosomal dominant, dystopia canthorum, SNHL, iris pigmentary disorder, hair hypopigmentation • WS2: Autosomal dominant, no dystopia canthorum, SNHL, iris pigmentary disorder, hair hypopigmentation • WS3: Autosomal dominant, dystopia canthorum, upper limb abnormalities, iris pigmentation disorder, hair hypopigmentation • WS4: Autosomal recessive, no dystopia canthorum, Hirschprung disease, SNHL, iris pigmentary disorder, hair hypopigmentation
169	What are the three most common causes of autosomal recessive syndromic SNHL?	Usher, Pendred, Jervell and Lange-Nielsen
170	Describe the three subtypes of Usher syndrome.	• Type 1: Bilateral profound deafness and vestibulopathy at birth; "night blindness," from retinitis pigmentosa, before teens (most severe form) • Type 2: Moderate to severe hearing loss at birth, worsening vision in young adulthood, and normal vestibular function • Type 3: Normal hearing at birth with progressive hearing loss and retinopathy by teens, variable vestibular involvement (mild form)
171	What is the most common cause of deaf-blindness in the United States?	Usher syndrome
172	Alport syndrome involves faulty synthesis of what protein(s)?	Type IV collagen
173	Describe the clinical manifestations of Norrie disease.	X-linked recessive syndrome that results in early rapidly progressive blindness. Progressive SNHL occurs in approximately a third of patients and usually ensues in the second to third decades of life.
174	Describe the classic head and neck manifestations of Pendred syndrome.	SNHL (often associated with enlarged vestibular aqueducts and mondini malformations) and euthyroid goiter
175	Describe the thyroid pathology typically seen in Pendred syndrome.	Patients often develop a multinodular goiter in the second decade of life but are usually euthyroid and rarely require intervention.
176	What specific precaution should patients diagnosed with enlarged vestibular aqueduct syndrome take to prevent further hearing loss?	Stepwise progression of hearing loss can be seen after minor head trauma. Participation in contact sports or activities associated with "minor head trauma" should generally be avoided.
177	Describe the typical presentation of enlarged vestibular aqueduct syndrome.	SNHL generally begins in childhood and often progresses in a stepwise manner. Vestibular symptoms and mixed hearing loss may also develop.
178	What gene mutation is responsible for approximately 50% of all cases of genetic hearing loss?	*GJB2* encodes connexin 26, located on chromosome 13, autosomal recessive inheritance pattern
179	What does the *GJB2* gene code for?	Gap junction β-2, responsible for potassium ion exchange of the inner ear
180	Describe the clinical manifestations of Jervell and Lange-Nielsen syndrome.	• An autosomal recessive syndrome characterized by congenital profound bilateral SNHL and arrhythmia • Patients may have syncopal episodes provoked by stress or exercise. • Sudden cardiac death from arrhythmia may occur if untreated. • Caused by a defect in potassium channels within the stria vascularis

181	Descrie the electrocardiographic findings in Jervell and Lange-Nielsen syndrome.	Long QTc (> 500 ms) with potential for arrhythmias
182	Describe the constellation of findings seen in MELAS syndrome.	**ME** Mitochondrial encephalopathy **LA** Lactic acidosis **S** Stroke Manifestations are variable and include hearing loss, limb weakness, partial paralysis, vision loss and seizures.
183	Describe the clinical features of Michel aplasia.	Michel aplasia is characterized by complete failure of inner ear development resulting in congenital anacusis.
184	Describe the radiographic findings with Mondini malformations.	Mondini malformation accounts for more than 50% of cochlear malformations. The characteristic findings include an incomplete or absent partition and less than 2.5 turns.
185	Describe the imaging findings of a common cavity malformation.	The cochlea and vestibule are joined as a single large confluent space. These patients typically have severe to profound SNHL.
186	What inner ear abnormalities are seen in Scheibe dysplasia?	*Scheibe dysplasia* (also called *cochlearsaccular dysplasia* or *pars inferior dysplasia*) includes a poorly developed organ of Corti and sacuule, whereas the bony labyrinth, semicircular canals, and utricle are preserved.
187	What is the most common form of membranous labyrinth dysplasia?	Scheibe dysplasia
188	What frequencies are most commonly affected by Alexander dysplasia?	High frequencies resulting from malformation of the cochlear duct and basal turn of the cochlea

Adult Hearing Loss

189	Where is the site of damage in chronic noise-induced SNHL?	Outer hair cells are damaged with chronic exposure to loud noise. With brief exposure to extremely loud sound (e.g., explosions), the impulse can lead to trauma of the cochlear membranes.
190	Describe the characteristic audiogram findings with noise-induced hearing loss.	4-kHZ notch. Hearing loss is almost always bilateral and is greater in the high frequencies compared with lower frequencies.
191	Describe the Occupational Safety and Health Administration (OSHA) sound level requirements.	If workplace noise levels are > 85 dB averaged over an 8-hour period, a hearing-conservation program is required with regular testing. Permissible noise exposure levels are based on duration: 8 hours at 90 dB; 6 hours at 92 dB; 4 hours at 95 dB; 3 hours at 97 dB; 2 hours at 100 dB; 1.5 hours at 102 dB; 1 hour at 105 dB; 0.5 hours at 110 dB; 0.25 hours at 115 dB
192	What is the definition of *sudden sensorineural hearing loss*?	Greater than 30 dB loss over three contiguous pure-tone frequencies occurring within a 3-day period
193	What percentage of patients with sudden SNHL can expect to experience some degree of spontaneous recovery?	Approximately two-thirds of patients
194	Describe the evaluation of sudden SNHL.	Patients should be evaluated for retrocochlear pathology (MRI with gadolinium), but routine laboratory testing should not be pursued unless there is clinical suspicion for an underlying cause based on history or physical examination.
195	Review the treatment of idiopathic sudden SNHL.	Options include early oral corticosteroid treatment and hyperbaric oxygen therapy within 3 months of diagnosis. Intratympanic steroid perfusion is offered to patients with incomplete recovery after initial therapy. Routine use of antivirals, thrombolytics, vasodilators, vasoactive substances, or antioxidants should be avoided.

196	What is the role of CT in evaluating patients with sudden SNHL?	Generally, MRI is preferred over CT. Relative exceptions include patients with focal neurologic findings, recent head trauma, severe claustrophobia, or devices that preclude MRI scanning (e.g., certain pacemakers).
197	What clinical variables are associated with a more favorable prognosis after sudden SNHL?	Young age, less severe hearing loss, absence of dizziness, low-frequency pattern of hearing loss, early treatment
198	Describe the diagnostic criteria for primary autoimmune inner ear disease.	Characterized by progressive (over weeks to months) bilateral SNHL loss that responds to immunosuppressive treatment (steroids). Other causes of progressive SNHL must be ruled out.
199	What is the first line of treatment for suspected autoimmune inner ear disease?	High-dose corticosteroids with a prolonged taper
200	What is the 68-kD inner ear antigen?	About 20 to 80% of patients with autoimmune inner ear disease will have a positive anti-68 kDa antibody test.
201	Describe the clinical manifestations of Susac syndrome.	An autoimmune small vessel disease characterized by the triad of encephalopathy, branch retinal artery occlusions and SNHL
202	Describe the clinical manifestations of Cogan syndrome.	A syndrome of nonsyphilitic interstitial keratitis and audio-vestibular symptoms. Most patients have bilateral sudden progressive SNHL. Dizziness is typically episodic. Although bilateral interstitial keratitis occurs, vision loss is rare. Systemic manifestations commonly include headache and fever.
203	What are the potential routes of communication that permit inner ear involvement in patients with meningitis?	Cochlear aqueduct and modiolus
204	Which organisms are associated with the highest risk of post-meningitic SNHL?	• *Streptococcus pneumoniae* • *Neisseria meningitidis* • *Haemophilus influenzae*
205	What percent aggeof patients with bacterial meningitis will develop SNHL?	15 to 20%; 5% have profound loss
206	Review the common otologic manifestations of Wegener granulomatosis?	Conductive hearing loss and chronic serous otitis media are most common; however, otalgia, facial palsy, vertigo, SNHL, and external ear involvement can also be seen.

Tinnitus

207	Describe the differential diagnosis of pulsatile "fluttering" tinnitus that is not synchronous with arterial pulse.	Myoclonus of the tensor tympani, stapedius, or palatal musculature
208	Provide a differential diagnosis for pulsatile tinnitus.	• Arterial: Aberrant internal carotid artery, carotid athero-sclerosis, persistent stapedial artery, arteriovenous mal-formations, aneurysm, carotid artery dissection, vascular compression of cranial nerve eight, vascular tumors (glomus) • Venous: Jugular bulb abnormalities (high-riding, dehis-cence, diverticulum), idiopathic intracranial hypertension, idiopathic pulsatile tinnitus (venous hum) • Nonvascular: Palatal, stapedial, and tensor tympani myoclonus
209	What is the prevalence of carotid artery dehis-cence within the middle ear?	Approximately 10%, but rarely does it follow an aberrant course placing it at risk during myringotomy
210	What otoscopic findings might make you suspect a dehiscent or high riding jugular bulb?	The most likely area to visualize a dehiscent jugular bulb in the middle ear is behind the posterior inferior quadrant of the tympanic membrane, where a dark blue and possibly pulsatile structure may be seen.

211	What is the clinical significance of an empty sella in a patient with pulsatile tinnitus?	Associated with elevated intracranial hypertension (idiopathic intracranial hypertension)
212	Describe the clinical manifestations of idiopathic intracranial hypertension syndrome.	The most common symptoms are headache (~ 90%) and then pulsatile tinnitus (~ 70%). Other signs and symptoms including extremity paresthesias, generalized weakness, hyposmia, abducens palsy, facial paresis, and incoordination are reported more rarely.
213	What constellation of symptoms is commonly associated with patulous eustachian tube?	Tinnitus, aural fullness, autophony, audible respiratory sounds, and vertigo
214	List common medications that may cause tinnitus.	Aspirin-containing products (most common), other non-steroidal anti-inflammatory drugs (or NSAIDs), aminoglycosides, proton pump inhibitors (omeprazole, esomeprazole), and certain antidepressants
215	What device (nonmedicinal) options are available for patients with subjective nonpulsatile idiopathic tinnitus?	Hearing aids, masking devices (deliver constant narrow-band white noise to "cover up" ringing), and tinnitus retraining therapy (pitch matched to the patient's tinnitus to theoretically habituate the central auditory system to the noise and eventually neglect it). Cochlear implants improve tinnitus in some patients, but tinnitus itself is not an indication for implantation.

Hearing Aids and Implantable Hearing Devices

216	What are assistive listening devices?	Auditory and nonauditory technologies that overcome limitations associated with the physical distance between the sound source and the patient
217	Provide examples of auditory and nonauditory assistive listening devices.	• *Auditory*: Microphone systems that capture the desired sound next to the sound source and transport the signal to the listener using FM, infrared, induction loop, Bluetooth, or hard-wired systems • *Nonauditory*: Alarm systems using vibrotactlile or visual signals to alert the patient of an event such as a phone ringing or doorbell activation
218	What conservative measures should be discussed with patients who have hearing impairment?	Strategic seating at meetings or events (better ear toward speaker, sitting close to the front), making eye contact with speakers, reducing competing background noise
219	Describe the basic components of a hearing aid.	Microphone, amplifier, receiver, power supply
220	Define *gain* as it pertains to conventional hearing aids.	*Gain* is the difference between the level of input and level of output at any given frequency.
221	What advantages do vented hearing aids provide?	Decrease in external auditory canal moisture, decrease in occlusion effect, dissipation of low frequency input (advantageous in patients with primarily high-frequency hearing loss).
222	What factors should be considered in predicting patient satisfaction with traditional hearing aids?	The best candidates are motivated patients who are receptive to the idea of hearing aid use. Those with predominantly high-frequency hearing loss generally do better than those with low-frequency hearing loss. Severe to profound hearing loss is often difficult to aid. Suprathreshold speech and speech recognition performance is important; patients with good word recognition when amplification is provided are more likely to report satisfaction and continued device use.
223	Describe the difference between the *speech reception threshold* and the *speech discrimination score*.	*Speech reception threshold* is the quietest volume (in dB) at which presented spondaic words can be identified at least 50% of the time, whereas the *speech discrimination score* is the percentage of time that a presented word is correctly identified.

224	Describe the advantages and disadvantages of the completely-in-canal and the in-the-canal hearing aid.	• *Advantages*: Discreet size offering enhanced cosmesis; takes advantage of the ear's innate shape assisting with natural sound amplification and limiting undesirable wind noise • *Disadvantages*: Power limitations, cerumen clogging, aural fullness and occlusion effect, difficult fit, fine dexterity requirements, cost, and external ear canal irritation
225	Describe the advantages and disadvantages of the in-the-ear hearing aid.	• *Advantages*: Delivers adequate power to rehabilitate mild to moderately severe losses, more powerful, and easier to manipulate than in-the-canal models • *Disadvantages*: Require some manual dexterity for placement and volume control. Less discreet than in-the-canal models
226	Describe the advantages and disadvantages of the behind-the-ear hearing aid.	• *Advantages*: Most adaptable hearing aid option; delivers enough power to rehabilitate moderately severe to severe hearing loss; generally offers more signal processing features; and is easier to handle than smaller devices in patients with poor manual dexterity • Disadvantages: Larger size, less discreet, pinna irritation
227	What is the primary advantage of a body aid?	With severe-to-profound hearing loss, feedback problems occur with ear-level devices because of the close proximity of the microphone to the receiver. The body aid places the microphone at a distant site from the amplifier, typically on a belt or in a pocket.
228	With regard to hearing aid technologies, what are the primary advantages of digital processing compared with analogue processing?	Beyond affording multiple programs, digital signal processors can selectively amplify specified frequencies, reduce acoustic feedback and background noise, automatically detect changes in listening environments to dynamically optimize signal, and offer enhanced connectivity to external sound sources.
229	What are directional microphones, and what advantages do they have over standard omnidirectional technologies?	Directional microphones selectively amplify sounds located in front of the listener, improving the signal-to-noise ratio. Adaptive directional microphones go one step further and are able to vary the direction of maximal amplification.
230	Describe the utility of a CROS and BiCROS aid.	The CROS (contralateral routing of signal) aid takes sound from the poorer ear and relays the signal to the better, contralateral ear. The BiCROS (bilateral contralateral routing of signal) aid similarly "throws" sound to the good ear but also amplifies sound in the receiving ear.
231	Which patients are candidates for bone-anchored hearing aid placement?	Currently, bone-anchored hearing aids are approved for children 5 years of age or older, patients with conductive or mixed hearing loss who can derive benefit from sound amplification, and patients with single-sided deafness and normal hearing in the contralateral ear.
232	What cells are directly stimulated by cochlear implant electrodes?	Spiral ganglion cells, found in the modiolus of the cochlea
233	If facial nerve stimulation occurs with cochlear implant use, how should this be managed?	The offending electrodes can be selectively deactivated or removed from the patient's programming strategy.
234	What are the Food and Drug Administration (FDA)'s audiometric candidacy criteria for cochlear implantation?	Severe to profound SNHL (> 70 dB PTA), with < 50% sentence testing in the ear to be implanted, and < 60% in the contralateral ear or best aided condition
235	List absolute contraindications to cochlear implantation.	Absent cochlea, congenitally absent cochlear nerve, deafness secondary to brainstem lesion, previously resected cochlear nerve

236	Describe clinical variables that are associated with good cochlear implant performance.	Age at implantation, prelingual versus postlingual deafness, duration of deafness, preimplant auditory performance, duration of cochlear implant use
237	What is the most common indication for revision cochlear implant surgery (reimplantation)?	Documented internal device failure
238	What conditions are associated with an unusually high prevalence of nonauditory stimulation (pain, vertigo, facial nerve activation) with cochlear implant use?	• *Otosclerosis*: Otic capsule bone is replaced with less dense otospongiotic bone, which may permit aberrant stimulation pathways, resulting in a higher prevalence of facial nerve stimulation. • *Temporal bone fracture*: Similarly, previous temporal bone fractures may allow abnormal electrical stimulation, frequently associated with pain.
239	Describe the benefits of bilateral cochlear implantation.	Improved speech understanding in noise and directional awareness, as well as the assurance that the "best performing ear" has been implanted
240	Theoretically, what is the ideal position of the cochlear implant electrode within the cochlea?	Perimodiolar within the scala tympani
241	Describe the potential advantages of implantable middle ear hearing aids.	Enhanced cosmesis, comfort, discrimination, minimized feedback, elimination of occlusion effect, permits amplification during bathing or swimming
242	Review the candidacy criteria for implantable middle ear hearing devices.	Candidates should be ≥ 18 years old, have moderate to severe SNHL, and have trialed conventional amplification before implantation. Pediatric patients, those with recurrent or chronic middle ear disease, patients with poor word discrimination, and subjects with fluctuating loss should not undergo implantation.
243	What is the mechanism behind implantable middle ear hearing aids?	They use either piezoelectric or electromagnetic platforms that transform sound signal into mechanical energy that is directly coupled to the ossicular chain.
244	Review the primary implant criteria for auditory brainstem implantation in the United States.	Bilateral eighth nerve schwannomas (neurofibromatosis type 2, or NF-2), age ≥ 12 years
245	What is the typical outcome with auditory brainstem implantation in patients with NF-2?	Most patients receive limited sound perception that augments lip reading. Few patients experience open-set speech understanding.

Disorders of the External Ear

246	What are risk factors for development of cerumen impaction?	Use of cotton-tip applicators, narrow canals, hearing aid use, earplug or earphone use, hair in the lateral external auditory canal, developmental delay, advanced age
247	Describe the function(s) of cerumen?	• Cleansing, lubrication, and antimicrobial (bacteria and fungus) activity • Lysozyme, saturated fatty acids, and lower pH of cerumen provide antifungal and antibacterial properties.
248	What audiometric findings would you expect to see in a patient with severe cerumen impaction?	• A predominantly high-frequency conductive hearing loss • Low-volume type B tympanograms
249	Describe the clinical presentation of chondrodermatitis nodularis chronica helicis.	Intensly painful nodule located on the helix or antihelix that is commonly pale gray or erythematous
250	What is the appropriate age for repair in patients with bilateral microtia and congenital aural atresia?	Generally, any repair for microtia or atresia is delayed until the patient is at least 6 years of age.
251	Review the common sequence of repair during microtia surgery.	1. Helix formation with rib cartilage 2. Lobule formation 3. Atresiaplasty 4. Formation of the tragus 5. Postauricular release

| 252 | What is the most appropriate initial treatment for an infant with bilateral congenital aural atresia? (▶ Table 6.1) | The most appropriate treatment is application of bone-conduction hearing aids. Providing amplification is crucial for early hearing and language development, although surgical procedures (bone-anchored hearing aid or atresia-plasty) are generally delayed until the patient is at least 5 years old. |

Table 6.1 Jahrsdoerfer grading scale score for congenital aural atresia.

Anatomical structure	Score
stapes bone	2
oval window open	1
middle ear space	1
facial nerve	1
malleus-incus complex	1
mastoid pneumatization	1
incus-stapes connection	1
round window	1
external ear	1
Total Possible Score	10

Data from Jahrsdoerfer RA, Yeakley JW, Aguilar EA, Cole RR, Gray LC. Grading system for the selection of patients with congenital aural atresia. Am J Otol. 1992;13(1): 6–12.

253	What are the indications for surgical treatment of external auditory canal exostoses?	In patients with chronic or recurrent otitis externa, trapping of debris, or if a conductive hearing impairment develops, surgical treatment is indicated.
254	How can exostoses be differentiated from osteomas on clinical examination?	Exostoses are most commonly multiple, medial, and frequently bilateral, as opposed to osteomas, which exist as single lesions.
255	Where are osteomas of the ear canal most likely to develop?	The bony cartilaginous junction
256	Review the indications for otomicroscopic removal of an ear canal foreign body (as opposed to blind removal with lavage).	Foreign-body type (e.g., sharp edges, disk battery, vegetable matter), location adjacent to the tympanic membrane, time > 24 hours in the ear canal, failed previous attempts at removal, in children younger than 4 years
257	What is the most appropriate initial treatment for patients with severe frostbite of the auricle?	Rapid rewarming of the ear with warm (38 to 42°C) saline-soaked gauze
258	Describe the examination findings of keratosis obturans.	Keratosis obturans demonstrates a dense plug of keratin that completely blocks and may widen the EAC. An important distinction between keratosus obturans and canal cholesteatoma is that keratosis obturans involves the entire circumference of the ear canal while cholesteatoma often has focal erosion.
259	Describe the treatment for psoriasis of the EAC.	This condition is treated in a similar fashion to psoriasis elsewhere. First-line treatments include simple warm-water soaks, application of occlusive ointments (e.g., petrolatum), avoidance of trauma, and use of topical corticosteroids. Other specialized topical or systemic treatments (e.g., methotrexate, cyclcosporin, retinoids) are generally reserved for those with extensive disease.

260	What are clinical manifestations of relapsing polychondritis?	Most common initial symptom is inflammation of the auricle that spares the lobule. Additional organ systems include the joints, nose (nasal chondritis), eyes (conjunctivitis, scleritis, iritis, keratitis), respiratory tract (laryngeal or tracheal inflammation), inner ear, cardiovascular system, and skin.
261	Describe the appearance of seborrheic dermatitis of the auricle.	• Inflammatory condition of the skin, generally limited to oil-rich regions • It occurs with a wide range of severity, from mild dandruff and flaking to a generalized exfoliating erythroderma. • It can be restricted to the ears but more often involves additional areas such as the scalp, face, upper trunk, and axillae.
262	Describe the clinical presentation of auricular tophi.	Moderately painful pink nodules most commonly involving the helix that contain chalky white material.
263	What is the most commonly cultured organism from the EAC of patients with otitis externa?	*Pseudomonas aeruginosa*
264	Why is water exposure a risk factor for acute otitis externa?	It can lead to loss of the acidic enviroment of the EAC. In addition, unclean water may carry a high bacterial load.
265	In the presence of a tympanostomy tube or tympanic membrane perforation, how should therapy for acute otitis externa be modified?	Potentially ototoxic medications should be avoided. Specifically, alcoholic and acidic drops should not be used, as well as antibiotics with known cochlear toxicity including aminoglycosides.
266	What is considered first-line therapy for uncomplicated acute otitis externa?	• Pain control, aural toilet, application of ototopical treatments (acidifying/drying agents, antibiotic preparations with or without corticosteroids), and avoidance of risk factors such as water exposure and ear canal trauma • Systemic antibiotics are not indicated for uncomplicated acute otitis externa in an otherwise healthy patient.
267	Describe common initial treatments for fungal otitis externa.	• Acidifying (aluminum sulfate-calcium acetate) or drying agents (boric acid) • Antifungal creams such as clotrimazole may also be used.
268	What treatment may be used for patients with chronic hypertrophic otitis externa refractory to maximal medical therapy?	Canaloplasty with split-thickness skin graft resurfacing of the EAC and a generous meatoplasty
269	Describe the clinical features of infectious perichondritis and chondritis of the auricle.	Otalgia and pruritus are the most common symptoms. The auricle is tender, erythematous, and may have flaking/weeping over the cartilaginous portions of the auricle with sparing of the fatty lobule. Risk factors include trauma and otitis externa.
270	What is the most commonly cultured fungus in cases of otomycosis?	*Aspergillus* spp.
271	Define *malignant* (or *necrotizing*) *otitis externa*.	Malignant otitis externa is progressive osteomyelitis of the temporal bone that has spread from the external auditory canal. The causative organism is most often *Pseudomonas aeruginosa,* and this condition ccurs almost exclusively in immunocompromised individuals (commonly elderly diabetics).
272	What nuclear medicine study is most helpful in establishing the diagnosis of necrotizing otitis externa?	Technetium-99 m bone scan detects osteoblastic activity and is useful for initial diagnosis of osteomyelitis. However, even after the infection has resolved, the scan remains positive, making it less useful for monitoring response to therapy.

273	What nuclear medicine study is most helpful in evaluating treatment response in patients with necrotizing otitis externa?	Gallium-67 nuclear medicine scan is useful for detection of inflammation, although its spatial resolution is poor. It is a useful adjunct to MRI for the diagnosis of necrotizing otitis externa. It is also useful in following response to treatment.
274	Describe the mangement of malignant otitis externa.	Malignant otitis externa is managed primarily with medical therapy, including 6 + weeks of broad-spectrum antibiotics (covering *Pseudomas* spp.), aggressive aural toilet, and strict glucose control for diabetics. Hyperbaric oxygen therapy is useful for patients with refractory or advanced disease. Surgical intervention is reserved for patients with refractory disease or associated abscess.
275	What is the treatment of bullous myringitis?	• Decompression of painful vesicles, oral pain medication, and systemic antibiotics • Steroids may be used in cases of sensorineural hearing loss.

Disorders of the Middle Ear

276	What antibiotic is considered first-line therapy for an otherwise healthy child with acute otitis media?	Amoxicillin, 90 mg/kg daily, divided into two doses each day for 10 days
277	What predisposing factors may put young children at risk for recurrent otitis media?	• Second-hand smoke exposure, group day care, nasal allergy, immunodeficiency, craniofacial abnormalities, adenoid hypertrophy, gastroesophageal reflux, vaccination status, supine bottle feeding, and pacifier use • Breastfeeding in the first 6 months of life is likely protective against recurrent acute otitis media.
278	What factors impact a child's candidacy for surgery to treat otitis media with effusion?	Hearing status, associated symptoms, duration of effusion (> 4 months), structural damage to the TM or middle ear, developmental delays or risk factors for delay (syndromic children, autism-spectrum disorders, uncorrectable visual impairment, etc.), craniofacial abnormalities/cleft palate
279	What condition must be excluded in all adult patients with a unilateral persistent middle ear effusion?	• Nasopharyngeal carcinoma should be ruled out by nasopharyngoscopy. • Examination of the oropharynx, hypopharynx, and larynx should also be performed if otalgia is present.
280	Define *atticotomy*, and describe the typical indications of this approach in the context of chronic ear disease.	Atticotomy involves removal of a portion of the scutum (lateral epitympanic wall) to visualize and access the epitympanum. This technique is often used in patients with limited cholesteatoma or retraction pockets and small contracted mastoids and can be performed in conjuction with tympanoplasty and ossicular chain reconstruction.
281	Define *congenital cholesteatoma*.	Caused by a persistent embryonic rest of epithelial tissue within the middle ear space. Patients should have a normal-appearing pars tensa and pars flaccida, no history of prior otorrhea, and no prior otologic surgery.
282	Differentiate *primary acquired* and *secondary acquired cholesteatoma*.	*Primary* acquired cholesteatoma arises from a tympanic membrane retraction pocket most commonly involving the pars flaccida; *secondary* acquired cholesteatoma results from an injury to the tympanic membrane (e.g., tympanostomy tube, surgery, accidental trauma) with implantation of skin into the middle ear space.
283	Describe the invagination theory of primary acquired cholesteatoma formation.	Infantile sterile otitis media develops shortly after birth. Before resorption occurs, mucosal fibrosis occurs, resulting in blockage of the epitymanum and localized negative pressure. This results in poor pneumatization of the mastoid and retraction of the pars flaccida.

284	Describe the metaplasia theory of acquired cholesteatoma formation.	Columnar epithelium of the middle ear space undergoes squamous metaplasia, resulting from inflammation associated with recurrent otitis media.
285	Describe the proposed mechanisms of bony erosion by cholesteatoma.	• Pressure erosion: Caused by mechanical pressure from the growing cholesteatoma sac • Biochemical erosion: Bacterial products, inflammation from granulation tissue, and enzyme products of the cholesteatoma itself • Cellular-mediated erosion: Osteoclastic activity
286	Define *Prussak space*.	Prussak space is a recess, bordered laterally by the pars flaccida, superiorly by the scutum and lateral malleolar ligament, inferiorly by the short process of the malleus, and medially by the neck of the malleus.
287	Describe the three most common sites of origin for cholesteatoma.	Posterior and anterior epitympanum and the posterosuperior mesotympanum
288	Describe the anatomical limits of the sinus tympani.	Ponticulus superiorly, subiculum inferiorly, the mastoid segment of the facial nerve laterally, and the posterior semicircular canal medially
289	What is the most common site of labyrinthine fistula formation secondary to chronic ear disease?	The horizontal semicircular canal
290	Describe the signs and symptoms of labyrinthine fistula secondary to chronic otitis media.	Labyrinthine fistula most commonly involves the lateral semicircular canal. Classically, patients show mixed hearing loss, intermittent dizziness, and potentially sound-induced vertigo (Tullio phenomenon), although in practice a large number of patients may lack such findings.
291	Describe the likely mechanism of dizziness associated pneumatic otoscopy in a patient with cholesteatoma.	Cholesteatoma eroding into the bony labyrinth has most likely led to an inner ear fistula. With the labyrinth exposed, increased middle ear pressure can be translated to perilymphatic fluid movement and subsequent vertigo.
292	How should a lateral semicircular canal fistula associated with chronic ear disease be managed?	In an "only hearing ear" or "better hearing ear," a canal wall–down procedure is often recommended, with exteriorization of the matrix overlying the erosion. If the other ear has good hearing, same-surgery repair with fascia or a second-look procedure with matrix removal may be considered if an intact canal wall is desired. Large or complex fistulae have a high risk of SNHL and are generally best managed with a canal wall–down procedure.
293	What is the difference between a *radical* and *modified radical mastoidectomy*?	With a *radical mastoidectomy*, there is complete removal of the malleus, incus, tympanic membrane, and middle ear mucosa, and the cavity is left open. With a *modified radical mastoidectomy*, the middle ear space is reconstructed. A *Bondy modified radical mastoidectomy* implies a canal wall–down procedure where the middle ear space is not entered or reconstructed.
294	Describe the Wullstein classification system for tympanoplasty.	• Type 1: All ossicles are present and mobile. • Type 2: The tympanic membrane is grafted to an intact incus and stapes. • Type 3: The tympanic membrane is grafted to the stapes superstructure. • Type 4: The tympanic membrane is grafted to the stapes footplate. • Type 5: Semicircular canal fenestration procedure
295	What are common indications for canal wall–down mastoidectomy?	Advanced cholesteatoma with significant canal wall erosion, labyrinthine fistula, cholesteatoma in an only hearing ear

296	What are the most common causes of persistent otorrhea after a canal wall–down mastoidectomy?	Inadquate meatoplasty, failure to lower the facial ridge, mucosalization, exposed eustachian tube
297	Describe the histologic appearance of cholesteatoma.	A sac of keratinizing squamous epithelium with a central core of keratinaceous debris
298	In a healthy patient with cholesteatoma and no history of other otologic procedures, what are the primary indications for surgery?	There is no effective medical therapy for cholesteatoma; surgical removal and exteriorization are the only effective treatments. The primary goal of surgery is to create a safe and dry ear. Surgery is almost universally recommended for healthy patients.
299	What are the advantages and disadvantages of lateral graft tympanoplasty?	The choice to use a lateral graft technique is based largely on the surgeon's preference. It is commonly used for total, near-total or anterior perforations. The main disadvantages are technical difficulty and the possibility of blunting (loss of the acute anterior canal angle) and lateralization (separation of the graft from the malleus).
300	Why is the temporomandibular joint potentially at risk for injury during lateral graft tympanoplasty?	Classically, lateral graft tympanoplasty involves temporary removal of the anterior canal wall skin with canalplasty, removing the bony overhang such that the entire drum can be seen through the canal. Overly aggressive drilling risks entry into the glenoid fossa.
301	Describe the mechanism of hearing loss in a patient with a tympanic membrane perforation.	There is a decrease in the ratio of the tympanic membrane to stapes footplate surface area (transformer ratio). In addition, sound striking the oval window and round window simultaneously (through the perforation) may result in phase cancellation.
302	What is the rate of persistent tympanic membrane perforation after tympanostomy tube placement?	Approximately 2 to 5%
303	Describe the advantage of cartilage grafts when used in repair of tympanic membrane perforations.	Cartilage is more rigid than other graft materials, making it more resistant to retraction and resorption. Long-term studies have demonstrated hearing results to be similar to those obtained with fascia.
304	Describe the Sade grading system for tympanic membrane retraction.	• Grade I: Simple, shallow, generally self-cleaning and nonadherent • Grade II: Contacting the incus or stapes • Grade III: Contacting the promontory without adhesion • Grade IV: Adhesion to promontory • Grade V: Grade III or IV with perforation
305	Why is the posterior superior quadrant of the pars tensa particularly susceptible to retraction?	This area is highly vascular, which may lead to increased inflammation with infection resulting in thinning. The middle fibrous layer in this area is also incomplete and often absent and therefore has less support.
306	What pathogens are most commonly cultured in chronic otitis media?	Polymicrobial, involving *Pseudomonas aeruginosa*, *Staphylococcus aureus*, *Escherichia coli*, *Klebsiella* spp., and *Proteus* spp.
307	In addition to antibiotics, what adjunctive treatments should be considered for a pediatric patient with facial paralysis in the setting of acute otitis media?	• Wide myringotomy or myringotomy with tympanostomy tube insertion is generally recommended. • Adjunctive use of systemic corticosteroids is also advocated by some.
308	If appropriately treated, what is the prognosis for facial nerve recovery in children with facial paralysis secondary to acute otitis media?	Generally, outcomes are excellent; greater than 95% of patients will have a full recovery. Treatment consists of systemic antibiotics with a low threshold for ventilation tube placement. Coritcal mastoidectomy should be considered for coalescent mastoiditis; however, facial nerve decompression is not indicated.

309	What are the three primary mechanisms of developing intracranial infection from otitis media?	• Direct extension after bone erosion or through existing congenital of acquired defects • Propagating thrombophlebitis of venous channels originating within the mastoid • Hematogenous seeding
310	What intracranial complication of otitis media is associated with "picket fence" spiking fevers?	• Lateral sinus thrombophlebitis • Septic emboli from the thrombus are believed to cause the spiking fevers associated with this entity.
311	What is the Tobey-Ayer or Queckenstedt's test?	To evaluate for lateral sinus thrombosis, the internal jugular vein is compressed on one side while intracranial pressure is being monitored. In the event of a positive test, compressing on the side ipsilateral to the thrombosis should result in no change, whereas compression on the contralateral side will cause a rapid rise in pressure.
312	What is the most appropriate initial management of noncoalescent mastoiditis with an intact tympanic membrane?	Systemic antibiotics with myringotomy and tympanostomy tube placement
313	What is the most common complication of pressure equalization tube placement	Post-tympanostomy tube otorrhea (up to ~ 75%)
314	What lumbar puncture findings would you expect in a patient with otitic hydrocephalus, presumably a result of lateral sinus and possibly concomittant superior saggital sinus thrombosis?	Elevated opening pressure, but otherwise normal CSF composition
315	What is *Gradenigo syndrome*?	Triad of otorrhea, retro-orbital pain from trigeminal nerve irritation, and abducens nerve palsy from edema within the Dorello canal. It is a classic presentation of petrous apicitis.
316	Why is the abducens nerve the most commonly affected cranial nerve in cases of petrous apicitis?	The adbucens nerve travels through the Dorello canal at the petrous apex, rendering it susceptible to compression if there is surrounding inflammation.
317	How does a subperiosteal abscess of the mastoid develop?	Acute coalescent mastoiditis leads to erosion of the mastoid cortex, and pus can track into the subperiosteal plane, presenting as an area of fluctuance.
318	What is the *Griesinger sign*?	Postauricular edema and tenderness thought to result from septic thrombosis of the mastoid emissary vein
319	What is the most common intracranial complication of acute otitis media?	• Meningitis is the most common complication, although the incidence has declined significantly with advances in antibiotics. • Brain abscess is the most common lethal intracranial complication of otitis media.
320	What is the incidence of malleus fixation?	0.5 to 2%
321	In reference to stapes surgery, what is a *perilymph gusher*?	Excessive flow of perilymph encountered when opening the vestibule during stapes surgery
322	What conditions place a patient at high risk for perilymph gusher at the time of stapedotomy or cochlear implantation?	Patients with cochlear and labyrinthine malformations, particularly enlarged vestibular aqueduct and Mondini malformations, are at highest risk. A young male patient with mixed hearing loss should raise concern for X-linked stapes gusher syndrome.
323	Review the differential diagnosis of *otosclerosis*.	Any disease process that can result in conductive hearing loss, including tympanosclerosis, malleus fixation, congenital stapes footplate fixation, osteogenesis imperfecta, tympanic membrane perforation, cholesteatoma, and superior semicircular canal dehiscence, to name a few

324	What genetic disorder of bone development can cause a clinical presentation similar to that of otosclerosis?	Osteogenesis imperfecta
325	What findings are typically seen on immittance audiometry for patients with otosclerosis?	It may not impact tympanometry, although a type A(s) tympanogram may be seen. Acoustic reflexes, however, will most likely be abnormal, with absent responses in the affected ear when sound is presented on either side.
326	What are the most common otoscopic findings with otosclerosis?	Normal examination. The goal of the examination is to try to exlcude other causes, including tympanosclerosis, malleus fixation, cholesteatoma, perforation, and other causes of conductive hearing loss.
327	What is a *Schwartze sign*?	A rosy hue seen through a transparent tympanic membrane resulting from increased blood around the promontory during active otospongiosis
328	Describe the pattern of hearing loss with otosclerosis?	Initially, otosclerosis manifests with a low-frequency conductive hearing loss and may progress to involve all frequencies. An artificial bone threshold shift is often seen centered at 2 kHz (Carhart notch). Mixed hearing loss is less common and may represent so-called retrofenestral or cochlear otosclerosis.
329	Describe the management of a prolapsed and dehiscent facial nerve during stapedectomy?	Treatment depends on the experience and comfort level of the performing surgeon. Poststapedectomy hearing results are similar in patients with ~ 50% prolapse compared with those without prolapse, and there is not a statistically increased risk of facial nerve weakness when performed by an experieneced team. The safest option, however, is to discontinue surgery and provide a hearing aid.
330	What is the *Carhart notch*?	The Carhart notch is an artificial depression in bone conduction thresholds centered at 2 kHz that is thought to result from disruption of ossicular resonance from stapes ankylosis. It is not a true measure of cochlear reserve because it usually reverses after stapedectomy. It is not specific to otosclerosis.
331	With respect to stapedectomy, what is meant by "overclosure" of the air-bone gap?	After stapedectomy with good result, artificially depressed bone conduction will often resolve, potentially resulting in air conduction that is better than the preoperative bone conduction level.
332	Is the Carhart notch specific to otosclerosis?	No. An identical 2-kHz notch can commonly be seen in other conditions, such as incudostapedial joint erosion or malleus and incus fixation. It can also be present with tympanic membrane perforation and otitis media.
333	Describe the phenomenon of *paracusis of Willis*.	In this condition, subjects with conductive hearing loss hear better in noise. It is thought to result from the dampening of background noise by a conductive hearing deficit and the fact that people tend to speak louder and more directly when competing with background noise.
334	What preoperative conditions place a patient at high risk for SNHL with stapedectomy?	Obliterative otosclerosis, otitis media, cochlear malformation, endolymphatic hydrops
335	What is the primary advantage of small fenestra stapedotomy versus stapedectomy?	Improved air-bone gap closure at higher frequencies (3 to 8 kHz)
336	What is the overall incidence of signficant SNHL after stapedectomy?	0.5 to 1%
337	What is the sensitivity of high-resolution CT in diagnosing otosclerosis?	~95%

338	What is the most common cause of early stapedectomy failure?	Displacement or slippage of the prosthesis
339	How is a depressed footplate (into the vestibule) addressed during stapedectomy?	If the footplate is deeply depressed and/or no longer visible, removal should not be attempted. If the footplate is readily visible and accessible, a small hook may be used to deliver the footplate from the stapedectomy. A vein or fascia graft can then be used to seal the oval window, and a prosthesis can be placed.
340	Describe the timing and symptoms of reparative granuloma after stapedectomy.	Most commonly, it occurs 1 to 2 weeks after surgery and manifests with dizziness, SNHL, and tinnitus.
341	What is the treatment of otosclerosis in a patient's only hearing ear?	Stapedotomy is generally contraindicated because of the risk of severe SNHL in the patient's dependent ear. Amplification is first-line treatment.
342	Why is appropriate sizing of a stapes prosthesis important?	If it is too short, the prosthesis may become displaced or not resolve the conductive hearing loss. An overly long prosthesis may impinge on the membranous labyrinth, causing vertigo or SNHL.
343	If encountered during stapedectomy, how should a persistent stapedial artery be managed?	A very fine persistent stapedial artery may be managed by bipolar or laser coagulation. If the footplate is fixed and the vessel occupies only a portion of the footplate, stapedectomy can proceed if the visualized portion of the footplate is clearly sufficient for fenestration. In cases of a larger-caliber vessel, however, aborting the procedure may be prudent.
344	What are the guidelines for skydiving and scuba diving after stapedectomy?	There is no obvious risk to inner ear function provided the patient has good eustachian tube function.
345	What is the natural history of dysgeusia after chorda tympani nerve injury resulting from otologic surgery?	More than 90% of patients will have complete symptomatic recovery by 1 year.

Disorders of the Inner Ear and Lateral Skull Base

346	What is the difference between *stereotactic radiosurgery* and *stereotactic radiotherapy*?	*Stereotactic radiosurgery* implies a single fraction treatment (all at once), whereas *stereotactic radiotherapy* implies delivery of mutliple fractions.
347	For what does the *NF-2* gene code?	The *NF-2* gene is a tumor suppressor gene located on chromosome 22q12.2, and it codes for the schwannomin or Merlin protein.
348	What are the diagnostic criteria for NF-2?	• Bilateral vestibular schwannomas • First-degree relative with NF-2 and the occurrence of a unilateral vestibular schwannoma or any two of the following: meningioma, neurofibroma, schwannoma, glioma, or posterior subcapsular lenticular opacities • Unilateral vestibular schwannoma and any two of the following: meningioma, neurofibroma, schwannoma, glioma, or posterior subcapsular lenticular opacities • Multiple meningiomas and a unilateral vestibular schwannoma or any two of the following: schwannoma, glioma, neurofibroma, cataract
349	What percent age of patients with NF-2 have a family history of disease?	Approximately 50% of cases are inherited, and 50% develop as a result of a new spontaneous mutation.
350	What are the two subtypes of NF-2?	• Gardner (mild) phenotype: Development of a limited number of intracranial tumors at a later age with slow progression • Wishart (severe) phenotype: Development of innumerable intracranial and spinal tumors early in life with rapid progression

351	What are current treatment options for patients wtih NF-2?	Observation with serial imaging, stereotactic radiation (focused radiation), microsurgical resection (gross total, near total or subtotal), or bevacizumab (monoclonal antibody targeting vascular endothelial growth factor)
352	What are the three surgical approaches commonly used during vestibular schwannoma resection? (▶ Fig. 6.6)	• Translabyrinthine • Middle fossa • Retrosigmoid

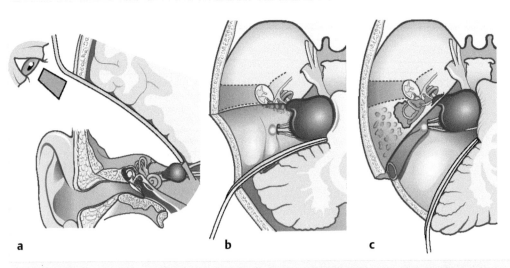

Fig. 6.6 Surgical approaches to the lateral skull base: (a) middle cranial fossa; (b) translabyrinthine; (c) retrosigmoid craniotomy. (Used with permission from Behrbohm H, Kaschke O, Nawka T, Swift A. Ear, Nose, and Throat Diseases: With Head and Neck Surgery. New York, NY: Thieme; 2009.)

353	What are the common indications for a translabyrinthine approach for resection of a vestibular schwannoma?	Patients with nonserviceable hearing (American Academy of Otolaryngology–Head and Neck Surgery [AAOHNS] class C or D), or with tumors > 2 cm where the prospect of hearing preservation is low. The primary advantages include minimal brain retraction, less risk of prolonged headache, and reliable early facial nerve identification at the fundus.
354	Describe the *Trautmann triangle*.	The dura of the posterior fossa located between the bony labyrinth anteriorly, the sigmoid sinus posteriorly, the superior petrosal sinus superiorly, and the jugular bulb inferiorly
355	What is the initial treatment of a venous air embolism supplied by a large rent in the sigmoid sinus?	Irrigate the wound, and place wet Gelfoam over the opening to block "air sucking." Place the patient in the left lateral decubitus (Durant maneuver) and Trendelenburg position to trap the air pocket in the right heart. Administer 100% oxygen. Perform cardiopulmonary resuscitation if cardiorespiratory collapse ensues.
356	Describe the orientation of the seventh to eighth nerve bundle at the fundus of the IAC. (▶ Fig. 6.7)	• Facial nerve (VII): Anterior superior • Superior vestibular: Posterior superior • Cochlear: Anterior inferior • Inferior vestibular: Posterior inferior

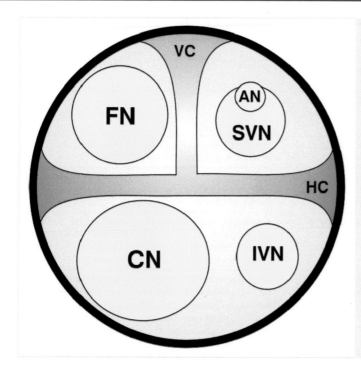

Fig. 6.7 Cross section of the distal internal auditory canal. Facial nerve (FN), anterior superior; superior vestibular (SVN), posterior superior; cochlear nerve (CN), anterior inferior; inferior vestibular (IVN), posterior inferior. Also shown, the vertical crest (VC); horizontal crest (HC); and superior ampullary nerve (AN) overlapping the superior vestibular nerve. (Used with permission from Sanna M, Mancini M, Russo A, Taibah A, Falcioni M, Di Trapani G. Atlas of Acoustic Neurinoma Microsurgery. New York, NY: Thieme; 2011.)

357	Describe *Mike's dot*.	The origin of the superior vestibular nerve in the medial wall of the vestibule
358	What are the common indications for a middle fossa approach for resection of a vestibular schwannoma?	Patients with serviceable hearing who have intracanalicular tumors or no more than 0.5 to 1 cm extension into the CPA. Advantages include ~ 50% chance of hearing preservation; disadvantages include a potentially unfavorable location of the facial nerve with respect to the tumor and temporal lobe retraction.
359	In middle cranial fossa surgery, what landmarks are used to locate the IAC?	The IAC is typically oriented parallel to the axis of the EAC, approximated by the line bisecting the angle between the greater superficial petrosal nerve and the arcuate eminence (superior semicircular canal).
360	To minimize greater superficial petrosal nerve injury during a middle fossa approach, in which direction should dural elevation proceed?	From posterior to anterior
361	What are the common indications for a retro-sigmoid approach for resection of a vestibular schwannoma?	It may be considered for patients with serviceable hearing and medial-based tumors. Tumors extending to the fundus of the internal auditory canal may be difficult to remove given restricted access around the posterior semicircular canal and vestibule. Larger, medial-base tumors can also be removed, even if hearing preservation is not attempted. Disadvantages include cerebellum retraction, headache, and potentially limited access into to the lateral IAC when hearing preservation is attempted.
362	Describe the superficial landmarks for approximating the transverse and sigmoid sinus.	The asterion approximates the location of the junction of the transverse sinus and sigmoid sinus and is often used during retrosigmoid craniotomy. Asterion is defined by the junction between the lambdoid, parietomastoid, and occiptomastoid sutures.

363	What percentage of patients with a vestibular schwannoma and "useful" hearing will ultimately lose their hearing after stereotactic radiosurgery?	Less than 25% of patients will retain useful hearing after stereotactic radiosurgery at 10 years after treatment.
364	What percentage of vestibular schwannoma are associated with NF-2?	5%
365	What percentage of intracanalicular vestibular schwannomas will remain stable in size for the first 5 years after diagnosis?	50 to 80%
366	Where along the eighth nerve are vestibular scwhannomas hypothesized to arise from?	Obersteiner-Redlich zone, near the porus acousticus, 1 cm from the brainstem
367	What is the Hitselberger sign?	Loss of sensation in the posterosuperior part of external auditory meatus and conchal bowl supplied by the sensory division of CN VII
368	What is the most common histologic classification for vestibular schwannomas?	Antoni type A or B. Type A tissue demonstrates dense cellularity with nuclear palisading and associated Verocay bodies, whereas type B has a loose arrangement with a less cellular reticular pattern in a myxoid stroma.
369	How are CPA meningiomas radiographically differentiated from vestibular schwannomas?	Meningiomas are sessile, demonstrating a broad base along the petrous ridge, and they have dural "tails." They often cause hyperostosis of the adjacent underlying bone and may have intratumoral calcifications. In contrast, vestibular schwannomas have a globular appearance and are centered over the IAC.
370	From what meningeal layer do meningiomas originate?	The arachnoid cap cells of the outer surface of the arachnoid mater
371	What percentage of paragangliomas will prove to be malignant?	Approximately 4%
372	From what cells do glomus tympanicum tumors originate?	Cells of neural crest origin arising from the tympanic branch (Jacobson nerve) of the glossopharyngeal nerve
373	Describe the Fisch classification system for paragangliomas of the temporal bone.	(▶ Table 6.2; ▶ Table 6.3; ▶ Table 6.4)

Table 6.2 Fisch classification of glomus tumors of the temporal bone.

Class	Description
A	Limited to the middle ear cleft
B	Limited to the tympanomastoid compartment of the temporal bone
C	Tumor involving the infralabyrinthine compartment of the temporal bone and extending into the petrous apex
C1	Limited involvement of the vertical portion of the carotid canal
C2	Invasion of the vertical portion of the carotid canal
C3	Invasion of the horizontal portion of the carotid canal
D	Tumor with intracranial extension
D1	<2 cm intracranial intradural extension
D2	>2 cm intracranial intradural extension
D3	Inoperable intracranial intradural involvement

Data from Fisch U. Infratemporal fossa approach for glomus tumors of the temporal bone. Ann Otol Rhinol Laryngol 91:474–479, 1982; and Fisch U, Mattox D: Classification of glomus temporal tumors. In Fisch U, Mattox D (eds): Microsurgery of the Skull Base. Stuttgart and New York, Georg Thieme, 1988, pp 149–153.

Table 6.3 Glasscock-Jackson classification of glomus tumors: Glomus Tympanicum.

Type	Description
I	Small mass limited to promontory
II	Tumor completely filling middle ear space
III	Tumor filling middle ear and extending into mastoid
IV	Tumor filling middle ear, extending into mastoid or through tympanic membrane to fill external auditory canal; may extend anterior to carotid

Data from Jackson CG, Glasscock ME, Harris PF. Glomus tumors: Diagnosis, classification, and management of large lesions. Arch Otolaryngol 108:401–410, 1982.

Table 6.4 Glasscock-Jackson classification of glomus tumors: Glomus Jugulare.

Type	Description
I	Small tumor involving jugular bulb, middle ear, and mastoid
II	Tumor extending under internal auditory canal; may have intracranial extension
III	Tumor extending into petrous apex; may have intracranial extension
IV	Tumor extending beyond petrous apex into clivus or infratemporal fossa; may have intracranial extension

Data from Jackson CG, Glasscock ME, Harris PF. Glomus tumors: Diagnosis, classification, and management of large lesions. Arch Otolaryngol 108:401–410, 1982.

374	Describe a positive Brown's sign.	• Blanching of a middle ear mass when performing pneumatic otoscopy • May be seen with glomus tympanicum or glomus jugulare tumors
375	What is the most appropriate management of a growing glomus tympanicum tumor that is limited to the promontory?	Transcanal tumor removal
376	What is the most appropriate management of a glomus tympanicum that fills the middle ear and extends into the mastoid air cells?	Tympanomastoidectomy with extended facial recess approach and tumor removal
377	How frequently would you expect a patient with a glomus tumor to have elevated catecholamine levels on laboratory workup?	About 1 to 3% of glomus tumors will have a secretory component with elevated catecholamine levels.
378	Describe the classic radiographic findings of a glomus jugulare on temporal bone CT.	Homogeneous soft tissue mass centered over an enlarged jugular foramen with "moth-eaten" irregular bony margins.
379	What nuclear medicine scans can be used to evaluate for head and neck paragangliomas?	Metaiodobenzylguanidine scan (MIBG), PET scan, and 111 In-pentetreotide scintigraphy
380	What is the general approach to treatment of petrous apex cholesterol granulomas?	Rather than excision, cholesterol granulomas are treated by drainage procedures. Transcanal (infracochlear), transmastoid (retrolabyrinthine, infralabyrinthine, subarcuate), and transsphenoidal endoscopic approaches are all methods of drainage that spare inner ear function.
381	How can a cholesterol granuloma be differentiated from an epidermoid cyst on imaging?	Classically, cholesterol granulomas appear as T1 and T2 hyperintense expansile lesions of the petrous apex that do not enhance with gadolinium. Epidermoids, on the other hand, most commonly demonstrate low intensity on T1 and high intensity on T2. Furthermore, diffusion-weighted MRI will reveal diffusion restriction with epidermoids. CT results are often similar.

382	What should be considered when determining the best surgical approach for drainage of a petrous apex cholesterol granuloma?	The location of the lesion in relationship to the jugular bulb, sphenoid sinus, eustachian tube, otic capsule, and most importantly the ICA should be considered. The patient's preoperative hearing status is also to be considered. Extended endonasal approaches are now being used with increasing frequency, but lesions in the posterior inferior petrous apex (between the carotid foramen and jugular foramen) are usually best approached by a transcanal infracochlear approach.
383	What is the key radiologic feature of a petrous apex epidermoid?	The key distinguishing feature between epidermoids and other lesions is the high-signal intensity of diffusion-weighted images. Epidermoids exhibit markedly restricted diffusion and therefore are bright on diffusion-weighted MRI.
384	How can you radiographically differentiate an IAC/CPA lipoma from a vestibular schwannoma or meningioma?	A lipoma is hyperintense on precontrast T1-weighted MRI and will subtract with fat-supression techniques.
385	Describe the management approach for a CPA/IAC lipoma?	Most CPA/IAC lipomas do not grow, and generally a "watch-and-scan" approach is used. Surgical resection is reserved for patients with intractable symptoms that are clearly attributable to mass effect.
386	From where do skull-base chondrosarcomas most commonly arise?	Chondrocytes of the foramen lacerum at the petroclival synchondrosis
387	What is the most common location from which a skull base chordoma arises?	Chordomas are tumors that arise from remnants of the notochord. These can occur anywhere along the axial skeleton, but at the skull base, they are almost invariably found at the clivus.
388	What percentage of patients with Von Hippel-Lindau disease will develop endolymphatic sac tumors?	Approximately 10%
389	What is the primary management strategy for endolymphatic tumors?	Complete surgical excision

Facial Nerve Disorders

390	What are the most common cranial neuropathies seen with neurosarcoidosis?	• Optic nerve, facial nerve, eighth nerve • Up to 50% of patients will have a least one cranial nerve palsy.
391	What are the classic features of Melkersson-Rosenthal syndrome?	• Recurrent orofacial edema, recurrent facial nerve paralysis, and lingua plicata (fissured tongue) • The classic triad is seen in only a minority of patients.
392	Describe the House-Brackmann grading scale for facial paralysis.	(▶ Table 6.5)

Table 6.5 House-Brackmann (HB) grading scale for facial paralysis.

Grade	Description
I	Normal function
II	Mild dysfunction: symmetric at rest with slight weakness and asymmetry with movement
III	Moderate dysfunction: able to close eye completely; symmetric at rest with an obvious difference between sides with expression; some synkinesis
IV	Moderately severe dysfunction: disfiguring asymmetry, incomplete eye closure
V	Severe dysfunction: barely perceptible movement
VI	Total paralysis

Data from House JW, Brackmann DE. Facial nerve grading system. Otolaryngol Head Neck Surg 1985;93(2):146–147.

393	What is Bell phenomenon?	A reflexive upward and outward movement of the globe during attempts at eye closure. Patients with incomplete eye closure resulting from facial palsy with an absent Bell phenomenon are at higher risk for corneal complications.
394	What is the organism responsible for Lyme disease?	*Borrelia burgdorferi*
395	How does treatment for facial paralysis secondary to Lyme disease differ from treatment of idiopathic facial paralysis (Bell palsy)?	Treatment with antibiotics (IV ceftriaxone or IV/PO doxycycline) has been found to improve outcomes in cases of facial paralysis associated with Lyme disease.
396	How does the prognosis for facial nerve recovery in Ramsay Hunt syndrome compare with that of Bell palsy?	The long-term facial nerve outcomes of Ramsay Hunt syndrome are generally worse, with more severe paralysis and a lower rate of full recovery.
397	Which sensory ganglion is believed to harbor latent varicella virus that becomes reactivated in cases of herpes zoster oticus (Ramsay Hunt syndrome)?	The geniculate ganglion
398	What is the prognosis for facial nerve recovery in patients with idiopathic facial paralysis (Bell palsy)?	80 to 90% of patients who receive no treatment experience full recovery. Among those who do not progress to complete paralysis, the prognosis is even better; 95% or greater of these patients have complete recovery. Evidence suggests that corticosteroids with or without antivirals provide improved outcomes, although the data are not conclusive, particularly for antivirals.
399	Where is the narrowest point in the fallopian canal?	At the meatal foramen, which marks the start of the labyrinthine segment
400	Describe how electroneuronography is performed.	Electronueronopgraphy (evoked electromyography) assesses the motor response to supramaximal stimulation of the facial nerve and compares the peak to peak difference between the abnormal side and the normal side. A bipolar stimulating electrode is placed at the stylomastoid foramen and surface electrodes are placed at the nasolabial fold. Increasing stimulation levels are provided until a maximal amplitude in the compound muscle action potential is reached. The difference between the abnormal and normal side provides the "percent drop."
401	At what critical electroneurogrphy (ENoG) value is facial nerve decompression considered in patients with Bell palsy?	Greater than 90% reduction compared with the opposite unaffected side
402	What is the significance of polyphasic motor unit action potentials during EMG testing?	Neural regeneration
403	What is the significance of fibrillation potentials during EMG testing?	Fibrillation potentials are spontaneous action potentials that arise from denervated muscle fibers and are generally not seen until after 21 days beyond denervation.
404	Describe how maximal stimulation testing is performed.	Transcutaneous electrical stimulation at the stylomastoid foramen is provided at a level that elicits maximal facial movement in an attempt to interrogate all functioning nerves. The response on the side with facial nerve paralysis is compared with the normal side and graded.
405	Describe how nerve excitability testing is performed.	Surface electrodes are placed near the stylomastoid foramen. Fixed-current pulses of increasing strength are delivered to the unaffected side until facial twitching is noted. The process is repeated on the affected side, and the difference in current required for stimulation is calculated.
406	What is the expected rate of neural regeneration following axonal injury?	1 mm/day

407 Describe the five levels of neural injury according to the Sunderland classification. (▶ Table 6.6; ▶ Fig. 6.8)

- Conduction block without axonal degeneration (neuropraxia)
- Isolated axonal injury that results in wallerian degeneration (axonotmesis)
- Axonal injury with loss of endoneurium, but the perineurium and epineurium remain intact.
- Axonal injury with loss of the endoneurium and perinerium, but the epineurium remains intact.
- Axonal injury with loss of all surrounding structures (transection)

Table 6.6 Seddon and Sunderland classification systems of nerve injuries and prognosis.

Seddon	Sunderland	Disrupted	Prognosis
Neuropraxia	Class I	Axon block	Complete recovery (days/months)
Axonotmesis	Class II	Axon injury (Wallerian degeneration)	Complete return (months)
Neurotmesis	Class III	Axon, endoneurium	Mild/moderate reduction in function
Neurotmesis	Class IV	Axon, endoneurium, perineurium	Moderate reduction in function
Neurotmesis	Class V	All structures	Marked reduction in function

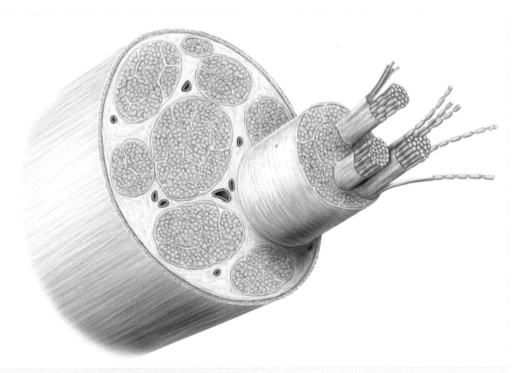

Fig. 6.8 Structure of peripheral nerves. (Used with permission from Thieme Atlas of Anatomy: Head and Neuroanatomy, © Thieme 2007, illustration by Markus Voll.)

408	Describe the three levels of neural injury according to the Seddon classification.	• Neuropraxia: Axons remain intact but have a temporary conduction block. Full recovery is expected. • Axonotmesis: Axons are damaged, but endoneurium remains intact. Wallerian degeneration will occur, but a full recovery without synkinesis is expected. • 3. Neurotmesis: Axons and surrounding support (endoneural tubules) are disrupted. Wallerian degeneration will occur, and recovery is variable.
409	What are the primary indications for rehabilitation of facial paralysis using dynamic muscle procedures such as temporalis tendon transfer?	Long-standing facial paralysis (> 2 years) is not amenable to primary reanastamosis, cable grafting, or jump grafts because facial motor endplates are no longer viable. Patients in these groups who desire dynamic facial rehabilitation may be candidates for muscle transfer techniques (temporalis transfer, masseter transfer, free gracilis, etc.).
410	What are the primary indications for rehabilitation of the eye in facial paralysis?	The primary goal is to protect the eye and vision from damage caused by chronic exposure and dryness. Corneal abrasion, ulceration, clouding, and epiphora can occur with facial paralysis and may result in vision loss if not aggressively managed.
411	What subset of patients with facial nerve paralysis are candidates for rehabilitation with facial-hypoglossal transfer?	Direct reinnervation (either primary anastomosis or cable grafting) is preferable, but when the proximal nerve stump is not available and the target facial motor endplates are still viable (within 12 to 18 months), facial-hypoglossal transfer is a viable treatment option.
412	What medical therapies are indicated for patients with delayed complete facial nerve paralysis after temporal bone trauma?	Eye care (drops, ointment, nocturnal moisture chamber) and corticosteroids
413	What is the significance of a completely unresponsive facial nerve after high-level proximal eletrical stimulation at the end of a surgery?	It denotes a complete conduction block, but without a subsequent examination to determine whether wallerian degeneration has occurred, a single test at the time of injury cannot differentiate between a simple neuropraxia and a transected nerve.
414	What is the mechanism of gustatory lacrimation after facial nerve injury?	Caused by a lesion proximal to the geniculate ganglion where fibers destined for the submandibular/sublingual glands reinnervate the lacrimal gland
415	How can synkinesis after traumatic facial nerve injury be managed?	Botulinum toxin injections or selective myectomy of affected muscles
416	During tympanomastoidectomy, the facial nerve is partially severed, with approximately 75% of its cross section still intact. What is the next step that should be performed?	With most of the nerve still intact, no further intervention should be undertaken. Limited proximal and distal facial nerve decompression could be considered to decrease ischemia associated with swelling.
417	What is the best outcome one could expect with primary tension-free nerve anastomosis after traumatic facial nerve injury?	House-Brackmann grade III function. Patients can achieve symmetric resting tone, good eye closure, and oral sphincter competence.
418	When awakening from a tympanomastoidectomy for cholesteatoma, a patient has an unexpected complete facial paralysis. What is the next step in care?	Consider observing the patient for 4 to 6 hours to allow local anesthetic injection to wear off.
419	What is the most common presentation of an intraparotid facial nerve schwannoma?	Asymptomatic enlarging mass
420	What are the common initial symptoms of an intratemporal facial nerve schwannoma?	Approximately 50% have slowly progressive or intermittent facial nerve paresis, and roughly 75% have some degree of hearing loss.

Osseous Dysplasias

421	Describe the histologic appearance of fibrous dysplasia.	Replacement of normal bone with benign fibrous tissue and irregular trabeculae of immature woven bone ("Chinese characters" appearance)
422	What are indications for surgical treatment of fibrous dysplasia of the skull base or craniofacial skeleton?	Generally, only symptomatic patients should undergo surgery (cranial neuropathies, vision loss, disfigurement). Some advocate optic canal decompression for asymptomatic patients with radiographic evidence of optic canal impingement, but this is debated.
423	What clinical findings are seen in McCune-Albright syndrome?	Polyostotic fibrous dysplasia, abnormal skin pigmentation (such as café-au-lait spots), and endocrine dysfunction (such as precocious puberty in girls)
424	What is the cause of hearing loss in patients with autosomal recessive osteopetrosis?	Most commonly, hearing loss is conductive, with disordered ossicular chain bony overgrowth, external auditory canal stensosis, stapes fixation, loss of temporal bone pneumatization, and recurrent otitis media resulting from eustachian tube narrowing. SNHL can also occur, likely from narrowing of the bony internal auditory canal.
425	What are the cause and the most common treatment for patients with recurrent facial palsy in the setting of osteopetrosis?	Compression of the facial nerve throughout its bony canal secondary to greatly increased bone density seen in osteopetrosis can lead to episodic, recurrent facial weakness. Complete facial nerve decompression can be attempted to manage this, because some residual and slowly progressive weakness are often seen after each episode.
426	What is the treatment for hearing loss secondary to Paget disease of bone involving the temporal bone?	Medical therapy consisting of bisphosphonates and calcitonin is the mainstay of therapy. Amplification may also be considered. Generally, hearing loss from bony abnormalities attributable to Paget disease is not correctable by surgical means.

Temporal Bone Malignancies

427	What is the most common cutaneous malignancy involving the auricle?	Basal cell carcinoma is both the most common auricular malignancy as well as the most common skin cancer in general.
428	What is the most common ceruminous gland malignancy of the external auditory canal?	Adenoid cystic carcinoma
429	You suspect a malignancy in a patient with an irregular, pigmented, and ulcerated lesion of the left lobule. Which biopsy techniques are acceptable in ascertaining a diagnosis?	A full-thickness biopsy is necessary for diagnosis. This should include epidermis, dermis, and some underlying subcutaneous tissue. Shave biopsies or fine needle aspiration of pigmented cutaneous malignancies are inappropriate because they may make tumor staging impossible.
430	List common risk factors associated with the development of temporal bone malignancy.	Fair complexion, sun exposure, immunocompromised status, recurrent otitis externa, previous radiation
431	List the most common types of temporal bone malignancy.	Approximately 70% squamous cell carcinoma, ~ 11% basal cell carcinoma, 4% adenocarcinoma, 4% adenoid cystic carcinoma
432	Describe the clinical presentation of squamous cell carcinoma of the external auditory canal?	Approximately 80% otorrhea and otalgia, ~ 70% hearing loss, 30% facial nerve disturbances
433	Describe the T staging of EAC carcinoma?	• T1: Limited to EAC without bony erosion • T2: Limited to the EAC with limited (not full thickness) bony erosion • T3: Tumor eroding through the EAC, involvement of the middle ear or mastoid, or facial nerve weakness • T4: Tumor invading otic capsule, jugular foramen, carotid canal, or dura (Pittsburgh staging system)

434	When is radiation indicated for patients with EAC squamous cell carcinoma?	T3–T4 disease, close margins, multiple positive lymph nodes, extracapsular spread, and perineural invasion
435	When is lateral temporal bone resection indicated in management of squamous cell carcinoma of the EAC?	Disease that is limited to the external auditory canal without significant extension into the mastoid, middle ear, or beyond (T1 and T2 disease).
436	What is the most common malignancy of the petrous apex?	Metastasis (breast). The low-flow marrow of the petrous apex is particularly susceptible to hematogenous metastasis.
437	What is the most common malignant tumor of the temporal bone in children?	Rhabdomyosarcoma, embryonal subtype
438	What is the appropriate initial management strategy for a carcinoid tumor of the middle ear?	A recent review (Ramsey et al, 2005) identified this rare tumor as a low-grade malignancy with the potential for local recurrence and regional metastasis. Complete excision of this tumor with long-term surveillance is recommended.
439	In cases of penetrating facial trauma where branches of the facial nerve are suspected to be transected, why should they be explored within 3 days?	The distal branches of the nerve can still be stimulated for approximately 3 days after they are transected, before wallerian degeneration takes place.
440	Describe the two most common classifications for temporal bone fractures. (▶ Fig. 6.9)	Orientation of the fracture line (longitudinal, transverse, or mixed) or by involvement of the otic capsule

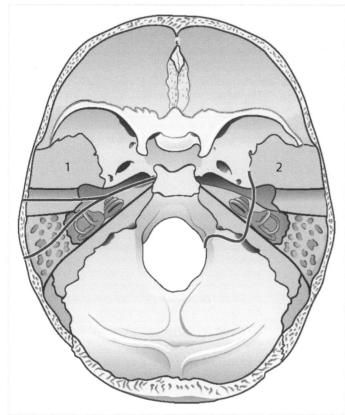

Fig. 6.9 Illustration of temporal bone fractures: (1) longitudinal fractures; (2) transverse fracture. (Used with permission from Behrbohm H, Kaschke O, Nawka T, Swift A. Ear, Nose, and Throat Diseases: With Head and Neck Surgery. New York, NY: Thieme; 2009.)

441	Describe associated sequelae of a longitudinal temporal bone fracture.	CSF otorrhea, tympanic membrane perforation, EAC laceration, conductive hearing loss from hemotympanum or ossicular discontinuity, bloody otorrhea, facial nerve injury uncommon (20%)

442	Describe associated sequelae of a transverse temporal bone fracture.	Vertigo, SNHL, facial nerve injury more common and often more severe (30 to 50%)
443	What type of head blow is likely to cause a longitudinal temporal bone fracture?	Temporal (lateral) blows are more likely to cause a longitudinal fracture, whereas frontal or occipital blows may cause a transverse fracture.
444	Describe the initial management of a traumatic CSF leak.	Most traumatic leaks resolve with conservative measures, including bed rest, head of bed elevation, and stool softeners. Generally, surgical repair is pursued if an active leak persists beyond a week from injury.
445	Review the role of antibiotics with traumatic temporal bone CSF leaks.	Controversial. A recent Cochrane Database review does not support the use of prophylactic antibiotics to reduce the risk of meningitis after basilar skull fractures.
446	Review the role of perioperative antibiotics in otologic and neurotologic surgery.	Available data do not support the use of perioperative antibiotics in routine otologic surgery. In cases with active infection, the role of antibiotics is more controversial. A single dose of perioperative antibiotics is generally recommended in cochlear implantation and skull base procedures, with many surgeons extending this to a 24-hour-long postoperative course.
447	What is the initial management of a temporal bone fracture with an intact otic capsule, intact tympanic membrane, and hemotympanum with conductive hearing loss?	Audiogram in 4 to 8 weeks. Otic drops can be considered if there is a laceration or blood in the ear canal. Persistent conductive hearing loss may suggest the presence of ossicular chain disruption.
448	Where is the most common site of ossicular chain disruption in the setting of temporal bone fracture?	The incudostapedial joint
449	What is the most common site of facial nerve injury in temporal bone fractures?	The perigeniculate region (80%+)
450	Describe the initial management of a tympanic membrane perforation related to a nonexplosive blast injury, such as a slap to the side of the head?	Conservative management and observation. The vast majority of these perforations will heal spontaneously.
451	What is the most common otologic sequelae of lightning strike?	Tympanic membrane perforation
452	What needs to be done before burying a traumatically avulsed portion of the pinna in a postauricular subcutaneous pocket?	The skin of the avulsed segment should be dermabraded to remove the surface epithelium while it is buried in the subcutaneous pocket.
453	What is the mechanism for SNHL resulting from decompression sickness?	Nitrogen, which was made temporarily soluble in blood by increased ambient pressure, comes out of solution in the form of bubbles during rapid depressurization. These "microbubble emboli" can involve the microcirculation of the ear and cause hearing loss, and they may be difficult to distinguish from inner ear barotrauma.
454	What are the symptoms of perilymphatic fistula?	Fluctuating hearing loss and intense vertigo that worsens with Valsalva or exertion
455	Describe the clinical presentation and radiologic findings of labyrinthine concussion.	Brief loss of consciousness associated with transient (days to weeks) vestibular symptoms, possible hearing loss and tinnitus. Dix-Hallpike maneuver does not elicit symptoms. CT scan does not show acute intracranial complications or otic capsule fracture.
456	Describe the most common mechanism of malleus handle fracture.	It is often caused by placing wet finger in ear canal. When the finger is withdrawn under a seal, this creates negative pressure in the ear canal that can result in fracture of the malleus. Patients often report a "pop" with sharp pain and immediate hearing decline.

457	How should bloody otorrhea after temporal bone fracture in a stable and awake patient be managed?	Otomicroscopy to debride the EAC. Irrigation or occlusion (except in cases of massive bleeding) of the EAC should not be performed because of the risk of ascending meningitis.
458	Describe the utility of the "halo" or "ring" sign when evaluating for traumatic CSF leak.	Not sensitive or specific. The halo sign may be seen when blood is mixed with CSF, saline, nasal mucus, and tap water. Futhermore, the concentration of CSF and blood must be correct for a halo to be seen.
459	In what body fluids can β-2 transferrin can be found?	CSF, perilymph of the inner ear, and vitreous humor of the globe
460	What initial screening tests should be performed when a CSF leak is suspected?	β2-transferrin and a fine cut CT of the entire skull base should be obtained with dedicated coronal and axial acquisition.
461	How long is CSF (beta-2 transferrin) stable for at room temperature?	Approximately 4 hours at room temperature, and approximately 3 days when refrigerated (not frozen).
462	Describe the Dandy maneuver.	The patient leans forward while performing a Valsalva. This maneuver may provoke clear rhinorrhea in a patient with a CSF fistula. The nostril that the drainage comes from generally predicts the laterality of the defect.
463	How much CSF is contained within the subarachnoid space at any given time?	Approximately 150 mL, with daily production of approximately 500 mL, which means that the CSF volume is turned over approximately three times per day.
464	Describe a positive reservoir sign.	Intermittent CSF rhinorrhea associated with change in head position, which results from pouring of CSF collecting in a dependent location of a sinus.
465	Describe Hyrtl fissure.	A Hyrtl fissure is an embryonic anomaly that leaves a connection between the middle ear and posterior fossa (between the jugular bulb and otic capsule). It may be a conduit for CSF leak, meningitis, or tumor spread (also known as the *tympanomeningeal fissure*).
466	Review possible sources for congenital CSF leaks involving the temporal bone.	• Hyrtl fissure • Dilated cochlear aqueduct • Dilated fallopian canal • Enlarged petromastoid canal (subarcuate canal) • Abnormal communication between IAC and inner ear (cochlear malformations)
467	What is the preferred management strategy for traumatic carotid-cavernous fistula associated with skull base fracture?	Endovascular repair (Ballooning/stenting/coiling)

7 Head and Neck Surgical Oncology

Joshua J. Thom, William R. Schmitt, David G. Stoddard Jr., Kathryn M. Van Abel, and Daniel L. Price

Tumor Biology and Carcinogenesis

1	What are the five basic phases of the cell cycle, and what occurs during each phase?	• *Quiescent phase* (G0): Resting state • *Gap 1* (G1): Preparation for cell division; increase in transcription/translation and ~ doubling of macromolecules • *Synthesis phase* (S): Replication of chromosomes • *Gap 2* (G2): Continued cellular growth • *Mitosis phase* (M): Chromosomes are separated, and two daughter cells result
2	What is the term given to cells in permanent cell-cycle arrest?	Senescent
3	What are the key checkpoints within the cell cycle?	• *G1/S checkpoint* ("restriction point"): Prevent entry into S-phase, rate-limiting step • *Intra-S phase checkpoint*: Halt progression of S-phase if damaged DNA is detected • *G2/M checkpoint*: Prevent entry into M phase • *M checkpoint*: Ensure correct replication of DNA and avoid mitotic exit if errors exist
4	If a lesion (i.e., partially replicated DNA, strand breaks, or other errors) is identified at a checkpoint, what processes can be activated?	• Recruitment of DNA repair effector complexes • Temporary cell-cycle arrest, which can lead to senescence or apoptosis, depending on the cell and the lesion
5	What key tumor suppressor protein controls progression through the G1/S checkpoint (restriction point) and the G2/M checkpoint?	*p53* (activates p21 → inhibits cyclin and cyclin-dependent kinase (Cdk) complexes)
6	What two key classes of molecules regulate a cell's progress through the cell cycle?	• *Cdks*: Catalytic subunit; require cyclin for activation; result in phosphorylation (activates/inactivates molecules necessary for progression through the cell cycle) • *Cyclins*: Regulatory subunit that activates Cdk molecules when bound to form a heterodimer
7	Although more than 15 Cdks have been identified, four have key biologic functions within the cell cycle. What are they, and what do they do?	• *Cdk 1*: Controls G2 phase and M phase (prophase) → Cyclin A dependent • *Cdk 2*: Controls G1 to S transition and S phase → cyclin E (and A) dependent • *Cdk 4*: G0 to G1 transition → cyclin D dependent • *Cdk 6*: G0 to G1 transition → cyclin D dependent
8	Specific families of activators and inhibitors regulate functional activities of the Cdk complexes. Identify the primary activators and inhibitors.	• Activators: Cdk-activating kinase (CAK) and Cdc-25 • Inhibitors: Cdk inhibitors (CKI) → Inhibitor of kinase 4 (INK4a), Cdk Interacting protein/kinase inhibitory protein (Cip/Kip)
9	What type of gene helps to control cell growth or progression through the cell cycle?	Tumor suppressor gene (also called *antioncogenes*)
10	What type of gene promotes cell growth and progression through the cell cycle?	*Proto-oncogenes*. Once a proto-oncogene is mutated, it is known as an *oncogene*.
11	The classic retinoblastoma tumor suppressor protein (pRb) functions to inhibit what key transcription factors, effectively preventing formation of cell cycle–related proteins and arresting the cell in G0 phase?	E2F factors

12	Phosphorylation of pRb by what important cyclin-Cdk complex(es) results in dissociation of pRb from E2F and subsequent entrance into the cell cycle?	Cyclin D-Cdk4 and cyclin D-Cdk6
13	Release of E2F from pRb inhibition results in the transcription of multiple genes necessary for the function of the cell cycle. Transcription of what key cyclin protein results in activation of Cdk2, progression from G1 to S phase, additional pRb inactivation, and p27 degradation?	Cyclin E
14	What genes are considered members of the Cip/Kip family of tumor suppressor genes, and in what phase of the cell cycle do they inhibit cyclin-Cdk complexes?	• *p21, p27,* and *p57* • G1 phase
15	DNA damage results in activation of what key tumor-suppressor gene and proapoptotic factor, which in turn activates *p21* (a Cip/Kip Cdk complex inhibitor) and results in arrest of the cell cycle in G1 phase?	*p53*
16	Transforming growth factor-β is a growth inhibitor, which results in activation of which *INK4* tumor suppressor gene causing subsequent cell-cycle arrest in G1 phase?	*p27*
17	What genes are considered members of the INK4a family of tumor-suppressor genes, and in what phase of the cell cycle do they inhibit cyclin-Cdk complexes?	• *p16* and *p19* • G1 phase
18	Name the tumor suppressor gene that is a member of the INK4a family that prevents p53 degradation and therefore results in cell-cycle arrest at the G1-checkpoint.	*p19*
19	Name the tumor suppressor gene that is a member of the INK4a family that inhibits cyclin D-Cdk4/6 complexes and therefore results cell cycle arrest during the G1 phase.	*p16*
20	What important enzymes function to dephosphorylate the targets of cyclin-Cdk complexes, such as pRb?	PP1 and PP2A (phosphatases)
21	To promote an orderly progression through the cell cycle, cyclin-Cdk complexes must be degraded to allow the next phase of the cell cycle to progress uninterrupted. For example, S-phase complexes cannot be active during M phase and so forth. What important enzymatic process selectively targets these complexes for degradation?	Ubiquitin-dependent protein degradation (ubiquitylation)
22	The phases G1, S, and G2 are collectively referred to as what?	Interphase
23	What are the five stages of mitosis (M phase)?	• *Prophase*: Preparatory; cyclin A-Cdk1 active; condensation of chromatin, polarization of centrosomes, and initiation of mitotic spindle formation • *Prometaphase*: Nuclear envelope breaks down, mitotic spindle microtubules attach to chromosomes • *Metaphase*: Alignment of chromosomes at metaphase plate • *Anaphase*: Separation of sister chromatids • Telophase: Cytoplasmic division (cytokinesis) into two daughter cells; chromatid decondensation (expansion)

24	Describe the "two-hit" hypothesis (Knudson, 1971) for carcinogenesis.	Loss of two alleles for a tumor-suppressor gene is necessary to result in loss of function and tumorigenesis. This hypothesis is not applicable to proto-oncogenes and dominant negative tumor suppressor genes (e.g., *p53*).
25	In an effort to understand carcinogenesis, Fearon and Vogelstein (Cell, 1990) presented a model of tumor progression that involved which three hypotheses?	• Inactivation of tumor suppressor genes or activation of proto-oncogenes results in the formation of cancer. • A series of defined genetic events lead to the development of cancer. • This linear progression may vary, but ultimately it is the accumulation of genetic events that results in the development of a malignant phenotype.
26	What is the estimated average of time required for the accumulation of enough genetic alterations to produce traditional head and neck squamous cell carcinoma (Renan, 1993)?	20 to 25 years
27	Carcinogenesis models describe a linear progression from precancerous lesions to overtly malignant tumors. Describe the steps involved for each of the following models: 1. Genetic progression model for head and neck cancer 2. Multistep carcinogenesis	1. Hyperplasia → dysplasia (mild, moderate, severe) → carcinoma in situ → invasive carcinoma 2. Initiation → promotion → progression
28	In upper aerodigestive tract tumors, what term describes the histopathologic changes seen in mucosa surrounding invasive carcinoma and result in an increased incidence of second primary tumors?	Field cancerization (Slaughter, 1953)
29	What hypotheses focusing on the clonal abnormality required for tumor growth have been put forth to explain field cancerization?	• Abnormal, and genetically unique, clones form independently at multiple sites due to exposure to similar environmental carcinogens. • A single tumoral clone forms and subsequently migrates via lateral movement through the mucosa (shown in several studies to be accurate).
30	What are the two predominant environmental carcinogens that have been associated with head and neck cancer, show a dose response, and can function synergistically?	• Tobacco • Alcohol
31	Why might alcohol, in particular, function as a synergistic carcinogen with other environmental carcinogens?	It may decrease the effectiveness of both local and systemic detoxification enzymes (e.g., cytochrome P450 system).
32	Does cessation of smoking and alcohol consumption reduce the risk of head and neck cancer development? If so, how long does it take for the risk to reach the level of never-smokers?	Yes. Some studies have shown 20 years or longer.
33	How does diet impact the development of cancer of the upper aerodigestive tract?	A high intake of fruits and vegetables and low intake of red meat or processed meats has been associated with a decreased risk of head and neck cancer (INHANCE Consortium, 2012).
34	Describe the cell-cycle dysregulation that is commonly seen in patients with environmentally related head and neck cancer.	(Posner, Goldman's Cecil Medicine, 24th ed., Chp196) • Loss of *p16* (normally inhibits cyclin D) • Upregulation of cyclin D • Loss of *p53* (normally inhibits cell cycle progression and promotes apoptosis) • Upregulation of EGFR (enhances mitogenic signaling) • Upregulation of COX-2 (increased angiogenesis, decreased apoptosis) • Increased chromosomal instability (increased aneuploidy)

35	What genetic conditions are related to an increased risk of head and neck cancer?	• Fanconi anemia (AR; DNA repair gene mutation) • Cowden syndrome (AD: PTEN hematoma tumor syndrome; PTEN is a tumor suppressor gene) • Mutations in the cytochrome P450 enzymes (CYP1A1 mutations in Asian populations)
36	What circular, double-stranded DNA virus commonly infects the basal layer of cutaneous of mucosal squamous epithelium and is spread by sexual contact?	Human papilloma virus (HPV)
37	What two HPV strains are considered "low-risk" for the development of cancer and are frequently associated with papillomas and warts?	HPV 6 and 11
38	What two HPV strains are considered "high-risk" for the development of cancer and have been associated with cervical, anogenital, and head and neck (predominantly oropharyngeal) carcinomas?	HPV 16* and 18 *90% of HPV(+) head and neck carcinomas
39	The HPV DNA encodes nine open reading frames (genes) on a single strand of its double-stranded circular DNA. Seven of these are considered early phase genes (E), and two are considered late-phase genes (L). What are the general functions of the E and L genes, respectively?	• E genes: Regulate the transcription viral DNA • L genes: Encode capsid proteins involved in viral spread
40	Name the two viral onco-proteins in HPV-related tumorigenesis, and identify the two genes, that control the transcription of these viral proteins.	• E6/E7: Onco-genes • E1/E2: Transcriptional regulators
41	When HPV DNA integrates into host DNA, the process can result in deletion or loss of function of the E1 and E2 viral genes. This in turn results in what?	Loss of regulation of E6 and E7 and subsequent increased transcription of these viral genes
42	What HPV protein functions to inhibit the function of p53 by targeting it for ubiquitin-dependent degradation? What is the result?	• E6 • Progression through G1 checkpoint and inhibition of apoptosis
43	What HPV protein phosphorylates pRb and thus targets it for ubiquitin-dependent degradation? What is the primary result?	• E7 • Release of *pRb* inhibition of E2F, activation of cell cycle-related transcription, progression through the G1 checkpoint
44	In addition to E2F-related transcription, the degradation of p53 results in over expression of what important protein? What impact does this have on cell-cycle progression?	• *p16* • Normally inhibits Cdk4/6, but with the los of p53 and pRb, does not meaningfully result in cell cycle control. Can be used as a biomarker of HPV activity.
45	In addition to HPV, what viruses have been associated with head and neck cancer?	• Epstein-barr virus (EBV): Nasopharyngeal carcinoma • Human immunodeficiency virus (HIV): Increased risk of head and neck cancers • Merkel cell polyomavirus: Merkel cell carcinoma • Human T-lymphotrophic virus (HTLV-1): Human T-Cell lymphoma/leukemia • Kaposi sarcoma associated herpesvirus (KSHV): Kaposi sarcoma
46	Whereas the epidermal growth factor receptor (EGFR) is normally expressed in the epithelium of several organ systems (dermis, gastrointestinal tract, kidney), it has been found to be dysfunctional in what percentage of head and neck (squamous cell) cancers?	80 to 90%

47	EGFR is a transmembrane glycoprotein that, when activated by binding an extracellular ligand, results in dimerization, tyrosine kinase activation, and a complex downstream pathway that ultimately results in what major outcomes?	• Cellular growth and proliferation • Apoptosis • Angiogenesis • Invasion • Metastasis
48	How does EGFR expression relate to prognosis in head and neck squamous cell carcinoma?	Increased expression and amplification are related to decreased recurrence-free survival and cancer-specific survival rates.
49	What strategies have been used to target aberrant signaling in head and neck squamous cell carcinoma based on a better understanding of EGFR signaling?	• Tyrosine kinase inhibitors (geftinib) • Monoclonal antibodies inhibiting dimerization (cetuximab) • Antisense oligodeoxynucleotide or small interfering mRNA inhibition of mRNA expression
50	What immune cell is primarily responsible for identifying normal cells that have been altered by viral or tumor activity? What is the general function of these cells in patients with head and neck cancer?	T cells Decreased: T cells demonstrate increased apoptosis, decreased recruitment from the thymus, and poor proliferation. Overall immunosuppression
51	What important normal immune system function is designed to prevent the recognition of "self" through processes such as anergy, suppression, and ignorance, which makes stimulating the immune system to target self-derived tumor cells challenging?	Tolerance
52	What cell-based therapeutic model has been studied in head and neck cancer with promising (although early) results that focuses on using the immune system to target cancer cells specifically?	Immunotherapy focused on manipulation of the following: • Cell signaling (i.e., cytokines such as interleukin-2) • Vaccination (i.e., Gardasil, whole-cell vaccines, dendritic-cell vaccines, etc.) • T cells, dendritic cells, or antibodies
53	What type of therapy has the potential to prevent head and neck cancer from occurring, recurring, or progressing?	Chemoprevention
54	What prominent chemopreventive agents have been studied for use in patients with head and neck cancer?	• Retinoids and vitamin A (betacarotene) • COX-2 inhibitors • Aspirin • Selenium • Vitamin D • Interpheron-α2a • α-tocopherol (Vitamin E) Many others are being studied. There is great controversy surrounding most of these agents as studies have demonstrated conflicting results.
55	What chemopreventive effects are retinoids purported to have on head and neck cancer?	They can retard progression of premalignant oral lesions (leukoplakia and erythroplakia) and have also been associated with lower rates of second primary tumors. Subsequent studies have called these results into question.
56	True or False. The risk of head and neck cancer increases in the setting of vitamin A toxicity.	False. The risk increases with vitamin A deficiency.
57	What inflammatory mediator is elevated in head and neck cancer cells?	Prostaglandins as a result of the upregulation of COX-1 and -2

Principles of Staging Evaluation and Prognosis

58	What oncologic staging system was devised in 1959 by the American Joint Committee on Cancer (AJCC) to describe the extent of the primary tumor, involvement of regional lymph nodes, and metastases to distant sites in an effort to form a	Tumor, node, metastasis (TNM) staging system

	cohesive system providing the clinician with an important tool to predict prognosis, counsel the patient, chose an intervention, and perform more consistent clinical research?	
59	Using the TNM staging system, how can you differentiate a *clinical stage* from a *pathologic stage*?	• *Clinical stage* is designated with a "c" and is based on physical examination or imaging (e.g., cT, cN, or cM). • *Pathologic stage* is designated with a "p" and is based on pathologic analysis of a specimen (e.g., pT, pN, pM).
60	Which subsites share the following criteria (in addition to subsite specific criteria) for T staging: • T1:< 2 cm • T2:> 2 cm, < 4 cmT3:> 4 cm	• Lips and oral cavity • Oropharynx • Hypopharynx (plus additional criteria) • Major salivary gland (plus additional criteria) • Well-differentiated thyroid cancer and medullary thyroid cancer (plus additional division of T1a, T1b)
61	In the 7th edition of the AJCC, the terms *resectable* and *unresectable* were changed to mean "moderately advanced local disease (T4a)" and "very advanced local disease (T4b)" in an effort to predict better the prognosis using current management strategies. What does "very advanced local disease" generally represent?	Very advanced disease correlates with extension into surrounding critical structures which are largely viewed as unresectable or incurable.
62	The following head and neck subsites share what nodal (N) staging system? • Oral cavity • Oropharynx • Hypopharynx • Larynx • Nasal cavity and paranasal sinuses • Major salivary glands	(▶ Table 7.1)

Table 7.1 AJCC neck (N) staging for head and neck tumors (excluding nasopharynx and thyroid).

Stage	Description
NX	Cannot assess
N0	No regional metastasis
N1	Single ipsilateral lymph node, ≤ 3 cm
N2a	Single ipsilateral lymph node, > 3 cm but ≤ 6 cm
N2b	Multiple ipsilateral lymph nodes, ≤ 6 cm
N2c	Bilateral or contralateral lymph nodes, ≤ 6 cm
N3	Lymph node > 6 cm

Data from Edge SB, Byrd DR, Compton CC, Fritz AG, Greene FL, Trotti A, eds. AJCC Cancer Staging Manual 7th Edition. New York, NY: Springer; 2010.

63	What two head and neck subsites have a unique nodal staging system compared with the majority of subsites?	• Nasopharynx • Thyroid
64	Using the TNM staging system, the lips, oral cavity, oropharynx, hypopharynx, larynx, nasal cavity, paranasal sinuses, and salivary glands can all be staged based on what system?	(▶ Table 7.2)

Table 7.2 TNM staging system for most head and neck cancers (lips, oral cavity, oropharynx, hypopharynx, larynx, nasal cavity, paranasal sinuses, and salivary glands).

Stage	TNM description
I	T1N0M0
II	T2N0M0
III	T3N0M0, T1–3N1M0
IVA	T4aN0–2M0, T1–3N2M
IVB	T4bAnyNM0, AnyTN3M
IVC	AnyTAnyNM1

Data from Edge SB, Byrd DR, Compton CC, Fritz AG, Greene FL, Trotti A, eds. AJCC Cancer Staging Manual 7th Edition. New York, NY: Springer; 2010.

65	Tumor invasion of what subsites are considered by some as unresectable?	• Nasopharynx • Prevertebral fascia • Base of skull • Intracranial extension • Mediastinum • Subdermal lymphatics • Carotid artery encasement (generally > 270 degrees)
66	Describe how the American Joint Committee on Cancer reports the presence or absence of residual tumor (R) following treatment.	• RX: Residual tumor cannot be assessed • R0: No residual tumor • R1: Microscopic residual tumor • R2: Macroscopic residual tumor
67	How does the AJCC recommend reporting tumor grade?	• GX: Grade cannot be assessed • G1: Well differentiated • G2: Moderately differentiated • G3: Poorly differentiated • G4: Undifferentiated
68	Patients with head and neck cancer will have symptoms related to the location and extent of their tumor that are often subsite specific. What "red flag" signs or symptoms should be reviewed with all patients who have concerns for head and neck cancer?	Pain, cranial neuropathy, bleeding, unintentional weight loss, lymphadenopathy, malaise, anorexia
69	What risk factors should be elicited when taking a history on a patient with potential head and neck cancer?	• Tobacco* (smoked and smokeless) and alcohol* exposure • Viral infection (EBV and HPV*) • Radiation exposure • Diet low in fruits and vegetables and high in red meats and processed meats • Occupational risk factors such as woodworking, textile exposure, and nickel refining • Sun exposure • Personal history of head and neck cancer • Family history of cancer • Poor dentition, chronic inflammation, or chronic irritation • Immunosuppression • Use of betel (quid or panna) (Asia) * Major risk factors in developed countries
70	What risk factors are associated with advanced head and neck cancer at presentation?	• Low income • Black race • Poorly differentiated tumors • Patient neglect

71	Define the Eastern Cooperative Oncology Group (ECOG) performance status system.	• Grade 0: Fully active, able to carry on all predisease performance without restriction • Grade 1: Restricted in physically strenuous activity but ambulatory and able to carry out work of a light or sedentary nature • Grade 2: Ambulatory and capable of all self-care but unable to carry out any work activities. Up and about > 50% of waking hours • Grade 3: Capable of only limited self-care; confined to bed more than 50% of waking hours. • Grade 4: Completely disabled; cannot carry out any self-care. Totally confined to bed or chair. • Grade 5: Deceased
72	During a head and neck examination in an adult patient, you note unilateral serous otitis media. On flexible endoscopic examination, to what anatomical region(s) should you pay particular attention?	Posterior nasal cavity, nasopharynx, fossa of Rosenmuller and eustachian tube orifice
73	During fiberoptic or mirror laryngoscopy, what maneuvers are critical for a complete oncologic head and neck examination?	• Phonation → assess vocal cord mobility • Tongue protrusion → full view of the epiglottis and vallecula • Puff out cheeks → full view of pyriform sinuses and postcricoid region
74	You perform an otoscopic examination on a patient complaining of otalgia but note no obvious source of pain. Which nerve(s) might be implicated in *referred otalgia*?	CN V3, IX (via Jacobson nerve), X (via Arnold nerve), and VII (via the Ramsay Hunt branch of VII), as well as branches from C2 and C3 through the great auricular nerve
75	On evaluation of a primary head and neck tumor, in addition to the location and size of the tumor, what information can be gained from palpation that is critical to the workup?	Fixation of the tumor *Note:* fixation of nodal metastases should also be noted.
76	What premalignant lesion can present as a thickened white patch that can't be scraped off on physical exam of the upper aerodigestive tract mucosa that can progress to invasive carcinoma in up to 30% of patients over a variable number of years?	Leukoplakia
77	What premalignant mucosal lesion can appear as a flat red patch with a malignant potential of up to 60% over a variable number of years?	Erythroplakia
78	What common initial screening test evaluates for pulmonary disease (metastases or primary lung cancer)?	Chest radiograph. PET/CT is also often ordered now as the initial screening test for distant metastases.
79	Which imaging modality is used most often in the initial workup of head and neck cancer patients?	Contrast-enhanced CT
80	CT scan of the head and neck is often ordered as a first-line imaging modality to evaluate the size, extent, and location of the primary tumor; status of the vasculature; and nodal disease. Should this scan be ordered with or without contrast?	With contrast (as patient's allergies and renal status permits). In the initial workup of differentiated thyroid carcinoma, avoidance of iodinated contrast should be considered.
81	What are frequently used as radiographic criteria for a nodal malignancy on CT scan?	• Size > 1 cm • Evidence of central necrosis (~100% specificity) • Spherical shape (suggestive) • Nodal grouping in the predicted drainage pathway, with nodes > 1 cm

82	What is a key disadvantage of CT scans when evaluating an oral cavity or oropharyngeal neoplasm in a patient with tooth fillings?	Dental artifact often obscures anatomy/pathology.
83	In what situations is evaluation with MRI most useful during the workup for head and neck cancer?	• Soft tissue tumor (e.g., base of tongue, infratemporal fossa, parapharyngeal space, parotid) • Intracranial extension or skull base involvement • Paranasal sinus disease (e.g., inspissated secretions vs. tumor) • Nasopharyngeal tumors • Temporal bone • Assessment of perineural invasion
84	When is a PET/CT scan indicated during the treatment of a patient with head and neck cancer?	• Evaluation of equivocal disease • Workup of an unknown primary tumor (can identify up to a third of primary tumors) • Evaluate nodal disease (studies argue against its use in the cN0 neck) • Evaluate for distant metastases (may see a high number of false-positives but has a very high negative predictive value) • Surveillance after treatment
85	True or False. All head and neck tumors are PET avid because of their high metabolic activity.	False. Several head and neck tumors have either variable/inconsistent or no FDG-avidity. These include • Well-differentiated thyroid cancer • Medullary thyroid cancer • Indolent lymphomas • Neuroendocrine tumors • Teratomas • Soft tissue sarcomas
86	Why is it difficult to use a PET/CT scan to determine the extent of a skull base tumor?	Brain metabolism is high, which can obscure skull-base tumors, or tumors with intracranial invasion.
87	What might result in a false-positive result on a PET/CT scan?	• Infection • Normal physiologic activity • Inflammation (e.g., after radiation, surgical resection or biopsy, aspiration) • Osteoradnionecrosis • Granulomatous disease • Patient movement
88	What is one of the major limitations of PET/CT scanning, which can result in a false-negative scan?	It is unreliable for lesions < 1 cm in diameter (some scanners can reportedly detect suspicious lymph nodes as small as 5 mm).
89	What is the sensitivity of PET scan for detecting squamous cell carcinoma recurrence less than 1 month after completion of radiation therapy? More than 1 month afterward?	55%, 95% *Key issue*: Waiting 3 months after completion of radiation minimizes false-positives resulting from inflammation and continued tumor regression. Patients should be clinically assessed for tumor progression during or after therapy, and patients with progression or bulky (N3) disease may require restaging and salvage sooner.
90	In addition to a CT scan, what imaging modality can be helpful for preoperative planning in a patient with a tumor invading the mandible that will require mandibulectomy or in a patient undergoing radiation therapy?	Panorex
91	Although ultrasound is not often used for the workup of nodal or primary head and neck cancer (other than thyroid disease), it is often used to assist in what important diagnostic procedure?	FNA biopsy. CT-guided biopsy can also be considered.

92	When should an excisional lymph node biopsy be considered?	It is not indicated for most head and neck cancers (e.g.,, squamous cell carcinoma). If there is concern for hematoproliferative malignancy, excisional biopsies are often necessary to provide adequate tissue for evaluation.
93	Incisional biopsies are routinely performed in the office setting for accessible tumors, such as oral cavity or oropharyngeal, to obtain a tissue diagnosis. Some clinicians recommend delaying this until after what key step in the workup?	Imaging
94	What is the most common pathologic type of cancer in the head and neck (excluding salivary and thyroid tumors)?	Squamous cell carcinoma (>90%)
95	Which immunohistochemical marker is most commonly associated with neural/cartilaginous tumors, melanoma, and Langerhans cell histiocytosis?	S-100
96	Which immunohistochemical marker is associated with carcinomas and papillomas?	Cytokeratin
97	Which immunohistochemical marker(s) is/are associated with melanoma?	• S-100 • HMB-45 • Melanoma-associated antigen recognized by T cells (MART-1) (diagnostic)
98	Which immunohistochemical marker is associated with neuroendocrine tumors (e.g., Merkel cell carcinoma, paraganglioma)?	• Neuron-specific enolase (NSE) • Chromogranin • Synaptophysin
99	Which immunohistochemical marker is most commonly associated with lymphoma?	• Leukocyte common antigen (LCA/CD45) • CD-20 → B-cell specificity • CD-3 → T-cell specificity
100	Which tumors stain positive for vimentin on immunohistochemistry? For desmin?	• Vimentin → sarcomas, lipomas, myomas • Desmin → sarcomas, myomas
101	Describe the World Health Organization (WHO) classification of *mild*, *moderate*, and *severe* dysplasia.	(▶ Table 7.3)

Table 7.3 The World Health Organization (WHO) classification of dysplasia.

Grade	Description
mild	nuclear atypia and architectural abnormalities of epithelial maturation confined to the basal third of the epithelium
moderate	abnormalities extend to the middle third of the epithelium
severe	abnormalities extend into the superficial third of the epithelium
carcinoma in-situ	full-thickness abnormalities without invasion beyond the basement membrane

102	What subtypes of squamous cell carcinoma of the head and neck have distinct clinical behaviors?	• Basaloid • Verrucous (<5%) • Spindle cell • Adenosquamous

103	What subtype of squamous cell carcinoma is commonly seen in HPV-positive oropharyngeal tumors (tonsil and base of tongue) and are more likely to present at an advanced stage owing to early nodal and distant metastases?	Basaloid carcinoma. *Note:* Despite the early regional metastases, these tumors are fairly sensitive to treatment and therefore have a better prognosis than conventional squamous cell carcinoma.
104	Describe the histopathology for spindle cell carcinoma.	Spindle cell carcinoma is also called carcinosarcoma or pseudosarcoma because it includes a squamous cell lesion on the surface and a more notable underlying malignant spindle cell component. Currently, it is thought that the tumor arises from epithelial cells and then undergoes mesenchymal differentiation.
105	Why are spindle cell carcinomas, which are a subtype of squamous cell carcinoma, most commonly found in the oral cavity and larynx, also known as sarcomatoid, carcinosarcoma, or pseudosarcoma?	• Contains a superficial squamous cell lesion and a deeper malignant spindle cell component. • Stain positive for both cytokeratin (epithelial cells) and vimentin (mesenchymal cells). • Arises from epithelial cells and then undergoes mesenchymal differentiation.
106	What is the management strategy of choice for spindle cell carcinomas?	The strategy is controversial because of the limited numbers of case reports in the literature. Most recommend surgery. There is controversy about the radiosensitivity of the tumor.
107	How can adenosquamous carcinoma be distinguished from mucoepidermoid carcinoma?	Mucoepidermoid carcinoma does not include a mucosal component. Adenosquamous carcinoma has a predominant mucosal squamous cell component and a deeper adenocarcinoma component.
108	What squamous cell carcinoma subtype manifests as a slow-growing, velvety, exophytic, and warty mass in elderly patients, and what pathologic feature determines their prognosis?	• Verrucous carcinoma • Focal areas of high-grade squamous cell carcinoma
109	What is the preferred management for localized verrucous carcinoma?	Complete surgical resection. Surgery was superior to primary radiation in 5-year survival (89 vs. 58%).
110	What are the most common sites of metastasis for head and neck squamous cell carcinoma?	• Lungs (66%) • Bone (22%) • Liver (10%) • Less often skin, mediastinum, and bone marrow
111	Traditionally, what single prognostic factor has been shown to decrease overall survival by as much as 50%?	Regional nodal disease (N +)
112	When considering nodal disease, what factors have been considered negative prognostic features?	• Presence of nodal disease (decreases survival by as much as 50%) • Increasing nodal size • Extracapsular spread • Bilateral neck disease • Matted lymph nodes • Disease in levels IV and V • "Skipped" levels • Invasion of local structures by nodal disease • Confluence of primary disease and nodal disease • Total number of involved lymph nodes
113	During the radiologic workup for a patient with head and neck cancer, in addition to the information needed to provide a TNM stage, what specific radiologic feature regarding the primary tumor size has been identified as negative prognosticator?	Gross tumor volume (poorer locoregional control and overall survival). *Note:* Standardized uptake values (SUVs) for PET/CT scans have been investigated but results are inconclusive.

114	What tumor biomarkers can be used to help determine prognosis in head and neck cancer?	• EGFR amplification and overexpression • HPV status • Loss of heterozygosity (suggests a loss of tumor suppressor gene function) • Aneuploidy
115	When considering head and neck cancer as a whole, what are the most important contributors to overall cancer specific mortality?	• Locoregional recurrence (50 to 60%) • Distant metastases (20 to 30%) • Second primary disease (10 to 20%)
116	What comorbidities most commonly impact the choice of therapeutic intervention in head and neck cancer patients (*therapeutic comorbidity*)?	• Severe lung disease and poor pulmonary function (e.g., not a candidate for a supraglottic laryngectomy) • Renal failure, hearing loss, neurologic disorder (e.g., choice of chemotherapeutic agents or therapy) • Severe atherosclerotic disease (e.g., may not be a candidate for free tissue transfer reconstruction)
117	What comorbidities have been found to negatively impact prognosis in head and neck cancer (*prognostic comorbidity*)?	• Recent myocardial infarction or ventricular arrhythmia • Severe hypertension • Severe hepatic disease • Recent severe stroke

Overview of Oncologic Therapy

118	What defines the ratio of therapy resulting in therapeutic effect to the amount that results in toxicity or mortality?	Therapeutic ratio or index
119	What type of treatment regimen uses only surgery or radiation therapy for curative intent?	Single-modality treatment. Any approach using more than one treatment modality is considered *multimodality* or *combined modality*.
120	What treatment approach uses chemotherapy and/or radiation therapy before definitive therapy?	Neoadjuvant/Induction therapy
121	What treatment approach uses chemotherapy and radiation therapy together as the primary treatment modality?	Concurrent (concomitant) therapy
122	What treatment approach uses radiation therapy with or without chemotherapy after primary surgical management?	Adjuvant therapy
123	What treatment approach uses surgery, chemotherapy, and/or radiation for patients with recurrent or metastatic disease without the intent to cure? With the intent to cure?	• Palliative therapy • Salvage therapy
124	Define the three types of clinical trials.	• Phase I: Defines the maximum tolerated dose or safety of a drug or invasive medical device • Phase II: Includes more patients than phase I; assesses the efficacy and side effects or toxicity associated with the intervention of interest • Phase III: Randomized prospective trial comparing the intervention of interest with the standard of care; at termination, can be considered for Food and Drug Administration approval for the intervention of interest.
125	What tumors are considered by the National Comprehensive Cancer Network (NCCN, 2011) to be very advanced and therefore managed with a unique algorithm regardless of tumor subsite?	T4b, any N, M0 or unresectable nodal disease

126	The NCCN (2011) recommends either a clinical trial or standard therapy for patients diagnosed with very advanced head and neck cancer. How is standard therapy individualized, and what does it include?	ECOG performance status (PS): • PS 0–1: Concurrent chemoradiation therapy with cisplatin or induction chemotherapy followed by radiation or chemoradiation therapy • PS 2: Definitive radiation therapy or concurrent chemoradiation therapy • PS 3: Radiation therapy vs. single-agent chemotherapy vs. best supportive care Note: With improvement in surgical management reconstructive techniques, some authorities suggest that surgical management should be considered for some T4b tumors.

127	Patients with recurrent or persistent head and neck cancer after primary management are considered by the NCCN (2011) to have very advanced head and neck cancer. For patients who do not have distant metastases, what are the treatment options?	• Locoregional recurrence without prior radiation therapy
		   ○ Resectable: Surgery ± adjuvant therapy (for adverse risk features) vs. primary chemoradiation therapy
		   ○ Unresectable: individualized based on performance status to nonsurgical treatment
		 • Locoregional recurrence or second primary with a history of prior radiation therapy
		   ○ Resectable: Surgery ± reirradiation ± chemotherapy
		   ○ Unresectable: Reirradiation ± chemotherapy vs. palliative care

128	What is the standard therapy recommended by the NCCN (2011) for metastatic head and neck cancer?	Based on ECOG performance status (PS): • PS 0–1: Combination or single agent chemotherapy → best supportive care • PS 2: Single-agent chemotherapy or best supportive care → best supportive care • PS 3: Best supportive care
129	What percentage of patients with locally advanced head and neck squamous cell carcinoma die from recurrent locoregional disease within five years of initial treatment?	30 to 50%
130	What is the median length of survival for a patient diagnosed with locally advanced or metastatic head and neck squamous cell carcinoma?	6 to 9 months
131	What are the primary goals of palliative therapy?	• Improve quality of life • Prolong life
132	What prognostic factors predict poor outcome for patients with incurable head and neck squamous cell carcinoma?	• Poor performance status • Extensive tumor burden • Malnutrition • Prior history of extensive definitive therapeutic intervention • Rapid recurrence or progression
133	What is the general surveillance schedule for history of physical examination and imaging as recommended by the NCCN (2011) for head and neck cancer?	History and physical examination • Year 1: Every 1 to 3 months • Year 2: Every 2 to 4 months • Year 3 to 5: Every 4 to 6 months • >5 years: Every 6 to 12 months Imaging • Within 6 months of treatment end for T3–4 or N2–3 cancers of the oropharynx, hypopharynx, glottic larynx, supraglottic larynx, and nasopharynx • Additional imaging based on concerning signs and symptoms
134	When should you evaluate a patient's thyroid-stimulating hormone (TSH) level after completion of treatment for head and neck cancer?	If the neck was irradiated, check a TSH every 6 to 12 months.

135	What are the three functional outcomes that are most commonly assessed for head and neck cancer?	• Airway • Speech • Swallowing
136	What focuses on a patient's perception of the impact of illness before, during, and after treatment?	Health-related quality of life
137	What domains are generally included in health related quality of life?	• Physical/somatic • Functional • Social • Psychological/emotional

Overview of Surgical Therapy

138	What are the three major categories that should be considered when determining candidacy for surgical intervention for head and neck cancer patients?	• Physiologic: Cardiorespiratory fitness, coagulation status, immune status, and weight loss (> 10% body weight considered poor prognosticator for surgical intervention) • Anatomical: Surgical access to the subsite of interest (e.g., trismus in oropharyngeal cancer, brittle cervical spine or large osteophytes in laryngeal cancer) • Oncologic: Ability to achieve surgical margins, acceptable morbidity with complete resection
139	When considering surgical management of a primary head and neck tumor, what is a critical component of successful management?	Ability to achieve negative margins
140	For upper aerodigestive tract tumors, what is the minimum width of tissue that must be taken to achieve a negative margin?	Controversial. The presence of invasive carcinoma in the margin specimen is the only factor that indicates a positive margin. In many subsites, width cutoffs have been abandoned for narrow margin analysis resulting from the proximity of critical adjacent structures.
141	True or False. En bloc tumor resection is the only oncologically sound method for surgical management of a primary head and neck tumor.	False. Narrow-margin analysis, "bread-loafing," or tumor mapping with frozen pathologic analysis of margins does not compromise oncologic outcomes (Hinni, 2013).
142	When a tumor invades a sensory or motor nerve, what is the recommended surgical approach?	Dissect proximally and distally along the nerve, take margins at either end and with the goal of obtaining negative margins on frozen section analysis.
143	In a patient with biopsy-proven squamous cell carcinoma metastases to the cervical lymph nodes, what are the most likely site and subsite of origin?	Unknown primary: • Site: Upper aerodigestive tract • Subsite: Oropharynx
144	Why is it clinically important, from both a prognostic and management standpoint, to identify the site of origin for an unknown primary tumor?	Failure to identify the site of origin results in • Significant decrease in 5-year overall survival (50%) • Need for wide-field radiation therapy with an increase in associated morbidity
145	What imaging modality can be helpful in identifying the unknown primary in as many as 30% of TX head and neck cancer patients?	PET/CT scan
146	Describe the surgical approach for a patient with an unknown primary tumor.	• Manual palpation of the upper aerodigestive tract • Visual inspection using naked-eye evaluation, rigid endoscopy, laryngoscopy and microscopy • Directed biopsies and frozen-section analysis. If negative, proceed. • Palatine and lingual tonsillectomy with frozen-section pathology ipsilateral to the cervical adenopathy. If negative, proceed. • Contralateral palatine and lingual tonsillectomy with frozen-section pathology. If negative, proceed.

		• Nasopharyngeal biopsies with frozen-section pathology. If negative, proceed. • Neck dissection and permanent serial sectioning of the biopsy specimens *Note*: If tumor is identified at any step, complete resection is advised. (Karni, 2011; Nagel, 2013).

Overview of Radiation Therapy

147	Why might tumor cells exposed to an increased concentration of growth factors, nutrients, and oxygen be more susceptible to radiation and chemotherapy?	A larger number will transition from G0 to G1 and enter the cell cycle, during which their DNA is more susceptible to antineoplastic therapy.
148	At what point during the cell cycle are cells most radiosensitive? Radioresistant?	• Radiosensitive: M phase and G2 • Radioresistant: S phase *Note*: The two most important checkpoints in relation to radiation damage are G1 and G2.
149	Does the proliferation rate of a tumor determine its radiosensitivity?	Controversial. Both proliferating and nonproliferating tissues can be radiosensitive, but the effects in nonproliferating or slowly proliferating tissues are often delayed. Radiosensitivity is unique to each tumor.
150	How does radiation result in cell killing?	Radiation therapy produces intracellular ionization → breaks chemical bonds, creates free radicals → DNA damage → cell death. Double-strand breaks are the most important and deadly injury imposed by radiation.
151	What generally determines the maximum dose of radiation that can safely be delivered to a tissue?	Ability of adjacent normal tissue to withstand the radiation and effectively repair damage
152	Although radiation can result in rapid cell death (*apoptosis*), some cells do not die until they attempt mitosis, and others continue to divide several times before cell death. What is this delayed cell killing called?	Mitotic cell death. This is why tumors do not shrink immediately after radiation and may take weeks to demonstrate the full effects of radiation treatment (simplified explanation).
153	Describe the basic principles involved in clinical radiobiology, which is often described as the four Rs of radiotherapy.	• Repair: Sublethal damage between fractions • Redistribution: Into radiosensitive phases of the cell cycle • Repopulation: With increased time between fractions • Reoxygenation: Response to ionizing radiation is increased 1.5–3x in well-oxygenated cells; fractionation allows for increased oxygen delivery to previously hypoxic cells.
154	What is the unit used to describe the absorbed radiation dose?	• Gray (Gy) = 1 Joule of energy per kilogram of material • 1 Gy = 100 centigray (cGy) = 100 rads (old unit) *Note*: The energy of radiation delivered determines the depth of tissue penetration.
155	What are the two general forms of ionizing radiation?	• *Particulate*: Kinetic energy is carried by a particle that has a resting mass, such as electrons, protons, or neutrons. • *Electromagnetic*: Massless, chargeless packets of energy (photon) that move through space at the speed of light, including X-rays and gamma rays
156	What are the three main radiotherapeutic modalities used clinically in head and neck cancer?	• *Electrons*: Produced by a linear accelerator; travel shorter distances within tissue • *Photons/X-ray*: Produced by linear accelerator; travel further within tissue; most widely used (e.g., intensity-modulated radiation therapy, or IMRT) • *Protons*: Produced by a cyclotron; charged particles; pronounced peak of energy deposition with little dose deposited beyond it (Bragg peak) *Note*: Can use a mix of photons and electrons

157	What device accelerates electrons to a high level of energy and then allows them to (1) exit the machine as an electron or (2) collide with a specific target that results in the emission of photons (both of which can be used for treatment)?	Linear accelerator
158	In what type of radiation treatment is the radiation source located outside the patient?	External-beam radiation therapy (EBRT)
159	What radiation strategy attempts to match the target volume (defined by high-resolution imaging, such as CT or MRI) with a high dose of radiation while limiting the amount of radiation given to adjacent normal tissue?	Conformal therapy (three-dimensional conformal radiation therapy) *Note*: IMRT is preferentially used to accomplish these goals in the head and neck.
160	What type of radiation therapy dynamically alters the intensity of radiation across a field during treatment delivery?	IMRT
161	What type of radiation therapy delivers a full dose of radiation in a single (or very few) fraction(s) using photons generated by a cobalt-60 source or by a linear accelerator?	Stereotactic radiation therapy, referred to as *stereotactic radiosurgery* for intracranial and skull base applications
162	What type of radiation therapy makes use of radionuclides that decay within specific anatomical subsites, resulting in very specific targeting?	Targeted radionuclide therapy (e.g., thyroid cancer and iodine-131)
163	Which form of radiation energy is better able to deposit most of its energy at a specific target, minimizing the dose to surrounding tissues based on the Bragg peak?	Protons
164	You are planning to treat a patient with a superficial head and neck cancer using photon radiation. To ensure that sufficient dose is deposited superficially, you create a material with a similar density to skin to place over the tumor. What is this called?	Bolus
165	What type of fractionation schedule uses radiation given in multiple daily doses without changing the overall treatment time compared with traditional daily radiotherapy, and why does this potentially result in decreased late morbidity despite a higher total dose?	Hyperfractionation. Normal tissue is more sensitive to the size of each individual dose. Therefore, if you decrease the size of each individual dose while increasing the total dose given over the entire course, there should be increase tumor cell killing and decreased impact on normal tissues.
166	What type of fractionation schedule relies on multiple daily treatments using larger doses of radiation and a shorter overall treatment time compared with standard daily radiation therapy?	Accelerated fractionation
167	What are the three primary radiosensitizing strategies currently available?	• Decreasing hypoxemia (due to increased interstitial pressure within the tumor or comorbid anemia): Hyperbaric oxygen therapy*, inhaled carbogen, hypoxic cell sensitizers (nimorazole, tirapazamine), recombinant human erythropoietin** • Concomitant chemotherapy: Additive (kills micrometastasis, toxicity profiles do not overlap) vs. synergistic effect (increased cytotoxic activity) • Targeted therapy: Goal is to decrease side effects and improve radiation efficacy; monoclonal antibody against EGFR (cetuximab). * No change in 5-year outcomes **Worse locoregional control and overall survival

168	What are the five basic steps involved in radiation treatment?	• Simulation • Treatment planning (defining target volumes, imaging, dose, schedule) • Verification • Dose delivery • Quality assurance
169	Imaging the patient to delineate targets and treatment volumes is done using CT or MRI. Is this typically done before or after the patient is immobilized?	After. It allows for better accuracy of treatment.
170	When planning radiation targets, what three volumes must be considered?	• Gross tumor volume: Delineates tumor boundaries • Clinical target volume: Identifies regions at high risk for harboring microscopic disease • Planning target volume: Includes a "margin" to allow and fraction to fraction variability in patient positioning
171	What types of tissues are at risk for acute radiation related toxicity? Delayed toxicity?	• Acute: Rapidly dividing cells; skin, mucous membranes, bone marrow, tumor cells. Related to *total treatment time, dose per fraction, total dose, time between treatments* • Delayed: More slowly dividing cells; neural and connective tissue. Related to *total dose and dose per fraction*
172	Acute radiation toxicity occurs over days to weeks following treatment. What are some of the most common toxicities associated with treatment of the head and neck?	• Mucositis • Dermatitis • Xerostomia • Hoarseness • Odynophagia • Dysphagia • Weight loss
173	Delayed or late radiation toxicity occurs months to years after treatment. What are the most common toxicities?	• Xerostomia • Dental caries/decay • Osteoradionecrosis, chondronecrosis • Fibrosis • Hypothyroidism • Neurologic damage
174	Compared with two- or three-dimensional conformal techniques, intensity-modulated radiation therapy may spare what organs within the head and neck?	• Salivary glands • Pharyngeal musculature • Otic structures • Optic structures • Temporomandibular joints (TMJs) • Brain
175	In an effort to reduce the incidence of osteoradionecrosis, when should decayed and nonrestorable teeth be extracted in relation to radiation therapy?	Before radiation
176	What are the theoretical advantages to preoperative radiation therapy?	• Reduction of unresectable tumors to the point of resectability • Reduces the extent of necessary surgery • Microscopic disease is usually more radiosensitive preoperatively because it has a better blood supply. • Cells disseminated during the course of surgery may be less viable after radiation therapy. • Requisite treatment volumes are smaller preoperatively than postoperatively.
177	What are the theoretical advantages to postoperative radiation therapy?	• Surgery allows for definition of the extent of tumor. • Surgery is easier before radiation. • Dosing can be adjusted depending on residual tumor after surgery. • Fewer wound-related complications

178	What type of fractionation regimen has been shown to result in better local control and overall survival compared with conventionally fractionated radiation therapy?	Hyperfractionated *Note*: With concurrent chemoradiation therapy, there is no benefit. This is a complex issue.

Overview of Chemotherapy

179	What is the role of chemotherapy in the treatment of head and neck cancers?	• For patients undergoing treatment with curative intent, chemotherapy is used concurrent with radiation therapy to improve locoregional control of disease, either as definitive chemoradiation therapy or as chemoradiation therapy after complete surgical resection (adjuvant therapy). Induction chemotherapy (multidrug regimen given before definitive chemoradiation) is another accepted use of chemotherapy for head and neck cancer. • For patients with recurrent or metastatic disease not amenable to curative therapy, chemotherapy is used as a palliative treatment to help control disease and improve cancer-related symptoms.
180	True or False. Head and neck squamous cell carcinoma is unusually sensitive to chemotherapy for a solid tumor.	True
181	For squamous cell carcinoma of the head and neck, chemotherapy (5-fluorouracil [5-FU]) and cisplatin) has been demonstrated to result in overall response rates up to 90%. What percentage of patients will have complete responses, and what percentage of these complete responses can be considered a cure?	• Complete response: 20 to 50% • Cure: ~ 0%; chemotherapy cannot be used with curative intent.
182	Studies have shown that patients who have not been treated with prior surgery and/or radiation respond to chemotherapy almost twice as often as patients who had. What might explain this?	• Better performance status before treatment • Intact blood supply to the tumor • Prior radiation may select for clonal populations of chemo-resistant cells.
183	What class of chemotherapeutic agents target DNA and cause cross-linking, double-strand breaks, or substitutions, thereby interfering with DNA replication and ultimately causing mutation and/or cell death?	Alkylating agents
184	What inorganic platinum chemotherapeutic agent results in DNA cross-links, denaturation of strands, covalent bonds with DNA bases, and DNA intra-strand cross-links?	Cisplatin
185	What common side effects are associated with cisplatin administration?	Nephrotoxicity, ototoxicity, neurotoxicity, nausea/vomiting, electrolyte disturbances, myelotoxicity
186	Name the second-generation platinum agent that binds with DNA to create interstrand and intra-strand cross-links and protein-DNA cross-links that ultimately result in interruption of the cell cycle and apoptosis.	Carboplatin
187	What class of chemotherapeutic agents inhibits accurate DNA replication by imitating naturally occurring metabolites imperative to DNA replication? What are some examples?	Antimetabolites • Methotrexate: Binds to dihydrofolate reductase, which is necessary for de novo synthesis of thymidine and purine synthesis • 5-FU: Irreversibly binds to thymidylate synthetase, blocking conversion of uridine to thymidine, thereby preventing DNA synthesis

188	Cultured *Streptomyces* spp. produce compounds that function as antibiotic chemotherapeutic agents. What agent in this class results in (1) intercalation between base pairs; (2) forms complexes with iron, thus reducing oxygen to superoxide and hydroxyl radicals which result in DNA strand breaks; (3) DNA cross-linking, alkylation, and oxygen radicals?	Antitumor antibiotics • Doxorubicin • Bleomycin • Mitomycin
189	What class of chemotherapeutic agents binds to free tubulin dimers and therefore results in disruption of microtubule polymerization or de-polymerization and ultimate disruption of the cell cycle? What are some examples?	Alkaloids • Vincristine: Binds irreversibly to microtubules and spindle proteins in S phase and interferes with the mitotic spindle → arrest in metaphase • Vinblastine: Binds to tubulin and inhibits microtubule formation, disrupts mitotic spindle → arrest in M phase
190	What class of chemotherapeutic agents causes stabilization of microtubules, thereby inhibiting the normal cell cycle by preventing microtubule disassembly and arrest at the G2/M phase and apoptosis? What are some examples?	Taxanes • Docetaxel • Paclitaxel
191	What chimeric monoclonal antibody targeting EGFR, which is overexpressed in head and neck squamous cell carcinoma, has proven to be effective for this pathology?	Cetuximab
192	What recombinant humanized monoclonal antibody targets EGFR and is currently being investigated in head and neck cancer?	Bevacizumab
193	What are the potential pros and cons of induction or chemotherapy followed by definitive treatment in head and neck squamous cell carcinoma?	Pros: • Decrease the size of the tumor prior to definitive management • Increase the response to locoregional definitive management (both radiation and surgery may be more effective for smaller tumors) • Theoretically decreases the risk for distant metastases • Assess tumor response to chemotherapy (also a surrogate marker for radiosensitivity) Cons: • Difficulty identifying tumor extent • Inability to tolerate definitive management due to toxicities • Increased cost and complexity of treatment • Decreased compliance with treatment
194	Phase II trials demonstrated considerable promise for the use of an induction/neoadjuvant approach to head and neck squamous cell carcinoma. What were the results of subsequent phase III trials?	Controversial. Initial phase III studies demonstrated no survival advantage. However, more recent phase III trials, including agents such as docetaxel, cisplatin, and 5-FU, demonstrated both a progression-free survival and overall survival advantage (European Organization for Research and Treatment of Cancer [EORTC] 24971; TAX 324).
195	The Head and Neck Contracts Program, run by the National Cancer Institute, and the Head and Neck Intergroup Study 0034 both demonstrated that adjuvant chemotherapy after primary surgery or radiation has the potential to reduce what key oncologic outcome measure?	• Distant metastases • Did not impact overall survival • Can be considered "maintenance" chemotherapy

196	What are some of the attributes that define *high-risk disease* in head and neck cancer patients that benefits from adjuvant chemotherapy?	• Positive surgical margins • Extracapsular extension • T3/T4 primary disease • Higher nodal stage • Perineural invasion • Angiolymphatic invasion • Involvement of level IV or V lymph nodes
197	What is the rationale for using chemotherapy and radiation therapy together to treat head and neck squamous cell carcinoma?	Each modality functions independently from the other, but together they result in synergistic chemotherapeutic radiosensitization.
198	Phase III trials have demonstrated improved disease-free survival for patients undergoing adjuvant chemoradiation therapy for high-risk disease. What factors conferred a high-risk status for these studies?	• Positive surgical margins • Extracapsular extension
199	Which agents have shown a survival advantage for concurrent chemotherapy as single agents?	• Cisplatin (low-dose daily; high-dose every 3 weeks) • Carboplatin • 5-FU
200	Aggressive, multiagent chemotherapy has been added to radiation therapy for head and neck cancer and has resulted in a locoregional control rate in some studies of > 90%. In this cohort of patients, what is the most likely oncologic failure?	Distant metastases. May suggest a role for induction chemotherapy. *Note:* Controversy is ongoing as to whether the benefit of multiagent chemotherapy outweighs the risks. Therefore, single-agent chemoradiation therapy remains the standard of care for this approach.
201	What clinical outcome has driven research into definitive chemoradiation strategies for head and neck cancer? Name two studies that provided evidence to usport this approach.	Organ preservation Department of Veterans Affairs Laryngeal Cancer Study Intergroup Radiation Oncology Group (RTOG) 91–11

Neck Anatomy

202	How are the lymph node levels divided in the neck? (▶ Fig. 7.1)	They are separated into levels based on anatomic or surgical and radiographic criteria. The following are the most commonly involved groups:
		• Level I (IA/IB)
		  ○ IA: Submental triangle
		  ○ IB: Submandibular triangle
		• Level II (IIA/IIB)
		  ○ IIA: Upper jugular chain
		  ○ IIB: Submuscular recess
		• Level III: Middle jugular chain
		• Level IV: Lower jugular chain
		• Level V (VA/VB): Posterior triangle
		  ○ VA: Spinal accessory chain
		  ○ VB: Supraclavicular and transverse cervical chain
		• Level VI: Anterior jugular chain

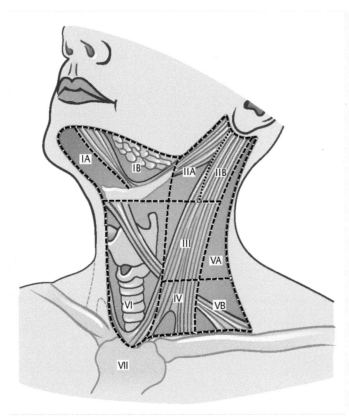

Fig. 7.1 Lymph node levels of the neck. (Used with permission from Bradley P, Guntinas-Lichius O. Salivary Gland Disorders and Diseases: Diagnosis and Management. New York, NY: Thieme; 2011.)

203	In addition to the six nodal levels, there are additional, unclassified nodal groups that are important in the surgical management of the neck. What are these, and where are they found?	• Suboccipital nodes: Deep to the insertion of the trapezius muscle • Retroauricular nodes: Superficial postauricular region • Parotid nodes: Can be superficial to, within or deep to the parotid gland • Retropharyngeal nodes: Between the prevertebral fascia and the pharyngeal constrictor muscles • Facial nodes: Superficial and deep to the facial artery and vein
204	What lymph node levels in the neck are unpaired?	Level IA. Level VI is often considered to have a right and a left but may also be considered as a single compartment.
205	How is level IB distinguished from level IIA surgically and radiographically?	Posterior edge of the submandibular gland
206	How is the lateral border of level IIA defined radiographically?	Posterior border of the internal jugular vein
207	What anatomical structure divides lymph node level II into IIA and IIB surgically?	Spinal accessory nerve (CN XI)
208	How are the superior and inferior boundaries of level IIA surgically defined?	• Superior: Skull base • Inferior: Carotid bifurcation
209	What are the radiographic and surgical landmarks that separate neck levels II and III?	Inferior border of the hyoid bone (radiographic) and carotid bifurcation (surgical)

210	What are the superior and inferior borders of level III radiographically?	• Superior: Horizontal plane from the inferior border of the hyoid bone • Inferior: Horizontal plane from the inferior border of the cricoid cartilage
211	What are the radiographic and surgical landmarks that separate neck levels III and IV?	Inferior border of the cricoid cartilage (radiographic) and the omohyoid muscle (surgical)
212	What anatomical structure divides lymph node level V into VA and VB?	A horizontal plane from the inferior border of the cricoid cartilage *Note*: Level VA includes the spinal accessory nodes, VB includes the transverse cervical nodes and supraclavicular nodes. Just inferior to the clavicle lies the sentinel node or Virchow node.
213	What are the surgical landmarks that define level VI (central compartment) lymphatics?	Hyoid bone superiorly, suprasternal notch inferiorly, and common carotid arteries laterally
214	Level VI lymph nodes are at greatest risk for metastasis from which primary locations?	• Glottic and subglottic larynx • Pyriform sinus • Cervical esophagus • Thyroid gland
215	What are the major divisions of cervical fascia in the neck?	• Superficial cervical fascia • Deep cervical fascia: Superficial (investing), middle (visceral), and deep layers
216	What layer of cervical fascia covers the superficial surface of the platysma muscle and is continuous with the superficial muscular aponeurotic system (SMAS) superiorly in the face and fascia overlying the chest, shoulder, and axilla?	Superficial cervical fascia
217	Which layer of cervical fascia arises from the vertebral spinous processes, wraps around the SCM and trapezius muscles, covers the mylohyoid muscle and anterior bellies of the digastric muscle, attaches to the hyoid bone, forms the floor of the submandibular and posterior triangle, wraps around the submandibular gland and parotid glands, and splits at the mandible into the internal layer, which lies over the medial surface of the medial pterygoid muscle and inserts onto the skull base, while the outer layer passes over the masseter muscle and inserts onto the zygomatic arch?	Superficial (investing) layer of the deep cervical fascia
218	What are the two subdivisions of the middle layer of the deep cervical fascia?	• Muscular division: Surrounds infrahyoid strap muscles, attached superiorly to the hyoid bone and thyroid cartilage and inferiorly to the sternum • Visceral division: Surrounds the thyroid, trachea, and esophagus and extends into the mediastinum to connect with the fibrous pericardium. Superiorly, the fascia may blend with the buccopharyngeal fascia (controversial).
219	Name the fascial layers that line the inner (pharyngeal) and outer (cervical) surface of the pharyngeal constrictor muscles.	• Inner: Pharyngobasilar fascia • Outer: Buccopharyngeal fascia
220	What are the two named divisions of the deep layer of the deep cervical fascia?	• *Prevertebral fascia*: Fused to the transverse processes of the vertebral bodies with extension medially to cover the prevertebral musculature and vertebral bodies. Continues posteriorly to cover the extensor muscles and insert onto the vertebral spinous processes • *Alar fascia*: Located between the prevertebral fascia and the visceral division of the middle layer of the deep cervical fascia

221	What layer(s) of cervical fascia form the carotid sheath?	The superficial (investing), middle (visceral), and deep layers of the deep cervical fascia
222	What is enveloped by the superficial (investing) layer of the deep cervical fascia?	• Two muscles (SCM and trapezius) • Two glands (parotid and submandibular gland) • Two spaces (Posterior triangle, suprasternal space of Burns)
223	What is the vascular supply and innervation of the platysma muscle?	• *Innervation*: Cervical branch of the facial nerve (CN VII) • *Arterial supply*: Submental branch of the facial artery and suprascapular artery

224	The SCM extends from the mastoid process of the temporal bone to the clavicle and manubrium, where it inserts as two separate heads (medial/sternal and lateral/clavicular) forming the lesser supraclavicular fossa. What is the innervation and blood supply to this muscle?	• Innervation: Spinal accessory nerve (CN XI), ventral rami of C2–4
		• Arterial supply:
		  ○ Occipital and posterior auricular arteries
		  ○ Superior thyroid artery
		  ○ Suprascapular artery

225	Describe the innervation and arterial supply to the anterior and posterior bellies of the digastric muscle.	• Innervation
		  ○ Anterior: mylohyoid branch of the inferior alveolar nerve (CN V$_3$)
		  ○ Posterior: facial nerve (CN VII)
		• Arterial supply
		  ○ Anterior: submental branch of the facial artery
		  ○ Posterior: posterior auricular and occipital arteries

226	Name the four paired infrahyoid strap muscles in order from superficial to deep.	• Superficial: sternohyoid and omohyoid • Deep: sternothyroid and thryohyoid
227	What is the predominant innervation and vascular supply to the infrahyoid strap musculature?	• Innervation: Ansa cervicalis (C1–3) • Arterial supply: Superior thyroid artery and lingual artery
228	What muscle can be found in the lateral neck extending from the transverse processes of C3 through C6 to the first rib, passing just posterior to the phrenic nerve, just anterior to the subclavian artery, and just medial to the brachial plexus?	Anterior scalene muscle
229	What spinal nerves provide sensory innervation to the cervical skin?	Ventral rami of C2–4 from the cervical plexus • Lesser occipital nerve (C2): Posterior scalp and ear • Great auricular nerve (C2, C3): Anterior branch → skin over parotid gland; posterior branch → mastoid area, lower ear and lobule • Transverse cutaneous nerve (C2, C3): Ascending/descending branches → anterolateral neck skin • Supraclavicular nerve (C3, C4): Medial, intermediate and lateral (posterior) branches → supraclavicular skin from second rib to shoulder
230	What anatomical location describes the point where the cutaneous nerves of the cervical plexus exit posterior to the sterncleidomastoid muscle, and what is the relationship between this point and the spinal accessory nerve (CN XI)?	Erb's point The spinal accessory nerve (CN XI) passes approximately 1 cm superior and deep to the sternocleidomastoid muscle and Erb's point.
231	What are the muscular branches that constitute the cervical plexus?	• Phrenic nerve (C3–5) • Inferior branch of ansa cervicalis (C1–3) • Segmental branches including cervical branches of the spinal accessory nerve (C1–4)

232	What structure travels deep to the deep cervical fascia and superficial to the anterior scalene and can be found when dissecting levels III and IV?	Phrenic nerve (C3–5)
233	The submandibular duct passes between what two nerves?	Lingual nerve and hypoglossal nerve
234	The sympathetic trunk travels deep and medial to the carotid sheath and is just superficial to the prevertebral fascia and what muscle?	Longus colli
235	What structure branches off the vagus nerve (CN X) at approximately T1–2, wraps around the subclavian artery from anterior to posterior, ascends in the neck along the tracheoesophageal groove, generally posterior to the inferior thyroid artery, and enters the larynx at a 30- to 45-degree angle by passing under the inferior constrictor muscle and through the cricothyroid joint space?	Right recurrent laryngeal nerve
236	The left recurrent laryngeal nerve wraps around the aortic arch before passing superiorly in the neck in the tracheoesophageal groove to enter the larynx at a 0- to 30-degree angle by passing under the inferior constrictor muscle and through what laryngeal space?	Cricothyroid
237	Describe the classic relationship between the inferior thyroid artery and the recurrent laryngeal nerve.	• 50%: Nerve passes deep to artery. • 25%: Nerve passes between arterial branches. • 25%: Nerve passes anterior to artery. Note: This relationship is extremely variable and may not represent a reliable landmark for identifying the nerve.
238	What is the incidence of a right nonrecurrent inferior/recurrent laryngeal nerve?	0.5 to 1%
239	What anomaly is associated with a right aberrant retroesophageal subclavian artery? Situs inversus?	• Right nonrecurrent inferior/recurrent laryngeal nerve • Left nonrecurrent inferior/recurrent laryngeal nerve
240	What structure is formed by the anastomoses of the posterior (dorsal) recurrent laryngeal nerve fibers and the posterior (dorsal) fibers of the internal branch of the superior laryngeal nerve, and what is its function?	Galen anastomosis (aka ramus anastomaticus)
241	What artery branches from the aortic arch, passes over the trachea from left to right and branches into the right common carotid artery and right subclavian artery?	Innominate (brachiocephalic) artery
242	What are the major divisions of the right subclavian artery?	• First part: Right, from innominate artery just posterior to the sternoclavicular joint to the medial border of the anterior scalene muscle; may rise 2 cm above the clavicle. Left, from aortic arch at T3–4 to the medial border of the anterior scalene muscle • Second part: Highest point, spans the width of the anterior scalene muscle. • Third part: Lateral border of anterior scalene muscle to outer border of the first rib → axillary artery

243	What artery branches off the first part of the subclavian artery, ascends in the neck by passing through the foramina of the transverse processes of C1–C6, and enters the foramen magnum and joins with its paired contralateral vessel to form the basilar artery?	Vertebral artery
244	What are the three arteries that arise from the first part of the subclavian artery?	• Vertebral artery • Thyrocervical trunk • Inferior thoracic artery
245	Name the branches of the thyrocervical trunk that branch off the first part of the subclavian artery at approximately the medial border of the anterior scalene muscle?	• Inferior thyroid artery • Suprascapular artery • Superficial/transverse cervical artery
246	On the left, the costocervical trunk arises from the first part of the subclavian artery, and on the right it arises from the second part. To what vessels does it give rise?	• Deep cervical artery • Superior intercostal artery
247	What structures are contained within the carotid sheath?	• Carotid arteries: Medial • Internal jugular vein: Lateral • Vagus nerve: Posterior
248	At what vertebral level(s) is the carotid bifurcation in the majority of people?	C3–4 (~ at the level of the superior border of the thyroid cartilage)
249	What bony skull base structure runs between the internal and external carotid arteries?	Styloid process
250	What are the branches of the external carotid artery, and to what named branches do these arteries give rise? (▶ Fig. 7.2)	• Superior thyroid artery → infrahyoid, superior laryngeal, cricothyroid and sternocleidomastoid arteries • Ascending pharyngeal artery → pharyngeal, inferior tympanic, and meningeal arteries • Lingual artery → suprahyoid, dorsal lingual, and sub-lingual arteries • Facial artery → ascending palatine, tonsillar, submental and glandular arteries • Occipital artery → Upper and lower branches to the sternocleidomastoid muscle • Posterior auricular artery → stylomastoid artery • Internal maxillary artery → see below • Superficial temporal artery → frontal and parietal branch

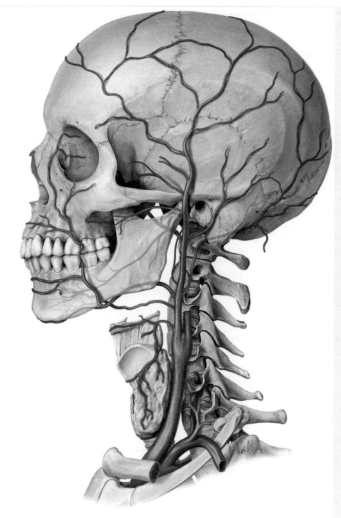

Fig. 7.2 Branches of the external carotid artery. (Used with permission from Thieme Atlas of Anatomy: Head and Neuroanatomy, © Thieme 2007, illustration by Karl Wesker.)

251	What artery arises at the level of the greater cornu of the hyoid bone from the external carotid, runs deep to the posterior belly of the digastric muscle and stylohyoid muscle, turns at the middle constrictor to follow the posterior boundary of the submandibular gland and medial border of the medial pterygoid muscle, and then winds around the mandible at the level of the facial notch?	Facial artery
252	What artery, or branch of this artery, often transverses level IIB in the neck and "tethers" the hypoglossal nerve in level IIA?	Occipital artery
253	What are the three parts of the internal maxillary artery?	• First part/mandibular portion: Arises between the ramus of the mandible and the sphenodmandibular ligament, passes the posterior to the lateral pterygoid muscle • Second part/pterygoid portion: Within the lateral pterygoid muscle • Third part/pterygopalatine portion: Pterygopalatine fossa

254	What are the branches of the first part (mandibular portion) of the internal maxillary artery?	• Deep auricular artery • Anterior tympanic artery • Middle meningeal artery • Accessory meningeal artery • Inferior alveolar artery • Mylohyoid artery
255	What are the branches of the second part (pterygoid part) of the internal maxillary artery?	• Anterior deep temporal artery • Posterior deep temporal arteries • Pterygoid branches • Masseteric artery • Buccinator/buccal artery
256	What are the branches of the third part (pterygopalatine part) of the internal maxillary artery?	• Posterior superior alveolar artery • Infraorbital artery • Sphenopalatine artery • Artery of the pterygoid (vidian) canal • Pharyngeal artery
257	What sensory organ(s) is located at the bifurcation of the common carotid artery, and what is the innervation?	• Carotid sinus → internal carotid artery, baroreceptor, glossopharyngeal nerve (IX), vagus nerve (X), sympathetics • Carotid body → posterior or between the carotid bifurcation, chemoreceptor, same innervation
258	What veins give rise to the external jugular vein, what structures does it drain, and where does it drain into?	• Retromandibular vein and postauricular vein • Scalp and face • Subclavian vein
259	What superficial veins drain the anterior neck by emptying into the external jugular vein or the subclavian vein and are at risk during thyroidectomy and tracheostomy?	Anterior jugular veins
260	What structures exit the skull base through the jugular foramen with the internal jugular vein?	Glossopharyngeal nerve (IX), vagus nerve (X), accessory nerve (XI), inferior petrosal sinus, and internal jugular vein
261	The internal jugular vein drains most of the head and neck into what venous structure?	Subclavian vein → brachiocephalic vein
262	What structure most commonly passes from the superior mediastinum, through the thoracic inlet on the left into level IV, passing anterior to the phrenic nerve and anterior scalene muscle, posterior to the carotid sheath, and most commonly terminates at the confluence of the left subclavian vein and internal jugular vein?	Thoracic duct
263	What is the incidence of right-sided thoracic duct in the neck? Bilateral?	• Right-sided only: 4% • Bilateral thoracic ducts: 12 to 15%

Evaluation and Management of the Neck

264	Malignancies involving the neck primarily arise as metastatic lesions (most commonly from the upper aerodigestive tract). What percentage of neck malignancies will arise primarily in the neck, and what are the most common sites of origin?	15%. Thyroid, salivary gland, and lymphoma
265	What percentage of neck masses in pediatric patients are benign?	>90%, most commonly inflammatory
266	Approximately what percentage of neck masses in adult patients are neoplastic?	~ 80%
267	What is the most common head and neck malignancy in the pediatric population and the second most common head and neck malignancy in the adult population after squamous cell carcinoma?	Lymphoma

268	What are common sites of origin for locoregional metastatic disease to cervical lymph nodes?	• Upper aerodigestive tract • Head and neck skin • Major and minor salivary glands • Thyroid gland
269	What are the most common sites of origin for distant metastatic disease to cervical lymph nodes?	• Lung • Thoracic esophagus • Ovary • Prostate • Kidney
270	What is the most likely site of origin for squamous cell carcinoma metastatic to cervical lymph nodes with an unknown primary?	Oropharynx (tonsil and tongue base)
271	What are the most common symptoms associated with nodal metastases to the neck?	• Palpable neck mass • Symptoms resulting from compression (e.g., dysphagia, dysphonia) • Symptoms resulting from invasion (e.g., recurrent laryngeal nerve paralysis, accessory neuropathy, pain)
272	What is the most common anterior neck mass diagnosed on physical examination?	Thyroid nodule
273	What are important features of lymphadenopathy that can be detected on a careful physical examination?	• Location • Mobility on palpation and with swallowing • Potential deep involved structures • Firm (i.e., not rubbery) • Involvement of the skin
274	True or False. Nodal cervical metastases from locoregional tumors are generally extremely painful.	False
275	When malignant lymphadenopathy is immobile and invasion or adherence of the nodal disease to underlying structures is suspected, what is the neck referred to as, and what implications does this have on management?	Fixed. It may be unresectable.
276	What is the best diagnostic test for determining the cause of a neck mass without a known primary tumor?	FNA biopsy
277	What diagnostic test is indicated if an FNA biopsy is performed on a suspicious cervical lymph node with an unknown primary and the pathology demonstrates lymphoid cells?	Excisional lymph node biopsy, most commonly in the operating room
278	Although there has been a significant amount of research into the application of sentinel lymph node biopsy for head and neck cancer, currently the literature supports its routine use for what types of cancer?	Cutaneous malignancies (especially melanoma). May also be used for known oral cavity cancer in patients with cN0 neck disease.
279	What are the general steps involved with performing a sentinel lymph node biopsy?	• Primary tumor is injected with technetium-99 sulfur colloid in the radiology suite. • Lymphoscintigraphy is performed, and the sentinel node is identified. • Patient is brought to the operating room (generally within 4 hours). • Use the gamma probe to confirm the location of the sentinel node and design surgical incision. • *Slowly* inject ~ 0.3 mL of isosulfan blue *intradermally* (not subcutaneously). This should result in a lacelike pattern under the skin. This should be done at least 10 minutes *before* any local anesthetic is injected if any is injected at all.

- Expose the tissue suspected of harboring the sentinel lymph node.
- Using the gamma probe (pointing away from the primary site if possible to avoid shine-through), identify the area containing the node. Visual confirmation of a blue node is supportive but not required if the gamma probe is suggestive.
- Excise the node and perform a 10-second gamma count in the dissection field to confirm that the sentinel node(s) was (were) removed.
- With the node placed away from the primary site and sentinel biopsy site, perform a confirmatory gamma count for 10 seconds to ensure you have removed the correct node.
- Excise the primary with appropriate margins. This may be done first if the primary is in close proximity to the sentinel lymph nodes.
- Depending on the pathology report results, the wound can be closed or a formal neck dissection is performed.

Note: It is not unusual for multiple lymph nodes to be identified. If the dissection bed after sentinel node excision contains > 10% of the gamma count detected before the node was removed, further exploration for remaining nodes is warranted.

280	In patients with common carotid artery or internal carotid artery invasion with tumor, which test should be employed before surgical resection of the involved carotid artery?	Carotid artery balloon occlusion test
281	What imaging modality is most commonly used for the initial workup of an adult neck masses?	CT with contrast
282	What imaging modality is best for evaluation of perineural spread associated with neck masses?	MRI
283	What imaging modality is best used to determine distant metastatic spread of disease and as an adjunct in patients with an unknown primary tumor?	PET/CT
284	What is the AJCC node (N) staging system for head and neck cancer (including salivary gland; excluding nasopharynx and thyroid)?	• Nx: Regional lymph nodes cannot be assessed • N0: No regional lymph node metastases • N1: One lymph node involved ≤ 3 cm • N2a: One ipsilateral lymph node involved > 3 cm and ≤ 6 cm in size • N2b: More than one ipsilateral involved lymph node, none > 6 cm • N2c: Contralateral or bilateral lymph node involvement ≤ 6 cm • N3: Lymph node > 6 cm
285	What is the AJCC lymph node (N) staging system for nasopharyngeal cancer?	• Nx: Regional lymph nodes cannot be assessed. • N0: No regional lymph node metastases • N1: Unilateral metastases in one of more lymph node ≤ 6 cm, above the supraclavicular fossa • N2: Bilateral metastases in lymph nodes ≤ 6 cm, above the supraclavicular fossa • N3a: Tumor > 6 cm • N3b: Tumor extends to the supraclavicular fossa.
286	What is the AJCC lymph node (N) staging system for soft tissue sarcomas?	• Nx: Regional lymph nodes cannot be assessed. • N0: No regional lymph node metastases. • N1: Regional lymph node metastases

287	What is the AJCC lymph node (N) staging system for thyroid cancer?	• Nx: Regional lymph nodes cannot be assessed. • N0: No regional lymph node metastases • N1a: Metastases to level VI (pretracheal, paratracheal, and prelaryngeal/Delphian node(s)) • N1b: Metastases to unilateral, bilateral, or contralateral cervical or superior mediastinal lymph nodes
288	For a patient with squamous cell carcinoma of the head and neck, the presence of nodal disease traditionally results what 5-year overall survival?	50%
289	In well-differentiated thyroid cancer, for what patient population does the presence of nodal metastases not influence their overall stage or prognosis?	Patients younger than 45 years
290	What pathologic nodal features have been associated with poor prognosis in head and neck cancer?	• Extracapsular spread (may not be true for HPV positive tumors) • Skipped nodal levels • Involvement of levels IV and V • Number of involved nodes • Size of involved nodes • Bilateral nodal disease • Matted lymph nodes
291	What is the difference between a *therapeutic* and an *elective* neck dissection?	• *Elective*: Performed in a clinically N0 neck owing to high risk (> 20%) for occult metastases • *Therapeutic*: Performed in a clinically N(+) neck
292	What type of neck dissection is delayed after primary chemoradiation therapy?	Staged neck dissection
293	What type of neck dissection is performed for recurrent disease after primary therapeutic intervention?	Salvage neck dissection
294	What is removed in a radical neck dissection?	• Lymph node levels I–V • SCM muscle • Spinal accessory nerve • Internal jugular vein
295	What are the three types of a modified radical neck dissection?	All three include dissection of levels I–V. Each type varies from a radical neck dissection by preserving the sternocleidomastoid (SCM), internal jugular vein (IJV) and/or spinal accessory nerve (SAN): • Type I: Preserves SAN • Type II: Preserves SAN + IJV • Type III (complete): Preserves SAN + IJV + SCM
296	The NCCN (2011) recommends using the term comprehensive neck dissection instead of radical or modified radical. How does the NCCN define a comprehensive neck dissection?	Resection of nodal levels I–V, regardless of preservation of SCM muscle, spinal accessory nerve, or IJV
297	In a select neck dissection, the surgeon will remove the lymphatic basins at highest risk for disease, which may vary according to the tumor, subsite, and individual patient. What is the most accurate way to refer to a select neck dissection?	Select neck dissection, levels X–X (detailing which levels were removed). However, the most common select neck dissections have associated terminology with which it is important to be familiar (see below).
298	In what type of neck dissection are levels I–III dissected, preserving the nonlymphatic structures of the neck?	Supraomohyoid neck dissection. Select neck dissection (levels I–III)
299	In what type of neck dissection are levels I–IV dissected, preserving the non-ymphatic structures of the neck?	Lateral neck dissection. Select neck dissection (levels I–IV)

300	In what type of neck dissection are levels III–V dissected, preserving the nonlymphatic structures of the neck?	Posterolateral neck dissection. Select neck dissection (levels II–IV)
301	In what type of neck dissection is level VI dissected, preserving the nonlymphatic structures of the neck?	Anterior/central neck dissection. Select neck dissection (level VI)
302	In what type of neck dissection are lymph node basins in addition to the more common I–V dissected?	• Extended neck dissection. This can include a radical neck dissection, modified neck dissection, or select neck dissection. • May designate using the type of dissection followed by the levels and additional lymph nodes dissected in parenthesis.
303	What type of neck dissection is generally recommended for oral cavity cancer?	Select neck dissection (level I-III) at minimum, with level IV for oral tongue cancers. Bilateral dissection should be considered for those with floor of mouth, ventral tongue, or midline tongue involvement in those undergoing elective ipsilateral neck dissection with no plans for postoperative radiation therapy.
304	What type of neck dissection is generally recommended for oropharyngeal cancer?	Select neck dissection (level II-IV). Bilateral dissection should be considered for base of tongue tumors, posterior oropharyngeal tumors, and those that cross midline. Dissection of retropharyngeal nodes should be considered. Routinely dissecting level IIB in cN0 necks is controversial.
305	What type of neck dissection is generally recommended for hypopharyngeal and laryngeal cancer?	Select neck dissection (level II–IV) and occasionally VI
306	In what type of neck dissection does the surgeon attempt to identify the first-echelon lymph node or nodes draining a particular subsite in an effort to determine whether the cancer has metastasized locally?	Sentinel lymph node biopsy
307	A meta-analysis of the EORTC (no. 22931) and RTOG (no. 9501) showed a benefit to postoperative concurrent chemoradiation in patients with locally advanced oral cavity, oropharynx, larynx, and hypopharynx squamous cell carcinoma when what risk factors were present?	Positive surgical margins and/or extracapsular spread
308	What branches of the vagus nerve are at highest risk for injury during neck dissection for head and neck cancer?	Recurrent laryngeal nerve and superior laryngeal nerve and its branches
309	After a select neck dissection (levels IA, IB, IIA, IIB, III), you note weakness in your patient's ipsilateral depressor anguli oris and depressor labii inferioris and resultant asymmetry during smiling. What structure was likely injured?	Marginal mandibular branch of CN VII
310	Describe the surgical techniques that can be used to decrease the risk of injury to the marginal mandibular nerve during neck dissection.	• Place incisions 3 to 4 cm (or two fingerbreadths) below the mandible. • Ligate the common facial vein under the superficial layer of the deep cervical fascia with a long tie. Lift this with the skin flap (this may limit oncologic dissection). • Elevate plane between the submandibular gland and superficial layer of the deep cervical fascia (this may limit oncologic dissection). • Identify marginal mandibular nerve as it branches from the cervical branch of the facial nerve.

311	What is the reported rate of marginal mandibular nerve injury after neck dissection (particularly level IB and occasionally level IIA), and what is the most common postoperative House-Brackmann score associated with neural injury?	Immediate: ~ 20%. Permanent: < 5% House-Brackmann grade II–III/VI
312	What sequelae results from resection of the spinal accessory nerve?	Shoulder syndrome: Denervation of the trapezius muscle resulting in destabilization of the scapula and inability to abduct the shoulder > 30 degrees, pain and shoulder girdle deformity. Injury from dissection around spinal accessory nerve in levels IIB and VA may also result in shoulder syndrome.
313	What nerve can be injured during dissection in level IV, which can result in paralysis of the ipsilateral hemidiaphragm?	Phrenic nerve
314	What factors increase the risk of postoperative wound infection or breakdown after neck dissection?	• Previous radiation therapy • Pharyngocutaneous or pharyngocervical fistula with salivary contamination • Chylous fistula • Hematoma • "Tight" wound closure with compromised vascular function • Comorbidities: Immunocompromised, malnourished, peripheral vascular disease, poorly controlled diabetes, and so forth
315	When planning a neck incision, why should you place any "T-limb" at 90 degrees to the main incision?	To maximize vascular supply and minimize skin flap necrosis
316	How should carotid artery exposure after neck dissection be dealt handled?	Coverage with vascularized tissue, preferably a myocutaneous flap (e.g., pectoralis major flap)
317	What are the risk factors for carotid blowout, which include rupture of any component of the carotid system, after management of head and neck cancer?	• Radiation therapy (≥ 70 Gray to the neck; accelerated fractionation schedule) • Neck dissection (radical = 8x increased risk) • Wound infection, breakdown, pharyngocutaneous fistula with salivary contamination • Mobile foreign material (wet to dry dressing) • Tumor involvement of the vessel • Malnutrition
318	What are the incidence and mortality rates associated with carotid blowout after management of the neck?	• Incidence: < 4% (occurs months to years after intervention/diagnosis) • Mortality: 3 to 50%
319	Why might patients receiving endovascular management for an acute carotid blowout fare better (less neurologic sequelae) than those undergoing emergent surgical intervention?	Patients going to surgery are more likely to have acute hemorrhage, common carotid rupture, and hemodynamic instability.
320	What sequelae can result from sacrifice of both internal jugular veins?	Facial and cerebral edema, increased intracranial pressure, altered mental status, syndrome of inappropriate antidiuretic hormone secretion, abducens palsy, and blindness have all been associated.
321	What is the prevalence of a persistent chylous fistula after neck dissection in area IV?	1 to 3%. Most are in the left neck, but 25% have been reported in the right neck.
322	What is the normal volume of chyle that passes through the lymphatic duct per day, and what does it contain?	2–4 L/day. Fat (chylomicrons, long-chain fats), protein, electrolytes, and lymphocytes

323	What are the possible sequelae of a persistent chyle leak?	Hypovolemia, electrolyte disturbances, hypoalbuminemia, coagulopathy, immunosuppression, infection (sepsis, wound infection), peripheral edema, possible chylothorax (50% mortality if left untreated), mortality (now 0.25% with treatment)
324	Suspected chylous fluid can be tested for what components to confirm that it is in fact chyle?	• Chylomicrons • Triglycerides (> 5 g/L) • Sudan III stain positive
325	What steps can initially be used to treat persistent chyle leaks less than 500 mL per day (low-output) after neck dissection?	• Low-fat, medium-chain fatty acid–only diet • Suction wound drainage • Pressure dressing • Consult dietician or nutritionist and follow laboratory results closely. If not successful, consider total parenteral nutrition (TPN). Some recommend for output < 500 mL/day x 5 days or longer.
326	In a patient with a high-output chyle leak after neck dissection, despite maximal medical therapy or in the presence of complications, what treatment is recommended?	Neck exploration and ligation of the thoracic duct. Other surgical options should also be considered (thoracoscopic or laparoscopic approach).
327	What laboratory test should be checked yearly in patients treated with neck radiation therapy?	Thyroid function tests (TSH)
328	What is the difference in impact on quality of life between a radical neck dissection and a modified radical neck dissection?	Radical neck dissection results in significantly worse shoulder function and a trend toward increased pain. No difference in subjective appearance, activity, recreation, chewing, swallowing, or speech occurs.

Oral Cavity Anatomy

329	What are the boundaries of the oral cavity?	• Anterior: Vermilion border of the lip • Posterior/superior: Hard and soft palate junction • Posterior/inferior: Circumvallate papillae • Lateral: Anterior tonsillar pillars and glossotonsillar folds

330	What are the anatomical subsites that constitute the oral cavity?	• Lips: Upper and lower, from vermilion border to buccal mucosa
		• Buccal mucosa: Mucosa lining cheeks and posterior lip from maxillary and mandibular vestibular folds to the pterygomandibular raphe (or anterior tonsillar pillars)
		• Retromolar trigone: *See below*
		• Alveolar ridges
		  ○ Upper (maxillary): Horizontal hard palate to maxillary vestibule and superior pterygopalatine arch posteriorly
		  ○ Lower (mandibular): Transition to floor of mouth to mandibular vestibule to ascending mandibular ramus posteriorly
		• Hard palate: Soft palate to upper (maxillary) alveolar ridge
		• Floor of mouth: Lower alveolar ridge to oral tongue and anterior tonsillar pillar, divided by the lingual frenulum anteriorly
		• Oral tongue: Anterior two thirds, from circumvallate papillae to tip

331	What are the anatomical boundaries of the retromolar trigone?	Mucosa over the ascending mandibular ramus: • Superior: Maxillary tuberosity • Anterior: Posterior aspect of the second mandibular molar • Lateral: Buccal mucosa • Medial: Anterior tonsillar pillar

332	Primary oral cavity tumors of which two subsites have the highest risk for bony invasion?	• Alveolar ridges • Retromolar trigone
333	Describe the course of the Stensen duct (parotid duct) from the gland to the oral cavity.	Anterior parotid gland → superficial to the masseter muscle and buccal fat pad → 90-degree turn to pierce the buccinator muscle → between the oral mucosa and buccinators muscle → papilla in buccal mucosa across from the second maxillary molar
334	Describe the course of the Wharton duct (sub-mandibular duct) from the gland to the floor of the mouth and its relationship to the lingual nerve along its course.	Anterior "deep lobe" of the submandibular gland → between the lingual and hypoglossal nerves over the hyoglossus muscle → anterior and superior ascent between the genioglossus and sublingual glands → over the lingual nerve → sublingual papilla just lateral to the lingual frenulum.
335	What is the arterial supply to the oral cavity?	External carotid artery • Lingual artery → oral tongue • Greater palatine artery→ hard palate • Superior alveolar arteries (anterior, middle, and posterior) → gingival of the maxilla, alveolar ridge, teeth, buccal mucosa • Transverse facial artery (superficial temporal artery) → buccal mucosa • Facial artery → lips (labial arteries) • Buccal artery (maxillary a) → buccal mucosa • Inferior alveolar artery → mandible, mandibular teeth • Ascending pharyngeal artery + lesser palatine arteries → retromolar trigone, posterior floor of mouth • Submental (facial artery) and sublingual (lingual artery) arteries → floor of mouth
336	Describe the venous drainage of the oral cavity.	All sites drain ultimately to the jugular system. The hard palate drains first through the pterygoid plexus.
337	What is the relationship between the lingual artery and vein, hypoglossal nerve, and the hyoglossus and mylohyoid muscles?	From superficial to deep (or lateral to medial): • Mylohyoid muscle • Hypoglossal nerve and lingual vein • Hyoglossus muscle • Lingual artery • Genioglossus
338	What nerves provide sensation to the upper and lower lips?	• Upper lip: Infraorbital nerve (CN V_2) • Lower lip: Mental nerve (CN V_3)
339	What is the sensory innervation of the retromolar trigone?	• Lesser palatine nerves • Glossopharyngeal nerve (CN IX)

340	What is the *sensory innervation of the tongue*?	• Anterior two-thirds
		  ○ General sensory: Lingual nerve (CNV_3)
		  ○ Special sensory: Chorda tympani nerve via the lingual nerve (CNV_3)
		Posterior third
		• General and special sensory: Glossopharyngeal nerve (CN IX).

341	What provides the sensory innervation of the floor of mouth?	Lingual nerve (CN V_3)
342	What provides sensory innervation to the hard palate?	Nasopalatine nerve (CN V2) via the incisive canal
343	What are the four intrinsic and four extrinsic tongue muscles?	All muscles are paired and separated in the midline by the lingual septum:

- Intrinsic tongue musculature: Change the shape of the tongue
  - Superior longitudinal
  - Inferior longitudinal
  - Transverse
  - Vertical muscles
- Extrinsic tongue musculature
  - Genioglossus
  - Hyoglossus
  - Palatoglossus
  - Styloglossus

344	Which tongue muscle is not innervated by the hypoglossal nerve (CN XII), and by what is it innervated?	Palatoglossus muscle is innervated by the pharyngeal branch of the vagus nerve (CNX).
345	What space is defined medially by the buccinators muscle and its fascia, the mandible inferiorly, the zygomatic arch superiorly, the risorius, zygomaticus major, and levator labii superioris muscles laterally, the orbicularis oris muscle anteriorly, and the anterior border of the masseter muscle and the parotid gland posteriorly?	Buccal space
346	What space is defined (1) by the layers of the deep cervical fascia as they split around the mandible and come back together at the ventral and dorsal borders of the mandibular ramus, thus enclosing the lateral pterygoid muscle; and (2) by the fascia surrounding the medial pterygoid, masseter and temporalis muscles?	Masticator space
347	Which lymph node areas usually drain the oral cavity?	Levels I, II, and III. Drainage pathways to level IV have also been described.
348	What lymph node basins drain the lips?	• Submandibular lymph nodes (level IB) → upper and lower lip • Submental lymph nodes (level IA) → lower lip, primarily midline lesions • Other: preauricular, parotid, perifacial → upper lip
349	What is the typical lymphatic drainage of the oral tongue?	• Tip → submental lymph nodes (level IA) • Ventral tongue → submental and submandibular lymph nodes (level IA and IB) • Lateral tongue → submandibular (level IB), jugulodigastric nodes (level IIA), directly to levels III and IV *Note:* Laterality of lymphatic drainage of the oral tongue due to the lack of lymphatic anastomoses across the fibrous lingual septum is unique from the base of tongue.
350	What lymph node basin(s) is primarily responsible for draining the retromolar trigone?	Upper jugular nodes (level IIA)
351	What is the lymphatic drainage for the floor of mouth?	• Anterior → Level IA and IB (often bilateral) • Posterior → Level IIA (ipsilateral)
352	What lymphatic basins preferentially drain the buccal mucosa?	Levels IA and IB
353	Which lymph nodes preferentially drain the hard palate?	Levels I and II

Evaluation and Management of Oral Cavity Cancer

354	What environmental risk factors act synergistically in the formation of oral cavity squamous cell carcinoma and are the most common risk factors in the Western world?	Tobacco and alcohol

355	In addition to tobacco and alcohol use, what risk factors place a patient at higher risk for developing oral cavity cancer?	• Betel nut chewing • Chewing tobacco or other oral tobacco • Chronic periodontal disease or irritation • History of head and neck radiation • History of head and neck cancer • Immunodeficiency • Sun exposure (lip) • Other: Plummer-Vinson syndrome, chronic syphilis
356	Is HPV infection considered a major risk factor in the development of oral cavity carcinoma?	No. Although it is a risk factor, it is not considered a major risk factor, and its role in carcinogenesis in the oral cavity is unclear.
357	What is the most common malignancy of the oral cavity?	Squamous cell carcinoma (~95%) *Note*: For the hard palate, tumors most commonly arise in the minor salivary glands.
358	What are the most common squamous cell carcinoma subtypes found within the oral cavity?	• Sarcomatoid carcinoma • Basaloid carcinoma • Verrucous carcinoma
359	What are the most common malignancies of the oral cavity, excluding squamous cell carcinoma?	• Lymphoma • Minor salivary gland tumors: Adenoid cystic carcinoma, mucoepidermoid carcinoma, polymorphous low-grade adenocarcinoma, adenocarcinoma • Sarcoma: Osteosarcoma, chondrosarcoma, malignant fibrous histiosarcoma, rhabdomyosarcoma, liposarcoma, Kaposi sarcoma • Melanoma: Malignant mucosal melanoma
360	What common premalignant lesions are associated with an increased risk of developing an oral cavity squamous cell carcinoma?	• Leukoplakia: White plaque, cannot be wiped off; lower risk of malignant conversion (<30%) • Erythroplakia: Red plaque, not associated with obvious cause; higher risk of malignant conversion (<60%) • Lichen planus: Lacy white pattern on mucosa or atrophic lesions (red and smooth) or erosive lesions (depressed margins, covered with fibrinous exudate), more common in women (40s), <1% 10-year conversion rate • Submucosal fibrosis: Thickened and fibrotic buccal mucosa and deeper structures; associated with betel quid chewing, poor oral hygiene
361	What premalignant lesion can be mistaken for verrucous carcinoma but is differentiated on pathology because it does not invade the lamina propria?	Verrucous hyperplasia. Most commonly occurs on the buccal mucosa of men in their fourth decade of life.
362	What benign lesion manifests as a butterfly-shaped ulceration commonly found at the hard–soft palate junction and is associated with pressure injuries?	Necrotizing sialometaplasia
363	What benign lesion is commonly found in mucosal or salivary tissue and may resemble squamous cell carcinoma?	Pseudoepitheliomatous hyperplasia
364	What are common benign exostoses that appear as firm submucosal masses on the anterior lingual mandible and midline hard palate?	Torus mandibularis and torus palatini, respectively
365	What are the most common initial signs and symptoms associated with oral cavity cancer?	Bleeding, pain, halitosis, dysphagia, and dysarthria
366	What is the most common site of oral verrucous carcinoma?	Buccal mucosa

367	What is the most common location of oral tongue squamous cell carcinoma?	Posterolateral oral tongue
368	What is the most common location of buccal mucosa squamous cell carcinoma?	Adjacent to the thirrd mandibular molar
369	When does the NCCN (2013) recommend PET/CT scan in the workup of patients with oral cavity cancer?	Consider for stage III–IV disease
370	Name four common features of patients with early stage (stage I or II) oral cavity cancer. (▶ Table 7.4)	• Primary tumor < 4 cm (T1–2) • No evidence of invasion into adjacent structures • No evidence of cervical metastases (N0) • No distant metastases (M0)

Table 7.4 AJCC tumor (T) staging of the oral cavity (superficial erosion alone of bone/tooth socket by gingival primary is not sufficient to classify as T4).

Stage	Description
TX	cannot be assessed
T0	no evidence of primary tumor
Tis	carcinoma in situ
T1	≤ 2 cm
T2	> 2 cm and ≤ 4 cm
T3	≥ 4 cm
T4 (lip)	invades through cortical bone, inferior alveolar nerve, floor of mouth, or skin of face
T4a (oral)	invades adjacent structures only (e.g., through cortical bone, into deep muscles of tongue)
T4b (oral)	invades masticator space, pterygoid plates, or skull base and/or encases the internal carotid artery

Data from Edge SB, Byrd DR, Compton CC, Fritz AG, Greene FL, Trotti A, eds. AJCC Cancer Staging Manual 7th Edition. New York, NY: Springer; 2010.

371	How is a T4a oral cavity tumor defined?	Moderately advanced local disease: • Lip: It invades through the cortical bone, inferior alveolar nerve, floor of mouth, or skin of face. • Oral cavity: Tumor invades adjacent structures (e.g., through cortical bone, extrinsic (deep) tongue musculature, maxillary sinus, skin of face).
372	True or False. Superficial erosion bone or tooth socket alone meets the criteria for staging a tumor as T4a.	False
373	How are T4b oral cavity tumors defined?	• Very advanced local disease • Tumor invades masticator space, pterygoid plates, or skull base, and/or encases the internal carotid artery.
374	What pathologic factors directly relate to prognosis in oral cavity cancer?	• Tumor thickness (> 5 mm = increased risk of occult nodal disease, decreased recurrence free and overall survival rates) • Differentiation • Angiolymphatic invasion
375	Which has a worse prognosis: upper or lower lip cancer?	Upper lip cancer tends to be more aggressive and to have early metastatic potential.

376	What are the adverse risk features considered by the NCCN (2011) in their algorithm for oral cavity cancer management?	• Extracapsular nodal spread • Positive margins • pT3 or pT4 primary • N2 or N3 nodal disease • Nodal disease in levels IV or V • Perineural invasion • Vascular embolism
377	What treatment strategy recommended by the NCCN (2013) for early stage (stage I and II) oral cavity cancer?	• Surgical resection ± neck dissection as indicated by tumor thickness and location (preferred): ○ No adverse risk factors→ Surveillance ○ One positive node without adverse risk features→ Optional adjuvant radiation ○ Extracapsular spread and/or positive margin→ Chemoradiation (preferred) versus reexcision versus radiation therapy ○ Other adverse risk features→ Radiation therapy versus chemoradiation therapy. • Radiation therapy ± brachytherapy
378	For patients with advanced stage disease (T1–3N1–3; T3N0; T4a, any N), excluding T4b or unresectable nodal disease, what is the primary treatment strategy recommended by the NCCN (2013)?	• Surgical resection with ipsilateral or bilateral neck dissection (N2c or high risk to contralateral neck) • No adverse features: Radiation therapy (optional) • Extracapsular spread and/or positive margin: Chemoradiation therapy (preferred) vs reexcision versus radiation therapy • Other risk features: Radiation therapy versus chemoradiation therapy • Multimodality clinical trials
379	How can the mandible be managed if an oral cavity cancer appears to invade the periosteum, cortex, or medullary space, either intraoperatively or on preoperative workup?	• Marginal or rim mandibulectomy: Periosteum or superficial cortical invasion • Segmental mandibulectomy: More than superficial cortical invasion, medullary invasion, invasion from perineural spread via the mandibular or mental foramen, hypoplastic/atrophic/edentulous mandible making rim mandibulectomy unsafe, invasion of periodontal ligament or tooth socket
380	When performing osteotomy for mandibulotomy, which is preferable: straight or stepwise osteotomy? Median or paramedian placement?	• Stepwise mandibulotomy: Provides better alignment and stability • Paramedian: Minimizes trauma to the genioglossus, geniohyoid, and digastric muscles
381	Describe the extent of neck dissection recommended by the NCCN (2013) for oral cavity cancer based on clinical nodal staging.	• No neck dissection: It can be considered for T1N0 lower-lip cancer, T1–T2N0 oral tongue with < 2 mm of invasion, T1–T2N0 upper alveolar ridge and hard palate tumors. For lesions 2- to 4-mm thick, elective neck dissection is used when appropriate (patient reliability, other risk factors, and so forth). • N0: Select neck dissection. Supraomohyoid (levels I–III) recommended for oral cavity tumors > 4 mm; level IIB dissection is controversial; can consider preserving for early stage disease. Consider suprahyoid dissection (levels IA and IB) for T2 lower-lip tumors. • N1–N2c: Select or comprehensive neck dissection as indicated • N3: Comprehensive neck dissection

382	What is regimen is recommended by the NCCN (2013) for definitive radiation therapy for oral cavity cancer with gross lymphadenopathy?	• Conventional fractionation: 66–74 Gy, Monday through Friday for 7 weeks
		• Altered fractionation:
		  ○ Six fractions/week accelerated: 66 to 74 Gy (gross disease), 44 to 64 Gy (subclinical disease)
		  ○ Concomitant boost accelerated: 72 Gy for 6 weeks (boost given during a second daily fraction for the last 12 days of treatment)
		  ○ Hyperfractionation: 81.6 Gy x 7 weeks given twice daily Monday through Friday.

383	What radiation dose is typically given to uninvolved nodal levels at risk for occult disease in oral cavity cancer undergoing definitive radiation?	44 to 64 Gy
384	When should adjuvant radiation or chemoradiation begin after surgical resection for oral cavity cancer?	Six weeks or less (often around 3 to 4 weeks). Ideally all treatment will be completed within 12 weeks from diagnosis. Given 6 weeks of typical adjuvant therapy, this gives 6 weeks from diagnosis to initiation of adjuvant therapy.
385	What is the recommended adjuvant radiation recommended for oral cavity cancer?	• Primary site: 60 to 66 Gy, daily Monday through Friday for 6 weeks • N(+) levels: 60 to 66 Gy • N(-) levels: 44 to 64 Gy
386	What chemotherapeutic regimen is recommended when adjuvant chemoradiation therapy is planned for oral cavity cancer?	Concurrent cisplatin (100 mg/m^2 every 3 weeks)
387	What is the reconstruction of choice for lower-lip defects smaller than one-third the length of the lip, between one-third and two-thirds, greater than two-thirds? (▶ Fig. 7.3)	• Less than one-third: Primary closure • One-third to two-thirds: Abbe-Estlander flap • More than two-thirds: Karapandzic flap, Webster-Bernard flap, or radial forearm free flap with palmaris longus tendon

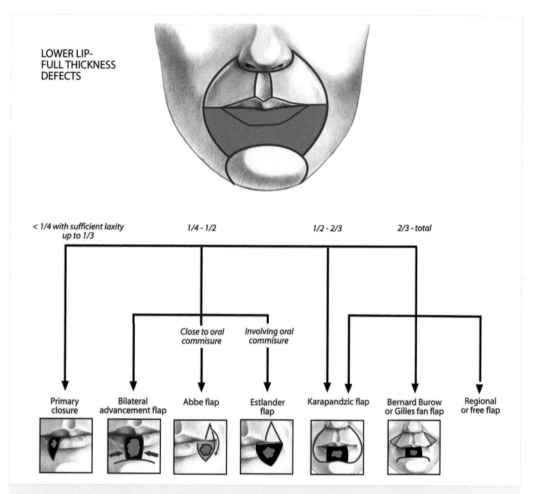

Fig. 7.3 Reconstruction algorithm for full-thickness defects of the lower lip. (Used with permission from Sherris DA, Larrabee WF. Principles of Facial Reconstruction 2nd Edition. New York, NY: Thieme; 2010.)

388	What local flap using the facial artery can be used to close intraoral defects?	Facial artery musculomucosal (FAMM) flap
389	In a patient with a floor of mouth or oral tongue tumor, resection followed by primary closure of a large defect can result in what long-term complication?	Tethered tongue
390	What reconstructive options are best used to avoid trismus in defects of the buccal mucosa larger than 3 cm in diameter?	Skin graft or free tissue transfer
391	What is the reconstruction of choice for patients with segmental resection of the anterior mandible?	Free tissue transfer with vascularized bone (i.e., fibula free flap)

392	What is the reconstruction of choice for patients who have greater than 50% of the oral tongue resected?	Fasciocutaneous free flap, radial forearm free flap
393	What reconstruction options are best in patients with segmental mandibulectomy who are not candidates for free tissue transfer?	Soft tissue pedicled flap with or without a reconstruction bar. Reconstruction bars should be used with caution without underlying bone. They are prone to fracture, exposure, and infection.
394	What is an adequate nonsurgical method for rehabilitation of speech and swallow function after resection of a hard palate or maxillary alveolar ridge tumor with resultant oronasal or oroantral fistula?	Prosthetic obturator

Oropharynx Anatomy

395	What head and neck subsite is defined by the posterior pharyngeal wall, lateral pharyngeal constrictors, superiorly by the hard palate, inferiorly by the vallecula and hyoid bone, and anteriorly by the circumvallate papilla and palatoglossal muscles?	Oropharynx
396	What are the anatomical subsites of the oropharynx, and how are they defined?	• Tonsil*: Bordered by the anterior and posterior tonsillar pillars, glossotonsillar sulcus, confluence of the soft palate and tonsillar pillars, and superior pharyngeal constrictor muscle • Base of tongue*: Circumvallate papillae anteriorly, glossotonsillar sulci laterally, hyoid bone/floor of the vallecula inferiorly • Soft palate: Hard palate anteriorly, palatopharyngeus muscle and uvula posteriorly, superior constrictor muscle laterally, confluence of the anterior and posterior tonsillar pillars inferiorly and nasopharynx superiorly • Posterior oropharyngeal wall: Level of the hyoid bone/floor of vallecula inferiorly, soft palate superiorly, posterior tonsillar pillars and piriform sinuses laterally * Most commonly involved subsites
397	What anatomical site is considered a part of the oropharynx and is defined as the space anterior to the lingual/oropharyngeal surface of the epiglottis, posterior to the base of tongue, medial to the glossoepiglottic fold and piriform sinus, and superficial to the hyoepiglottic ligament (which denotes the superior extent of the pre-epiglottic space)?	Vallecula
398	Lymphatic tissue of the nasopharynx and oropharynx, including the pharyngeal tonsil, palatine tonsil, and lingual tonsil, constitute what important complex?	Waldeyer ring
399	What anatomical structures enter the pharynx between the superior and middle pharyngeal constrictor muscles, just inferior to the tonsil?	Stylopharyngeus muscle, styloglossus muscle, stylohyoid ligament, glossopharyngeal nerve (CN IX).
400	What important fascial layer separates the tonsillar region from the parapharyngeal space?	Buccopharyngeal fascia.
401	Name the layers of the posterior pharyngeal wall.	Mucosa → superior pharyngeal constrictor muscle → buccopharyngeal fascia → retropharyngeal space (contains lateral fat pads and retropharyngeal nodes) → alar fascia → prevertebral fascia → prevertebral muscles (laterally)/anterior longitudinal ligament (medially) → vertebral bodies
402	Name the muscular components of the soft palate and their innervation.	• Superior pharyngeal constrictor muscle (CN IX, X) • Palatopharyngeus muscle (CN X) • Palatoglossus muscle (CN X)

		• Tensor veli palatini muscle (CN V₃)
		• Levator veli palatini muscle (CN X)
		• Uvular muscle (CN X)
403	Describe the arterial supply to each oropharyngeal subsite.	External carotid system: • Tonsil: Tonsillar branch of the ascending pharyngeal artery, descending palatine artery, tonsillar branch of the facial artery,* dorsal lingual artery, and ascending palatine artery • Base of tongue: Lingual artery* and its branches (suprahyoid branch, dorsal lingual artery, and arteria profunda linguae) • Soft palate: Lesser palatine artery,* ascending pharyngeal artery, tonsillar branches from the dorsal lingual artery, ascending palatine artery • Posterior pharyngeal wall: Ascending pharyngeal artery* * Denotes primary arterial supply.
404	Describe the location of the internal carotid artery in relationship to the tonsil.	• Posterolateral to the lateral oropharyngeal wall • Separated from tonsil by superior constrictor and buccopharyngeal fascia • On average, it is 1.4 cm from the tonsillar fossa in a 1-year-old and 2.5 cm in an adult.
405	Describe the venous outflow from the oropharynx.	Drains to the jugular venous system: • Tonsil: Tonsillar and pharyngeal plexus, lingual and facial veins • Base of tongue: Lingual and retromandibular veins • Soft palate: pharyngeal and pterygoid plexus, external palatine vein • Posterior pharyngeal wall: pharyngeal venous plexus
406	What nerve is at risk during base of tongue surgery if resection of the hyoglossus muscle to the level of the hyoid bone is required? (▶ Fig. 7.4)	Hypoglossal nerve (CN XII)

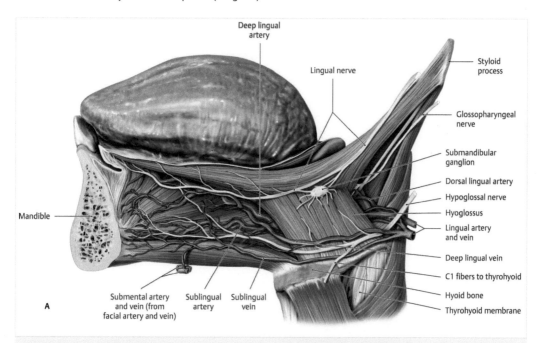

Fig. 7.4 Anatomy of the tongue and floor of mouth. (Used with permission from Thieme Atlas of Anatomy: Head and Neuroanatomy, © Thieme 2007, illustration by Karl Wesker.)

407	Which nerves supply the pharyngeal plexus?	Vagus nerve (CN X), glossopharyngeal nerve (CN IX), and sympathetic fibers from the superior cervical ganglion
408	Which lymph node basins are common sites of spread of oropharyngeal carcinoma? (▶ Fig. 7.5; ▶ Fig. 7.6)	Levels II, III, and IV most commonly

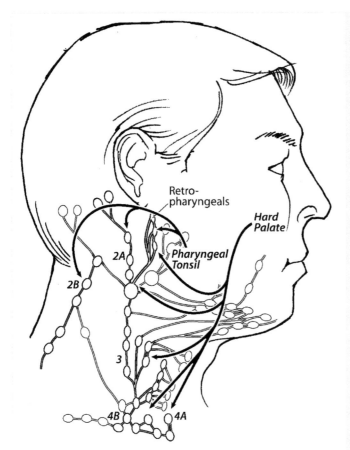

Fig. 7.5 Lymphatic drainage of the tonsil and hard palate. (Used with permission from Genden EM, Varvares MA, eds. Head and Neck Cancer: An Evidence-Based Team Approach. New York, NY: Thieme; 2008.)

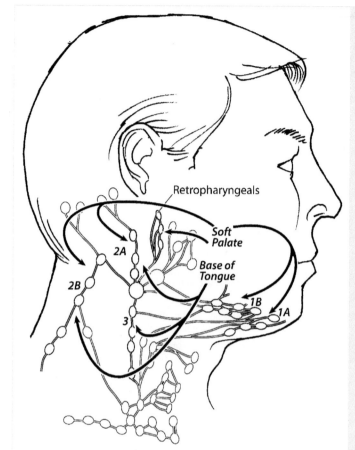

Fig. 7.6 Lymphatic drainage for the soft palate and the base of the tongue. (Used with permission from Genden EM, Varvares MA, eds. Head and Neck Cancer: An Evidence-Based Team Approach. New York, NY: Thieme; 2008.)

409	In addition to levels II, III, and IV, what other lymph node group is at risk with tonsil, soft palate, and posterior pharyngeal wall cancer?	Retropharyngeal nodes
410	Why do tumors of the base of tongue have a high risk of bilateral nodal disease?	Precollecting lymphatic channels on each side cross the midline to drain to the contralateral side (up to 30% at presentation). Level II is at highest risk for bilateral disease.
411	Describe the three lymphatic systems associated with the soft palate.	• Medial → middle one-third of the jugular chain (level III) • Lateral → retropharyngeal lymph nodes • Anterior → hard palate → submental and submandibular nodes (levels IA and IB) *Note*: Uvular lymphatics drain primarily to level IIA.
412	Describe the lymphatic drainage of the posterior pharyngeal wall.	Retropharyngeal nodes (up to 44%), levels II and III

Evaluation and Management of Oropharyngeal Carcinoma

413	What are the two most important risk factors associated with the development of oropharyngeal squamous cell carcinoma?	HPV infection and tobacco smoking. Traditional risk factors for head and neck squamous cell carcinoma are still relevant (see Oncology section).
414	Which HPV subtypes are associated with an increased risk of oropharyngeal squamous cell carcinoma?	HPV 16 (predominant), 18, 31, and 33

415	What is the most common malignancy of the oropharynx?	Squamous cell carcinoma
416	What rare malignancy arising in the oropharynx (most commonly in the tonsil and base of tongue) is a poorly differentiated squamous cell carcinoma or undifferentiated carcinoma associated with a reactive lymphoplasmacytic infiltration?	Lymphoepithelial carcinoma
417	What is the most common type of lymphoma found in the oropharynx?	Non-Hodgkin lymphoma. Diffuse large B-cell lymphomas are the most common subtype.
418	What percentage of extranodal head and neck lymphomas are found in the Waldeyer ring?	36%
419	What locally aggressive oral and cutaneous vascular malignancy can be found in the oropharynx (primarily soft palate) in AIDS patients?	Kaposi sarcoma
420	What are the two most common salivary gland malignancies that arise in the oropharynx?	They arise from minor salivary glands most commonly in the soft palate, tonsil, and base of tongue: • Adenoid cystic carcinoma (cylindromatous or cribriform) • Mucoepidermoid carcinoma
421	What malignant tumor can rarely arise from melanocytes in the mucosa of the oropharynx?	Malignant mucosal melanoma
422	What are common initial symptoms of oropharyngeal malignancy?	Odynophagia, referred otalgia, dysphagia, speech distortion, globus, bleeding, painless neck mass
423	Why might patients with oropharyngeal cancer often be initially diagnosed with stage III or IV disease?	Vague symptoms that are often experienced in benign disease processes
424	If a patient with oropharyngeal cancer develops severe trismus, what might this indicate?	Invasion into the masseteric space with involvement of the pterygoid musculature
425	A patient has a palpable mass centered in the right base of the tongue. On tongue protrusion, you note hemitongue atrophy and fasciculations on the right. Which nerve is likely involved by the tumor?	Hypoglossal nerve
426	What adjuvant physical examination tool should be used when there is concern for an oropharyngeal malignancy?	Flexible endoscopy; evaluate for tumor extension, status of the larynx, etc. Mirror should be considered if flexible endoscopy is not available or as an adjunct to flexible endoscopy.
427	In addition to direct visualization of the anatomy, what important physical examination maneuver should be performed in patients with possible oropharyngeal cancer?	Digital palpation for submucosal disease, friability, and mobility. Palpation of the neck is also imperative.
428	What structure(s) are potentially involved if a patient presents with an immobile oropharyngeal tumor?	• Medial pterygoid muscle • Mandible • Maxillary tuberosity • Hyoid bone • Parapharyngeal structures
429	Tumors in which oropharyngeal subsite is most commonly diagnosed by visual inspection at earlier stages?	Soft palate. They generally occur on the anterior oropharyngeal surface of soft palate.
430	What patient specific/anatomical factors identified on physical examination may indicate that a patient with an oropharyngeal tumor is a poor candidate for a transoral procedure?	• Severe trismus due to tumor invasion or fibrosis • Narrow mandibular arch • Crowded oral cavity, making displacement of the soft tissues challenging • Long incisor teeth • High body mass index

		• Retrognathic
		• High Mallampati score
		• Mandibular tori
431	What tumor specific factors can be identified on physical examination, which would suggest that a patient is a good candidate for transoral surgery?	• Exophytic • Mobile • Proximal oropharynx • No evidence of involvement of deep structures such as the mandible, pterygoid musculature, maxillary tuberosity, hyoid bone, or parapharyngeal structures • Predicted resection < 50% of the base of tongue or < 75% of the soft palate
432	Describe the tumor specific contraindications to transoral tumor resection for an oropharyngeal tumor.	• Invasion of the skull base • Invasion or encasement of the great vessels • Invasion of the mandible • Confluent primary tumor and neck metastasis • Tumor extension potentially necessitating an R1 or R2 resection.
433	How is T4a oropharyngeal cancer defined? (▶ Table 7.5)	Moderately advanced local disease: Tumor invades larynx, extrinsic tongue musculature (genioglossus, hyoglossus, styloglossus, palatoglossus), medial pterygoid muscle, hard palate, or mandible

Table 7.5 AJCC tumor (T) staging of the oropharynx.

Stage	Description
T1	≤ 2 cm
T2	> 2 cm and ≤ 4 cm
T3	≥ 4 cm
T4a	invades the larynx, deep/extrinsic muscle of the tongue, medial pterygoid, hard palate, or mandible
T4b	invades the lateral pterygoid muscle, pterygoid plates, lateral nasopharynx, or skull base or encases the carotid artery

Data from Edge SB, Byrd DR, Compton CC, Fritz AG, Greene FL, Trotti A, eds. AJCC Cancer Staging Manual 7th Edition. New York, NY: Springer; 2010.

434	How is T4b oropharyngeal cancer defined?	Very advanced local disease: Tumor invades lateral pterygoid muscle, pterygoid plates, lateral nasopharynx, skull base, or encases the carotid.
435	With regard to tongue-base tumors, does mucosal extension of a tumor to the lingual surface of the epiglottis constitute invasion of the larynx and T4a status?	No
436	True or False. Nodal metastases to level VII (superior mediastinal lymph nodes: between the common carotid arteries laterally, superior border of manubrium, and innominate artery) are not considered distant metastases.	True
437	Currently, there is no widely accepted staging system that takes into account HPV status of an oropharyngeal tumor. However, the NCCN (2013) does recommend HPV testing to better define prognosis. What test is currently recommended?	Immunohistochemical staining for p16 *Note*: The best test to diagnose HPV status is controversial.

438	What prognostic role does HPV positivity play in oropharyngeal squamous cell carcinoma?	Improved disease-free survival and overall survival when compared with HPV-negative oropharyngeal squamous cell carcinoma
439	What are the adverse features identified by the NCCN (2013) for oropharyngeal cancer?	• Extracapsular nodal spread • Positive margins • pT3 or pT4 primary • N2 or N3 nodal disease • Nodal disease in levels IV or V • Perineural invasion • Vascular embolism

440	What treatment modalities does the NCCN (2013) recommend for patients with T1–2, N0–1 oropharyngeal cancer?	• Definitive radiation therapy
		• Surgical resection of the primary ± ipsilateral or bilateral neck dissection as indicated; additional intervention based on adverse features:
		  ◦ None → no additional intervention
		  ◦ One positive node, no adverse features consider radiation therapy
		  ◦ Positive margin → Reexcision or radiation therapy (CRT for T2)
		  ◦ Extracapsular spread→CRT
		  ◦ Other risk feature → radiation therapy ± concomitant chemotherapy
		  ◦ T2N1: Consider primary chemoradiation therapy

441	What treatment modalities does the NCNN (2013) recommend for patients with T3–4a, N0–1 oropharyngeal cancer?	• Concurrent chemoradiation therapy with cisplatin (category 1, preferred)
		• Surgical resection of the primary ± ipsilateral or bilateral neck dissection as indicated; additional intervention based on adverse features:
		  ◦ None → Radiation therapy
		  ◦ Extracapsular spread and or positive margin → Chemoradiation therapy
		  ◦ Other risk feature → radiation therapy ± concomitant chemotherapy
		  ◦ Induction chemotherapy + radiation therapy ± concomitant chemotherapy
		  ◦ Multimodality clinical trials

442	What treatment modalities does the NCCN (2013) recommend for patients with any T, N2–3 oropharyngeal cancer?	• Concurrent chemoradiation therapy with cisplatin ± neck dissection for residual nodal disease
		• Induction chemotherapy + radiation therapy ± chemotherapy
		• Surgical resection of the primary ± ipsilateral or bilateral neck dissection as indicated; additional intervention based on adverse features:
		  ◦ None → no additional intervention (N1 only)
		  ◦ Extracapsular spread and/or positive margin → chemoradiation therapy
		  ◦ Other risk feature → radiation therapy ± concomitant chemotherapy
		  ◦ Multimodality clinical trials

443	For all stages of oropharyngeal cancer, if there is residual disease with radiation therapy ± concomitant chemotherapy, what intervention is recommended?	Salvage surgery
444	What radiation technique or modality is recommended for management of oropharyngeal tumors?	Intensity modulated radiation therapy (IMRT)

445	What does the NCCN (2013) recommend for definitive radiation therapy for oropharyngeal cancer?	• Conventional fractionation: 66 to 74 Gy, daily Monday through Friday for 7 weeks
		• Altered fractionation:
		  ○ Accelerated: 66 to 74 Gy to gross disease, 44 to 64 Gy to occult disease; six fractions/week
		  ○ Concurrent boost accelerated: 72 Gy, daily + twice daily for last 12 treatments, for 6 weeks
		  ○ Hyperfractionation: 81.6 Gy, twice daily, Monday through Friday, for 7 weeks

446	When considering concurrent chemoradiation therapy, what amount of energy does the NCCN (2013) recommend for (1) primary disease, (2) gross adenopathy, and (3) occult adenopathy?	Conventional fractionation • ≥ 70 Gy • ≥ 70 Gy • 44–64 Gy
447	What does the NCCN (2013) recommend for adjuvant radiation therapy after primary surgical intervention for oropharyngeal cancer?	Conventional fractionation • 60 to 66 Gy to the primary and gross nodal disease • 44 to 64 Gy to occult nodal disease for 6 weeks
448	What is the recommended radiation target volume of the neck in patients with oropharyngeal squamous cell carcinoma and ipsilateral N2a or N2b disease?	Levels IB-V and retropharyngeal lymph nodes
449	What chemotherapy regimen is recommended for concurrent chemoradiation therapy in oropharyngeal squamous cell carcinoma?	Cisplatin: 100 mg/m^2 every 3 weeks x three doses
450	What surgical approach can be used for most early and some advanced oropharyngeal malignancies?	Transoral approach, including laser microsurgery or robotic surgery
451	What surgical approach can be used for more extensive inferiorly located oropharyngeal tumors not amendable to transoral approaches and does not require mandibulotomy?	• Lateral pharyngotomy • Transhyoid pharyngotomy • Lingual release and pull-through technique
452	What surgical approach can be used for the most advanced oropharyngeal lesions often requiring reconstruction?	Mandibulotomy with mandibular swing
453	Similar to the management recommendations for oral cavity cancers, what options are available for surgical management of oropharyngeal tumors that invade the mandible?	• Periosteal or superficial cortical invasion only: Rim mandibulectomy • Medullary invasion: Segmental mandibulectomy See oral cavity malignancy for additional discussion of mandibulectomy indications.
454	How should retropharyngeal lymph nodes be addressed in patients with advanced oropharyngeal squamous cell carcinoma?	Retropharyngeal lymph node dissection and/or radiation therapy
455	When performing transoral lateral oropharyngectomy or base-of-tongue resection, in addition to clipping named vessels in the operative field with two or three clips and meticulous hemostasis, what additional procedures should be considered to decrease the risk of postoperative hemorrhage?	Ligation of vessels at risk for bleeding into the oropharynx (lingual, facial, and superior laryngeal arteries; some authorities consider tying off the external carotid system). This can be done during concomitant neck dissection or as a separate procedure.
456	What is the most common method used for reconstruction of oropharyngeal defects after transoral procedures?	None: The wound is allowed to heal by secondary intention.
457	If a patient undergoes transoral tumor extirpation for a primary base-of-tongue or tonsil tumor at the same time as a neck dissection, and the decision is made to allow the wound to heal by second intention, what should be carefully ruled out before closure of the neck?	Orocervical fistula

458	What is the best reconstructive option for large oropharyngeal defects involving the tonsillar fossa, pharyngeal wall, and tongue base?	Fasciocutaneous free flap (radial forearm free flap is used most commonly)
459	What are the most important goals of tongue base reconstruction?	• Maintenance of the airway with prevention of aspiration • Preservation of swallowing • Preservation of speech
460	When considering a pectoralis major myocutaneous flap or a fasciocutaneous free flap for reconstruction of the oropharynx, which reconstructive option provides the best functional outcome with respect to swallowing?	Free flap reconstruction (decreased percutaneous endoscopic gastrostomy tube dependence)
461	Although multiple reconstructive options are available for soft palate reconstruction, including primary closure, local mucosal flaps, and free tissue transfer, what additional option should be considered for smaller defects, and what healing process may contribute to decreased velopharyngeal insufficiency over time?	• Healing by second intention • Cicatricial scarring
462	What might result if a large portion of the soft palate is resected and *not* reconstructed after surgery for oropharyngeal tumors?	Velopharyngeal insufficiency with nasopharyngeal reflux and hypernasal speech

Hypopharynx Anatomy

463	What are the anatomical boundaries of the hypopharynx?	• *Superior*: Hyoid bone/floor of vallecula, pharyngoepiglottic folds • *Inferior*: Plane at the lower border of the cricoid cartilage; esophageal introitus or cricopharyngeus muscle • *Anterior*: Junction of the pyriform sinuses in the postcricoid region • *Posterior*: Level of the superior surface of the hyoid bone/floor of the vallecula to the inferior border of the cricoid cartilage and from the apex of one piriform sinus to the other
464	Which paired subsite of the hypopharynx extends from the pharyngoepiglottic fold to the upper end of the esophagus or lower border of the cricoid cartilage and is referred to as an *inverted pyramid* (base at pharyngoepiglottic fold, apex at level of cricoid)?	Pyriform sinus
465	What subsite of the hypopharynx extends from the level of the superior surface of the hyoid bone or floor of the vallecula to the inferior border of the cricoid cartilage and from the apex of one piriform sinus to the other?	Posterior hypopharyngeal wall
466	What subsite of the hypopharynx extends from the anterior hypopharyngeal wall from below the posterior arytenoid cartilage to the inferior border of the cricoid cartilage?	Postcricoid area
467	What subsite forms a transition point between the supraglottis and hypopharynx, is considered a part of the supraglottis, and often results in aggressive disease when involved by tumors?	"Marginal area": Lateral wall of the aryepiglottic folds
468	What is the distribution of hypopharyngeal tumors arising in the three subsites?	Varies geographically. In the United States: Pyriform sinus (up to 86%) > posterior pharyngeal wall (10 to 23%) > postcricoid area (less than 5%). In Egypt: Postcricoid area (50.1%) > pyriform sinus (26.5%) > posterior pharyngeal wall (23.4%)

469	Between the area of transition of the inferior pharyngeal constrictor muscle and the cricopharyngeus muscle is a potential area of weakness and spread of posterior hypopharyngeal wall tumors beyond the hypopharynx. What is the name of this area?	Killian triangle
470	What is the arterial supply to the hypopharynx?	• External carotid artery: • Superior laryngeal artery* • Branches of the lingual artery • Branches of the ascending pharyngeal artery *Denotes primary blood supply; venous drainage is through the pharyngeal plexus, adjacent named veins, and jugular system.
471	Describe the sensory and motor innervation of the hypopharynx.	• Sensory: Glossopharyngeal (IX) and vagus (X) nerves via the pharyngeal plexus; additionally, sympathetics from the pharyngeal plexus may also contribute. • Motor: Vagus (X) nerve via pharyngeal plexus
472	Which aerodigestive tract primary site has the highest prevalence of cervical nodal metastasis?	Hypopharynx (approximately 70%)
473	What is the primary lymphatic drainage of the hypopharynx?	Primarily drain to levels II–IV, also level VI (especially with inferior hypopharyngeal and post cricoid disease). Other nodal basins at risk include retropharyngeal nodes.

Evaluation and Management of Hypopharyngeal Carcinoma

474	What risk factors are associated with hypopharyngeal carcinoma?	• Tobacco smoking • Alcohol use • Chewing tobacco • Male sex • Fifth to seventh decade of life • Plummer-Vinson syndrome or Patterson-Brown-Kelly syndrome • Black race
475	What syndrome with the triad of hypopharyngeal/esophageal webs, glossitis, and iron deficiency anemia can cause an increased risk of cervical esophageal and hypopharyngeal cancer, especially in nonsmoking women from the United States, Wales, or Sweden in their third to fifth decade of life?	Plummer-Vinson syndrome
476	Tumors in which hypopharyngeal subsite(s) are associated with Plummer-Vinson syndrome?	Postcricoid region
477	Approximately what percentage of hypopharyngeal tumors are squamous cell carcinoma?	95%
478	Describe three of the most common nonepithelial tumors that form within the hypopharynx.	• Adenocarcinoma • Lymphoma • Sarcoma
479	Where do adenocarcinomas of the hypopharynx arise?	Minor salivary glands or ectopic gastric mucosa
480	What pathologic growth characteristics of hypopharyngeal cancer can make assessment of the primary tumor challenging?	• Submucosal spread • Skip lesions • Multifocal disease
481	What is the risk of finding a second primary tumor in a patient with hypopharyngeal cancer?	Up to 18%
482	What are the most common initial symptoms in patients with hypopharyngeal cancer?	• All stages: Dysphagia, neck mass, sore throat • Early stage (I/II): Gastroesophageal reflux, sore throat, dysphagia

		• Advanced stage (III/IV): Neck mass, shortness of breath, dysphagia, odynophagia, referred otalgia, hemoptysis, gastroesophageal reflux, hoarseness
483	Approximately what percentage of hypopharyngeal tumors manifest at advanced stage (stage III–IV)?	70 to 75%
484	Explain why patients with hypopharyngeal tumors, particularly those located in the pyriform sinus, develop referred otalgia.	Sensory fibers from the superior laryngeal nerve (particularly the internal branch) and Arnold nerve both synapse within the jugular ganglion.
485	Why is in-office flexible endoscopy imperative in any patient with suspected hypopharyngeal cancer?	It is essential to evaluate the larynx to assess the presence of laryngeal invasion, cricoarytenoid joint fixation, and/or recurrent laryngeal nerve involvement.
486	During flexible endoscopy, what maneuver can allow improved visualization of the pyriform sinuses and postcricoid space?	Asking the patient to puff out the cheeks or perform a Valsalva maneuver
487	What signs are suggestive of hypopharyngeal cancer on flexible endoscopy?	• Mucosal fullness • Ulceration • Pooling of secretions • Hyperkeratotic lesions • Erythematous or friable lesions
488	Aside from pathologic staging, what diagnostic imaging modalities are most commonly used for the workup of hypopharyngeal cancer, and what advantages do they provide for this subsite in particular?	• MRI: Staging accuracy is 85%; better at detecting submucosal spread • CT with contrast: Best for assessing cartilage and bone invasion • PET/CT: Recommended for stage III/IV disease; 10% of patients have distant metastatic disease; identification of an unknown primary; primary staging *Note*: At minimum, a chest X-ray is recommended to evaluate pulmonary metastases.
489	During the workup for hypopharyngeal cancer, what test is occasionally ordered to work up second primaries in the esophagus?	Barium swallow (not an imaging modality of choice)
490	What additional test should be ordered for any patient with hypopharyngeal cancer if the treatment plan includes partial laryngeal surgery or conservative hypopharyngectomy?	Pulmonary function tests
491	Describe T1–3 hypopharyngeal tumor staging according to the AJCC, 7th edition. (▶ Table 7.6)	• T1: Limited to one subsite of hypopharynx and/or ≤ 2 cm • T2: One or more subsites of hypopharynx or an adjacent site or measures > 2 cm and < 4 cm without fixation of the hemilarynx • T3: > 4 cm or with fixation of the hemilarynx or extension to the esophagus

Table 7.6 AJCC tumor (T) staging of the hypopharynx.

Stage	Description
T1	Limited to one subsite of hypopharynx and/or ≤ 2 cm
T2	≥ 1 subsite of hypopharynx or an adjacent site, or measures > 2 cm and < 4 cm without fixation of the hemilarynx
T3	> 4 cm or with fixation of the hemilarynx or extension to the esophagus
T4a	invades thyroid/cricoid cartilage, hyoid bone, thyroid gland, esophagus, or central compartment soft tissue
T4b	invades prevertebral fascia, encases the carotid artery, or involves mediastinal structures

Data from Edge SB, Byrd DR, Compton CC, Fritz AG, Greene FL, Trotti A, eds. AJCC Cancer Staging Manual 7th Edition. New York, NY: Springer; 2010.

492	Describe the criteria for a T4a hypopharyngeal tumor.	Moderately advanced local disease: Invades thyroid/cricoid cartilage, hyoid bone, thyroid gland, or central compartment soft tissue (prelaryngeal strap muscles and subcutaneous fat)
493	Describe the criteria for a T4b hypopharyngeal tumor.	Very advanced local disease: Invades prevertebral fascia, encases carotid artery, or involves mediastinal structures
494	Which head and neck aerodigestive tract primary site has the lowest 5-year survival rate?	Hypopharynx (20 to 47%)
495	What is the most common cause of mortality in patients with hypopharyngeal cancer?	• Locoregional recurrence • Distant metastases (bone, lungs, liver), second primary tumors, comorbid disease
496	What clinical factors are associated with poor prognosis in hypopharyngeal cancer?	• Increasing age • Male sex • Black ethnicity • Poor performance status (ECOG or Karnofsky) • Traditional risk factors for head and neck cancer
497	What tumor specific factors are associated with improved prognosis in hypopharyngeal cancer?	• Primary tumor located on the aryepiglottic fold or medial wall of the pyriform sinus • Low T or N stage, early overall stage • Smaller primary tumor volume
498	Describe the adverse features highlighted by the NCCN (2013) for hypopharyngeal cancer.	• Extracapsular nodal spread • Positive surgical margins • pT3 or pT4 • N2 or N3 nodal disease • Perineural invasion • Vascular embolism
499	What primary treatment modalities does the NCCN (2013) recommend for the management of most T1N0 and select T2N0 (not requiring total laryngectomy) tumors?	• Definitive radiation therapy • Partial laryngopharyngectomy (open or endoscopic) with ipsilateral or bilateral neck dissection as indicated • No adverse features → surveillance • Extracapsular spread ± positive margin → chemoradiation therapy • Positive margins → re-excision or radiation therapy • Other risk features → radiation therapy ± chemotherapy • Multimodality clinic trials
500	What primary treatment modalities does the NCCN (2013) recommend for the management of selected T2N0 (those requiring total laryngectomy), T1N+, T2–3 any N (if total laryngectomy is required)?	• Induction chemotherapy • Complete response → radiation therapy ± chemotherapy • Partial response → chemoradiation therapy • < partial response → surgery • No adverse features → radiation therapy • Extracapsular spread ± positive margin → chemoradiation therapy • Other risk features → radiation therapy ± chemotherapy • Laryngopharyngectomy + neck dissection (includes level VI) • No adverse features → surveillance • Extracapsular spread ± positive margin → chemoradiation therapy • Other risk features → radiation therapy ± chemotherapy • Concurrent chemoradiation therapy (cisplatin) • Multimodality clinical trial
501	What are the options available for managing T4a (any N) hypopharyngeal tumors according to the NCCN (2013)?	• Surgery + neck dissection (preferred) → adjuvant radiation therapy ± chemotherapy • Induction chemotherapy ○ Complete response → radiation therapy ± chemotherapy

		○ Partial response → chemoradiation therapy ○ <Partial response → surgical salvage + neck dissection as indicated → radiation therapy ± chemotherapy • Concurrent chemoradiation therapy • Multimodality clinical trials
502	What levels should be addressed in an elective neck dissection for hypopharyngeal cancer?	Select neck dissection levels II–IV with inclusion of level VI in pyriform apex tumors and retropharyngeal lymph nodes in pharyngeal wall tumors
503	For patients undergoing surgical treatment for hypopharyngeal squamous cell carcinoma, what is the recommended extent of therapeutic neck dissection of the clinically N + ipsilateral neck?	Comprehensive neck dissection including levels I-V and inclusion of level VI with pyriform apex tumors and retropharyngeal lymph nodes with pharyngeal wall tumors
504	What are the most common surgical approaches used for the management of hypopharyngeal tumors?	• Laryngeal conservation approach (T1, T2, and some T3 tumors): • Partial pharyngectomy: Lateral pharyngotomy, partial pharyngectomy via lateral pharyngeal approach, anterior transhyoid pharyngotomy • Partial laryngopharyngectomy • Supracricoid hemilaryngectomy • Transoral laser microsurgery • Total laryngectomy with partial/total pharyngectomy (T3, T4) • Total pharyngo-laryngo-esophagectomy (T4)
505	An open partial pharyngectomy can be considered in patients with T1 or T2 hypopharyngeal tumors of the pyriform sinus. What are the contra-indications to this procedure?	• Tumor extension to more than one wall of the pyriform sinus • Involvement of the pyriform apex • Involvement of the larynx including the medial wall of the pyriform sinus
506	An open partial laryngopharyngectomy combines a classic hemilaryngectomy with a partial pha-ryngectomy and is used for what specific hypo-pharyngeal tumors?	Medial wall pyriform sinus tumors
507	What are the advantages of transoral laser microsurgery and endoscopic resection of hypo-pharyngeal tumors when compared with open approaches?	• No tracheostomy • No reconstruction • Preservation of the suprahyoid musculature improving postoperative swallowing • Earlier return to an oral diet • Shorter hospital stay
508	What is the surgical treatment of choice for most T3 and T4 hypopharyngeal squamous cell carci-nomas?	Total laryngectomy with partial or total pharyngectomy with neck dissection as indicated by clinical nodal disease
509	What are the contraindications for conservation laryngeal surgery in patients with hypopharyngeal malignancy?	• Thyroid or cricoid cartilage invasion • Pyriform apex involvement • Postcricoid region involvement • Impaired vocal cord mobility
510	What is the recommended definitive radiation therapy for primary hypopharyngeal cancer and gross lymphadenopathy according to the NCCN (2013)?	• Conventional fractionation: 66 to 74 Gy, daily (Monday through Friday) for 7 weeks • Altered fractionation: ○ Accelerated: 6 fractions/week, 66 to 74 Gy to gross disease, 44 to 64 Gy to subclinical disease ○ Concomitant boost accelerated radiation therapy: 72 Gy/6 weeks with a boost given as a second daily dose for the last 12 days of treatment ○ Hyperfractionation: 81.6 Gy, twice daily (Monday through Friday) for 6 weeks

511	What dose of radiation is generally recommended for subclinical hypopharyngeal nodal disease when given as definitive management?	44 to 64 Gy
512	What dose of radiation is recommended for hypopharyngeal cancer when given as primary concomitant chemoradiation?	Conventional fractionation: • Gross disease: ≥ 70 Gy • Subclinical disease: 44 to 64 Gy
513	What does the NCCN (2013) recommend for adjuvant radiation therapy after primary surgical intervention for hypopharyngeal cancer?	Conventional fractionation: 60 to 66 Gy to the primary and gross nodal disease, 44 to 64 Gy to occult nodal disease for 6 weeks
514	What chemotherapy regimen is recommended for concurrent chemoradiation therapy in hypopharyngeal squamous cell carcinoma?	Cisplatin: 100 mg/m^2 every 3 weeks in three doses
515	What chemotherapy regimen is recommended for induction chemotherapy in patients with hypopharyngeal cancer?	Cisplatin and 5-FU (up to three cycles)
516	What is the reconstruction of choice after an open conservation procedure for an early stage hypopharyngeal tumor?	Primary closure. Exception is for endoscopic tumor resection → healing by secondary intention
517	What are the reconstructive options for circumferential defects of the hypopharynx?	• Tubed fasciocutaneous free flap • Gastric transposition (gastric "pull-up") • Colonic transposition • Jejunal free flap
518	In terms of function, what are the differences between chemoradiation (organ sparing) therapy and surgery with adjuvant radiation therapy for hypopharyngeal cancer?	Although data are sparse, there are no studies that have shown a clear advantage in terms of function for one treatment algorithm over the other. Eating, aesthetics, and speech are comparable in most studies.
519	What factors correlate with higher complication rate in patients with hypopharyngeal cancer treated with laser excision?	Surgeon inexperience Tumor size Diagnosis of diabetes mellitus
520	What are the most common complications associated with CO$_2$ laser excision of hypopharyngeal carcinoma?	• Hemorrhage (8% in one series) • Pneumonia (6%) • Fistula (1%) • Less commonly local infection and dyspnea

Esophagus Anatomy

521	What anatomical structures form the superior and inferior limits of the cervical esophagus?	• Superior: Cricopharyngeus muscle • Inferior: Thoracic inlet (sternal notch)
522	What are the layers of the cervical esophagus?	• Squamous epithelium • Submucosa • Inner circular muscle layer • Outer longitudinal muscle layer • Adventitia *Note*: There is no distinct serosal layer.
523	Which section of the esophagus contains striated muscle? Smooth muscle?	• Upper one-third: Striated • Middle one-third: Mixed • Distal one-third: Smooth
524	What structure(s) make up the upper esophageal sphincter?	• Posterior surface of thyroid and cricoid cartilage • Hyoid bone • Cricopharyngeus muscle • Inferior constrictor muscle (thyropharyngeus muscle) • Cervical esophageal muscles Extends 3 to 4 cm in total.
525	True or False. The upper esophageal sphincter is tonically contracting.	True. Tonically contracting resulting from discharges from the vagus nerve (X)

526	What potential space lies posterior to the cervical esophagus and communicates superiorly with the retropharyngeal space and inferiorly with the posterior mediastinum?	Retroesophageal space
527	Describe the arterial supply to the esophagus.	• Segmental blood supply: • Upper esophageal sphincter and cervical esophagus: Inferior thyroid artery • Thoracic esophagus: Aortic esophageal arteries, terminal bronchial arteries • Distal esophagus and lower esophageal sphincter: left gastric artery, branch of the left phrenic artery
528	Describe the venous drainage of the cervical esophagus.	Segmental drainage: submucosal plexus → superior vena cava

529	Describe the innervation of the esophagus.	• Sensory: Vagus (X), glossopharyngeal (IX), and spinal afferent nerves
		• Motor: Vagus (X) nerve, parasympathetic and sympathetic nerves
		• Intrinsic innervation:
		  ○ Auerbach plexus: Between the inner circular and outer longitudinal muscle layers
		  ○ Meissner plexus: Submucosa

530	What lymph node basins drain the cervical esophagus?	Primarily levels II–IV. Also drains to level VI, retroesophageal, retropharyngeal, and superior mediastinal nodes (level VII).

Evaluation and Management of Esophageal Cancer

531	What are the risk factors for cervical esophageal squamous cell carcinoma?	• Tobacco • Alcohol • Gastroesophageal reflux • Plummer-Vinson syndrome
532	What is the most common type of cervical esophageal cancer?	Squamous cell carcinoma (approximately 80%)
533	What is the most common type of distal esophageal cancer?	Adenocarcinoma. Increasing incidence related to gastroesophageal reflux disease
534	What are common initial symptoms in patients with cervical esophageal cancer?	Progressive dysphagia (solids, then solids and liquids) and weight loss. Other symptoms include hematemesis, pain, hoarseness or cough.
535	What are the typical nasopharyngoscopy findings in patients with cervical esophageal cancer?	Negative findings unless esophagoscopy is performed or tumor extends to the hypopharynx.
536	According to the AJCC, 7th edition, the cervical esophagus begins at approximately what distance from the incisors?	15 cm to less than 20 cm
537	What imaging modality is most accurate at identifying the extent of cervical esophageal cancer and its relationship with adjacent soft tissues?	MRI
538	What procedure is generally required for direct visualization, biopsy, and staging of an esophageal tumor?	EGD
539	What procedure or diagnostic test is the most sensitive for T and N staging for esophageal cancer?	Endoscopic ultrasonography
540	What is the new T staging system for cervical esophageal squamous cell carcinoma according to the AJCC 7th edition?	(▶ Table 7.7)

Table 7.7 AJCC tumor (T) staging of the cervical esophageal squamous cell carcinoma (SCC).

Stage	Description
T1a	invades lamina propria or muscularis mucosa
T1b	invades submucosa
T2	invades muscularis propria
T3	invades adventitia
T4a	resectable tumor; invades pleura, pericardium, or diaphragm
T4b	invades adjacent structures such as aorta or vertebral body and considered unresectable

Data from Edge SB, Byrd DR, Compton CC, Fritz AG, Greene FL, Trotti A, eds. AJCC Cancer Staging Manual 7th Edition. New York, NY: Springer; 2010.

---

541   What is the N staging system for cervical esophageal squamous cell carcinoma according to the AJCC 7th edition?   (▶ Table 7.8)

Table 7.8 AJCC neck (N) staging for cervical esophageal squamous cell carcinoma.

Stage	Description
N0	no regional metastasis
N1	1–2 regional lymph nodes
N2	3–6 regional lymph nodes
N3	≥ 7 lymph node metastasis

Data from Edge SB, Byrd DR, Compton CC, Fritz AG, Greene FL, Trotti A, eds. AJCC Cancer Staging Manual 7th Edition. New York, NY: Springer; 2010.

542	Describe the staging system used to classify esophageal cancer based on the TNM stage.	• Stage IA: T1N0 • Stage IA: T2N0 • Stage IIA: T3N0 • Stage IIB: T1-T2N1 • Stage IIIA: T4aN0, T3N1, T1–2N2 • Stage IIIB: T3N2 • Stage IIIC: T4aN1–2, T4bAnyN, AnyTN3 • Stage IV: M1
543	What tumor characteristics have been recently added to the AJCC, 7th edition, staging of esophageal cancer?	• Histologic type (squamous cell carcinoma versus adeno-carcinoma) • Histologic grade (1–3) • Tumor location (upper, middle, or lower esophagus)
544	Although cervical esophageal and hypopharyngeal squamous cell carcinomas are commonly grouped together, what is an important difference in staging at presentation?	Hypopharyngeal squamous cell carcinoma has a higher incidence of advanced T and N stages at presentation compared with cervical esophageal squamous cell carcinoma.
545	True or False. Comparing stages, esophageal squamous cell carcinoma, and adenocarcinoma have similar survival rates.	True
546	What imaging modality may play a role in predicting prognosis in esophageal cancer, and what is the unit of measurement that is used to predict prognosis?	PET scans. Standardized uptake values (SUV). This has not borne out in other head and neck cancer thus far, despite intense evaluation.

547	What overexpression or gene amplification of what molecular marker has been associated with poor outcome in esophageal cancer?	Human epidermal growth factor receptor (HER-2)
548	What treatment modalities are recommended for esophageal cancer based on stage?	• Stage I: Endoscopic resection vs surgical resection • Stage II–III: Chemoradiation followed by surgery • Stage IV: Chemotherapy or best supportive care *Note:* Increasing stage is associated with poorer prognosis.
549	What surgical technique is used for primary cervical esophageal tumors or hypopharyngeal tumors with involvement of the cervical esophagus?	Total pharyngo-laryngo-esophagectomy and total pharyngolaryngectomy with cervical esophagectomy
550	What are the reconstructive options after surgery for cervical esophageal cancer when resection includes the esophagus below the thoracic inlet?	• Gastric transposition (gastric "pull-up") • Colonic transposition
551	What are some of the disadvantages of the gastric transposition (gastric "pull-up") reconstruction for pharyngeal and esophageal defects?	• High incidence of morbidity and mortality • Inability to close some defects with oropharyngeal or nasopharyngeal extension • Frequent pulmonary complications • Risk of hypoparathyroidism • Gastric dumping syndrome • Gastric outlet obstruction • Regurgitation
552	What are the reconstructive options after surgery for cervical esophageal cancer when resection does not include the esophagus below the thoracic inlet?	• Gastric transposition (gastric "pull-up") • Colonic transposition • Jejunal vascularized free flap • Tubed fasciocutaneus vascularized free flap
553	What is the major functional disadvantage for patients undergoing jejunal free flap reconstruction for pharyngeal defects?	Poor speech and swallowing function. See also dysphagia and donor-site morbidity. Relatively low rate of stenosis.

Larynx Anatomy

| 554 | Describe the boundaries of the larynx according to the AJCC. | • *Superior*: Oropharynx; tip and lateral borders of the epiglottis
• *Inferior*: Trachea; plane passing through the inferior limit of the cricoid cartilage
• *Posterior/lateral*: Hypopharynx; laryngeal surface of the aryepiglottic folds, arytenoid region, interarytenoid space, mucous membrane covering the posterior surface of the cricoid cartilage
• Anterior: Anterior/lingual surface of the suprahyoid epiglottis, thyrohyoid membrane, anterior commissure, thyroid cartilage, cricothyroid membrane, anterior arch of the thyroid cartilage |
| 555 | What are the subsites of the larynx according to the AJCC? | • *Supraglottis*: Lingual and laryngeal surfaces of the epiglottis, laryngeal surface of aryepiglottic folds, arytenoids, false vocal folds; divided from glottis by a horizontal plane passing through the lateral margin of the ventricle at its junction with the superior surface of the vocal cord.
• *Glottis*: Superior and inferior surface of the true vocal fold, anterior and posterior commissure; extends 1 cm below the plane dividing supraglottis and glottis; lateral margin defined by the junction of the lateral aspect of the ventricle at its junction with the superior surface of the true vocal fold.
• *Subglottis*: inferior margin of the glottis to inferior border of the cricoid cartilage. |

556	What subsite of the larynx arises from the buccopharyngeal primordium (third or fourth branchial arches) and therefore derives its arterial supply from the superior laryngeal arteries and lymphatic drainage is to levels II and III?	Supraglottis
557	What subsites of the larynx arise from the tracheobronchial primordium (sixth branchial arch) and therefore derives its arterial supply from the inferior laryngeal arteries and lymphatic drainage is to levels IV and VI?	Glottis and subglottis
558	What branchial arch structures give rise to the hyoid bone?	• Second branchial arch: Lesser horn and upper portion of the hyoid bone • Third branchial arch: Greater horn and lower portion of the hyoid bone
559	What are the five subsites of the supraglottis?	• Suprahyoid epiglottis • Infrahyoid epiglottis • Aryepiglottic fold (laryngeal surface) • False vocal fold (also called the *ventricular bands*) • Arytenoid
560	What are the subsites of the glottis?	True vocal folds (superior and inferior surface), including the anterior and posterior commissures
561	What are the subsites of the subglottis?	None
562	What is the normal histology of the supraglottis?	• Pseudostratified columnar respiratory epithelium. The lateral surface of the aryepiglottic folds and epiglottis are stratified squamous epithelium. • Numerous mucous glands
563	What is the normal histologic structure of the glottis, proceeding medial to lateral through the true vocal fold?	• Stratified squamous epithelium • Superficial lamina propria (Reinke space) • Vocal ligament (intermediate and deep lamina propria) • Thyroarytenoid muscle • Paraglottic fat • Thyroid cartilage
564	What is the normal histology of the subglottis?	Pseudostratified columnar epithelium
565	What are the natural barriers to spread of laryngeal cancer? (► Table 7.9)	• Quadrangular membrane* • Conus elasticus* • Thyrohyoid membrane* (aperture for superior laryngeal neurovascular bundle allows spread) • Laryngeal cartilages • Hyoepiglottic ligament • Anterior commissure tendon • Cricothyroid membrane *Most commonly considered

Table 7.9 AJCC tumor (T) staging of the larynx.

Stage	Description
Supraglottis	**Suprahyoid epiglottis, Infrahyoid epiglottis, Aryepiglottic folds (laryngeal aspect), Arytenoids, False vocal cords (VCs)**
T1	one subsite of supraglottis, normal VC mobility
T2	> 1 adjacent subsite of supraglottis or glottis or region outside supraglottis
T3	limited to larynx with VC fixation and/or invades any of the following: postcricoid area, pre-epiglottic tissues, paraglottic space, and/or minor thyroid cartilage erosion
T4a	invades through thyroid cartilage and/or invades tissues beyond larynx
T4b	invades prevertebral space, encases carotid artery, or invades mediastinal structures
Glottis	**True VC, including anterior and posterior commisures, including region 1 cm below plane of true VCs**
T1a	limited to one VC, normal mobility
T1b	involves both VCs, normal mobility
T2	extends to supraglottis and/or subglottis, and/or with impaired VC mobility
T3	limited to larynx with VC fixation and/or invades paraglottic space, and or minor thyroid cartilage erosion
T4a	invades through thyroid cartilage and/or invades tissues beyond larynx
T4b	invades prevertebral space, encases carotid artery, or invades mediastinal structures
Subglottis	**Region extending from 1 cm below true VC to cervical trachea**
T1	limited to subglottis
T2	extends to VC(s), with normal or impaired mobility
T3	limited to larynx, with VC fixation
T4a	invades cricoid or thyroid cartilage and/or invades tissues beyond larynx
T4b	invades prevertebral space, encases carotid artery, or invades mediastinal structures

Data from Edge SB, Byrd DR, Compton CC, Fritz AG, Greene FL, Trotti A, eds. AJCC Cancer Staging Manual 7th Edition. New York, NY: Springer; 2010.

566	What sheet of fibroelastic tissue stretches from the epiglottis to the arytenoid and corniculate cartilages, contributes to the aryepiglottic fold superiorly, and defines the free margin of the false cord inferiorly?	Quadrangular membrane
567	What sheet of fibroelastic tissue stretches from the vocal ligament to the superior margin of the cricoid laterally and inferior margin of the thyroid cartilage anteriorly (where it forms the cricothyroid membrane)?	Conus elasticus
568	What 1 × 10-mm fibrous tissue band connects the vocal ligaments to the midline of the thyroid cartilage, is associated with a lack of perichondrium at the insertion point, and serves as a strong barrier to spread of laryngeal cancer (Kirchner, 1987)?	Anterior commissure tendon (the Broyles ligament)

569	Broyles ligament, or the anterior commissure tendon, is often sited as a pathway for spread of laryngeal cancer through the thyroid cartilage. However, studies have shown that this structure actually serves as a strong barrier to spread in the absence of what tumor characteristics?	Significant supraglottic (petiole, pre-epiglottic space) or subglottic extension (ossified thyroid cartilage, lymphatics, cricothyroid membrane)
570	Name the funnel-shaped space formed by the thyrohyoid membrane and thyroid cartilage anteriorly; the epiglottis posteriorly; the hyoepiglottic ligament, vallecula, and hyoid bone superiorly; and the thyroepiglottic ligament inferiorly. The space communicates laterally with the paraglottic space and acts as an avenue for tumor spread.	Pre-epiglottic space.
571	Name the paired spaces that are defined by the thyroid cartilage laterally, the conus elasticus inferomedially, the ventricle medially, the quadrangular membrane superomedially, and the pyriform sinus mucosa posteriorly. It is an avenue for spread of laryngeal cancer and communicates anteriorly with the pre-epiglottic space.	Paraglottic space
572	What important feature of the infrahyoid epiglottic cartilage allows easy tumor growth into the pre-epiglottic space?	Fenestrations
573	Transglottic tumors by definition cross the ventricle and involve the supraglottis and glottis and may involve the subglottis. Define the theoretical methods by which a laryngeal tumor can become transglottic.	• Directly crossing the ventricle • Crossing at the anterior commissure • Via the paraglottic space (all three subsites of the larynx are accessible) • Spread along the arytenoid cartilage to the posterior ventricle
574	Why do lateralized supraglottic tumors drain bilaterally?	The supraglottis is formed embryologically from a single structure (i.e., no midline fusion), and therefore its lymphatics cross midline, allowing for bilateral spread of disease.
575	What is the inferior limit of the supraglottic lymphatic system within the larynx?	Inferior false vocal fold (barrier is the quadrangular membrane)
576	What nodal levels are most commonly involved by supraglottic tumors?	Levels II, III, and IV. Bilateral disease is common, especially with midline tumors.
577	What is the pathway for nodal spread from a supraglottic tumor to level II?	Along the superior laryngeal neurovascular bundle
578	What supraglottic subsite presents a high risk for aggressive behavior and early nodal metastases?	The "marginal zone": suprahyoid epiglottis and superior aspect of the aryepiglottic folds
579	What is the rate of occult nodal disease in supraglottic malignancies (considering all stages)?	Up to 40%. Increases with increasing T stage (10% T1 to 57% T4)
580	Why do lateralized glottic tumors drain unilaterally?	They are formed embryologically by paired structures that fuse in the midline. Lymphatics within this subsite are minimal and do not communicate across midline.
581	What is the risk of occult nodal metastases in glottic carcinoma?	18%. Increases with T stage
582	What nodal levels are at risk for disease in glottic carcinoma?	Levels II, III, IV, and VI (prelaryngeal, pretracheal, and paratracheal nodes)
583	What nodal levels are at highest risk for disease in subglottic carcinoma?	Level VI. Commonly present with contralateral or bilateral disease and mediastinal lymphadenopathy below level VII (distant metastases)

Evaluation and Management of Laryngeal Cancer

584	What patient demographic is at highest risk for laryngeal cancer?	• Males (3.8:1) • Associated with tobacco exposure • Age younger than 40 years
585	What are the strongest risk factors for laryngeal carcinoma?	• Tobacco smoking (packs per day and years of use) • Alcohol use (amount consumed and duration of use)
586	What is the role of laryngopharyngeal reflux in laryngeal cancer?	Controversial. It is unclear whether it is an independent or associated risk factor.
587	What percentage of laryngeal cancers have been associated with high-risk HPV (HPV 16 > HPV 18)?	~ 25%. Clinical significance is unclear.
588	What are four primary premalignant laryngeal lesions as defined by the WHO?	• Hyperplasia • Keratosis • Dysplasia: Mild, moderate, severe • Carcinoma in situ
589	What significance does laryngeal leukoplakia have?	Leukoplakia means "white plaque" and without a biopsy gives no information relevant to management.
590	What is the approximate rate of dysplasia in laryngeal leukoplakia?	40%
591	What is the approximate rate of malignant transformation of mild dysplasia? Severe dysplasia or carcinoma in situ?	• 11% • 30% *Note*: It may take up to 10 years for malignant conversion (average 3 years).
592	What percentage of laryngeal tumors are squamous cell carcinomas?	85 to 95%
593	According to WHO, what are the possible subtypes of squamous cell carcinoma found in the larynx?	• Verrucous • Spindle cell carcinoma (also called sarcomatoid carcinoma, carcinosarcoma, pseudosarcoma) • Adenoid (acantholytic) Basaloid squamous cell carcinoma • Clear cell carcinoma • Adenosquamous carcinoma • Giant cell carcinoma • Lymphoepithelial carcinoma
594	What laryngeal lesion is characterized by proliferation of the squamous mucosa, elongated rete ridges that appear worrisome for carcinoma and show no evidence of cytologic abnormalities consistent with malignancy?	Pseudoepitheliomatous hyperplasia. It can be associated with infection (e.g., tuberculosis, syphilis, blastomycosis), trauma, granular cell tumor, and chronic irritation. It is easily mistaken for squamous cell carcinoma and requires proper orientation of specimens and periodic-acid Schiff stain.
595	What pathology in the larynx is associated with trauma and infarction of salivary gland tissue (ducts and acini of seromucinous glands), is often misdiagnosed as squamous cell carcinoma or mucoepidermoid carcinoma, and requires immunohistochemistry for diagnosis?	Necrotizing sialometaplasia
596	What subtype of squamous cell carcinoma results in largely exophytic growth, pushing margins, does not metastasize, is associated with HPV-16 and -18, and has an indolent course?	Verrucous carcinoma. It is the second most common site in the head and neck (to oral cavity).
597	What epithelial laryngeal cancer contains both basaloid and squamous components (biphasic), cystic spaces, results in frequent regional and distant metastases, occurs most commonly in the supraglottis, and has a worse prognosis than standard squamous cell carcinoma?	Basaloid squamous cell carcinoma

598	What epithelial laryngeal cancer contains malignant squamous epithelium on its surface associated with a deeper malignant spindle cell carcinoma (biphasic), is associated with tobacco and alcohol use, results in common regional metastases, and is relatively radioresistant?	Spindle cell carcinoma
599	What is the most common location for adenosquamous carcinoma, a biphasic tumor arising from the basal layer of the epithelium and demonstrating behavior more aggressive than conventional squamous cell carcinoma, in the upper aerodigestive tract?	Larynx
600	What is the key pathologic difference between laryngeal verrucous carcinoma and papillary squamous cell carcinoma, which demonstrates exophytic papillary growth with cores of fibrovascular stroma?	Significantly abnormal cytology
601	According to the WHO, what are the possible subtypes of malignant salivary gland tumors found in the larynx, which make up less than 1% of all laryngeal tumors?	• Mucoepidermoid carcinoma • Adenoid cystic carcinoma • Adenocarcinoma • Acinic cell carcinoma • Carcinoma ex-pleomorphic adenoma • Epithelial-myoepithelial cell carcinoma • Salivary duct carcinoma
602	What are the cells of origin for supraglottic adenocarcinoma?	Minor salivary glands
603	Are salivary gland carcinomas of the larynx more common in men or women?	Men (2:1). However, adenoid cystic carcinoma has no gender bias.
604	What are the two most common laryngeal malignant salivary gland cancers?	Mucoepidermoid carcinoma and adenoid cystic carcinoma, constituting one-third of malignant laryngeal salivary gland tumors
605	What laryngeal tumor is composed of squamous, mucin-secreting, and intermediate-type cells and likely forms in the intercalated ducts of seromucinous glands?	Mucoepidermoid carcinoma
606	What percentage of supraglottic cancers arising from minor salivary glands will be mucoepidermoid carcinoma on pathological analysis?	35%. They are less common than adenoid cystic (46%), more common than adenocarcinoma (12%).
607	Adenoid cystic carcinoma is defined by uniform basaloid cells that grow in what three distinct patterns?	• Cribriform • Tubular • Solid
608	According to the WHO, what are the possible subtypes of neuroendocrine tumors found in the larynx, which are the second most common tumors of the larynx next to squamous cell carcinoma?	• Atypical carcinoid tumor (54%) • Small cell carcinoma (28%) • Malignant paraganglioma (12%) • (Typical) carcinoid tumor (7%)
609	What is the relative occurrence of supraglottic neuroendocrine tumors in men and women?	They occur three times more commonly in women than in men.
610	What is the 5-year survival rate for laryngeal neuroendocrine carcinoma?	Although it is one of the most common extrapulmonary sites for neuroendocrine carcinoma, laryngeal neuroendocrine carcinoma is extremely rare. It is also most often lethal, with 2- and 5-year survival rates of 16% and 5%, respectively.

611	What subsite of the larynx is most commonly involved by both typical and atypical carcinoid tumors, which present as submucosal and poly-poid masses?	Supraglottis
612	To what unusual locations do atypical carcinoids commonly metastasize?	Skin and subcutaneous tissue
613	What percentage of patients with laryngeal small cell carcinoma will develop distant metastases?	90%
614	According to the WHO, what are the possible subtypes of malignant soft tissue tumors found in the larynx?	• Fibrosarcoma • Malignant fibrous histiocytoma • Liposarcoma • Leiomyosarcoma • Rhabdomyosarcoma • Angiosarcoma • Kaposi sarcoma • Malignant hemangiopericytoma • Malignant nerve sheath tumor • Alveolar soft part sarcoma • Synovial sarcoma • Ewing sarcoma
615	According to the WHO, what are the possible subtypes of malignant bone and cartilage tumors in the larynx?	• Chondrosarcoma (most common) • Osteosarcoma
616	What laryngeal tumors arise from ossified hyaline cartilage, most commonly from the cricoid carti-lage?	Chondrosarcomas
617	What is the distant metastasis rate in laryngeal chondrosarcoma?	8.5%
618	According to the WHO, what are the possible subtypes of malignant hematolymphoid tumors found in the larynx?	• Extramedullary plasmacytoma (most common) • Lymphoma
619	According to the WHO, what tumors most commonly metastasize from a distant site to the larynx?	• Kidney • Skin (melanoma) • Breast • Lung • Prostate • Gastrointestinal tract
620	What is the most common site of second primaries in patients with larynx cancer?	Lung. Consider a pulmonary lesion a second primary tumor until proven otherwise.
621	What are the clinical risk factors that may increase the likelihood of stomal recurrence?	• Primary subglottic tumor • Glottic tumor invading subglottis by > 1 cm • T4 glottic primary tumor
622	What are the proposed causes of stomal recur-rence after total laryngectomy for laryngeal cancer?	• Positive tracheal margin • Paratracheal nodal metastases • Thyroid gland invasion • Seeding of the stoma at initial operation
623	What is the most common initial symptom associated with supraglottic carcinoma?	Dysphagia. It can also manifest with dysphonia, odyno-phagia, otalgia, stridor, dyspnea, hemoptysis, and neck mass.
624	What is the most common initial symptom associated with early versus late glottic carcino-ma?	• Early disease: Dysphonia • Advanced disease: Stridor, dyspnea
625	What are the most common initial symptoms associated with subglottic carcinoma?	Dyspnea and stridor

626	Patients with what symptoms may require urgent or emergent management of their laryngeal tumor?	Dyspnea and stridor
627	On endoscopy, which of the following lesions may be suspicious for a laryngeal carcinoma: ulceration, sessile lesion, polypoid lesion, submucosal fullness, or exophytic friable mass?	All should suggest ppossible malignant process.
628	What laryngoscopy adjunct should be used in the clinic to evaluate a patient in whom you are concerned about a laryngeal malignancy?	Flexible fiberoptic laryngoscopy and/or video stroboscopy
629	To evaluate a patient with laryngeal carcinoma for posterior invasion of the prevertebral fascia, you grasp the larynx and rock it back and forth. Inability to rock the larynx and lack of what sound/tactile feedback suggest invasion?	Laryngeal crepitus (movement of laryngopharyngeal framework across the prevertebral and vertebral structures)
630	What is the most commonly used imaging modality for the initial workup of laryngeal cancer?	CT with contrast using fine cuts through the larynx (~ 1 mm)
631	Which offers better evaluation of cartilage invasion: CT or MRI?	MRI
632	When using MRI for the evaluation of a patient with laryngeal cancer, what modality or sequences would be most useful to determine invasion of the preepiglottic and/or paraglottic spaces?	T1-weighted gadolinium enhanced MRI with fat suppression. High negative predictive value. False-positive results are caused by inflammation.
633	During direct endoscopic examination of the upper aerodigestive tract in the operating room for laryngeal cancer, what maneuver should be performed if there is concern for fixation of the larynx or immobility of a vocal cord?	Palpation of the laryngeal structures
634	Describe microflap excision for laryngeal biopsy.	Microflap surgery requires dissection of the superficial lamina propria as opposed to excision. This allows for sparing of the vocal ligament and affords a better postoperative mucosal wave.
635	Why is detection of recurrence after radiation more difficult in laryngeal cancer?	Persistent edema and fibrosis are common post-treatment sequelae that obscure visualization of (often submucosal) tumor growth.
636	Although deep biopsies are often necessary to diagnose a recurrent laryngeal tumor after radiation therapy, what adverse outcomes are associated with biopsy in this setting?	Increased risk of infection, perichondritis, and chondroradionecrosis
637	Describe the "T" staging system for epithelial supraglottic malignancies according to the AJCC. (▶ Fig. 7.7)	• T1: Tumor limited to one supraglottic subsite, normal vocal cord mobility. • T2: Tumor invasion of more than one subsite of the supraglottis or glottis or region outside the supraglottis (e.g., mucosa of base of tongue, vallecula, medial wall of pyriform sinus) *without* fixation of the larynx • T3: Tumor limited to the larynx *with* vocal cord fixation and/or invades any of the following: postcricoid area, preepiglottic tissues, paraglottic space, and/or minor thyroid cartilage erosion (e.g., inner cortex). • T4a: Moderately advanced local disease: tumor invades through the thyroid cartilage and/or invades tissue beyond the larynx (e.g., trachea, soft tissues of neck including deep extrinsic muscles of the tongue, strap muscles, thyroid, or esophagus).

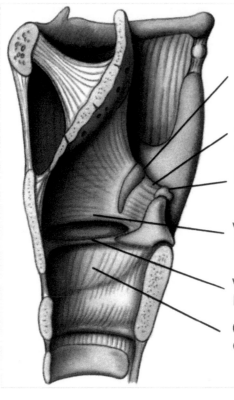

Corniculate
cartilage

Quadrangular
membrane

Cuneiform
cartilage

Vestibular
ligament

Vocal
ligament

Conus
elasticus

Fig. 7.7 Midsagittal section through the larynx illustrating some of the natural barriers to spread of laryngeal cancer: Quadrangular membrane, conus elasticus, thyrohyoid membrane (not labeled), laryngeal cartilages, hyoepiglottic ligament (not labeled), anterior commissure tendon (not labeled), cricothyroid membrane (not labeled). (Used with permission from Donald PJ, ed. The Difficult Case in Head and Neck Cancer Surgery. New York, NY: Thieme; 2010.)

		• T4b: Very advanced local disease: Tumor invades prevertebral space, encases carotid artery, or invades mediastinal structures.
638	What differentiates T2 from T3 supraglottic tumors?	T2 tumors do not invade the parilaryngeal spaces; T3 tumors present with vocal cord fixation.
639	What differentiates T1 from T2 supraglottic tumors?	• T1 tumors are limited to one subsite with normal vocal cord mobility. • T2 tumors may involve multiple supraglottic subsites or adjacent regions (tongue base, glottis).
640	Describe the "T" staging system for epithelial glottic malignancies according to the AJCC).	• T1: Tumor is limited to the vocal cord(s); may involve anterior or posterior commissure; normal vocal cord mobility. • T1a: Tumor is limited to one vocal cord. • T1b: Tumor involves both vocal cords. • T2: Tumor extends to supraglottis and/or subglottis or with impaired vocal cord mobility (some authors divide T2 into T2a and T2b; see below). • T3: Tumor is limited to the larynx with vocal cord fixation and/or invades the paraglottic space, and/or minor thyroid cartilage erosion (e.g., inner cortex). • T4a: Moderately advanced local disease: Tumor invades through the thyroid cartilage and/or invades tissues beyond the larynx (e.g., trachea, soft tissues of neck including deep extrinsic muscle of the tongue, strap muscles, thyroid or esophagus). • T4b: Very advanced local disease: Tumor invades prevertebral space, encases carotid artery, or invades mediastinal structures.

641	Although the AJCC, (7th edition) does not differentiate T2 into T2a and T2b, some authorities do. How are these stages defined?	Tumor extends to the supraglottis and/or subglottis: • T2a: Without impaired vocal cord mobility • T2b: With impaired vocal cord mobility
642	What is the rate of nodal metastases in T1 glottic carcinoma?	5%
643	What differentiates T3 from T4 glottic tumors?	T3 tumors are confined to the larynx, whereas T4 have spread extralaryngeally (into strap musculature, thyroid gland, trachea, esophagus).
644	Describe the "T" staging system for epithelial subglottic malignancies according to the AJCC.	• T1: Tumor is limited to the subglottics. • T2: Tumor extends to vocal cord(s) with normal or impaired mobility. • T3: Tumor is limited to the larynx with vocal cord fixation. • T4a: Moderately advanced local disease. Tumor invades cricoid or thyroid cartilage and/or invades tissues beyond the larynx (e.g., trachea, soft tissues of the neck including deep extrinsic muscles of the tongue, strap muscles, thyroid or esophagus) • T4b: Very advanced local disease: Tumor invades prevertebral space, encases carotid artery, or invades mediastinal structures.
645	Describe the stages of stomal recurrence after total laryngectomy for laryngeal cancer (Sisson, 1989).	• Stage I: Superior to the stoma, at 9 to 3 o'clock position. Normal swallowing and esophagoscopy • Stage II: Above or below the stoma, 9 to 3 o'clock. Most have dysphagia and esophageal invasion. • Stage III: Below the stoma, at 9 to 3 o'clock. Esophagus is always involved. High risk of upper mediastinal disease • Stage IV: Lateral extension of the tumor under the clavicle, dysphagia, and esophageal invasion
646	What is the overall 5-year survival rate for laryngeal cancer, and what subsite has the best overall survival?	• 64% • Glottic (79%) > supraglottic (47%) > subglottic (30 to 50%)
647	During the initial workup of a patient with laryngeal cancer, you identify cartilage invasion. How does this impact prognosis and management?	• Upstages tumor (T3 or T4a) • Poorer response to radiation therapy • Decreased local control rates • Higher risk of chondroradionecrosis
648	What is the incidence of distant metastasis in glottic carcinoma?	4%
649	What are the most important clinical prognostic factors in order of importance?	• Clinical stage (most important to least: M > N > T) • Location of the primary (best to worst: glottic > supraglottic > subglottic)
650	Why does involvement of the anterior commissure decrease prognosis (local control rates) for both surgery and radiation therapy?	Inadequate recognition of deep extension
651	What factors increase the risk of peristomal recurrence after laryngectomy for laryngeal cancer?	• T3 or T4 tumors • Subglottic tumor extension
652	What histologic characteristics decrease local control and overall survival?	• Extracapsular spread* • Positive surgical margins* • Histologic subtype • Histologic grade (well, moderate, poor) • Pattern of invasion (pushing vs infiltrative) • Perineural invasion* • Vascular embolus (invasion)* *Considered adverse features impacting management decisions by the NCCN (2013)

653	In addition to primary oncologic management, what behavioral modifications should be recommended to maximize treatment benefit and decrease the risk of recurrence for premalignant and malignant laryngeal cancer?	• Tobacco and alcohol cessation • Reflux control
654	What is the wavelength and chromophore of the CO_2 laser?	• Wavelength: 10,600 nm • Chromophore: water
655	What is the wavelength and chromophore of the potassium-titalyl-phosphate (KTP) laser?	• Wavelength: 532 nm • Chromophore: Oxyhemoglobin
656	What treatment modality makes use of photo-reactive chemicals (5-aminolevulinic acid, Photofrin, hematoporphyrin, foscan), which are preferentially absorbed by premalignant or malignant cells and then subsequently activated by light of a specific frequency?	Photodynamic therapy
657	What is the treatment of choice for premalignant laryngeal lesions?	• Complete excision with pathologic analysis (microflap, vocal cord stripping; higher risk for poor voice outcomes, laser resection) • Close follow-up • Can consider laser ablation (pulsed dye laser or KTP) once pathologic diagnosis is established
658	What are the management options for carcinoma in situ?	Complete surgical excision or radiation therapy. *Note:* Recurrence is higher after surgical excision than after radiation therapy, but local control is equivalent with repeat excision.
659	For a patient with significant airway obstruction from a laryngeal tumor, should you perform an emergent laryngectomy or tracheostomy?	High tracheostomy. No evidence has been established that tracheostomy increases the risk of peristomal recurrence, and emergent laryngectomy does not allow time for complete workup and counseling.
660	In the Veterans Affairs' (VA) laryngeal cancer study, what groups were compared?	• Induction chemotherapy and radiation for responders and surgery followed by postoperative radiation therapy for responders • Surgery and postoperative radiation
661	What were the laryngeal preservation rates and overall survival figures in the VA laryngeal cancer study?	For patients with advanced resectable laryngeal cancer (stage III or IV, excluding T1N1), induction chemotherapy and radiation allow for laryngeal preservation in 64% of patients and a similar 2-year overall survival (68%) compared with total laryngectomy and postoperative radiation therapy.
662	What proportion of patients in the VA laryngeal cancer study preoperatively had mobile vocal cords? Cartilage invasion?	44% and 9%, respectively
663	In the RTOG 91–11 organ preservation in advanced laryngeal cancer study, what groups were compared?	• Concurrent cisplatin and radiation • Induction cisplatin/5-FU followed by radiation therapy for complete and partial responders or surgery and adjuvant radiation therapy for non responders • Radiation alone
664	What was the laryngeal preservation rate for concurrent chemoradiation, induction chemotherapy/radiation, and radiation alone in RTOG 91–11?	• CRT: 88% • Induction chemotherapy/radiation + radiotherapy: 75% • Radiotherapy alone: 70%
665	What was the grade 3/4 mucositis rate for concurrent chemoradiation, induction chemotherapy/radiation, and radiation alone in RTOG 91–11?	• CRT: 43% • Induction chemotherapy + radiotherapy: 24% • Radiotherapy: 24%

666	What patients with advanced laryngeal cancer were excluded from RTOG 91–11?	Patients were excluded if they were not eligible for total laryngectomy with curative intent, T1 primary tumors, and large-volume T4 disease (transcartilaginous or > 1-cm tongue base invasion).
667	What are the contraindications to transoral resection of laryngeal carcinoma?	• Subglottic extension (> 5 mm) • Postcricoid extension • Pyriform sinus invasion • Cartilage invasion • Tongue base involvemen *Note*: Restricted vocal cord mobility and extension onto the arytenoid are relative contraindications.
668	What factors are critical to transoral resection of laryngeal carcinoma?	Adequate exposure, accurate assessment of tumor extension, complete resection
669	Name the open conservation laryngeal procedure in which one vocal cord or one and a portion of the other vocal cord are removed in continuity with the adjacent paraglottic space and overlying thyroid cartilage.	Vertical partial laryngectomy. The vertical height of the larynx is maintained by the retained contralateral thyroid ala.
670	What contraindicates vertical partial laryngectomy?	• Cricoid cartilage involvement (1-cm subglottic extension anteriorly and 5 mm posteriorly) • Thyroid cartilage involvement (often the case for transglottic tumors because mucosal spread from the supraglottis to glottis across the ventricle brings tumor into close proximity to the inner thyroid perichondrium) • Poor pulmonary function
671	Name the operation and its subtypes in which the entire superior portion of the thyroid cartilage is removed along with the underlying laryngeal structures, reducing the vertical height of the larynx by the subsequent reconstruction.	Horizontal partial laryngectomy: • Supraglottic • Extended supraglottic • Supracricoid (with cricohyoidopexy or cricohyoiodoepiglottopexy)
672	What is the embryologic rationale behind horizontal hemilaryngectomy?	An embryologic boundary exists between the false and true vocal folds, resulting in independent lymphatic drainage from each. Therefore, in select (T1/T2) supraglottic tumors that do not extend into neighboring structures, horizontal supraglottic hemilaryngectomy may be considered an oncologically sound resection strategy.
673	What are the contraindications for supracricoid horizontal partial laryngectomy?	• Arytenoid fixation • Cricoid/thyroid cartilage involvement • Hyoid involvement • Significant pre-epiglottic space disease • Poor pulmonary function
674	What *patient* factors are critical to conservation laryngeal operations?	Excellent cardiopulmonary reserve and motivation to retain larynx
675	What *tumor* factors contraindicate conservation laryngeal surgery?	• Cartilage invasion • Extralaryngeal spread • Interarytenoid involvement • Postcricoid spread • Invasion to pyriform apex
676	What factors reduce the efficacy of radiation in laryngeal cancer?	• Cartilage invasion • T4 stage • Extralaryngeal spread
677	What site(s) are most commonly involved by distant metastases from the larynx?	Lung and mediastinum (not including level VII)
678	What subsite of the larynx has the highest risk for distant metastasis?	Supraglottis (up to 15%)

679	What factors increase the risk of distant metastasis for laryngeal cancer?	History of nodal metastasis
680	What is the management of choice for supraglottic carcinoma not requiring a total laryngectomy (mostly cT1–2, N0) according to the NCCN (2011)?	• Endoscopic resection → neck dissection • Open partial supraglottic laryngectomy → neck dissection • Definitive radiation therapy
681	For patients undergoing primary surgical management of cT1–2N0 supraglottic carcinoma not requiring a total laryngectomy, what are the adjuvant treatment recommendations according to the NCCN (2011)?	• N0 → observation • One positive node, no adverse features → consider radiation therapy • N+, positive margin → re-excision, radiation therapy, or chemoradiation therapy • N+, extracapsular spread → chemoradiation therapy or radiation alone
682	What is the treatment of choice for cT1–2N+ and select cT3N1 supraglottic carcinomas not requiring a total laryngectomy according to the NCCN (2011)?	• Concurrent chemoradiation therapy with cisplatin (preferred) → additional therapy dictated by response to therapy • Definitive radiation therapy → additional therapy dictated by response to therapy • Partial supraglottic laryngectomy and neck dissection(s) → adjuvant therapy as dictated by pathologic findings • Induction chemotherapy
683	What is the treatment of choice for a cT3N0 supraglottic carcinoma requiring a total laryngectomy according to the NCCN (2011)?	• Concurrent chemoradiation therapy with cisplatin (preferred) • Laryngectomy, ipsilateral thyroidectomy, with ipsilateral or bilateral neck dissection • Radiation therapy (if not a candidate for concurrent chemotherapy) • Induction chemotherapy
684	For patients undergoing primary surgical management of cT3N0 supraglottic carcinoma, what are the adjuvant treatment recommendations according to the NCCN (2011)?	• N0 or 1 positive node without adverse features → consider radiation therapy • Extracapsular spread or positive margin → chemoradiation • Other risk features → radiation therapy with or without chemotherapy
685	What is the management of choice for a cT3N2–3 supraglottic carcinoma requiring a total laryngectomy according to the NCCN (2011)?	• Concurrent chemoradiation therapy with cisplatin (preferred) → surgical salvage based on response to therapy • Laryngectomy, ipsilateral thyroidectomy with neck dissection(s) → radiation therapy → chemotherapy based on the presence of pathologic adverse features • Induction chemotherapy followed by chemoradiation therapy
686	What is the management of choice for a cT4aN0–3 supraglottic carcinoma requiring according to the NCCN (2011)?	• Laryngectomy, ipsilateral thyroidectomy, with ipsilateral or bilateral neck dissection: • N0, no risk features → radiation therapy • Extracapsular spread and/or positive margin → hcemoradiation therapy • Other risk features → radiation therapy → chemotherapy • *Note*: For those who decline surgery, concurrent chemoradiation therapy, enrollment in a clinical trial, or induction chemotherapy followed by primary chemoradiation therapy can be considered.
687	For patients undergoing primary induction chemotherapy for supraglottic carcinoma, what are the treatment recommendations based on response to induction according to the NCCN (2011)?	• Primary site: Complete response → radiation therapy with or without chemotherapy • Primary site: Partial response → chemoradiation therapy → if partial response → salvage surgery • Primary site < partial response → surgery → radiation therapy with or without chemotherapy based on presence of pathological adverse features

688	What dose of definitive radiation therapy is recommended by the NCCN (2011) for patients with T1–2N0 supraglottic squamous cell carcinoma?	• ≥ 66 Gy
689	What dose of definitive radiation therapy is recommended by the NCCN (2011) for patients with T2–3N0–1 supraglottic squamous cell carcinoma?	• Primary and cN + ≥ 70 Gy, conventional fractionation (Monday through Friday for 7 weeks), high-risk nodal basins 44 to 64 Gy • Accelerated fractionation: 66 to 74 Gy to gross disease, 44 to 64 Gy to high-risk regions for 6 weeks • Concomitant boost accelerated radiation therapy: 72 Gy/ 6 weeks, second daily dose for the last 12 days • Hyperfractionation: 81.6 Gy for 7 weeks
690	What dose of radiation therapy is recommended by the NCCN (2011) for patients undergoing concomitant chemoradiation therapy for supraglottic squamous cell carcinoma?	70 Gy for 7 weeks, conventional fractionation
691	What dose of radiation therapy is recommended by the NCCN (2011) for patients undergoing postoperative radiation therapy for supraglottic squamous cell carcinoma?	• Primary 60 to 66 Gy, conventional fractionation (Monday through Friday for 7 weeks), high-risk nodal basins 44 to 64 Gy • N + neck: 60 to 66 Gy • N0, high-risk neck: 44 to 64 Gy
692	What chemotherapeutic agent and dose are recommended by the NCCN (2011) for patients undergoing concomitant chemoradiation therapy for supraglottic squamous cell carcinoma?	Cisplatin 100 mg/m^2 every 3 weeks during radiation
693	What levels of the neck should be addressed during an elective neck dissection for an N0 supraglottic cancer according to the NCCN (2011)?	Level II-IV, level VI when appropriate
694	What is the initial local control achieved by radiation alone for T1 and T2 supraglottic carcinoma?	92 to 100%
695	What percentage of patients who undergo supracricoid partial laryngectomy with cricohyoidopexy for supraglottic cancer will never achieve decannulation?	1.5%
696	Which of the following has more influence on survival in supraglottic malignancies: histology of tumor (squamous vs. nonsquamous) or T/N-staging?	T and N staging
697	What is the management of choice for glottic carcinoma not requiring a total laryngectomy according to the NCCN (2011)?	• Radiation therapy • Partial laryngectomy/open or endoscopic resection as indicated • N0 → observe
698	What is the management of choice for T3 glottic carcinoma requiring total laryngectomy (N0–1) according to the NCCN (2011)?	• Concurrent chemoradiation therapy with cisplatin (preferred) • Radiation (if not a candidate for surgery) • Surgery
699	If a patient with T3 glottic cancer requiring a total laryngectomy (N0–1) undergoes concurrent chemoradiation therapy with cisplatin or primary radiation therapy alone, what are the recommended management steps based on the patient's response to therapy at the primary site?	• Complete response (N0 at initial staging) → observe • Complete response (N + at initial staging) • Residual nodal disease → neck dissection • Complete clinical response in neck → evaluation → if N + → neck dissection, if N0 → observe • Residual tumor at the primary site → salvage surgery + neck dissection as indicated

700	If a patient with T3 glottic cancer requiring a total laryngectomy (N0–1) elects to undergo primary surgical intervention, what are the recommended management steps based on the patient's nodal status?	• N0 → Laryngectomy with ipsilateral thyroidectomy • N1 → Laryngectomy with ipsilateral thyroidectomy, ipsilateral or bilateral neck dissection • No adverse features → observe • Extracapsular spread or positive margins → chemoradiation therapy • Other risk features → radiation therapy → chemotherapy
701	What is the treatment of choice for T3 glottic carcinoma requiring total laryngectomy (N2–3) according to the NCCN (2011)?	• Concurrent chemoradiation therapy with cisplatin (preferred) • Laryngectomy with ipsilateral thyroidectomy and ipsilateral or bilateral neck dissection • Induction chemotherapy
702	If a patient with T3N2–3 glottic carcinoma requiring a total laryngectomy undergoes concurrent chemoradiation therapy with cisplatin, what are the treatment options based on response to therapy?	• Primary site: complete response • Residual tumor in neck → neck dissection • Complete clinical response in neck → evaluation → if N0, observe, if N + then neck dissection • Primary site: residual tumor • Salvage surgery + neck dissection as indicated
703	If a patient with T3N2–3 glottic carcinoma requiring a total laryngectomy undergoes primary surgical treatment, what are the treatment options based on pathologic analysis?	• No adverse features → observe • Extracapsular spread and/or positive margins → chemoradiation therapy • Other risk features → radiation therapy → chemotherapy
704	If a patient with T3N2–3 glottic carcinoma requiring a total laryngectomy undergoes induction chemotherapy, what are the treatment options based on clinical response of the primary site?	• Complete response → definitive radiation therapy or chemoradiation therapy • N + → neck dissection • N0 → evaluation, if N + → neck dissection • Partial response → chemoradiation therapy • Complete response → observe • Residual disease → Salvage surgery • < Partial/no response → surgery • No adverse features → radiation therapy • Extracapsular spread and/or positive margin →chemoradiation therapy • Other risk features → radiation therapy → chemotherapy
705	What is the treatment of choice for T4aN0 glottic carcinoma according to the NCCN (2011)?	Laryngectomy with ipsilateral thyroidectomy → unilateral/bilateral neck dissection → chemoradiation therapy
706	What is the treatment of choice for T4aN1 glottic carcinoma according to the NCCN (2011)?	Laryngectomy with ipsilateral thyroidectomy and ipsilateral neck dissection → contralateral neck dissection → chemoradiation therapy
707	What is the treatment of choice for T4aN2–3 glottic carcinoma according to the NCCN (2011)?	Laryngectomy with ipsilateral thyroidectomy and ipsilateral or bilateral neck dissection → chemoradiation therapy
708	What is the definitive radiation therapy for T1N0 glottic carcinoma recommended by the NCCN (2011)?	63 to 66 Gy, conventional fractionation
709	What is the definitive radiation therapy for T1–2 glottic carcinoma recommended by the NCCN (2011)?	> 66 Gy, conventional fractionation
710	What is the definitive radiation therapy for > T2N + glottic carcinoma recommended by the NCCN (2011)?	66 to 74 Gy, conventional fractionation (accelerated fractionation schedules may be considered)Nodal levels at risk for disease: 44 to 64 Gy
711	What is the radiation dose for primary concurrent chemoradiation therapy for glottic carcinoma recommended by the NCCN (2011)?	• Primary and N + disease: ≥ 70 Gy • Nodal levels at high risk: 44 to 64 Gy

712	What is the radiation dose for adjuvant radiation therapy for glottic carcinoma recommended by the NCCN (2011)?	• Primary: 60 to 66 Gy • N+: 60 to 66 Gy • N0: 44 to 64 Gy
713	What is the chemotherapeutic agent and dose of choice for chemoradiation therapy for glottic carcinoma recommended by the NCCN (2013)?	Cisplatin 100 mg/m^2 every 3 weeks (generally for three cycles)
714	Describe *vestibulotomy* as a component of transoral laser resection of glottic carcinoma.	*Vestibulotomy* refers to removing those portions of the false cord that overlie the tumor. It affords lateral exposure and may facilitate postoperative surveillance.
715	What is the initial treatment of an airway fire?	First remove the endotracheal tube because it is providing the fuel (oxygen) for the fire. Irrigate with water, reintubate, and perform bronchoscopy to survey the injury.
716	What is the point of entrance into the larynx during laryngofissure?	The larynx is divided in the midline, with entry at the anterior commissure.
717	What are the benefits of transoral approach for cordectomy?	Avoidance of initial tracheostomy and external scar. The main disadvantage, of course, is poorer access.
718	What are the indications for cordectomy via transoral access or laryngofissure?	• Cordectomy can be considered for T1 tumors limited to the middle third of the vocal fold. • Contraindications include extension of tumor to vocal process or anterior commissure, subglottis, ventricle, or false cord.
719	What is the standard treatment for subglottic carcinoma?	Total laryngectomy with paratracheal node dissection followed by radiation therapy (including the mediastinum) ± chemotherapy
720	For carcinoma with unilateral subglottic extension, what additional surgery should be considered during total laryngectomy?	Ipsilateral thyroid lobectomy and paratracheal node dissection
721	What are the surgical options for primary subglottic squamous cell carcinoma?	When treated surgically, all require total laryngectomy with paratracheal node dissection.
722	What proportion of patients for whom radiation for advanced larynx cancer fails would be suitable candidates for salvage surgery?	Two-thirds
723	What are some of the common indications for salvage surgery after nonoperative primary management of laryngeal cancer?	• Residual or recurrent locoregional disease • Chondroradionecrosis • Severe aspiration • Laryngeal stenosis • Pharyngoesophageal stenosis
724	What are the contraindications to partial laryngectomy in the salvage situation for patients with recurrent laryngeal cancer (Biller et al, 1970)?	• Subglottic extension > 5 mm • Cartilage invasion • Contralateral vocal cord invasion • Arytenoid cartilage invasion (other than vocal process) • Vocal cord fixation • Recurrence not associated with the primary lesion
725	What complications are frequently associated with management of stomal recurrences?	• Vascular injury • Hypocalcaemia • Mediastinitis • Fistula
726	What laryngeal reconstructive technique used for supracricoid partial laryngectomy preserves the epiglottis?	Cricohyoidoepiglottopexy
727	What laryngeal reconstructive technique is used after horizontal partial laryngectomy and requires resection of the epiglottis?	Cricohyoidopexy

728	In a patient undergoing laryngopharyngectomy with primary closure, what additional procedure should be performed to decrease postoperative dysphagia?	Cricopharyngeal myotomy
729	What type of stitch is most frequently used for closure of laryngopharyngectomy?	Running modified Connell stitch, followed by one or two layers of interrupted 3-0 Vicryl to imbricate overlying layers. Flood the mouth to ensure closure is water tight.
730	What are the benefits of the artificial larynx for speech after total laryngectomy?	Inexpensive, relatively easy to learn, provides loud voice
731	After laryngectomy, what type of speech is being used if a patient injects (swallows) air into the esophagus, which acts as a reservoir for the expelled air used for voicing?	Esophageal speech. This produces a characteristic belching sound. Patients are usually limited to soft volume and short duration of utterance.
732	Name the one-way valve placed across the wall between the trachea and esophagus that allows exhaled air to pass through the neopharynx for voicing.	Tracheoesophageal prosthesis
733	Describe *primary tracheoesophageal puncture (primary TEP)*.	Before closing the pharyngeal defect, a hemostat is passed into the esophagus to the posterior tracheal wall, where a blade is used to create a small fistula. A catheter is placed through this to maintain patency until a prosthesis is fitted.
734	Describe the esophageal insufflation test in evaluating candidates for secondary TEP.	A catheter is placed transnasally into the esophagus, air is insufflated, and the patient is asked to count.
735	Describe two anatomical relative contraindications to TEP voice rehabilitation.	• Microstomia (< 1 cm) • Pharyngeal stricture
736	Why is a cricopharyngeal myotomy critical to total laryngectomy voice rehabilitation?	Cricopharyngeal muscle spasm diverts air passing through the TEP into the distal esophagus (instead of through the mouth), which prevents acquisition of alaryngeal speech.
737	What is the most common reason for TEP valve failure?	*Candida* fungal colonization
738	What is the definitive treatment for aspiration through the TEP site in the setting of a properly-functioning TEP valve?	A SCM flap or pectoralis major myofascial flap interposition (between the trachealis and esophagus) to reconstruct the party wall
739	How should a dislodged TEP temporary catheter be triaged?	Urgently. If not replaced within 24 hours, the fistula is likely to close, and the TEP would require surgical revision.
740	When factors imply that a patient has a functional larynx?	• Intelligible voice • Able to take in adequate calories by mouth with no/minimal aspiration • Avoidance of a stoma
741	What tumor factors most notably influence voice outcomes after surgery or radiation therapy?	Tumor extent and depth of invasion
742	What patient factors affect the functional outcome of total laryngectomy?	• Motivation for alaryngeal speech • Ability to communicate by writing • Manual dexterity for using voice prostheses • Family and social support
743	What are the functional effects after total laryngectomy?	• Loss of normal speech (not aphonia) • Inability to develop positive airway pressure (straining, coughing) • Loss of nasal airflow (anosmia, air filtration) • Presence of stoma (water precautions, body image)

744	True or False. Aggressive tumor surveillance with imaging and examinations improves the detection of asymptomatic recurrences and second primaries and therefore improves oncologic outcomes after primary management of laryngeal cancer.	False
745	What are the early complications of conservation laryngectomy?	• Tracheotomy tube obstruction • Hemorrhage • Aspiration pneumonia • Subcutaneous emphysema
746	What is the long-term incidence of hypothyroidism in patients treated primarily with radiation for laryngeal cancer?	70%
747	What is the appropriate sequence of actions in the event of an airway fire?	Extubation, then removal of supplemental oxygen and instillation of saline into the airway, then reintubation
748	What are the main risk factors for developing a pharyngocutaneous fistula after laryngectomy? *Comment:* Does history of neck radiation need to be included in the risk factors for fistula formation (or at least should we specify in patients who are not undergoing salvage)?	• Postoperative hemoglobin < 12.5 • Congestive heart failure • Extended laryngectomy • History of head and neck radiation
749	What is the best initial treatment for pharyngocutaneous fistula?	• Debridement • Wound dressing with antiseptic packing material • Nothing taken orally (NPO) • Antibiotics (if infected) • Consideration of hyperbaric oxygen therapy if initial measures are not successful
750	What complications are associated with tracheotomy placement during total laryngectomy?	• Pneumothorax • Hemorrhage via tracheoinnominate fistula • Subcutaneous emphysema.
751	What medical therapy would be most effective for a patient with persistent gastric inflation when attempting to use a transesophageal prosthesis?	Botulinum toxin injections to the cricopharyngeus muscle

Nasopharynx Anatomy

| 752 | What are the boundaries that define the nasopharynx? (▶ Fig. 7.8) | • Superior: Sphenoid bone
• Anterior: Choana
• Posterior: Clivus, C1 and C2 vertebrae
• Inferior: Soft palate
• Lateral: Torus tubarius, Rosenmuller fossa |

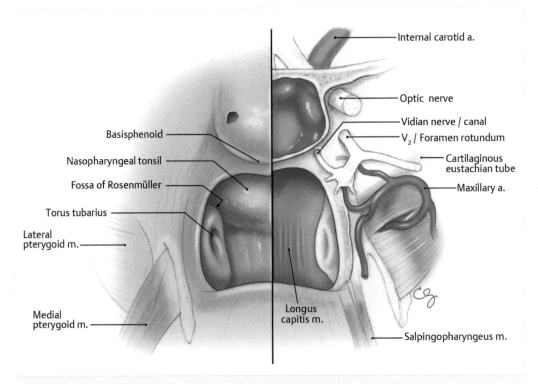

Fig. 7.8 Coronal section through the nasopharynx. (Used with permission from Kennedy DW, Hwang PH, eds. Rhinology: Diseases of the Nose, Sinuses, and Skull Base. New York, NY: Thieme; 2012.)

753	What skull base foramen defines the lateral roof of the nasopharynx?	Foramen lacerum
754	What space lies just posterior to the eustachian tube orifice and levator veli palatine muscle, at the junction of the lateral and posterior nasopharyngeal walls, inferior to the foramen lacerum and carotid canal within the sphenoid bone, medial to the foramen lacerum and spinosum, and superior to the upper border of the superior constrictor muscle?	Fossa of Rosenmuller
755	What space will be violated if a nasopharyngeal tumor extends laterally through the buccopharyngeal fascia? If it extends laterally through the anterior surface of the lateral pterygoid muscle?	• Parapharyngeal space • Masticator space
756	What is the relationship between internal carotid artery and the fossa of Rosenmüller?	Internal carotid artery lies immediately posterolateral to this space.
757	What functional structure, located on the posterior nasopharyngeal wall, is formed by the movement of the superior constrictor muscle and palatopharyngeus muscle?	Passavant ridge
758	What is the blood supply to the nasopharynx?	• Ascending pharyngeal artery (external carotid artery) • Sphenopalatine artery (internal maxillary artery) • Vidian artery (internal maxillary artery)
759	What is the venous drainage of the nasopharynx?	Pharyngeal plexus → jugular system

760	Sensation from the nasopharynx is conveyed by which nerve(s)?	• Glossopharyngeal nerve (CN IX) • Cranial nerve V_2
761	What are the three subsites of the nasopharynx?	• Lateral wall • Posterior wall • Soft palate
762	Where do most nasopharyngeal carcinomas originate?	Fossa of Rosenmüller
763	What is the most common site of distant metastases from nasopharyngeal carcinomas?	Bone
764	What nodal levels are at highest risk for metastases from a nasopharyngeal carcinoma? (▶ Fig. 7.9)	Retropharyngeal nodes and level II and VA. Bilateral disease is common.

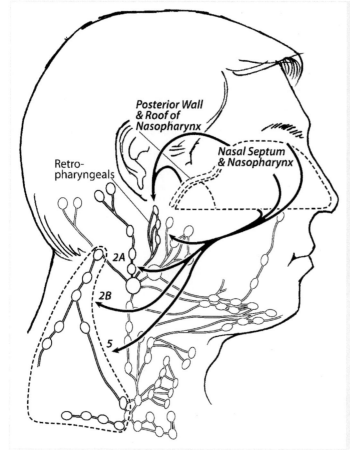

Fig. 7.9 Lymphatic drainage of the nose and nasopharynx. (Used with permission from Genden EM, Varvares MA, eds. Head and Neck Cancer: An Evidence-Based Team Approach. New York, NY: Thieme; 2008.)

765	What percentage of patients with nasopharyngeal carcinoma will develop nodal disease diagnosed either on physical examination or with imaging?	80%
766	What are the nodes of Rouviere?	Lateral retropharyngeal lymph nodes

Evaluation and Management of Nasopharyngeal Carcinoma

767	What are the primary risk factors associated with nasopharyngeal carcinoma?	• EBV • Genetics (including ethnicity and gender) • High intake of preserve foods (nitrosamines)

768	People of what ethnicity are most commonly affected by nasopharyngeal carcinoma?	Chinese. It is endemic in Southern China and Southeast Asia.
769	What food confers an increased risk for nasopharyngeal carcinoma?	Salted fish. Thought to be related to the volatile nitrosamines released in steam while cooking salt-cured foods and early exposure to these foods in childhood
770	What genetic factors have been associated with nasopharyngeal carcinoma?	• Family history (especially first-degree relatives) • Haplotype human leukocyte antigen (HLA) alleles • Genetic polymorphisms in CYP2A6 (nitrosamine metabolizing gene) • Male sex 3:1 ratio
771	Describe the basic structure of the herpes virus that represents a major risk factor for developing nasopharyngeal carcinoma.	Epstein-Barr virus (EBV): • Nuclear core early antigens (Ea) • Double-stranded DNA • Viral capsid antigen (VCA) • Lytic membrane proteins (LMP): LMP-1, -2, -3 • EBV nuclear antigens (EBNA): 1–6 • EBV encoded ribonucleic acids (EBER)
772	What is the primary mode of transmission of EBV infection?	Saliva
773	In which nasopharyngeal cell type is EBV infection a risk factor for the development of malignancy?	Pseudostratified columnar respiratory epithelium. It is carried for life by the infected person.
774	What is the most common nasopharyngeal malignancy?	Nasopharyngeal carcinoma
775	How does the WHO classify nasopharyngeal carcinoma?	• Type 1 (I): Squamous cell carcinoma • Type 2a (II): Keratinizing undifferentiated carcinoma • Type 2b (III): Nonkeratinizing undifferentiated carcinoma
776	In lymphoepitheliomas, does the lymphoid infiltrate give prognostic information?	No
777	In lymphoepitheliomas, what characterizes a Regaud pattern?	Tumor cells growing in well-defined aggregates admixed with a lymphoid infiltrate
778	What is the most common clinical manifestation for nasopharyngeal carcinoma?	Lymphadenopathy (60%)
779	In addition to cervical lymphadenopathy, what initial symptoms are common in nasopharyngeal carcinoma?	• Blood tinged/stained saliva/sputum; more common than epistaxis • Conductive hearing loss, serous otitis media • Epistaxis • Nasal obstruction • Tinnitus • Cranial nerve palsy
780	A patient with nasopharyngeal carcinoma has headache and cranial nerve deficits. What do these symptoms most likely indicate?	Intracranial extension
781	What syndrome is defined by tumor invasion of the base of skull with involvement of CN III–VI resulting in facial pain and diplopia?	Petrosphenoidal syndrome
782	What notochord remnant presents as a benign cystic nasopharyngeal mass?	Thornwaldt cyst
783	A patient has an ulcerative nasopharyngeal mass, bulky unilateral adenopathy, V1/V2 numbness, and ophthalmoplegia. This process has most likely invaded what structure?	Cavernous sinus

784	A middle-aged immigrant from the Guangdong province in Southern China presents with a unilateral middle ear effusion. What is the most important diagnostic maneuver?	Nasopharyngoscopy
785	A patient with locally advanced nasopharyngeal cancer complains of ipsilateral dry eye. Which nerve is most likely affected?	Vidian nerve
786	A patient with locally advanced nasopharyngeal cancer has a unilateral true vocal-fold paralysis, winged scapula, and uvular deviation. What is the name of this syndrome?	Vernet syndrome
787	A patient with locally advanced nasopharyngeal cancer has an ipsilateral constricted pupil and ptosis. What structure has been invaded?	Cervical sympathetic trunk
788	What blood test predicts survival in EBV-related nasopharyngeal carcinoma?	Polymerase chain reaction (PCR) of EBV DNA
789	What serologic test allows for screening and monitoring response to therapy in EBV-related nasopharyngeal carcinoma?	Anti-EBV viral capsid antigen (VCA) and early antigen (EA) immunoglobulin A (IgA)
790	What characterizes WHO type 1 nasopharyngeal carcinoma?	Keratinization
791	Which of the WHO subtypes for nasopharyngeal carcinoma is nonkeratinizing and undifferentiated?	WHO type 3
792	How do WHO type 3 tumors tend to fail treatment?	Distant metastases
793	Where do WHO type 1 tumors tend to fail treatment?	Locoregional recurrence is most common.
794	How often does nasopharyngeal carcinoma involve the skull base at the time of diagnosis?	35%
795	A nasopharyngeal malignancy extends into the nasal cavity but not the parapharynx. What is the AJCC T stage?	T1
796	A nasopharyngeal malignancy extends into the sphenoid sinus. What is the AJCC T stage?	T3
797	A nasopharyngeal malignancy causes a lateral rectus palsy. What is the AJCC T stage?	T4
798	A patient with nasopharyngeal carcinoma has a palpable 2-cm supraclavicular fossa lymph node. What is the AJCC N stage?	N3b
799	A patient with nasopharyngeal carcinoma has 3-cm bilateral retropharyngeal lymph nodes evident on MRI. What is the AJCC N stage?	N1
800	Which is more important prognostically in nasopharyngeal carcinoma: low nodes or bilateral nodes?	Low (supraclavicular fossa) nodes
801	How is the supraclavicular fossa defined for N staging nasopharyngeal carcinoma?	A triangle is bound by three points: the superior margin of the medial end of the clavicle, the superior margin of the lateral end of the clavicle, and the point where the neck meets the shoulder.
802	A patient with nasopharyngeal carcinoma has a 5-cm ipsilateral level II lymph node. What is the AJCC N stage?	N1

803	What is the least common WHO subtype of nasopharyngeal cancer in the Far East?	WHO type 1
804	Compared with its incidence in the Far East, is WHO type 1 nasopharyngeal carcinoma more or less common in North America?	More
805	What features of the primary tumor in nasopharygenal carcinoma predict poor outcomes?	cranial neuropathy, bone erosion, and extensive parapharyngeal space involvement
806	Does upper cranial neuropathy give a worse prognosis than lower cranial neuropathy in nasopharyngeal carcinoma?	No
807	What is the strongest predictor of regional failure in nasopharyngeal carcinoma?	Nodal stage
808	What predicts a worse prognosis in nasopharyngeal cancer: prestyloid or poststyloid parapharyngeal extension?	Prestyloid
809	What is the strongest predictor of overall survival in nasopharyngeal carcinoma?	M stage
810	What is the best treatment for stage III–IV nasopharyngeal carcinoma?	Concurrent chemoradiation therapy
811	What is the best treatment for stage I nasopharyngeal carcinoma?	External-beam radiation to the primary and bilateral necks
812	What doses are used to treat the nasopharynx in nasopharyngeal carcinoma?	~ 70 Gy
813	What is the best surgical treatment for regionally recurrent nasopharyngeal carcinoma?	Modified radical neck dissection
814	Local recurrence of nasopharyngeal carcinoma involving the lateral nasopharyngeal wall, with extension across the midline, is best suited for what salvage surgical approach?	Anterolateral, or maxillary swing, approach
815	What is the most sensitive imaging test for detecting nasopharyngeal carcinoma recurrence?	PET scan
816	What are treatment options for locally recurrent or residual nasopharyngeal carcinoma?	Nasopharyngeal carcinoma is unique in the head and neck in that reirradiation shortly after treatment is often used for residual or recurrent disease. Other options include stereotactic radiation therapy, brachytherapy, photodynamic therapy, endoscopic or open resection, chemotherapy, or combined regimens.
817	What are common acute side effects of external beam radiation for nasopharyngeal carcinoma?	Mucositis, xerostomia, cutaneous erythema, malaise
818	A patient is having seizures 4 years after primary radiation therapy for nasopharyngeal carcinoma. What is the likely cause?	Temporal lobe necrosis
819	Fatigue and amenorrhea 6 years after radiation therapy are likely due to what late complication?	Hypopituitarism
820	A patient develops hearing loss with normal immittance after treatment for nasopharyngeal carcinoma. What is the most common audiologic pattern?	Downsloping sensorineural hearing loss
821	A patient develops hypernasal speech after an anterior approach surgical salvage of locally recurrent nasopharyngeal carcinoma. What is the most likely cause?	Palatal fistula

822	What feature of tumor recurrence contraindicates nasopharyngectomy?	Cranial neuropathy

Paranasal Sinus Anatomy

823	The sphenopalatine artery enters the nasal cavity through the sphenopalatine foramen, which is located where?	Lateral nasal wall just posterior to the end of the middle turbinate
824	Which nerve originates in the pterygopalatine fossa and innervates the hard palate?	Greater palatine
825	The name of what line from the medial canthus to the angle of the mandible carries significant prognostic value in sinonasal malignancies? (▶ Fig. 7.10)	Öhngren line. It is largely of historical significance when plain X-rays were used to evaluate sinonasal malignancy.

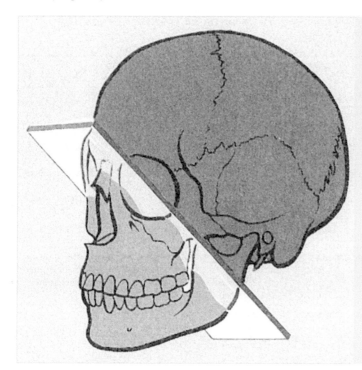

Fig. 7.10 Öhngren's line extends from the medial canthus to the angle of the mandible, dividing the maxillary sinus into a posterosuperior and an anteroinferior portion. Tumor limited to the anteroinferior portion portends better prognosis. (Used with permission from Becker W, Naumann HH, Pfaltz CR. Ear, Nose, and Throat Diseases: A Pocket Reference 2nd Edition. New York, NY: Thieme; 1994.)

826	What are the anatomical boundaries of the pterygopalatine fossa?	The pterygopalatine fossa is a pyramidal space beneath the orbit that is bounded anteriorly by the posterior wall of the maxillary sinus and posteriorly by the pterygoid plates.
827	Which nerves and what important vessel run through the pterygopalatine fossa?	Sphenopalatine, lesser and greater palatine nerves, Vidian; internal maxillary artery
828	What is the most common site of sinonasal malignancy?	Maxillary sinus
829	Tumors in which paranasal sinus are associated with the highest rate of neurological sequelae?	Sphenoid sinus
830	What is the most common lymph node basin involved by metastatic sinonasal malignancy?	Upper jugulodigastric

Evaluation and Management of Paranasal Sinus Malignancy

831	Which environmental risk factor is associated with adenocarcinoma of the ethmoid sinus?	Wood dust (wood workers)

832	Nickel exposure greatly increases which type of sinonasal cancer?	Squamous cell carcinoma
833	Inverted papilloma is associated with malignant transformation to what type of cancer?	Squamous cell carcinoma
834	What is the most common sinonasal malignancy?	Squamous cell carcinoma
835	Which histologic type of sinonasal malignancy is associated with exposure to wood dust?	Intestinal-type adenocarcinoma
836	What is the second most common sinonasal malignancy?	Adenoid cystic carcinoma
837	What histologic type of sinonasal adenoid cystic carcinoma is the most common and has the best prognosis?	Cribriform
838	What rare sinonasal tumor is thought to arise from the mucoserous glands of the sinonasal cavity and stains positive with mucicarmine?	Mucoepidermoid carcinoma
839	What is the most common location of sinonasal mucosal melanoma?	Lateral nasal wall including turbinates
840	Esthesioneuroblastoma arises from what location?	Olfactory mucosa along the cribriform plate
841	Which sinonasal tumor has the following histopathologic features: S100-positive sustentacular cells, Homer-Wright rosettes, and Flexner-Wintersteiner rosettes?	Esthesioneuroblastoma
842	What sinonasal tumors can be considered small, round blue cell tumors?	Sinonasal undifferentiated carcinoma, small cell carcinoma, esthesioneuroblastoma, poorly differentiated and nonkeratinizing squamous cell carcinoma, neuroendocrine carcinoma, plasmacytoma, lymphoma, mucosal melanoma, Ewing sarcoma, rhabdomyosarcoma, synovial sarcoma, desmoplastic small round blue cell tumor
843	What are common histopathologic features of sinonasal small cell carcinoma?	Small cells with scant cytoplasm and round hyperchromatic nuclei with absent or poorly visualized nucleoli. Cells grow in clusters and commonly display extensive necrosis and hemorrhage.
844	What is the most common pediatric malignant sinonasal tumor?	Rhabdomyosarcoma
845	Alveolar type rhabdomyosarcoma is associated with what chromosomal translocation?	t(2;13)(q35;q14), PAX3-FKHR gene fusion
846	Hemangiopericytomas arise from what cell types?	Extracapillary pericytes (of Zimmerman)
847	What are typical clinical features of sinonasal hemangiopericytomas?	Soft, slow-growing tumors typically arising in the nasal cavity that occasionally metastasize. The most common presentation is nasal obstruction and epistaxis.
848	In what anatomical site are sinonasal angiosarcomas most frequently found?	Nasal cavity
849	Which type of tumor is the most common to metastasize to the nose and paranasal sinuses?	Renal cell carcinoma
850	What is the most common sinonasal lymphoma in Western populations?	Diffuse large B-cell lymphoma
851	What is the most common sinonasal lymphoma in Asian populations?	Natural kill (NK)/T-cell lymphoma
852	What is the name of the syndrome in a patient who has epistaxis, diplopia, decreased visual acuity, and numbness above the eye?	Orbital apex syndrome

853	What is the name of the constellation of symptoms that includes ophthalmoplegia, periorbital numbness, ptosis, proptosis, and fixed dilated pupil?	Superior orbital fissure syndrome
854	A patient has unilateral nasal obstruction, eye proptosis, and decreased sensation of his cheek. Which cranial nerve is affected?	V2 (infraorbital nerve)
855	Which imaging modalities are most useful in sinonasal malignancies?	MRI and CT scan
856	How is CT superior to MRI in evaluation of paranasal sinus masses?	Better bone detail. Better evaluation of skull base and lamina papyracea erosion
857	How is MRI superior to CT in the evaluation of paranasal sinus masses?	• Better soft tissue detail • Differentiates tumor from inspissated secretions • Better evaluation of dural invasion • Differentiates brain invasion from brain edema • Better assessment of perineural invasion
858	TNM staging for sinonasal cancer includes what three primary anatomic sites?	Maxillary sinus, ethmoid sinus, and nasal cavity
859	A squamous cell carcinoma localized to which two sinonasal sites is automatically stage T4?	Frontal and sphenoid sinuses
860	What is unique about the AJCC staging of head and neck mucosal melanoma?	All lesions are considered T3 or T4, reflecting the aggressive behavior.
861	What is the Kadish staging system for esthesioneuroblastoma?	(► Table 7.10)

Table 7.10 Kadish staging system for esthesioneuroblastoma.

Type	Extent
A	tumor limited to the nasal cavity
B	tumor in nasal cavity but extending into paranasal sinuses
C	tumor extends beyond paranasal sinuses to involve cribriform, skull base, orbit or intracranial space
D	tumor with neck or distant metastasis

Data from Kadish S, Goodman M, Wang CC. Olfactory neuroblastoma. A clinical analysis of 17 cases. Cancer. 1976;37 (3): 1571–6.

862	The Hyams grading system of esthesioneuroblastoma has proven to provide significant prognostic information and includes what histologic features?	• Lobular architecture • Neurofibrillary background • Rosettes • Nuclear pleomorphism • Mitosis • Necrosis • Calcification
863	Which sinonasal sarcoma has the best prognosis?	Chondrosarcoma
864	Which sinonasal malignancy has the worst prognosis?	Mucosal melanoma
865	Which sinonasal malignancy has the best prognosis?	Minor salivary gland tumors
866	Invasion of which structure by a sinonasal malignancy has the worst prognosis?	Brain; 5-year survival is 26% in the largest series.
867	Which pathologic finding in sinonasal malignancy has the worst prognosis?	Positive margins are associated with a 24% 5-year survival.

868	What is the treatment of choice for advanced esthesioneuroblastoma?	Multimodality treatment including surgical resection and radiation therapy with or without chemotherapy
869	What is the treatment of choice for most sinonasal undifferentiated carcinomas?	Multimodality treatment including surgical resection and radiation therapy with or without chemotherapy
870	What is the treatment of choice for sinonasal diffuse large B-cell lymphoma?	Chemoradiation therapy (R-CHOP and IFRT)
871	What long-term complication can occur after resection of a frontal sinus tumor with osteoplastic flap and frontal sinus obliteration?	Frontal sinus mucocele
872	What is the surgical procedure best used to treat a sinonasal malignancy that has invaded through the cribriform plate?	Anterior craniofacial resection
873	What is the surgical procedure best used to treat a sinonasal tumor limited to the medial wall of the maxillary sinus?	Inferior medial maxillectomy
874	What is a common postoperative complication of medial maxillectomy?	Epiphora and/or recurrent dacryocystitis from division of the nasolacrimal duct
875	What locoregional flaps are commonly used to close large anterior skull-base defects after anterior craniofacial resection?	Vascularized pericranium and nasoseptal mucosa flaps
876	What free tissue flap is best for reconstruction of large anterior skull base defects after craniofacial resection?	Rectus abdominis
877	What free tissue flaps are best used for reconstruction of total maxillectomy defects?	Osteocutaneous free flaps for bone stock to reconstruct the orbital floor, orbital rim, and/or alveolar ridge

Sarcomas of the Head and Neck

878	What are the two most common head and neck locations for osteosarcoma?	Mandible and maxilla
879	Hemangiopericytomas arise most commonly from what head and neck site?	The sinonasal cavity
880	What is the most common head and neck site of origin of leiomyosarcoma?	The oral cavity
881	What is the most common head and neck site for chondrosarcoma?	The sinonasal cavity
882	What hereditary syndrome is caused by a mutation in the *p53* tumor suppressor gene resulting in a greatly increased risk of sarcomas as well as other cancers?	Li-Fraumeni syndrome
883	What condition is associated with half of all neurogenic sarcomas (malignant peripheral nerve sheath tumor)?	Neurofibromatosis type 1
884	What percentage of patients with head and neck fibrosarcomas report a history of prior radiation exposure?	10%
885	What are the four histologic subtypes of rhabdomyosarcoma?	• Embryonal • Alveolar • Anaplastic (previously pleomorphic) • Mixed

886	What histologic subtypes of rhabdomyosarcoma have the worst prognosis?	Alveolar and anaplastic
887	What is the most common head and neck sarcoma in children?	Rhabdomyosarcoma
888	Head and neck rhabdomyosarcoma can be divided into three sites that have staging and prognostic value; what are they?	• Orbit • Head and neck • Nonparameningeal • Parameningeal
889	What is the primary treatment for rhabdomyosarcoma?	Chemotherapy is the mainstay of treatment. It is typically used with radiation as an induction agent and then concurrently. Typically, vincristine is the main agent used with two other agents. These regimens have been established by the Intergroup Rhabdomyosarcoma Studies (IRS) now renamed the Children's Oncology Group (COG)
890	What soft tissue sarcoma has the highest response rate to adjuvant radiation therapy?	Liposarcoma
891	Synovial sarcoma is thought to be most likely derived from what cell type?	Pluripotent mesenchymal cells
892	What are the most common head and neck sites of origin for synovial sarcoma?	Hypopharynx and retropharynx
893	What recent chromosomal translocation has been identified in patients with epithelioid hemangioendothelioma?	t(1;3)(p36;q25)
894	What prognostic factor is included in the AJCC staging system for sarcomas in addition to the traditional TNM staging factors?	Histologic grade (G1–G3)
895	What is the T-staging system of soft tissue sarcomas according to the AJCC?	• Tx: Primary tumor cannot be assessed • T0: No evidence of primary tumor • T1: Tumor < 5 cm in greatest dimension (T1a, superficial; T1b, deep); • T2: tumor > 5 cm in greatest dimension (T2a, superficial; T2b, deep)
896	What prognostic factor at the time of surgical excision of head and neck osteosarcoma plays the most significant role in local control and survival rates?	Surgical margin status
897	What is the primary treatment modality for osteosarcoma of the head or neck?	Surgery
898	What is the treatment modality of choice for dermatofibrosarcoma protuberans?	Surgical resection
899	What is the classic initial symptom of angiosarcoma?	Unexplained bruising of the forehead or scalp, which may progress in a rapid fashion in an elderly patient.
900	What features are associated with most strongly associated with prognosis in angiosarcoma?	Size, grade, and depth. Tumors < 5 cm and superficial tumors have significantly better survival than tumors > 5 cm or deeply invasive tumors. High-grade tumors have also been associated with worse prognosis.
901	What percentage of angiosarcomas will occur in the head and neck region?	50%

902	What is the standard treatment for scalp angiosarcoma?	Wide local excision with postoperative radiation therapy
903	What areas of the head and neck are most likely to be involved with dermatofibrosarcoma protuberans?	Scalp and supraclavicular fossa
904	What is the long-term prognosis for patients with dermatofibrosarcoma protuberans?	If it is adequately managed, dermatofibrosarcoma protuberans commonly recurs locally, but it seldom metastasizes. Long-term survival is therefore excellent.
905	What modifications should be considered to Mohs surgery in the case of dermatofibrosarcoma, and why?	Because of the infiltrating growth pattern exhibited by dermatofibrosarcoma protuberans, some have advocated a "modified Mohs" procedure with paraffin sections as opposed to frozen sections, alternatively taking an extra border of tissue from around the tumor.
906	What options are available for treatment of unresectable or recurrent dermatofibrosarcoma protuberans or in patients who are not surgical candidates?	Imatinib, a tyrosine kinase inhibitor, has been shown to induce partial or complete remission in dermatofibrosarcoma protuberans.
907	What are the relative recurrence rates for dermatofibrosarcoma protuberans treated with Mohs surgery and wide local excision respectively?	1.6% versus 20% (favoring Mohs) in a large meta-analysis
908	Describe the common history and findings in patients with atypical fibroxanthoma.	A rapidly enlarging, red, ulcerated lesion within the field of prior radiation treatment.
909	What is the treatment of choice for atypical fibroxanthoma?	Simple excision with clear margins, often by Mohs surgery. Nodal metastasis is rare.
910	How commonly does malignant fibrous histiocytoma recur?	Recurrence is common in malignant fibrous histiocytoma and even more so in patients previously exposed to radiation. Local metastasis is uncommon, whereas distant metastasis is more frequent.
911	Pleomorphic undifferentiated sarcoma is formally known as what?	Malignant fibrous histiocytoma
912	To what site does pleomorphic undifferentiated sarcoma most often metastasize?	Lungs
913	What are common histologic features of pleomorphic undifferentiated sarcoma (malignant fibrous histiocytoma)?	A storiform pattern of pleomorphic and bizarre cells with foamy cytoplasm, marked atypia, and numerous mitotic figures in a collagenous background
914	What are the risk factors for Kaposi sarcoma?	All Kaposi sarcomas are caused by HHV-8, but the groups most at risk for the disease are patients with AIDS and those who are on immunosuppression medications. Patients with AIDS are 20,000 times more likely to have Kaposi sarcoma than the general population and 300 times more likely than renal transplantation patients.

Lymphomas of the Head and Neck

915	Where are the most common locations for extranodal lymphoma in the head and neck?	Waldeyer ring. Nasopharynx > tonsil > tongue base
916	What structures in the head and neck can be involved with lymphoma?	Essentially any; paranasal sinuses, salivary glands, thyroid, lymph nodes, Waldeyer ring, larynx, and the orbit are all possible sites.

917	In addition to the lymph nodes, what anatomical sites should be considered for involvement in a patient with extranodal tonsillar non-Hodgkin lymphoma?	About 20% of patients with tonsillar non-Hodgkin lymphoma have gastrointestinal tract involvement.
918	What percentage of patients with extranodal lymphoma will have associated nodal disease?	50%
919	Between Hodgkin lymphoma and non-Hodgkin lymphoma, which is more likely to involve extra-nodal disease at diagnosis?	Non-Hodgkin lymphoma (30% extranodal presentation) more than Hodgkin lymphoma (5%)
920	What is the primary risk factor for parotid mucosa-associated lymphoid tissue (MALT) lymphoma?	Sjögren syndrome
921	What is the primary risk factor for thyroid MALT lymphoma?	Hashimoto thyroiditis
922	What is the second most common malignancy in the head and neck?	Lymphoma; it makes up 15 to 20% of all head and neck cancers.
923	What are the indolent non-Hodgkin lymphomas?	Follicular, B-cell chronic lymphocytic lymphoma, marginal B-cell, lymphoplasmacytic (Waldenstrom macroglobuline-mia)
924	What are the aggressive non-Hodgkin lymphomas?	Diffuse large B-cell, peripheral T-cell, mantle cell
925	What are the highly aggressive non-Hodgkin lymphomas?	Burkitt, precursor T- and B-cell lymphoblastic
926	Describe the endemic form of Burkitt lymphoma.	A form of non-Hodgkin lymphoma that arises from EBV genomic integration and t(8;14) translocation that constitutively activates c-myc, causing mandible tumors among children of central Africa.
927	What are common markers for B-cell lymphoma?	CD20, CD22, and CD79a are strongly positive in most B-cell lymphomas.
928	What is the typical histopathology of Hodgkin disease?	Reed-Sternberg cells, which contain two large nuclear lobes with pale chromatin and distinct eosinophilic nucleoli
929	Describe *tumor lysis syndrome*.	The development of hypocalcemia, hyperkalemia, hyper-uricemia, hyperphosphatemia, and acute renal failure in the days after initiation of chemotherapy for aggressive lymphoma. Death from cardiac arrhythmias can result.
930	What are B-symptoms as they pertain to lympho-ma?	Fever > 38°C, > 10% weight loss in 6 months, night sweats
931	Are B-symptoms more common with Hodgkin lymphoma or non-Hodgkin lymphoma?	Hodgkin lymphoma
932	How common are B-symptoms in patients with extranodal non-Hodgkin lymphoma?	Approximately 20% of patients with extranodal non-Hodgkin lymphoma have B symptoms.
933	What are the findings for lymphoma on T1- and T2-weighted MRI with and without gadolinium enhancement?	T1-low signal intensity and T2-low to high signal intensity. Gadolinium uptake is variable but usually demonstrates low enhancement.
934	How is FNA limited in diagnosing lymphoma?	FNA results yield cytology, which does not provide information on nodal architecture (follicular vs. diffuse).
935	Describe the Ann Arbor staging system for lymphoma.	• Stage I: single lymph node region or single extralym-phatic organ • Stage II: Two or more lymph node regions or extra-lymphatic organs on one side of the diaphragm • Stage III: Involvement on both sides of the diaphragm • Stage IV: Diffuse or disseminated involvement of 1 or more extralymphatic organs with or without node involvement

936	What is the mechanism of action of rituximab?	A monoclonal antibody against CD20, which is a B-cell marker.
937	What agents are included in CHOP therapy?	• Cyclophosphamide (Cytoxan) • Hydroxydaunorubicin (doxorubicin) • Oncovin (vincristine) • Prednisone
938	What is the primary treatment modality for localized (stage I or II) low-grade lymphoma?	Radiation therapy, to which chemotherapy is often added in more advanced disease.
939	What is the primary role of surgery for head and neck non-Hodgkin lymphoma?	Surgery is useful for establishing diagnosis. Further treatment is better served with radiation and chemotherapy.

8 Cutaneous Malignancies

William R. Schmitt, Joshua J. Thom, David G. Stoddard Jr., Kathryn M. Van Abel, and Daniel L. Price

Cutaneous Squamous Cell Carcinoma

| 1 | What are the layers of the epidermis from superficial to deep? (▶ Fig. 8.1) | <ul><li>Stratum corneum (cornified layer)</li><li>Stratum granulosum (granular layer)</li><li>Stratum spinosum (spinous layer)</li><li>Stratum germinativum (basal layer)</li></ul>The dermis is immediately deep to this. |

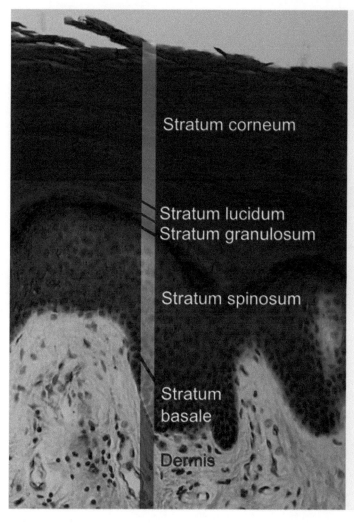

Fig. 8.1 Histological section with H&E stain of the epidermis showing the five strata, from superficial to deep: corneum, lucidum, granulosum, spinosum and basale. (Used with permission from Gantwerker EA, Hom DB. Principles to minimize scars. Facial Plastic Surg. 2012 Oct;28(5):473-486.)

| 2 | Name the four cell types of the epidermis. | <ul><li>Keratinocytes (80%)</li><li>Merkel cells (mechanoreceptors)</li><li>Langerhans cells (antigen processing and presenting cells</li><li>Melanocytes (pigmented dendritic cells)</li></ul> |

| 3 | What is the "H-zone" of the head and neck? (▶ Fig. 8.2) | This area extends vertically from the angle of the mandible through the ear and preauricular region to the temple and is connected horizontally through the periorbital skin, nasal skin, and upper lip. |

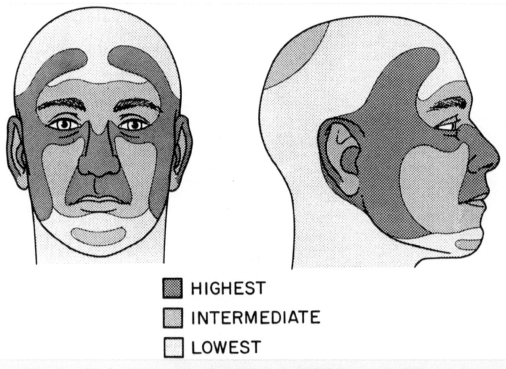

HIGHEST

INTERMEDIATE

LOWEST

Fig. 8.2 "H-zone" of the face where squamous cell carcinoma and basal cell carcinoma potentially demonstrate a more aggressive course. (Used with permission from Donald PJ, ed. The Difficult Case in Head and Neck Cancer Surgery. New York, NY: Thieme; 2010.)

4	Which skin cancer type is most common on the lower lip?	Squamous cell carcinoma
5	What risk factors are associated with lymphatic metastasis of cutaneous squamous cell carcinoma?	• Area > 20 mm (less in the H-zone) • Recurrent tumors • Site of prior radiation or scar • Rapidly growing tumor • Perineural invasion • Poorly differentiated tumors, high-grade tumors • Depth > 5 mm or subcutaneous fat • Lymphovascular invasion • Immunosuppression
6	Metastasis from cutaneous head and neck squamous cell carcinoma most commonly occurs in which lymphatics?	About 75% of cutaneous lymphatic metastases occur in the parotid bed; 40% occur in level II.
7	What are risk factors for cutaneous squamous cell carcinoma of the head and neck?	• Ultraviolet radiation is the number 1 risk factor • Light skin pigmentation • Ionizing radiation • Immunosuppression • Exposure to coal tar, asphalt, and arsenic consumption • Xeroderma pigmentosa, basal cell nevus syndrome

		• Tendency to burn or freckle (rather than tan) • Male sex
8	Describe the Fitzpatrick scale.	Classification schema for the color of skin. Associated with decreasing risk of cutaneous malignancy: • Type I: Pale white, blond, or red hair; blue eyes; always burns, never tans; freckles • Type II: White, fair, blond or red hair; blue, green, or hazel eyes; tans minimally, often burns • Type III: Fair skin; any hair and eye color; tans evenly, sometimes burns. • Type IV: Mediterranean skin, rarely burns, tans easily • Type V: Dark brown skin, rarely burns, tans easily • Type VI: Dark brown to black, never burns, tans very easily
9	What are the risk factors for development of solar keratosis, how many of these eventually undergo malignant transformation, and what percentage of squamous cell carcinomas can be traced to actinic keratosis?	Sun exposure is the most important risk factor, but immune suppression is also important (immune-suppressed individuals are 250 times more likely to develop solar keratoses). Fewer than 1/1,000 solar keratoses will go on to become squamous cell carcinoma; 60% of squamous cell carcinomas can be traced back to solar keratoses.
10	What is Marjolin ulcer?	Marjolin ulcer is a term used to describe an ulcerative squamous cell carcinoma at the site of prior trauma, inflammation, or scarring such as radiation or a burn.
11	What percentage of nonmelanoma cutaneous malignancies are made up of squamous cell carcinoma?	20%
12	Which pathologic finding in squamous cell carcinoma is associated with the highest recurrence rate and regional metastasis?	Perineural invasion. This is associated with metastasis in 47% of patients.
13	How many solar keratoses eventually undergo malignant transformation?	Fewer than 1 in 1,000 solar keratoses will become squamous cell carcinoma.
14	What percentage of squamous cell carcinomas can be traced to actinic keratosis?	60%
15	Describe the clinical and pathological characteristics of Bowen disease.	Bowen disease is an intraepidermal squamous cell carcinoma that manifests as an enlarging, well-demarcated erythematous plaque with surface crusting. Histologically, it resembles squamous cell carcinoma with atypical keratinocytes replacing epidermis. It appears more commonly in women (70 to 85%) and in the sixth or seventh decades of life. It can appear anywhere, but it is more common in the lower legs. The cause has been traced to sun exposure, arsenic, immune suppression, and viral infection. Treatment is most often provided with cryotherapy, curettage, excision, laser, photodynamic therapy and topical 5-fluorouracil (5-FU), with no treatment showing a clear superior effect.
16	What type of skin cancer is known for rapid progression of a swelling, dome-shaped lesion that eventually resolves by sloughing off and scarring?	Keratoacanthoma
17	Your patient, a 67-year-old farmer, has a rapidly expanding, symmetric, dome-shaped lesion on his neck. The lesion is surrounded by smooth, inflamed skin, but it has a central crater containing keratinous debris. What is the most likely diagnosis?	Keratoacanthoma
18	Describe the typical manifestation of a keratoacanthoma.	Keratoacanthomas are rapidly growing lesions that may then slowly spontaneously involute after a plateau phase.

19	Describe the typical manifestation of cutaneous squamous cell carcinoma.	Cutaneous squamous cell carcinoma can present in a number of ways: A thick, scaly patch, an ulcerated patch with rolled borders, a nodular lesion, or scale with pigmentation
20	What symptoms should be elicited in an history of present illness for a patient with newly diagnosed cutaneous squamous cell carcinoma?	Symptoms of advanced disease: numbness, pain, weakness or other perineural symptoms; weight loss, bone pain, shortness of breath to suggest distant disease; rapid growth, bleeding, fixation, neck mass to suggest locally advanced or aggressive disease
21	What features of cutaneous squamous cell carcinoma merit radiologic workup?	• Locally advanced disease: Fixation, numbness, weakness, pain or trismus, extensive lesions (>2 cm), or perineural or lymphovascular invasion • Regionally advanced disease: Palpable lymphadenopathy, intransit metastasis • Distant metastasis risk: Axillary adenopathy, bone pain, shortness of breath, unexplained weight loss, unexplained neurologic symptoms • High-risk patients: Recurrent lesions, immunosuppression, history of radiation
22	What is the most appropriate biopsy technique for deep ulcerated lesions of the skin of the head and neck?	• Punch of incisional biopsy at the thickest portion of the lesion • Full-thickness biopsy should be attempted and should involve the reticular dermis or subcutaneous fat when possible.
23	What features of head and neck nonmelanoma skin cancer are associated with American Joint Committee on Cancer (AJCC) T2 tumors?	Greater than 2 cm greatest dimension or Two or more high-risk features: • >2-mm invasion • Clark level ≥ IV • Perineural invasion • Primary site ear • Primary site non-hairbearing lip • Poorly or undifferentiated tumor *Note*: Excludes cutaneous squamous cell carcinoma of the eyelid
24	What features of head and neck nonmelanoma skin cancer are associated with T3 and T4 tumors (AJCC seventh edition)?	• T3: Invasion of the maxilla, mandible, orbit, or temporal bone • T4: Perineural invasion of the skull base
25	What are the high-risk features of head and neck cutaneous squamous cell carcinoma?	Deep lesions (<2 mm, Clark level IV) • Perineural invasion • H-zone lesions • Recurrent lesions Lesions arising in radiated fields or scar • Size >1.5 cm • Poorly differentiated lesions • Immunosuppression
26	What locations of head and neck cutaneous squamous cell carcinoma are more likely to exhibit recurrence and why?	High-risk sites for recurrence include the so-called H-zone along the preauricular and postauricular areas as well as across the midface, including the nose. This has been attributed to these sites being the location of embryologic fusion, affording tumors planes that provide avenues for spread.
27	True or False: Pathologic involvement of neck nodes with metastatic cutaneous squamous cell carcinoma is associated with worse survival in patients who also have parotid metastasis.	True. Andruchow et al 2006
28	What are appropriate margins for low-risk cutaneous squamous cell carcinoma?	4- to 6-mm clinical margins.

29	Although not yet approved by the Food and Drug Administration (FDA), imiquimod has shown some promise of utility for the treatment of cutaneous squamous cell carcinoma. What is the mechanism of action for imiquimod?	Imiquimod is a local immune response modifier that induces activity of interferon-α and other cytokines.
30	Describe the technique for electrodessication and curettage (EDC) used in cutaneous squamous cell carcinoma and basal cell carcinoma.	In EDC, a curette is used to scrape tumor off down to the dermis, following which an electrodessication is performed to denature any cells along the surface. This is repeated until a satisfactory depth of excision is reached.
31	When is Mohs surgery indicated for cutaneous squamous cell carcinoma of the head and neck?	• Anatomically or aesthetically sensitive areas where wide margins are not achievable (periorbital, nasal, periauricular and auricular, and perioral) • Positive margins after wide local excision and potential extension into an area fulfilling the first criteria
32	When is radiation indicated for cutaneous squamous cell carcinoma?	• Nonoperative candidates (surgical risk or unresectable) • Positive margins or incomplete excision • Solitary node ≥ 3 cm or with extracapsular extension • Multiple positive nodes • Multiple recurrent disease despite appropriate treatment • Perineural invasion of major (named) nerve or extensive perineural invasion • T4 disease
33	What is the appropriate treatment of keratoacanthoma?	• Wide local excision is preferred • Intralesional methotrexate, steroids, and 5-FU can be used for nonoperative cases.

Basal Cell Carcinoma

34	What proportion of basal cell carcinomas occur on the head and neck?	Four in five cutaneous basal cell carcinomas
35	Is upper lip cancer more common in men or women?	It is more common in women: 21% of lip cancers on the upper lip versus only 3% of lip cancer in men.
36	What percentage of cutaneous malignancies occur on the lower lip?	90%
37	What is the significance of basal cell carcinoma found in the folds of the face?	These tumors develop at the site of embryonic fusion plates, resulting in more likely recurrence and higher risk of spread. They therefore require close follow-up.
38	Is basal cell carcinoma more likely on the upper or lower lip?	Upper lip (13% vs. 1% of lower lip cancers)
39	What is the likelihood of regional nodal metastasis in basal cell carcinoma?	Nodal spread is rare, occurring in fewer than 0.0028 to 0.5% of patients.
40	What is the mechanism by which ultraviolet (UV) B-wave light damages skin?	UV light in the B-band (280 to 320 nm), which is the same wavelength responsible for sunburn, causes direct damage to DNA by exciting DNA molecules, resulting in covalent bonds between adjacent cytosine bases. These dimers are read as "AA" by DNA polymerase, and therefore the corresponding "TT" is added to the growing strand.
41	What are the risk factors for basal cell carcinoma?	Sun exposure is the most important risk factor, with other factors including lightly pigmented skin, blue or green eyes, and white ethnicity. Certain genetic conditions also predispose individuals to basal cell carcinoma, including basal cell nevus syndrome (also called Gorlin syndrome) and xeroderma pigmentosum. Exposure risks include tanning beds, arsenic, prior trauma, ionizing radiation, and immune suppressants.

42	What are the so-called high-risk features used in staging of basal cell carcinoma?	• Poor differentiation • Perineural spread • Origination in the ear or the hair-bearing lip • Depth > 2 mm • Clark level IV or V invasion
43	What percentage of nonmelanocytic cutaneous neoplasms are basal cell carcinoma?	80%
44	What are the most commonly described types of basal cell carcinoma?	There are 26 different subtypes of basal cell. The following are the most commonly described: • *Nodular* is the most common form of basal cell carcinoma (60 to 80%), often described as pearly with rolled borders and occasionally central ulceration. • *Morpheaform* (or *sclerosing* or *fibrosing*) has irregular borders on yellow plaques and is the most aggressive type of basal cell carcinoma, with higher recurrence and worse prognosis. • *Fibroepithelial* • *Superficial* is most common type on the trunk, irregularly shaped, waxy, and with an occasionally eczematous or psoriatic appearance. • Other commonly described types are *pigmented* and *micronodular*.
45	What percentage of basal cell carcinomas are nodular?	56 to 78%
46	Which subtype of basal cell carcinoma has the youngest average age at initial diagnosis?	Superficial, which is more common on the trunk
47	What aspect of morpheaform tumors render them able to spread along embryogenic fusion planes and therefore makes them more aggressive with worse prognosis?	Morpheaform tumors secrete collagenases, enabling movement between anatomic subsites.
48	Which subtype of basal cell carcinoma is much more common in patients of African and Chinese descent than those that are found in white patients?	Pigmented basal cell carcinoma
49	Describe the clinical constellation known as *nevoid basal cell carcinoma syndrome* (or *Gorlin syndrome*)	Patients are diagnosed at an early age with multifocal basal cell carcinomas, odontogenic keratocysts, and often also bifid ribs, scoliosis, developmental delay, and frontal bossing.
50	Describe the characteristic features of nodular basal cell carcinoma.	Classically, nodular basal cell carcinoma is described as a pearly lesion with rolled borders, central ulceration, and peripheral telangiectasias.
51	Describe the features associated with arsenic exposure.	• Truncal basal cell carcinoma • Keratoses of the palms and soles • Nail changes (Mees lines)
52	What type of biopsy should be performed for a suspected basal cell carcinoma?	Shave biopsy is appropriate for the vast majority of basal cell carcinomas. When lesions are pigmented, a punch biopsy should be performed to assess the depth of the lesion.
53	When is imaging required in basal cell carcinoma?	Rarely: Large tumors, suspicion of invasion of deeper structures (e.g., fixation, bone invasion), symptoms of perineural invasion, palpable lymphadenopathy
54	What parts of the head and neck are at highest risk of recurrence when affected by cutaneous malignancies?	The preauricular and postauricular regions, floor of nose/columella, medial and lateral canthi, nasolabial fold, aka the so-called H-zone

55	Under what circumstances should cryosurgery be considered for management of basal cell carcinoma?	Cryosurgery can be used in small (<1 cm) nonaggressive tumors.
56	In the management of basal cell carcinoma, what tumor attributes favor excisional curettage and electrodessication?	Small (<2 cm), nonaggressive tumors can be removed with excisional curettage with 90% success. Excisional curettage is not optimal for management of functionally and cosmetically important tumors.
57	What rate of cure can be expected with Mohs surgery in basal cell carcinoma?	96 to 99% cure rate in recurrent and primary resections, respectively
58	What are the advantages of Mohs surgery over simple excision with electrodessication?	Maximal preservation of normal tissue, optimization of functional/cosmetic outcomes, assessment, and clearing of entire margin, lower recurrence rates, immediate reconstruction (usually), only one practitioner involved at all phases of management
59	What are the nonsurgical options for management of basal cell carcinoma?	• Radiation therapy (most commonly used nonsurgical therapy, although waning in popularity) • Photodynamic therapy • Immunotherapy • Chemotherapy • Vismodegib, an agent that targets the hedgehog signaling pathway and was approved in 2012 for treatment of basal cell carcinoma
60	In patients with cutaneous basal cell carcinoma, when should neck dissection be considered?	Neck dissection should be used only in instances when there is clinical evidence of nodal metastasis because basal cell carcinoma metastasizes to the lymph nodes in only 0.5% of cases.
61	Why is it best to defer reconstruction in the morpheaform type of basal cell carcinoma?	Morpheaform basal cell carcinoma classically exhibits subdermal spread that results in more common recurrence than other variants of basal cell carcinoma. Reconstruction either with grafting or tissue rearrangement may cover this subdermal extension and delay diagnosis of recurrence, sometimes with devastating consequences for the patient.

Melanoma

62	What percentage of mucosal melanomas present in the head and neck?	55%
63	What is the most common head and neck site where mucosal melanoma is found?	Nasal cavity
64	Where do most melanomas arise?	• Most melanomas arise on the trunk and extremities. • Nodular melanoma and lentigo maligna melanoma more commonly occur in the head and neck than other subtypes.
65	What is the incidence of lymphatic metastasis in malignant melanoma?	Incidence varies by subtype, depth, and location. • <0.75 mm: <5% • 0.75 to 4.0 mm: 15 to 20% • 4.0 mm: 34% Incidence increases with ulceration, nodular type, Clark level IV or V, and elevated mitotic rate.
66	What is the metastatic rate of desmoplastic melanoma?	Pure desmoplastic melanoma displays regional lymph node involvement in 0 to 2.2% of cases, whereas mixed desmoplastic melanoma has regional lymph node involvement in 8.5 to 22%. Distant metastasis is similar in the two subtypes, at approximately 11 to 12%.

67	How has the incidence of melanoma changed in the United States in the last 30 years?	• It has seen a threefold increase in the white population. • The rate has been stable in the black population.
68	What are the risk factors for cutaneous melanoma?	Family history, lightly pigmented skin, tendency to burn, red hair, DNA repair defects (e.g., xeroderma pigmentosum), chronic and intense sun exposure, equatorial residence, tanning bed use, immunosuppression, > 100 melanocytic nevi, more than five atypical melanocytic nevi, multiple solar lentigines, personal history of cutaneous melanoma
69	What familial autosomal dominant disorder greatly increases the risk of melanoma?	Atypical mole syndrome
70	What are the common subtypes of cutaneous melanoma?	• Superficial spreading (57%) • Nodular melanoma (21%) • Lentigo maligna (9%) • Acral lentiginous (4%) • Unclassifiable (4%) • Other (5%)
71	What sizes of congenital nevus have an increased risk of developing into melanoma?	Giant congenital nevus (2 cm or larger)
72	What is the most common histologic subtype of melanoma?	Superficial spreading
73	What is the second most common histologic subtype of melanoma and the most aggressive subtype?	Nodular melanoma
74	What differentiates *lentigo maligna* from *lentigo maligna melanoma*?	Lentigo maligna melanoma has invasion into the dermis.
75	What subtype of melanoma is found on the soles of feet or palms of hands?	Acral lentiginous
76	Which melanoma subtype is considered the least aggressive?	Lentigo maligna melanoma. It displays a long radial growth phase relative to other subtypes.
77	What are the most common genetic aberrations found in melanoma?	• Chronic sun-damaged skin: KIT > KIT + NRAS = BRAF = NRAS • Nonchronic sun-damaged skin: BRAF > > NRAS • Mucosal: KIT > > NRAS
78	What are the ABCDEs of melanoma?	• A = asymmetry • B = border irregularity • C = color variability • D = diameter greater than 6 mm • E = evolving over time
79	What is the clinical evaluation that all patients with newly diagnosed melanoma should receive?	Full-body skin examination, including hair-bearing areas and intertriginous areas, and examination of the relevant lymph node basins
80	When should imaging be performed in malignant melanoma?	• Extensive primary (fixation, perineural symptoms) • Abnormal or equivocal adenopathy • Stage III or greater disease • Specific signs or symptoms to suggest metastatic disease
81	What is the most ideal method to obtain a biopsy of a lesion suspicious for melanoma?	Narrow-margin excisional biopsy with adequate depth to determine accurate Breslow depth
82	What histopathologic markers are commonly used to identify melanoma?	• Homatropine methylbromide (HMB-45) • S-100 protein • Melan-A (MART-1)

83	What is the preferred evaluation of suspicious lymphadenopathy in patients with cutaneous melanoma?	FNA with or without ultrasound. Equivocal adenopathy can be evaluated with ultrasound. Suspicious adenopathy should be biopsied. A normal ultrasound does not replace sentinel lymph node biopsy.
84	What are potential sites for occult primaries in patients with metastatic melanoma of the head and neck?	Ocular, mucosal, external auditory canal, hair-bearing areas, or tumor regression
85	Describe the Clark levels for melanoma staging. (▶ Fig. 8.3)	• Level I: Epidermis only • Level II: Through basal cell layer into papillary dermis • Level III: Fills papillary dermis, to junction with reticular dermis • Level IV: Involves reticular dermis • Level V: Subcutaneous tissue

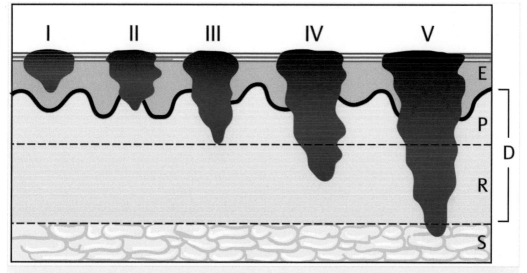

Fig. 8.3 Clark levels of invasion by cutaneous melanoma. Level I, limited to the epidermis; level II, into the underlying papillary dermis; level III, to the junction of the papillary and reticular dermis; level IV, into the reticular dermis; level V, into the subcutaneous fat. E, epidermis; D, dermis; P, papillary dermis; R, reticular dermis; S, subcutaneous tissue. (Used with permission from Behrbohm H, Kaschke O, Nawka T, Swift A. Ear, Nose, and Throat Diseases: With Head and Neck Surgery. New York, NY: Thieme; 2009.)

86	What is the stage of a 2-mm-thick melanoma without ulceration?	T2a, stage IB
87	What are the M stages of melanoma metastasis? (▶ Table 8.1)	• M1a: Metastatic melanoma to dermis • M1b: Metastatic melanoma to the lung • M1c: Metastatic melanoma to other visceral organs or abnormally elevated LDH

Table 8.1 Melanoma of the skin TNM staging. T (a) and (b) subcategories are assigned based on absence (a) or presence (b) of ulceration and number of mitoses.

Stage	Description
Primary Tumor (T)	
TX	primary cannot be assessed
T0	no evidence of primary tumor
Tis	melanoma in situ
T1 (a/b)	≤1.0 mm
T2 (a/b)	1.01–2.0 mm
T3 (a/b)	2.01–4.0 mm
T4 (a/b)	>4.0 mm
Regional Lymph Nodes (N)	
NX	regional nodes cannot be assessed
N0	no regional metastases detected
N1 (a,b)	1 node
N2 (a,b)	2–3 nodes
N3	4 or more metastatic nodes, matted nodes, or in transit met(s) or satellite(s) with metastatic node(s)
Distal Metastasis (M)	
M0	no detectable distant metastases
M1a	metastases to skin, subcutaneous, or distant nodal mets (LDH normal)
M1b	metastases to lung (LDH normal)
M1c	all other visceral metastases (LDH normal) any distant metastasis with elevated LDH

Data from Edge SB, Byrd DR, Compton CC, Fritz AG, Greene FL, Trotti A, eds. AJCC Cancer Staging Manual 7th Edition. New York, NY: Springer; 2010.

88	What is the most common site of melanoma metastasis?	Regional lymph nodes
89	How does mitosis impact T stage in cutaneous melanoma?	T1 lesions with one or more mitoses/mm^2 are T1b.
90	How does ulceration impact T stage in cutaneous melanoma?	Lesions ulceration are upstaged to b (i.e., T1a vs. T1b)
91	What differentiates Stage III A, B, and C disease in cutaneous melanoma?	• IIIA: Any T-a and N-a (i.e., T4aN2a) • IIIB: One of T or N is a, one is b (i.e., T4aN2b or T4bN2b) or any T1–4aN2c • IIIC: Any T1–4b and N1–2b or N2c or any TN3 (i.e., T1bN2b or T1aN3) • All must be M0 (M1 = stage 4)
92	What is the lifetime risk of developing a second primary melanoma?	4 to 8%
93	In localized melanoma, what is the most important prognostic factor?	Tumor thickness (Breslow depth of invasion)
94	What is the most significant prognostic factor in patients with stage III melanoma?	Presence of in-transit metastasis or in-satellite metastasis

95	What are the respective 5-year survival rates for melanoma patients with positive and negative sentinel lymph nodes?	56% vs. 90%
96	What is the 5-year survival for a patient with metastatic melanoma?	10 to 20%
97	What serum factor is an independent predictor of survival in stage IV metastatic melanoma?	LDH
98	What is the treatment of choice for superficial-thickness melanomas (<1.01 mm)?	Wide local excision with 1 cm margins
99	When should sentinel lymph node biopsy be considered in melanoma measuring 0.75 to 1.00 mm?	Tumors with ulceration or one or more mitosis/mm²
100	What is the treatment of choice for intermediate thickness melanomas (1.01 to 4.00 mm)?	Wide local excision with 2-cm margins and sentinel lymph node biopsy
101	What is the treatment of choice for deep thickness melanomas (>4.00 mm)?	Wide local excision with 2-cm margins and sentinel lymph node biopsy
102	Which chemotherapeutic agent is approved for treatment of stage IV melanoma?	Dacarbazine
103	What is the treatment of choice for melanoma involving the auricle?	Wide local excision
104	What adjuvant therapy is approved for use after surgery for stage III melanoma?	Interferon-α2b
105	What is the recommended treatment for Spitz nevus?	In many instances, Spitz nevus is difficult to distinguish from melanoma even for experienced pathologists. Therefore, complete excision is essential.
106	What are the contraindications to methylene-blue dye injection?	• Previous hypersensitivity • Pregnancy • Concurrent use of selective serotonin reuptake inhibitor or other serotonergic drugs (serotonin syndrome) • Glucose-6-phosphate dehydrogenase deficiency
107	What are the most common complications associated with Mohs surgery?	Complication rates in Mohs surgery are quite low, with hematoma and graft necrosis being among the most common.

Other Cutaneous Lesions

108	Merkel cell carcinoma is what type of tumor?	Neuroendocrine. It arises from Merkel cells, which are specialized touch receptors, found in the basal layer of the epidermis. They are very aggressive. Pathologic nodal staging (neck dissection) has been associated with better survival, as 23% of patients with no clinical evidence of nodal disease were found to have positive nodes on neck dissection.
109	What is the relationship between Merkel cell polyoma virus (MCV) and Merkel cell carcinoma (MCC)?	About 80% of Merkel cell carcinoma tumors have cells that exhibit MCV infection. MCV infection is widespread among humans, but it is thought to be an important factor in most MCCs.
110	What immunohistochemical stains are used for MCC?	Cytokeratin 20 (CK20), chromogranin, Cam5.2

111	A patient has a rapidly enlarging 6-cm cystic mass of the scalp. Excisional biopsy shows deep dermal and subcutaneous involvement, which histologically shows evidence of a squamous-lined cyst with extensive trichilemmal keratinization. What is the most likely diagnosis?	Proliferating trichilemmal cyst
112	What is the recurrence rate of microcystic adnexal tumors treated with wide local excision compared with those treated with Mohs surgery?	Wide local excision 60%, Mohs surgery 0 to 12%
113	A patient presents with an 8-mm lesion on the upper lateral eyelid. Biopsy shows neoplastic cells with sebaceous differentiation and cytoplasmic vacuolization. What is the preferred treatment?	Sebaceous carcinoma is an aggressive tumor with a proclivity for metastasis. Mohs surgical resection is associated with lower local and distant recurrence rates.
114	What are *syringomata*?	Syringomata are benign sweat gland tumors that commonly occur in multiples. They are more common in women and occur predominantly on the face at the eyelids, upper cheeks, and neck.
115	What is a *pilomatrixoma*?	Benign appendageal tumors that commonly affect the head and neck and contain a differentiation toward hair cells; rarely associated with carcinoma
116	What is the typical clinical presentation of a pilomatrixoma?	Single, firm, skin-colored or slightly bluish nodule occurring on the face, neck, and shoulders
117	What are *epidermoid cysts*?	Benign cutaneous cysts with epithelial lining that produce keratinized cellular debris. They usually occur after puberty and may rupture, drain, or become infected.
118	Which defects require immediate management?	• *Periocular defects* require early treatment to prevent ocular damage either with reconstruction or temporary eye closure. • *Perioral defects* with oral contamination should be reconstructed early to minimize oral contamination. • *Alar defects* should be reconstructed early to prevent tissue contraction.

Reconstruction After Excision of Cutaneous Malignancy

119	What is the appropriate management of a 1-cm skin only central cheek defect?	Primary closure
120	What is the appropriate management of a 2- to 4-cm skin only central cheek defect?	Local flap
121	What is the appropriate management of a >4 cm skin-only central cheek defect?	Facial or cervicofacial rotation flap
122	What is the appropriate closure of a skin only defect of less than half the lip (orbicularis intact)?	Primary closure
123	What is the appropriate closure of a full thickness defect of half to two-thirds of the lip (commissure intact)?	Abbe-Estlander flap
124	What is the appropriate closure of a full-thickness defect of one-half to two-thirds of the lip involving the commissure?	Karapandzic flap
125	What is the appropriate closure of a full thickness defect involving greater than two-thirds of the lip?	Radial forearm free flap with palmaris tendon or anterior lateral thigh and fascia lata flap
126	What is the vascular supply for the paramedian forehead flap used in nasal reconstruction?	Supratrochlear artery and vein

127	What components of the nose must be considered during reconstruction?	Skin, cartilage, bone, and mucosal lining. Failure to reconstruct each of these elements will lead to poor cosmetic and functional results.
128	What is the aesthetic subunit principle of nasal reconstruction?	The nose is made up of nine subunits: the dorsum, tip and columella, paired lateral sidewalls, ala, and soft tissue triangles. The best cosmetic result can be achieved when these are reconstructed separately, and when greater than half of a subunit is resected, resection of the remainder of the subunit is desirable for cosmesis.
129	What local flap is most commonly used for nasal sidewall defects when primary closure is not achievable?	Bilobed flap
130	What is the general reconstructive ladder for full thickness lower eyelid defects?	• <30%: Primary closure, with or without lateral cantholysis, for larger defects • 30 to 50%: Semicircular flap with or without periosteum • >50%: Tarsoconjunctival flap with flap or graft closure of the skin
131	What is a *Tenzel flap*?	Periorbital semicircular advancement flap for eyelid reconstruction
132	What is a *Hughes flap*?	A pedicled tarsoconjunctival flap used in reconstruction of large (>50 to 60%) full-thickness eyelid defects
133	What are limiting factors in using split-thickness skin grafts in scalp reconstruction?	• They require a vascular bed; if periosteum is absent, must drill to bleeding bone or rotate vascular tissue (periosteum, temporalis) into defect • Poor color, texture, thickness, and hair match • If postoperative radiation is required, a split-thickness skin graft on bone will very likely undergo necrosis.
134	What is the flap of choice for large (>100 cm^2) scalp defects	Latissimus dorsi myocutaneous free flap with split-thickness skin graft

9 Facial Plastic and Reconstructive Surgery

David J. Archibald, Cody A. Koch, Matthew L. Carlson, and Kathryn L. Hall

Wound Healing and Scar Revision

1	What are the layers of the skin from superficial to deep?	• Epidermis • Basement membrane • Dermis (papillary and reticular) • Subcutis
2	What are the layers of the epidermis from superficial to deep?	• Stratum corneum • Stratum lucidum • Stratum granulosum • Stratum spinosum • Stratum basale
3	What are *epidermal appendages*?	Skin-associated structures including hair follicles, apocrine glands, sebaceous glands, and eccrine (sweat) glands
4	What is the predominant type of collagen in the basement membrane?	Type IV collagen
5	What are the three phases of wound healing? (▶ Fig. 9.1)	Inflammation, proliferation, and remodeling. Some authors also include hemostasis as the first phase.

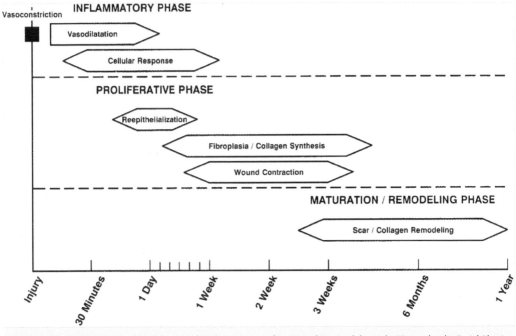

Fig. 9.1 The phases of wound healing. (Used with permission from Papel ID, Frodel J, Holt GR, et al, eds. Facial Plastic and Reconstructive Surgery 3rd Edition. New York, NY: Thieme; 2009.)

6	What are four general categories of wound healing?	• Healing by primary intention: Two wound edges are brought together as the primary intention of the surgeon. • Delayed primary healing: Two wound edges are not brought together immediately but are reapproximated and closed at a later time.

		• Healing by secondary intention: A full-thickness wound where the edges are not reapproximated and the wound is allowed to heal by granulation and contracture • Epithelialization Occurs in partial-thickness wounds as epithelial cells migrate and replicate over the wound.
7	What cell types are primarily involved in the inflammatory phase?	After vasoconstriction and subsequent vasodilation, polymorphonuclear neutrophils arrive and predominate for the first 24 to 48 hours after injury. Following this, monocyte migration occurs.
8	What cell type synthesizes collagen?	Fibroblasts
9	What cell type is responsible for wound contraction during healing?	Myofibroblasts containing microfilaments capable of producing contractile forces. These cells predominate the fibroblast population during the second week of wound healing.
10	What major events occur during the proliferative phase of wound healing?	Re-epithelialization, neovascularization, collagen deposition, and wound contraction
11	During which phase of healing are keratinocytes, fibroblasts, and endothelial cells recruited to the wound?	Proliferative phase
12	During the proliferative phase, which cytokine modulates angiogenesis and neovascularization?	Vascular endothelial growth factor (VEGF)
13	How does hyperbaric oxygen therapy encourage wound healing?	It promotes angiogenesis, fibroblast proliferation, leukocyte activity, and is synergistic with antibiotic therapy.
14	What is the predominant type of collagen in an early scar?	Type III collagen
15	What is the approximate tensile strength of a healing wound at 3 months?	50% of normal tissue
16	When is the remodeling phase of wound healing usually complete?	12 months
17	What are the *tenets of Halsted*?	• Gentle handling of tissues • Aseptic technique • Sharp anatomical dissection of tissues • Careful hemostasis, using fine, nonirritating suture materials in minimal amounts • The obliteration of dead space in the wound • Avoidance of tension
18	How can local tissue factors impact wound healing?	Wound healing is compromised by any tissue effect that decreases oxygenation, increases infection risk, prolongs inflammation, delays neovascularization, or otherwise alters the normal process of healing. Examples include local infection, ischemia resulting from pressure necrosis (e.g., diabetic neuropathy, hematoma), alteration in tissue structure resulting from radiation therapy, locally destructive processes (neoplasia, wound desiccation).
19	What patients should be counseled about increased risk for postoperative infection or wound breakdown?	Patients with medical comorbidities, medications, or history of recent treatments, which alter the normal healing process or suppress the immune system. For example, patients who have undergone chemotherapy and radiation therapy, are taking immunosuppressants, or have diseases that affect the vasculature (e.g., peripheral vascular disease, diabetes, tobacco dependence.) are at increased risk for wound complications.

20	What are *relaxed skin tension lines*?	They are the lines of minimal tension on the skin. They run parallel to natural wrinkle lines and are usually perpendicular to the force of action of the underlying muscles of facial expression.
21	What are some of the technique- and patient-related factors that may lead to an aesthetically unacceptable scar?	• *Patient variables*: Diabetes, chronic steroid use, systemic vasculitis, vitamin deficiency, poor overall nutrition, chronic renal disease, wound infection, collagen vascular disease, sun exposure • *Technical variables*: Failure to clean the wound adequately, excessive tension on epidermal sutures, step-off between wound edges, rough handling of tissue, prolonged suture retention, failure to orient incision parallel to relaxed skin tension lines, delayed wound closure
22	What are some of the performance differences between monofilament and braided suture?	Monofilament suture has "memory" and usually requires more knots to secure a tie. Braided suture has more tensile strength but creates more resistance through tissue, induces a stronger inflammatory response, and is more likely to serve as a reservoir for microorganisms.
23	What type of surface contour is most favorable for wound healing by secondary intention? (▶ Fig. 9.2)	Concave surfaces

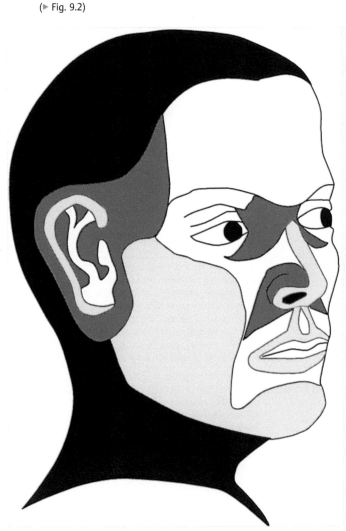

Fig. 9.2 Cosmetic results after wound healing by secondary intentention. Dark gray (concave surfaces of the nose, eye, ear, and temple) are usually associated with excellent results. White (forehead, antihelix, eyelids, rest of nose, lips, and cheeks) grant satisfactory results. Light gray (convex surfaces of the nose, lips, cheeks, chin and helix) provide variable results. (Used with permission from Papel ID, Frodel J, Holt GR, et al, eds. Facial Plastic and Reconstructive Surgery 3rd Edition. New York, NY: Thieme; 2009.)

24	What are some surgical options for scar revision?	Excision and closure with straight line, broken geometric line, W-plasty, Z-plasty, or local flap; excision and placement of a skin graft
25	What medications may be injected into a scar to improve its appearance?	Steroids (triamcinolone diacetate), antimitotic agents (5-FU and bleomycin)
26	What is the role of silicone in scar revision?	The mechanism by which silicone sheeting reduces the appearance of hypertrophic scars has not been clearly elucidated. One hypothesis is that direct pressure exerted by silicone sheeting on the wound decreases scar hypertrophy. Another theory is that silicone's ability to maintain a hydrated environment inhibits fibroblast production of collagen and glycosaminoglycans.
27	What is the primary difference between *keloid formation* and *hypertrophic scarring*?	*Keloids* spread beyond the boundaries of the original scar, whereas *hypertrophic scars* do not extend outside the wound perimeter.
28	Review some treatment options for keloids and hypertrophic scars.	Occlusive dressings, intralesional steroid injections, cryotherapy, radiation therapy, 5-FU, BOTOX injection, tacrolimus, retinoic acid, laser therapy, re-excision combined with above treatments

Resurfacing

29	What is dermabrasion, and what is its role in scar revision?	*Dermabrasion* is a mechanical method of removing the epidermis and creating a papillary to upper reticular dermal wound. Injuries to the epidermis and papillary dermis heal without scarring. Dermabrasion changes the depth of the scar to help it blend with surrounding normal tissue. It also seeks to create a wound with texture and color closely matching normal skin.
30	What layer of the dermis contains the predominant blood supply of the skin?	Reticular dermis
31	Dermabrasion injury to the papillary dermis results in production of what tissue elements?	Type I procollagen Type III procollagen Transforming growth factor-β1
32	Routine prophylaxis for what infection is typically offered to patients before they undergo dermabrasion?	Herpes simplex virus, typically beginning 24 hours preoperatively and continuing for 5 days
33	Which Fitzpatrick skin types have the greatest risk of pigmentary dyschromia (hyper-pigmentation or hypopigmentation) after resurfacing?	Fitzpatrick type III through VI
34	What is the mechanism of action of hydroquinone?	Hydroquinone blocks tyrosinase from developing melanin precursors, thereby impeding new pigment formation as the new epidermis heals after a chemical peel.
35	What are the major indications for a medium depth chemical peel?	• Destruction of epidermal lesions • Resurfacing of moderate photoaging skin • Correction of pigmentary dyschromias • Repair of mild acne scars • Blending of photoaging skin with laser resurfacing
36	Baker-Gordon phenol is used to achieve what level of chemical peeling?	Deep chemical peel
37	What toxicities are associated with phenol chemical peels?	• Cardiotoxicity • Hepatotoxicity • Nephrotoxicity

38	What methods may be used to limit the potential toxic effects of a phenol chemical peel?	• Administering intravenous hydration before and during the procedure • Increasing the duration of application • Electrocardiographic monitoring • Oxygen administration • Screening for patients with arrhythmias or hepatic/renal compromise or patients taking medications that may increase the risk of cardiac arrhythmias
39	What does the acronym *LASER* stand for?	Light amplification by stimulated emission of radiation
40	What is the role of lasers in scar revision?	Lasers create thermal injury leading to collagen retraction. They can also be used for skin resurfacing to correct pigmentary defects.
41	What is the role of pulsed dye laser in scar revision?	A 585-nm wavelength pulse dyed laser can decrease the vascularity of scar tissue and reduce scar redness. The laser may also decrease the number and activity of fibroblasts.
42	What is the wavelength of the CO_2 laser? (▶ Fig. 9.3)	10,600 nm, infrared spectrum

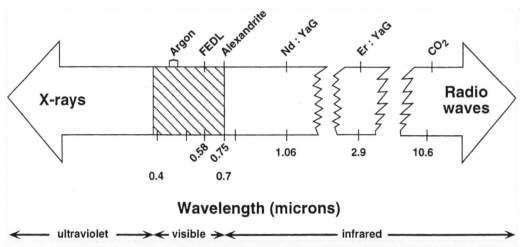

Fig. 9.3 The electromagnetic spectrum of surgical lasers. (Used with permission from Papel ID, Frodel J, Holt GR, et al, eds. Facial Plastic and Reconstructive Surgery 3rd Edition. New York, NY: Thieme; 2009.)

43	What characteristic of CO_2 lasers allows them to vaporize superficially and provide, for the most part, a what-you-see-is-what-you-get type of tissue interaction, similar to electrocautery?	They have increased absorption by tissues with high water content.
44	What is the primary chromophore for both the CO_2 and Er:YAG laser?	Water. Er:YAG has strong tissue water absorption, approximately 12 times that of the CO_2 laser.
45	What is the wavelength of the Er:YAG laser?	2940 nm, infrared spectrum
46	What is the definition of *laser fluency*?	The amount of energy (joules) that is applied to the surface area of tissue (centimeters squared), expressed as J/cm^2

47	The effect of a laser on specific tissue depends on what four factors?	• Laser wavelength • Laser energy density • Pulse duration • Tissue absorption
48	How is laser power density altered?	By changing the focal length of the lens or changing the working distance
49	How does the pulsed delivery of a laser allow a higher energy delivery with less thermal injury?	By using the heat sink effect of the adjacent tissue and blood flow during the interpulse intervals
50	What is the term used to describe the characteristic of a laser's ability to have photons move in the same temporal and spatial phase?	Coherence
51	What terms describe the laser-tissue surface interaction?	Absorption, transmission, reflection, scatter

Implants and Fillers

52	Which botulinum neuromodulator serotype demonstrates the longest duration of effect?	Serotype A (90 to 120 days)
53	What is the mechanism of action of BOTOX?	BOTOX prevents presynaptic neurosecretory vesicles from docking/fusing with the nerve synapse plasma membrane (degrades the SNAP-25 protein) and releasing acetylcholine into the neuromuscular junction.
54	Vertical glabellar furrows are most likely caused by which muscle?	Corrugator supercilii
55	What muscle arises in the medial end of the orbit/nasal prominence and interdigitates with the orbicularis oculi muscle laterally and the frontalis muscle superiorly?	Corrugator supercilii
56	What medication can be given to patients who develop botulinum toxin-related blepharoptosis, and what is its mechanism of action?	• Apraclonidine eye drops. An α2-adrenergic agonist, which causes Müller muscle to contract. • Phenylephrine can be used when apraclonidine is not available.
57	A patient does not appear to have further benefit after repeated botulinum toxin injections. What is the most likely cause?	Formation of neutralizing antibodies rendering resistance to the paralytic effect of the toxin. Often responds to switching to an alternate type.
58	What muscle may be treated with botulinum toxin to decrease the "peau d'orange" or dimpled chin appearance with facial animation?	The mentalis muscle
59	What is the role of fillers in scar revision?	To provide bulk to bring a depressed scar level with surrounding normal skin
60	List examples of tissue-derived injectable fillers?	• Bovine collagen (Zyderm, Zyplast) • Human particulate "dermal matrix" (Cymetra) • Cultured autologous fibroblasts (Isologen)
61	List examples of implantable soft tissue fillers.	• Human acellular dermis (AlloDerm) • Porcine acellular dermis (Surgisis)
62	List examples of synthesized selective bioactive (resorbable) injectable fillers.	• Calcium hydroxyapatite particles (Radiesse) • Polylactic acid particles (Sculptra)
63	What is an example of an implantable synthetic polymer?	Expanded polytetrafluoroethylene (Gore-Tex)
64	Which implant particle size is not readily phagocytized by macrophages?	20 to 60 µm. Particles smaller than this have been shown to precipitate a chronic inflammatory response, whereas larger particles cannot be easily phagocytized and therefore elicit minimal inflammatory reaction.

65	What are the challenges associated with the use of polymethylmethacrylate?	The final phase of polymerization is associated with an exothermic reaction that can cause tissue injury. It can become loose with time despite immobilization. The need for implant removal is higher if in contact with nasal or frontal sinus tissue.
66	What is the primary advantage of dermal fat grafts over free adipose grafts?	There is less resorption than with free adipose grafts, although even up to 70% of dermal fat grafts are resorbed.
67	Describe some uses of facial fat grafting in facial aesthetic surgery.	Lip augmentation, effacement of glabellar rhytids, tear trough deformity, and deep nasolabial folds; replacing volume in areas of facial fat atrophy and to fill in depressed scars
68	When using tissue expanders, as a general rule of thumb, how much larger should the surface area of the base of the expander be than the defect size?	2.5 times
69	In the context of tissue expanders, what is *mechanical creep*?	Rapid collagen and elastin realignment and dispersion of interstitial fluid and ground substance during applied soft tissue stretch
70	Review some complications from use of tissue expanders.	Hematoma, infection, extrusion, migration, necrosis of overlying tissue, loss of hair, pain, erosion of underlying bone
71	Why are gold and platinum the current metals of choice for eyelid-loading surgery?	Chemically inert and relatively dense

Brow and Forehead Lift

72	What muscles of facial expression are responsible for the horizontal rhytides of the glabella?	Procerus
73	What two dissection planes are commonly used during brow lift surgery?	• Subgaleal • Subperiosteal
74	What nonsurgical technique can be used for browplasty?	Selectively paralyzing the temporal brow depressors (lateral orbicularis muscle) with BOTOX type A which then allows unopposed elevation of the frontalis muscle
75	List the various surgical techniques used for brow rejuvenation	Temporal lift; direct brow, midforehead, temporal extension of rhytidectomy incision; coronal, pretrichial/trichophytic, endoscopic
76	What anatomical structure lies between the intermediate temporal fascia and the deep temporal fascia?	Intermediate fat pad
77	What surgical brow rejuvenation techniques involve subcutaneous tissue dissection?	Midforehead and direct brow
78	What is the *sentinel vein*?	A zygomaticotemporal vessel encountered between the deep temporal fascia and the temporoparietal fascia during dissection in the temporal region during brow lift surgery. It has been shown to point to the frontal branch of the facial nerve as it courses through the temporoparietal fascia.
79	What is the *Pitanguy line*?	A line that runs from the lobule to the lateral canthus. This line crosses the zygoma roughly at the midpoint from the helical root to the lateral canthus and approximates the location of the frontal branch of the facial nerve.
80	What is the aesthetic ideal for brow position in a man?	Horizontal, resting on the superior orbital rim

| 81 | What is the aesthetic ideal for brow position in a woman? (▶ Fig. 9.4) | The brow should arc above the orbital rim with its highest point centered over the lateral limbus. |

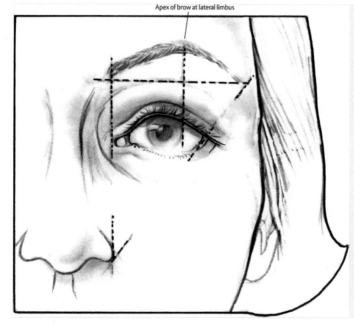

Apex of brow at lateral limbus

Fig. 9.4 The ideal female brow position rests just above the superior orbital rim with the apex tangent to the lateral limbus. (Used with permission from Papel ID, Frodel J, Holt GR, et al, eds. Facial Plastic and Reconstructive Surgery 3rd Edition. New York, NY: Thieme; 2009.)

82	What incision placement strategy should be used during midforehead brow-lift surgery?	Centering incisions over existing rhytids and selecting two different vertical forehead creases to stagger the incisions
83	What brow-lift surgery technique is best used in a man with a receding hairline?	Midforehead
84	Currently, what is the surgical technique of choice for correction of both brow ptosis and forehead and glabellar rhytids?	Endoscopic blepharoplasty
85	What are contraindications to a coronal lift for brow ptosis?	• High female hairline • Male-pattern baldness • Brow asymmetries
86	In what percentage of patients will the supratrochlear or supraorbital nerves arise from a true foramen, putting them at risk for transection?	10 to 30%
87	What muscle is considered the primary elevator of the brow?	Frontalis
88	The galea aponeurosis is contiguous with what two other anatomical structures?	The SMAS of the face below and the temporoparietal fascia (TPF) laterally.

Ptosis and Blepharoplasty

| 89 | What are the four standard clinical measurements used for evaluating someone with ptosis? | • Palpebral fissure height
• Marginal reflex distance
• Upper eyelid crease distance
• Levator excursion |

90	How does one assess eyelid ptosis?	Eyelid ptosis should be evaluated in primary gaze with the frontalis relaxed and the brow fixed. The average vertical palpebral fissure is approximately 10 mm. The levator function is tested by measuring the vertical excursion of the eyelid (normal 12 to 18 mm). The margin-to-reflex distance is the distance between the central corneal light reflex and the upper eyelid margin (normal ~ 4.5 mm).
91	What is the normal position of the upper eyelid relative to the limbus?	The upper eyelid margin typically rests 1.5 mm below the superior corneal limbus, with the highest point just medial to the pupil.
92	Describe the ideal upper eyelid configuration.	The lid crease is 6 to 8 mm from the lash line in a man and 8 to 10 mm in a woman. The upper lid covers approximately 1.5 mm of the iris and does not reach the level of the pupil during primary gaze.
93	What two muscles are responsible for elevation of the upper eyelid? (▶ Fig. 9.5)	Levator palpebrae superioris and Müller muscle

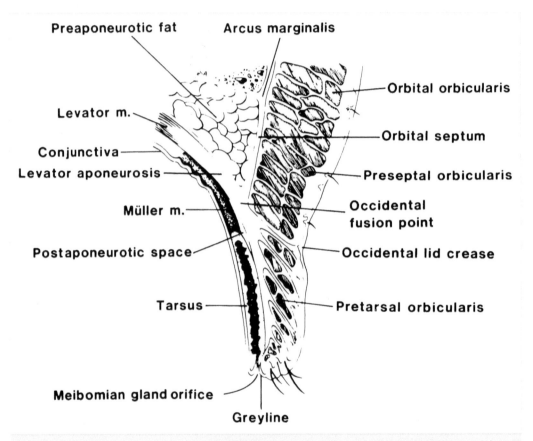

Fig. 9.5 Cross sectional anatomy of the upper eyelid demonstrating the position of the levator and Müller muscle. (Used with permission from Edelstein DR, ed. Revision Surgery in Otolaryngology. New York, NY: Thieme; 2009.)

94	Where does the levator palpebrae superioris originate and insert?	It originates from the lesser wing of the sphenoid and inserts on the superior tarsal plate.

95	What is the innervation of the levator palpebrae superioris?	The oculomotor nerve
96	Where does Müller muscle originate and insert?	It originates from the undersurface of the levator palpebrae superioris and inserts on the superior aspect of the tarsus.
97	What is the innervation of Müller muscle?	Sympathetic nervous system from the superior cervical ganglion to the carotid plexus and along the oculomotor nerve
98	Describe the *margin crease distance*.	The distance from the upper eyelid crease to the upper eyelid margin measured during downgaze
99	Where should the inferior incision be placed during upper eyelid blepharoplasty?	At the natural lid crease, which is at the upper margin of the underlying superior tarsal plate (8 to 10 mm above the lid margin in women and 6 to 9 mm in men)
100	What are *milia*?	*Milia* are 1- to 2-mm cysts that appear as white, smooth nodules on the face. Histologically, they are identical to epidermoid cysts except for their smaller size.
101	Describe the *marginal reflex distance-1*?	Distance from the center of the pupillary light reflex to the upper eyelid margin during primary gaze
102	What is the *marginal reflex distance-2*?	The space between the lower eyelid margin and the pupillary light reflex during primary gaze (normally ~ 5 mm)
103	What is the difference between *blepharoptosis* and *blepharochalasis*?	• *Blepharoptosis* (ptosis) refers to an abnormally low-lying upper eyelid margin during primary gaze. • *Blepharochalasis* refers to a condition of unilateral or bilateral episodic painless, periorbital edema that leads to lid redundancy.
104	What is *pseudoptosis*?	When the upper eyelid appears to be low as a result of malposition of the globe or brow rather than eyelid dysfunction
105	What is the cause of an undesirable hollowed-out appearance after cosmetic blepharoplasty?	Excessive resection of orbital fat
106	What is the anatomical basis for the difference between the Asian and white upper eyelid?	In the Asian eyelid, the orbital septum fuses with the levator aponeurosis below the superior tarsal border. The accompanying preaponeurotic or orbital fat is allowed to proceed to the anterior tarsal surface, resulting in a full, thickened or puffy eyelid. In the white eyelid, the levator aponeurosis penetrates the orbital septum and orbicularis muscle attaching to the overlying dermis, creating a superior palpebral fold.
107	What is the primary risk of epicanthoplasty in the Asian patient?	Web formation in the medial canthal region
108	What percentage of Asians demonstrate a "single-eyelid," and what percentage have an epicanthal fold?	50% and 90%, respectively; the size of the fold is usually relatively small.
109	What is the most common form of ptosis?	Acquired aponeurotic or senile ptosis
110	What is a common clinical sign of acquired aponeurotic ptosis?	Normal or near normal levator function with an abnormally elevated upper eyelid crease
111	What is the most common type of congenital ptosis?	Congenital myogenic ptosis. Caused by dysgenesis of the levator palpebrae superioris in which the muscle fibers are replaced by fibroadipose tissue.
112	What percentage of congenital ptosis is unilateral?	Approximately 75%
113	What coexisting ocular condition is present in a significant number of patients with congenital ptosis?	Amblyopia

114	Describe the phenylephrine test for evaluating ptosis?	This test involves placing dilute phenylepherine in the eye. After waiting 5 minutes, the palpebral fissure and marginal reflex distance are measured and compared with baseline. If there is a good response, then the Müller muscle conjunctival resection should be considered. If there was no response, the external levator advancement should be considered.
115	Describe the clinical manifestation of myogenic ptosis secondary to myasthenia gravis.	Nearly all patients with myasthenia gravis develop ocular symptoms, including ptosis and diplopia. Ptosis is generally bilateral and worsens throughout the day. Symptoms may alternate from one eye to the other.
116	What surgical technique can be used for treatment of ptosis with poor or absent levator function?	Frontalis sling
117	What are the clinical manifestations of Marcus Gunn jaw-winking ptosis?	Elevation of a ptotic eyelid during ipsilateral activation of the mandibular division of the trigeminal nerve (chewing, jaw opening)

Periocular Reconstruction

118	What are the most common causes for needing eyelid reconstruction?	Eyelid tumor excision followed by trauma
119	What are the *lamellae* of the eyelid?	Anterior, middle, and posterior
120	What structures make up the anterior, middle and posterior lamellae of the eyelid?	• Anterior: Skin and orbicularis oculi • Middle: Orbital septum, orbital fat, and the suborbicularis fibroadipose tissue • Posterior: Eyelid retractors, tarsal plate, and conjunctiva
121	Describe the anatomy of the medial canthus?	The medial canthus consists of the lacrimal drainage system and the medial canthal tendon. The medial canthal tendon surrounds the lacrimal sac (creating a "pump") and splits to form anterior and posterior heads attaching to the anterior and posterior lacrimal crests. The medical canthal tendon diverges to join the suspensory ligaments of the eyelid, the orbicularis oculi muscle, and the tarsal plate.
122	What types of defects of the upper eyelid can be allowed to heal by secondary intention with acceptable results?	Medial canthal region less than 1 cm and the upper eyelid when not involving the lid margin and less than 5 mm in diameter
123	What is the maximum defect size of an eyelid that can be closed primarily?	25% in an adult and up to 45% in elderly patients with significant lid laxity
124	What is the most commonly used reconstructive option for a defect that involves more than 50% of the upper eyelid?	Cutler-Beard flap
125	After a Cutler-Beard flap reconstruction of the upper eyelid, what will the newly reconstructed eyelid lack?	Eyelashes and tarsus. Tarsus can be reconstructed if desired, but this is not typically done.
126	Describe a Tenzel rotation flap?	Semicircular musculocutaneous rotation flap that recruits redundant skin from the lateral orbit and can be used to reconstruct defects up to 60% of the width of the upper or lower eyelids
127	Lower eyelid defects of 50% or greater are most commonly reconstructed with what type of flap?	Hughes tarsoconjunctival flap
128	What anatomical layer of the eyelid does the Hughes tarsoconjunctival flap reconstruct?	Posterior lamella

| 129 | When are Hughes tarsoconjunctival flaps and Cutler-Beard flaps most commonly divided after initial surgery? | 4 to 6 weeks |

Facial Analysis

| 130 | Describe the Fitzpatrick scale of skin typing. | (▶ Table 9.1) |

Table 9.1 Fitzpatrick skin types.

Type	Description
I	always burns, never tans (pale white skin)
II	always burns easily, tans minimally (white skin)
III	burns modestly, tans uniformly (light olive skin)
IV	burns minimally, always tans well (moderate brown skin)
V	rarely burns, tans profusely (dark brown skin)
VI	never burns (deeply pigmented brown to black skin)

Data from Fitzpatrick TB. Soleil et peau [Sun and skin]. Journal de Médecine Esthétique. 1975(2): 33–34.

| 131 | Describe the Glogau classification of photoaging skin. | • Class I: Little wrinkling, ages 28 to 35 years, mild pigment changes without keratosis
• Class II: Wrinkles with motion, ages 35 to 50 years, early pigment changes and early actinic keratosis
• Class III: Wrinkles at rest, ages 50 to 65 years, gross discoloration, visible keratosis, and telangiectasia
• Class IV: Severe wrinkling, 60 years and older, prior skin cancers, diffuse wrinkling with color changes |
| 132 | Describe the *Frankfort horizontal line*. (▶ Fig. 9.6) | An imaginary line that extends from the superior aspect of the external auditory meatus to the inferior orbital rim |

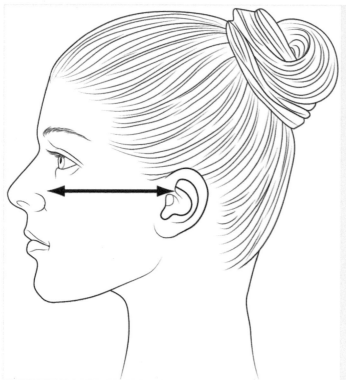

Fig. 9.6 The Frankfort horizontal plane. (Used with permission from Godin MS, ed. Rhinoplasty: Cases and Techniques. New York, NY: Thieme; 2012.)

133	How is the ideal facial height described?	The facial height can be divided into three equal parts. The superior third is measured from trichion to glabella, middle third from glabella to subnasale, inferior third from subnasale to menton.
134	How is the lower third of the face subdivided? (▶ Fig. 9.7)	The upper third is determined by the subnasale to stomion and lower two-thirds by the stomion to mentum.

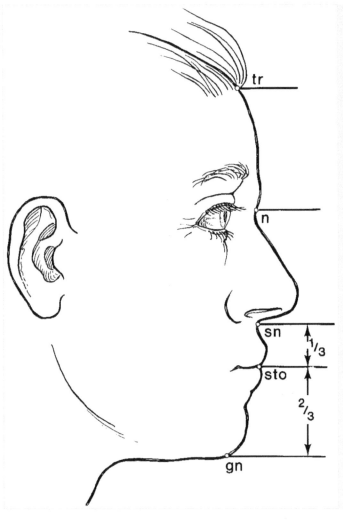

Fig. 9.7 The lower face is divided into two parts between the subnasale (sn), stomion (sto), and gnathion (gn). The ideal vertical ratio is 1:2 between the height of the upper lip and the lower lip/chin. The height of the lower third of the face should be similar to the height of the middle third [nasion (n) to subnasale (sn)] and upper third [trichion (tr) to nasion (n)]. (Used with permission from Papel ID, Frodel J, Holt GR, et al, eds. Facial Plastic and Reconstructive Surgery 3rd Edition. New York, NY: Thieme; 2009.)

135	Describe how the face is divided into vertical fifths.	On frontal view, the face is divided into five equal proportions using the lateral-most projection, the lateral canthi, and the medial canthi.

Facelift and Facial Implants

136	With what layer in the neck is the SMAS layer contiguous?	The platysma

137	What leads to jowl formation?	Relaxation of the masseteric cutaneous ligament and the parotid cutaneous ligament (Lore fascia) allows for infer-omedial migration of the buccal fat pad. The descent of the fat pad is halted when it reaches the mandibular cutaneous ligament, leading to formation of the jowl and deepening of the prejowl sulcus (Marionette line).
138	What structures are responsible for creating the nasolabial fold?	The distal portions of the zygomaticus major and zygomaticus minor muscles insert into the dermis at the lateral aspect of the upper lip, creating the nasolabial fold.
139	What is the process of aging that leads to the nasojugal/tear trough deformity?	Atrophy and descent of the suborbicularis oculi fat and malar fat pad collecting at the nasolabial fold, leaving the infraorbital region exposed and the infraorbital rim more prominent
140	What surgical approach is most common for malar implant placement?	Intraoral (canine fossa)
141	Anterior to the parotid gland, what layer separates the branches of the facial nerve from the SMAS?	The parotidomasseteric fascia
142	What is the vector of pull for the soft tissues of the face during rhytidectomy?	Posterior and superior
143	During rhytidectomy, what determines whether the preauricular incision curves into the hairline or stays below the inferior edge of the preauricular tuft?	The level of the hairline. If the preauricular tuft is 1 to 2 cm below the superior portion of the helical insertion, the incision can curve into the hairline. If there is a high preauricular tuft, the incision should be immediately below this.
144	Review some risk factors associated with skin necrosis following rhytidectomy.	Tobacco use, superficial dissection, excessive wound tension, untreated hematoma, systemic conditions associated with microvascular disease
145	Smoking increases the risk of flap necrosis following rhytidectomy by what factor?	Thirteen times
146	Which facelift technique is most prone to hypertrophic scarring?	Skin-only facelift
147	What is the most commonly injured nerve during rhytidectomy?	Greater auricular nerve (1 to 7%)
148	When elevating the cervical skin flap during rhytidectomy, the great auricular nerve is inadvertently transected. How should this complication be managed?	Direct suture anastomosis
149	During rhytidectomy, an uninterrupted bridge of tissue should be maintained between the temporal and preauricular elevations to protect what structure?	Frontal branch of the facial nerve
150	The temporal branch of the facial nerve lies within or immediately deep to what structure? (▶ Fig. 9.8)	Superficial temporal fascia, also known as the *temporoparietal fascia*

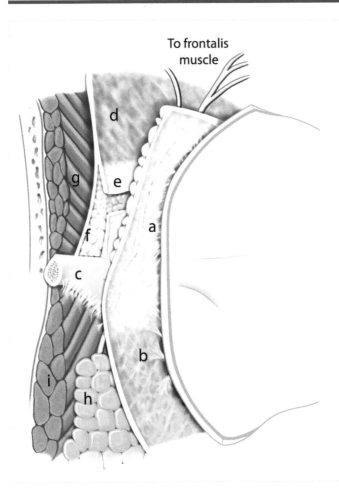

To frontalis muscle

Fig. 9.8 Frontotemporal branches of the facial nerve shown traveling immediately deep to the superficial temporal fascia (temporoparietal fascia). (a) superficial temporal fascia, (b) superficial muscular aponeurotic system, (c) zygomatic arch, (d) deep temporal fascia, (e) superficial layer of the deep temporal fascia, (f) deep layer of the deep temporal fascia with the overlying intermediate fat pad, (g) temporalis muscle, (h) parotid gland, and (i) masseter muscle. (Used with permission from Capone RB, Sykes JM, eds. Complications in Facial Plastic Surgery. New York, NY: Thieme; 2012.)

151	What is the cause of Satyr (devil's) ear after rhytidectomy?	Downward tension on the earlobe leading to inferior displacement of the lobule
152	What causes a cobra deformity after rhytidectomy?	Overaggressive submental lipectomy and/or inadequate platysmal plication
153	What is the cause of the "turkey gobbler" deformity?	Diastasis and ptosis of the platysma muscle with accumulation of submental and cervical fat
154	How is the mentocervical angle determined?	In lateral view, the angle created by a line drawn from the glabella to the pogonion and an intersecting line drawn from the menton to the junction of the neck and submental region
155	What percentage of women undergoing rhytidectomy will experience depression after surgery?	50%
156	How does liposuction lead to a decrease in subcutaneous fat?	By direct removal of adipocytes and induction of apoptosis
157	For what type of fat deposits, congenital or acquired, is liposuction most effective?	Congenital fat accumulations that do not shrink with weight loss
158	Describe the ideal chin position.	Draw a vertical line through the vermilion border of the lower lip. In men, the pogonion should touch this line and may lie up to 2 mm anterior. In women, the pogonion should touch this line and should not rest more than 2 mm posterior.

| 159 | What method is used to determine ideal chin projection? (▶ Fig. 9.9) | Gonzalez-Ulloa method: A line is made from the nasion perpendicular to the Frankfort horizontal. The ideal chin projection should be at this line. When the chin is posterior, and the patient has normal occlusion, a hypoplastic mentum is present. |

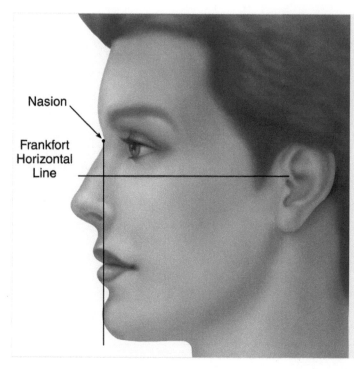

Fig. 9.9 The Gonzalez-Ulloa method for assessing ideal chin position: a line is made from the nasion perpendicular to the Frankfort horizontal. The ideal chin projection should be at this line. (Used with permission from Papel ID, Frodel J, Holt GR, et al, eds. Facial Plastic and Reconstructive Surgery 3rd Edition. New York, NY: Thieme; 2009.)

Nasion

Frankfort Horizontal Line

160	What is the difference between *microgenia*, *micrognathia*, and *retrognathia*?	• *Microgenia* is caused by an underdeveloped mentum with an otherwise normal mandible and normal occlusion. • *Micrognathia* implies a hypoplastic retruded mandible with class 2 occlusion. • *Retrognathia* implies a normal sized mandible with class 2 occlusion.
161	What is a useful landmark for identifying the mental foramina?	The mental foramina is variable but is usually found below the second premolar tooth.
162	Where should the pocket for a chin implant be created?	Inferior to the mental foramen but above the muscle insertions of the inferior mandibular border (generally 8 to 10 mm of space). It may be placed transorally or transcutaneously through a submental crease incision.
163	What are some of the indications for distraction osteogenesis of the mandible?	Hemifacial microsomia, syndrome-related micrognathia, severe obstructive sleep apnea, deformity of the mandibular angle, and mandibular hypoplasia causing malocclusion

Rhinoplasty and Nasal Reconstruction

| 164 | What are the subunits of the nose? (▶ Fig. 9.10) | Dorsum, root, sidewalls (two), tip, columella, soft tissue triangles (two), ala (two). If more than 50% of a subunit is injured or resected, the remaining portion should be removed before reconstruction. |

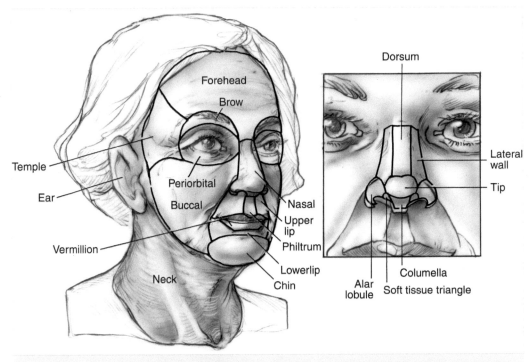

Fig. 9.10 Aesthetic units of the face (a) and aesthetic subunits of the nose (b). (Used with permission from Papel ID, Frodel J, Holt GR, et al, eds. Facial Plastic and Reconstructive Surgery 3rd Edition. New York, NY: Thieme; 2009.)

165	Which arteries supply the nasal septum? (▶ Fig. 9.11)

- Sphenopalatine artery
- Anterior and posterior ethmoid arteries
- Superior labial artery
- Greater palatine artery

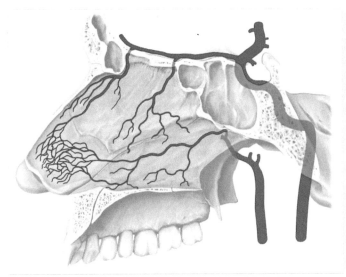

Fig. 9.11 The vascular supply of the nasal septum: sphenopalatine artery, anterior and posterior ethmoid arteries, superior labial artery, and greater palatine artery. (Used with permission from Thieme Atlas of Anatomy: Head and Neuroanatomy, © Thieme 2007, illustration by Karl Wesker.)

166	Which arteries supply the external nose?	• Facial artery • Angular artery • Superior labial artery • Infraorbital artery • Ophthalmic artery
167	What are some of the unique characteristics that may be found in the Asian nose?	Thick, sebaceous skin, low radix, weak lower lateral cartilages
168	What are some of the typical differences in the appearance of a child's nose compared with an adult's nose?	A child's nose displays a more obtuse nasolabial angle, more circular nares, shorter dorsum and columella, less defined and projected nasal tip, and decreased dorsal projection.
169	What is the primary concern of septal surgery in prepubertal children?	Underdevelopment of the nose and maxilla
170	How is the nasofrontal angle determined? (► Fig. 9.12)	A line tangent to the nasal dorsum is intersected with a line tangent to the glabella and nasion.

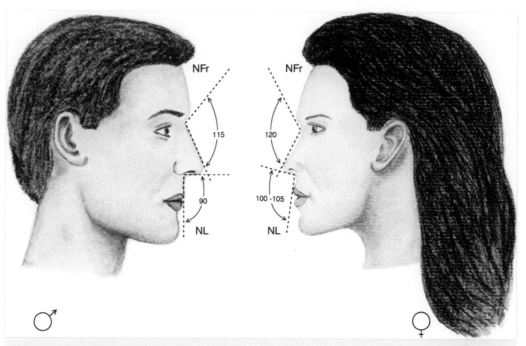

Fig. 9.12 Gender differences between the male and female nasofrontal (NFr) and nasolabial (NL) angles considered ideal. (Used with permission from Papel ID, Frodel J, Holt GR, et al, eds. Facial Plastic and Reconstructive Surgery 3rd Edition. New York, NY: Thieme; 2009.)

171	How is the nasofacial angle determined?	In lateral view, it is the angle created by the intersection of a line parallel to the nasal dorsum intersecting the tip and nasion and a vertical line from the glabella to the pogonion.
172	How is the nasolabial angle determined?	In lateral view, it is the angle created by a line drawn perpendicular to the Frankfort horizontal at the subnasale and a second line drawn through the midpoint of the nostril aperture.

173	What is meant by the term *tip-defining point* in the context of nasal analysis?	The anterior most projection of the domes, which are represented by two distinct light reflexes on the skin of the nasal undertip
174	Describe the Simons method of determining nasal projection.	A line drawn from the subnasale to the nasal tip is compared with a line drawn from the subnasale to the vermilion border of the upper lip. In an ideal nose, the length of these lines should be equal.
175	Describe the Crumley method for determining nasal projection.	In lateral view, the nose is seen as a 3–4–5 triangle with points at the alar facial crease, tip, and nasion. The shortest arm of the triangle is between the tip and the alar facial crease. The longest arm is between the tip and the nasion. Another alternative is to measure the distance from the subnasale to the nasal tip and compare it with the distance from the subnasale to the vermilion border of the upper lip. If the distance from the subnasale to the tip is greater than the distance from the subnasale to the upper lip, the nose is overprojected.
176	Describe the Goode method for determining nasal projection. (▶ Fig. 9.13)	A horizontal line drawn from the alar facial crease to the nasal tip is 0.55 to 0.6 the length of a line drawn from the nasion to the nasal tip. If the ratio is less than 0.55, the nose is underprojected. If the ratio is greater than 0.6, the nose is overprojected.

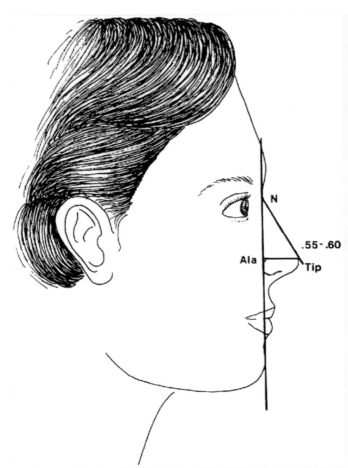

Fig. 9.13 Goode method of determining nasal tip projection. A horizontal line drawn from the alar facial crease (Ala) to the nasal tip is 0.55 to 0.6 the length of a line drawn from the nasion (N) to the nasal tip. (Used with permission from Papel ID, Frodel J, Holt GR, et al, eds. Facial Plastic and Reconstructive Surgery 3rd Edition. New York, NY: Thieme; 2009.)

177	How is the ideal width of the nasal base determined?	It should lie within vertical lines drawn inferiorly from the medial canthi.
178	What is the ideal ratio of the nasal lobule and columella on basal view of the nose?	The nasal tip should occupy the upper third and the columella the lower two-thirds. The nasal tip should be approximately 45% the width of the base of the nose.
179	What is the ideal ratio of nasal lobule to columella on base view?	1:2
180	On lateral view, what is the ideal amount of columellar show?	2 to 4 mm
181	Describe the anatomy of the nasal bones.	Superiorly, the nasal skeleton is composed of paired nasal bones. The premaxilla and palatine bones constitute the floor. The lateral wall of the nose is formed by the medial walls of the maxilla. The superior, middle, and inferior conchal bones are attached to the lateral nasal walls. The cribriform plate is the roof of the nose. The bony septum is formed by the vomer and the perpendicular plate of the ethmoid.
182	Describe the skeletal support of the nose.	The upper third of the nose is supported by the nasal bones and the medial portion of the frontal process of the maxilla. The dorsal septum and upper lateral cartilages are the framework for the middle third of the nose. The anterior septal angle and the lower lateral cartilages suspend the lower third of the nose.
183	What are the major tip-supporting structures of the nose?	• The intrinsic length and strength of the lower lateral cartilages • Attachment of the medial crura to the caudal aspect of the quadrangular cartilage • Attachment of the cephalic border of the lower lateral cartilages to the caudal aspect of the upper lateral cartilages
184	What are the minor tip-supporting structures of the nose?	Anterior nasal spine, attachment of the skin and soft tissue to the lower lateral cartilages, membranous septum, cartilagenous septal dorsum, sesamoid complex, interdomal ligament
185	What is the *rhinion*?	The rhinion is the point that corresponds with the junction of the bony and cartilaginous dorsum.
186	Which structures form the *internal nasal valve*?	• Medially, the nasal septum • Laterally, the caudal border of the upper lateral cartilage and piriform aperture • Inferiorly and posteriorly, the head of the inferior turbinate
187	What structures constitute the *external nasal valve*?	• Laterally, the pyriform aperture, lateral crus of the lower lateral cartilage, fibrofatty tissue, and alar rim • Superolaterally, the caudal aspect of the upper lateral cartilage • Medially, the septum and columella
188	What are some surgical techniques to correct external nasal valve collapse?	The technique chosen depends on the cause of valve compromise. Options include alar batten grafts, lateral crural strut grafts, narrowing of a wide columella, repair of caudal septal deflection, and alar flaring sutures.
189	What muscles constitute the *nasal compressor group*?	Procerus, quadratus (levator labii and nasi superioris), nasalis (pars tranversalis and pars alaris), depressor septi
190	What muscles constitute the nasal dilator group?	The dilator naris posterior and the dilator naris anterior

191	What muscle lowers the nasal tip?	Depressor septi nasi muscle. Results in the unfavorable appearance of a rounded, depressed, and lengthened tip, which can be corrected during rhinoplasty by transecting the insertions of these muscles at the base of the columella.
192	What is a marginal incision in rhinoplasty?	An incision made along the caudal aspect of the lower lateral cartilage
193	What is a rim incision in rhinoplasty?	An incision made along the alar rim. This approach has been largely abandoned secondary to subsequent alar notching.
194	What transcolumellar incisions may be used during external approach rhinoplasty?	V shaped, inverted-v, stair-step, or slightly curvilinear
195	Describe the surgical approaches to the nasal tip.	Endonasal approaches can be divided into *nondelivery* and *delivery* techniques. Nondelivery techniques include trans-cartilaginous and intercartilaginous with retrograde dissection. Delivery techniques include making intercartilaginous and marginal incisions to create a chondrocutaeous flap. An open (external) approach involves a midcolumellar and bilateral marginal incisions.
196	List some techniques to increase nasal projection. (▶ Fig. 9.14)	Lateral crural steal, shield graft, advancement of medial crura along the caudal septum, columellar strut graft, vertical dome division, interdomal suture placement, premaxillary graft

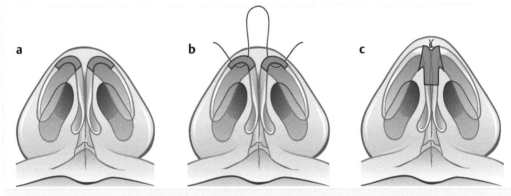

Fig. 9.14 The lateral crural steal technique increases nasal tip projection (a compared to c) and rotation by lengthening the medial crura at the expense of the lateral crura (b and c). (Used with permission from Georgalas C, Fokkens W, eds. Rhinology and Skull Base Surgery. New York, NY: Thieme; 2013.)

197	List some techniques to decrease nasal projection.	• Combined medial and lateral crural flap • Full transfixion incision • Reduction of the nasal septum
198	List some techniques to increase nasal rotation.	• Lateral crural steal • Tip graft • Vertical dome division
199	Describe the Goldman technique of vertical dome division.	The lower lateral cartilages are delivered through marginal and intercartilaginous incisions. A vertical incision is made through the dome, resulting in a transfer of cartilage from the lateral crus to the medial crus. The incision goes through the overlying vestibular skin and mucosa. This results in increased length of the middle leg of the tripod, in turn increasing projection and improving tip refinement.

200	Describe the Simons modification of vertical dome division.	It is performed the same way as the Goldman technique except for the following: • The vestibular skin and mucosa are not incised. • A triangular piece of cartilage is excised in the region of dome division. • The medial crura are resecured in a superiorly oriented vector.
201	What are some factors that might predispose a patient to the development of internal nasal valve obstruction after rhinoplasty?	• Weak upper lateral cartilages • Short nasal bones • Thin skin • History of prior surgery or trauma
202	What techniques should be used to decrease the likelihood of postsurgical middle vault deformities after rhinoplasty?	• Preservation of middle vault mucosa • Reattachment of the upper lateral cartilages with the nasal dorsum if disrupted • Conservative dorsal hump reduction • Avoidance of overaggressive osteotomies
203	What are some surgical techniques used to correct internal nasal valve narrowing?	The technique chosen depends on the cause of valve compromise. Options include spreader grafts, valvuloplasty, conchal cartilage butterfly graft, flaring sutures, septoplasty, and inferior turbinate reduction.
204	During rhinoplasty, how much lateral crural cartilage should be preserved after horizontal cephalic excision to minimize the risk of alar collapse?	6 to 8 mm
205	Review some causes of saddle-nose deformity.	Prior surgery resulting in inadequate support of the upper lateral cartilages or loss of adequate dorsal and caudal septal struts (each should have at least 1-cm height); history of trauma with septal hematoma/abscess and loss of septal support; self-inflicted from use of cocaine or neurotic nasal picking; medical condition, including Wegener granulomatosis, relapsing polychondritis, and syphilis.
206	What autologous tissues may be used for reconstruction of the dorsal nasal skeleton?	Rib cartilage, conchal cartilage, calvarial bone, iliac crest
207	What are some contraindications to repair of a saddle-nose deformity?	• Use of intranasal cocaine • Poor general health • Poorly controlled relapsing polychondritis
208	Describe the order in which medial, lateral, and intermediate osteotomies should be performed.	Medial osteotomies are performed first, followed by intermediate osteotomies (if needed), and finally lateral osteotomies. If lateral osteotomies are performed first, it is difficult for the osteotome to gain purchase for the medial osteotomies on a mobile segment of bone.
209	What is the cause of inverted-V deformity following rhinoplasty?	Collapse of the upper lateral cartilages with narrowing of the angle between the upper lateral cartilages and nasal septum, resulting in pinching of the middle nasal vault and internal nasal valve collapse
210	What is the cause of an open roof deformity following rhinoplasty?	Incomplete lateral osteotomies after osseous dorsum reduction that result in a gap between the bilateral nasal bones
211	What is the cause of a step deformity following rhinoplasty?	A step deformity occurs when the lateral osteotomy is placed too far medially, resulting in a visible step off in the nasal sidewall.

212	What is a *rocker deformity*?	If osteotomies are extended too far superiorly, the thicker frontal bone may be included in the fracture line. When the nasal bones are fractured in medially, the thicker superior frontal bone will "rock" out laterally.
213	What is a *pollybeak deformity*?	Excessive supratip fullness in relation to the tip.
214	What are some of the causes of pollybeak deformity?	Under-resection of the cartilaginous dorsal hump, over-resection of the nasal bones, loss of tip support, and excessive scar formation in the supratip region
215	What are *nasal bossae*?	Prominent, often sharply demarcated, protuberances of lower lateral cartilage in the domal region
216	What are some causes of alar retraction after rhinoplasty?	Over-resection of the lateral crura, excision of vestibular mucosa, rim incision
217	What is the most common donor site for composite grafts used in facial reconstruction?	The ear, incorporating auricular cartilage
218	What is a *tent pole deformity*?	Excessive length of the medial crura relative to the lateral crura leading to a visible step-off and an overprojected, pinched tip, which may occur secondary to over-recruitment of the lateral crura in a vertical dome division procedure
219	What are some of the physical examination findings associated with a retruded premaxilla?	Acute nasolabial angle, difficulty maintaining the lips in a closed position at rest, nasal tip ptosis
220	What are some of the materials that can be used for premaxillary augmentation?	• Autografts: Rib cartilage, split calvarial bone graft, iliac crest, conchal cartilage, septal cartilage • Homografts: Cadaveric acellular human dermis, irradiated rib • Synthetics: Silicone, hydroxyapatite, polytetrafluoroethylene
221	Describe two early signs of rhinophyma.	Dilated (patulous) pores and telangiectatic vessels on the distal nose
222	Rhinophyma may manifest as the final stage of what other skin disease?	Acne rosacea, although not all patients with rhinophyma have a history of rosacea
223	What nasal disorder results from hypertrophy of the sebaceous glands in the nasal skin and fibrosis?	Rhinophyma
224	What malignant condition can be associated with rhinophyma?	Basal cell carcinoma
225	Which patient population(s) is most commonly affected by rhinophyma?	Whereas acne rosacea is more common in women (3:1) compared with men, rhinophyma almost always affects men (30:1). The disease typically afflicts white men in their 50 through 70 s.
226	How is rhinophyma managed?	Inflammation can be managed conservatively, similar to rosacea. For significant hypertrophy, deformity, and nasal obstruction, surgical recontouring can be performed using, most commonly, a carbon dioxide laser with or without dermabrasion.

Otoplasty and Auricular Reconstruction

| 227 | Describe the ideal orientation of the auricle relative to the skull. | The distance from the mastoid skin to the lateral helical rim is 2 to 2.5 cm. The average height of the ear is 5.9 cm in women and 6.4 cm in men. On superior view, the ear should protrude 20 to 30 degrees from the skull (auriculocephalic angle). |

228   Describe the Mustarde technique of otoplasty.
(▶ Fig. 9.15)

A postauricular incision is made and supraperichondrial dissection performed. The ear is folded into the desired configuration, and sutures are passed from the posterior surface of the auricle through the anterior surface but not through dermis. The distance between the medial and lateral aspect of each mattress suture is 16 mm. The vertical distance between the superior and inferior aspect of each mattress suture is 10 mm. Individual mattress sutures are placed 2 mm apart.

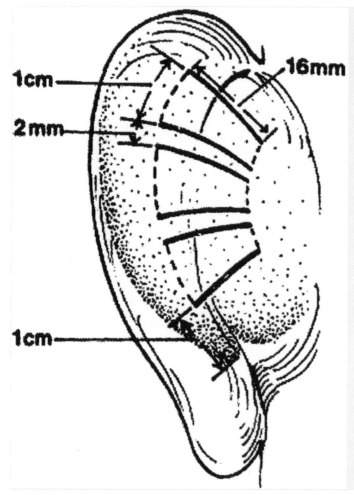

Fig. 9.15 Mustarde otoplasty technique. Posterior view of a left auricle demonstrating ideal suture placement. (Used with permission from Papel ID, Frodel J, Holt GR, et al, eds. Facial Plastic and Reconstructive Surgery 3rd Edition. New York, NY: Thieme; 2009.)

229   Describe the Furnas technique of otoplasty.

Permanent horizontal mattress sutures are used to tack the posterior conchal bowl to the mastoid periosteum, with or without trimming of conchal cartilage.

230   A patient undergoes a conchal setback procedure for treatment of prominent ear deformity. Postoperatively, the patient has narrowing of the external ear canal. What is the most likely cause of this complication?

The mastoid periosteal suture was placed too anteriorly, causing the conchal bowl to impinge on the external auditory meatus.

231	What are the causes of telephone ear deformity?	Over-correction of the middle third of the prominent ear during otoplasty
232	What are the subunits of the ear?	Helix, antihelix, scaphoid fossa, triangular fossa, concha cymba, concha cavum, tragus, anti-tragus, lobule
233	What embryonic structures give rise to the pinna?	The six hillocks of His. Hillocks 1 through 3 develop from the first branchial arch, hillocks 4 through 6 arise from the second branchial arch. • Hillock 1: Tragus • Hillock 2: Helical crus • Hillock 3: Helix • Hillock 4: Antihelix • Hillock 5: Antitragus • Hillock 6: Lobule
234	What arteries supply the auricle?	Superficial temporal artery, posterior auricular artery, and the deep auricular artery (minor contribution)
235	Describe the classification system for grading microtia.	• Class I: All structures of the external ear are present with slight underdevelopment. • Class II: Structures are smaller and more dysmorphic than in type I microtia. • Class III: Only a small vestigial structure (peanut) is present. • Class IV: The external ear is absent (anotia).
236	What congenital syndromes are associated with microtia?	Goldenhar syndrome, hemifacial microsomia, Treacher Collins syndrome, Robinow syndrome, and branchio-otorenal syndrome
237	At what age is a patient considered an acceptable candidate for microtia repair?	At 6 years old, when the ear has neared full adult size and the quantity of rib cartilage is sufficient
238	Describe the stages microtia repair using autologous costal cartilage.	• Stage 1: Harvest costal cartilage from the sixth, seventh, and eighth ribs; carve into auricular framework; and place in subcutaneous pocket posterior to the external auditory canal. • Stage 2: Auricular remnant is rotated inferiorly to recreate the lobule. • Stage 3: Elevation on neoauricle off mastoid and placement of a postauricular skin graft • Stage 4: Tragal reconstruction
239	When do most authorities recommend atresia repair in patients with microtia who desire autologous cartilage microtia repair?	Usually after the costal cartilage framework has been placed and elevated off the mastoid with a posterior skin graft. This sequence is preferred to optimize blood supply during initial microtia repair.

Lip Reconstruction

240	What are the treatment options for lower-lip actinic cheilitis?	Small areas may be treated with cryosurgery, whereas more extensive lesions may require vermilionectomy or CO_2 laser ablation.
241	What are some reconstructive options for a full-thickness defect involving less than 30% of the length of the lip?	Wedge or W-excision with primary closure
242	What are some reconstructive options for a full-thickness defect involving 50 to 75% of the length of the lip?	• Abbe flap • Estlander flap • Gillies fan flap • Karapandzic flap

243	What are some reconstructive options for a full-thickness defect involving more than 75% of the length of the lower lip?	• Bilateral nasolabial flaps • Karapandzic flap • Bernard-Burrow flap • Fujimori Gate flap • Microvascular reconstruction with radial forearm fascio-cutaneous flap
244	Describe the similarities and differences between an Abbe flap and an Estlander flap.	Both flaps involve transfer of a pedicled full-thickness flap between the upper and lower lip, both are used for defects involving 50 to 75% of the lip length, and both are based on a labial artery pedicle. The Estlander flap is used for defects of the oral commissure and lateral lip, whereas the Abbe flap is used for central defects.
245	Off what artery is the Gillies fan flap based?	Superior labial artery

Cleft Lip and Palate

246	Describe the embryologic development of the lip.	In the 4th week of gestation, the paired maxillary prominences, derived from the first branchial arch, are seen. Proliferation of mesenchyme ventral to the forebrain gives rise to the frontonasal prominences. Nasal placodes arise on each side of the frontonasal prominence. In week 5, invagination of the nasal placodes leads to development of nasal pits. The medial and lateral ridges of tissue around the pit are called the medial and lateral nasal prominences, respectively. Between weeks 5 and 7, the medial maxillary prominences grow medially to fuse with the medial nasal prominences, forming the upper lip. Fusion of the medial nasal prominences leads to formation of the philtrum, medial upper lip, columella and nasal tip. The lateral upper lip arises from the maxillary processes.
247	Maternal use of which medication has been linked to a significant increase in the incidence of cleft lip and palate?	Phenytoin
248	What are the classic physical examination findings in Pierre Robin sequence?	• Micrognathia • Glossoptosis • Cleft palate
249	What is van der Woude syndrome?	An autosomal dominant disorder characterized by lower-lip pits, cleft lip and palate, congenital heart disease, syndactyly, and ankyloglossia
250	What are some of the physical examination findings in velocardiofacial syndrome?	Facial asymmetry with a long midface, inferior displacement of the auricles, widened nasal base with bulbous nasal tip, micrognathia, microcephaly, medially displaced internal carotid arteries
251	What is the difference between a complete and incomplete cleft lip?	A *complete cleft* is a full-thickness defect of the entire height of the lip with extension into the nose. An incomplete cleft does not involve the entire vertical height of the lip and contains a web of bridging tissue across the nasal aperture.
252	Describe the anatomy of a bilateral cleft lip.	The orbicularis oris fibers travel parallel to the edges of the cleft. Medially, the muscle fibers insert into the columella, and laterally the fibers insert into the nasal ala. The prolabial segment is composed of nonfunctional fibrous tissue. The premaxilla and central maxillary alveolus are protruberant.
253	What physical examination findings are associated with a submucous cleft palate?	• Bifid uvula • Notching of the hard palate • Palpable or visible diastasis of the midline palatal musculature

254	Which muscles contribute to the velopharyngeal sphincter?	Levator veli palatini, tensor veli palatini, palatoglossus, palatopharyngeus, superior pharyngeal constrictor, and musculus uvulae
255	Which muscle is primarily responsible for providing velopharyngeal closure during speech production?	Levator veli palatini
256	In reference to cleft lip repair, describe "the rule of 10s."	Cleft lip repair can be performed when the child is at least 10 weeks old, has a hemoglobin greater than 10 g /dl, and weighs at least 10 pounds.
257	What are some techniques used to repair a unilateral cleft lip?	Millard rotation advancement flap, LeMesurier quadrilateral flap, Randall-Tennison triangular flap repair, Skoog and Kernahan-Bauer upper and lower lip Z-plasty repairs
258	What are some of the techniques described for cleft palate repair?	Primary veloplasty, double-opposing Z-plasty (Furlow palatoplasty), bipedicled flap palatoplasty (von Langenbeck), palatal lengthening (V-Y pushback palatoplasty)
259	What are some of the complications of palatoplasty?	Bleeding, infection, oronasal fistula, velopharyngeal insufficiency, wound dehiscence, airway obstruction, and obstructive sleep apnea
260	Describe the nasal deformities associated with a unilateral cleft lip.	There is an abnormally short medial crus, and an abnormally long caudally displaced lateral crus on the cleft side. The nasal floor is deficient, and the alar base is displaced posteriorly, laterally, and inferiorly. The tip, columella, and septum are deviated toward the non-cleft side.
261	Describe the nasal deformities associated with a bilateral cleft lip.	The nasal tip is flat and broad. There is deficient skin and cartilage in the columella. The nostrils assume a horizontal orientation, and the alae are displaced laterally, inferiorly, and posteriorly.
262	When should primary unilateral cleft lip rhinoplasty be undertaken?	At the same time as cleft lip repair, by 3 months of age

Hair Restoration

263	What are the layers of the scalp?	Skin, loose connective tissue, galea or epicranial aponeurosis, loose areolar tissue, periosteum
264	What are the five main arteries that supply blood to the scalp?	• Supratrochlear • Supraorbital • Superficial temporal • Occipital • Posterior auricular arteries
265	What makes up the hair bulb?	Papilla combined with surrounding epidermal cells
266	What is the function of the hair bulb?	Site of hair shaft formation
267	What is a follicular unit?	A group of one to four hairs with an accompanying neurovascular plexus, arrector pili muscle, and sebaceous glands
268	What are the phases of hair growth?	• Anagen • Catagen • Telogen
269	What is the primary growth phase of the hair growth cycle?	Anagen phase
270	What are some infectious and inflammatory causes of alopecia?	Dermatophytes, demodex folliculorum, foliculitis, secondary syphilis, seborrheic dermatitis, psoriasis, pityriasis amiantacea
271	What is the most common cause of male baldness?	Androgenic alopecia
272	What hormone plays the most significant role in androgenic alopecia?	Dihydrotestosterone

273	What is the most widely used classification system for hair loss?	Norwood classification (stages I through VII)
274	What classification system is most commonly used for grading female androgenic alopecia?	Ludwig classification (grades 1 through 3)
275	What is the mechanism of finasteride in the treatment of hair loss?	5α-Reductase inhibitor; blocks the conversion of serum testosterone into dihydrotestosterone
276	What is the most common topical medication prescribed for alopecia?	Minoxidil. Treatment results in a lengthening of the anagen phase and an increase in the blood supply to the follicle.
277	How long should balding patients use minoxidil before they can expect to see noticeable results?	4 to 6 months
278	What hair qualities yield better results with hair replacement surgery?	Hair color that matches skin color, coarse texture, high density, curly
279	What is follicular unit extraction?	The process by which follicular units are harvested individually as opposed to the strip method in which a strip of scalp is removed and then cut into individual follicular units
280	What are the advantages of follicular unit extraction?	Can be harvested from multiple different areas on the scalp. A long postoperative scar is avoided compared with the strip method of harvesting.
281	What is the difference between follicular unit *micrografts* and *minigrafts*?	*Micrografting* involves transplantation of one or two hair follicles per unit used predominantly at the hair line, whereas *minigrafts* are three or four hair follicles used to fill in bulk areas.
282	After transplantation, what phase of hair growth will transplanted hair enter?	Telogen phase. Patients should be told to expect that the transplanted hairs will fall out, with regrowth occurring by 3 to 4 months.
283	Where is the donor strip of hair typically taken for hair transplantation?	Occipital region near the inion
284	What are the primary advantages of scalp flaps over hair transplantation?	Scalp flaps maintain the blood supply to hair follicles, thus preventing them from entering the telogen phase; hair continues to grow immediately after the procedure; hair density is maximized with instantaneous results.
285	What is the Juri flap?	The Juri flap is an axial scalp flap based on the superficial temporal artery that allows for the entire frontal hairline to be covered with a single flap.
286	In the context of hair restoration treatments, what is scalp reduction?	Scalp reduction is a technique that reduces the surface area of the balding scalp using serial excisions. Areas of balding are excised and closed primarily or with various local flaps.
287	Review the role of tissue expanders in hair restoration.	Tissue expanders do not increase the number of follicles but increase the distance between follicles to cover a larger surface area. Usually, they can be expanded by a factor of 2 without noticeable thinning.

Skin Grafts

288	What are the benefits of a full-thickness skin graft over a split-thickness skin graft?	• Better color and texture match • Less scar contraction • No need for additional equipment (dermatome) for harvest • Easier donor-site wound care and less contour irregularity
289	What are the most common head and neck donor sites for full-thickness skin grafts used in facial reconstruction?	Upper eyelid, preauricular or postauricular, supraclavicular, melolabial fold, and forehead

290	How do full-thickness skin grafts survive initially during the first 24 to 48 hours?	Plasma imbibition: the diffusion of nutrition from the fluid at the recipient site, after which capillary inosculation takes place at 48 hours
291	What are the primary causes of skin graft failure?	Infection, shearing, fluid accumulation between the graft and recipient bed
292	What is the function of a bolster dressing over a skin graft?	It ensures maximal graft to recipient bed contact and decreases shearing forces that might affect graft survival.

Local Flaps

293	What are the two general categories of local flaps based on blood supply?	• Random (based on subdermal plexus) • Axial (based on named vessels)
294	Define the term *flap delay*, and review its importance.	*Surgical flap delay* is the technique of elevating a flap on a pedicle and then returning it to the donor site for days to weeks before final transfer. It is believed to condition the flap to ischemic conditions and/or improve vascular supply of the pedicle.
295	What are the four types of pivotal flaps used in head and neck reconstruction?	• Rotation • Transposition • Interpolated • Island
296	Defects of what shape are best suited for closure with rotational flaps?	Triangular defects
297	What is the definition of an *interpolated flap*?	It is a local flap whose pedicle passes over or under intervening tissue to reach a nonadjacent defect. Typically, it requires a second stage in which the pedicle is divided.
298	What is the definition of an *advancement flap*?	It is a flap with a linear configuration that closes a defect by sliding toward it.
299	What are the some advantages and disadvantages of a Z-plasty closure?	• Advantages: It can orient scar parallel to resting skin tension lines, requires minimal excision of normal skin, interrupts forces of scar contracture, and creates broken line which is less noticeable than a straight line • Disadvantage: Increases the overall scar length
300	What is the approximate lengthening of the central limb of a Z-plasty when using 30-degree, 45-degree, and 60-degree angles? (▶ Fig. 9.16)	25%, 50%, and 75% respectively

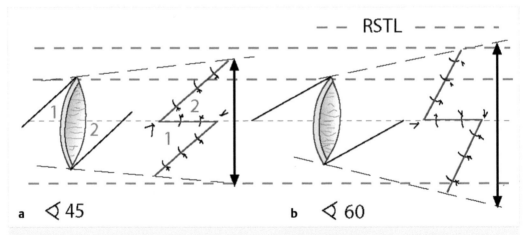

Fig. 9.16 Simple Z-plasty transposition flap. (a) 45° Z-plasty lengthens the central limb of the Z-plasty by 50%. (b) 60° Z-plasty lengthens the central limb of the Z-plasty by 75%. 30° Z-plasty lengthens the central limb of the Z-plasty by 25% (not shown). (Used with permission from Weerda H. Reconstructive Facial Plastic Surgery: A Problem-Solving Manual. New York, NY: Thieme; 2001.)

301	What are the internal angles of the rhombic flap?	60 degrees and 120 degrees
302	Describe the technique of performing a bilobed flap as originally described by Esser. (▶ Fig. 9.17)	A double transposition flap, with the first flap oriented 90 degrees to the defect and measuring the same size as the defect. The second flap is oriented 180 degrees to the defect and is slightly smaller than the first flap. The first flap is rotated into the primary defect, the second flap is rotated into the defect created by the first flap, and the defect created by the second flap is closed primarily.

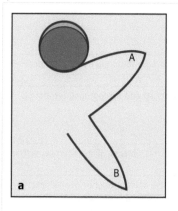 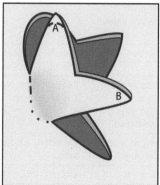 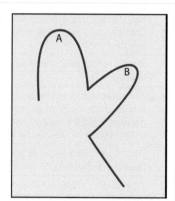

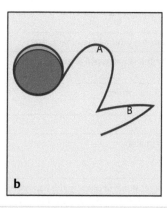 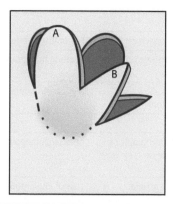 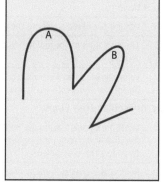

Fig. 9.17 Classic (Esser) bilobed flap (a), and Zitelli modification of the classic bilobed flap (b). (Used with permission from Sherris DA, Larrabee WF. Principles of Facial Reconstruction 2nd Edition. New York, NY: Thieme; 2010.)

303	Describe the Zitelli modification of the bilobed flap.	The angle of the first flap is oriented 45 degrees to the defect, and the second flap is oriented 90 degrees to the defect. It is designed to keep less tension on repair and reduce standing cone deformity.
304	Describe the indications for a nasolabial flap in nasal reconstruction.	Superiorly based flaps are best suited for reconstruction of the lower two-thirds of the nose, including the inferior dorsum, alae, and tip. Inferiorly based flaps are used for reconstruction of the columella and nasal floor.

305	What is the blood supply to the paramedian forehead flap?	Supratrochlear artery, located between 1.7 and 2.2 cm from the midline at the medial aspect of the brow
306	How long after the first stage of a paramedian forehead flap is the pedicle typically divided?	Three weeks; however, in patients who are smokers or have other comorbidities, pedicle division can be delayed

Regional Flaps

307	Why might regional control of oral cavity malignancies be of concern when using the submental island flap?	The flap incorporates a portion of the level I nodal basin, which can be involved with metastases
308	When raising the facial artery musculomucosal flap, the facial artery lies immediately superficial to what muscle, a portion of which is incorporated into the flap?	Buccinator muscle
309	What is the primary arterial supply to the temporalis flap?	Anterior and posterior deep temporal arteries, branches of the internal maxillary artery
310	The temporalis is commonly used in facial reanimation of the mouth in patients with facial paralysis. What are the two contrasting ways the temporalis can be used for facial reanimation?	Temporalis myofascial flap and orthodromic temporalis tendon transfer
311	What is the blood supply to the masseter when used as a pedicled flap in facial reanimation?	Masseteric artery, which is a branch of the internal maxillary artery
312	What arteries supply the sternocleidomastoid muscle?	Occipital artery (superior third), superior thyroid artery (middle third), suprascapular artery (inferior third)
313	What is the blood supply to the superior trapezius myocutaneous flap?	Paraspinous perforating branches of the intercostal vessels
314	Which type of trapezius pedicled flap can be successfully harvested after radical neck dissection?	Superior trapezius myocutaneus flap
315	What is the blood supply to the deltopectoral flap?	Perforator arteries from the internal mammary artery
316	The pectoralis major regional flap is based on what artery?	Pectoral branch of the thoracoacromial artery
317	What nerves must be transected to allow for atrophy of the pectoralis major regional flap?	Medial and lateral pectoral nerves

Microvascular Free Flaps

318	What are vessels leaving the axial blood supply of a free flap and passing through muscle on their way to supply the skin called?	Musculocutaneous perforators
319	Review the clinical findings of acute arterial thrombosis of a free flap in the early postoperative period.	Loss of implanted Doppler signal (if placed); the flap is cool, pale, and without capillary refill, and there is no bleeding after pinprick.
320	A free-flap arterial anastomosis is revised within the first 24 hours after surgery for presumed arterial thrombosis. Despite good blood flow through the artery after the revision, the flap's appearance at the skin level does not improve; subsequently, it undergoes necrosis. What is the most likely reason for failure after revision surgery despite good blood flow through the artery?	No-reflow phenomenon: Despite restoration of blood flow through the major artery, the prior occlusion and ischemia have detrimental effects on the microvasculature, which caused subsequent necrosis.
321	Review the clinical findings of venous congestion of a free flap in the early postoperative period.	Congestion and edema, violaceous color with brisk bleeding of dark blood on pinprick, loss of venous Doppler signal
322	What is the most common reason for venous occlusion of a free-flap vascular pedicle?	Mechanical obstruction from compression, twisting, or kinking

323	What nonsurgical therapy can be used to treat venous congestion after free-flap reconstruction?	Leech therapy
324	What is the most common free flap used for reconstruction of hemi-glossectomy defects?	Radial forearm free flap
325	Describe the Allen test.	The patient makes a fist and elevates the hand. The radial and ulnar arteries are compressed. The hand is then opened and should appear blanched. Pressure is released from the ulnar artery. The hand should have capillary refill and return to a normal color in 5 to 7 seconds, indicating a patent ulnar artery and palmar arches.
326	What is the vascular supply to an osteocutaneous radial forearm free flap?	Perforators from the radial artery
327	What nerves provide sensory innervation to the fasciocutaneous paddle of the osteocutaneous radial forearm free flap?	The medial and lateral antebrachial cutaneous nerves
328	What added complication can occur when using an osteocutaneous radial forearm free flap as opposed to a fasciocutaneous radial forearm free flap?	Pathologic fracture of the radius
329	What are some of the potential donor site complications of an osteocutaneous radial forearm free flap?	Incomplete skin graft take, radius fracture, hand and forearm weakness and contracture, numbness, and hematoma
330	What are some potential donor sites for osseocutaneous free tissue transfer for reconstruction of segmental mandibular defects?	Fibula, radius, scapula, iliac crest
331	Which osteocutaneous free flaps can accept dental implants?	Iliac crest and fibula. The scapula has a variable ability to accept dental implants.
332	Review relative candidacy requirements for osseointegrated dental implant placement?	Absence of poorly controlled autoimmune or small vessel disease, which could impair healing; no trismus; good tongue mobility; adequate bone stock
333	Describe the difference between *segmental* and *marginal mandibulectomy*.	In a *segmental mandibulectomy*, the entire vertical height of a portion of the mandible is removed. In a *marginal mandibulectomy*, at least 1 cm of the inferior border remains in continuity.
334	Review the general options for segmental mandibular defect reconstruction?	Reconstruction with hardware alone (large reconstruction bar for lateral defects), hardware combined with a local flap (large reconstruction bar with pectoralis muscle), hardware combined with free tissue transfer
335	What are the reconstructive goals when repairing a segmental mandibulectomy defect?	Maintenance of occlusion, restoration of bone continuity, oral competence, maintenance of facial symmetry, and ability to place a dental prosthesis
336	What are the major disadvantages to the use of a reconstruction plate alone for reconstruction of a segmental mandibulectomy defect?	Plate extrusion, plate fracture, development of mandible osteomyelitis
337	What is the vascular supply to the osteocutaneous fibular free flap?	The peroneal artery and the paired venae comitantes
338	What is the most effective test to evaluate the lower extremities for adequate vasculature prior to fibula free flap harvest?	CT angiogram with three-vessel runoff of the lower extremities. Angiography is probably the gold standard but has largely been replaced by CT angiography.
339	What are some of the potential donor site complications of an osteocutaneous fibular free flap?	Compartment syndrome, peroneal nerve weakness, hematoma, decreased range of motion, ankle instability, and foot ischemia

340	What is the vascular supply to the osteocutaneous scapular free flap?	Circumflex scapular branch of the subscapular artery
341	What are some of the potential complications of an osteocutaneous scapular free flap?	Potential donor-site complications include long thoracic nerve injury, winged scapula, upper-extremity weakness and decreased range of motion, wound dehiscence, hematoma, and seroma. Potential recipient-site defects include hematoma and flap necrosis.
342	What is the most common type of perforating vessels encountered in the anterolateral thigh free flap?	Myocutaneous perforators
343	The anterolateral thigh free flap is based on what artery?	Descending branch of the lateral femoral circumflex artery
344	The rectus abdominis free flap is based on what artery?	Deep inferior epigastric artery
345	The latissimus dorsi free flap is based on what artery?	Thoracodorsal artery from the subscapular system
346	What donor site nerve is used for neurorrhaphy when the gracilis free flap is used for facial reanimation?	The obturator nerve

Facial Reanimation

347	What are the intratemporal segments of the facial nerve?	Canalicular (within the internal auditory canal), labyrinthine, tympanic, and mastoid
348	What are the extratemporal branches of the facial nerve?	Posterior auricular nerve, nerve to the stylohyoid, nerve to the posterior belly of the digastric, temporal, zygomatic, buccal, marginal mandibular, and cervical branches
349	What is the primary blood supply to the facial nerve distal to the stylomastoid foramen?	Posterior auricular artery
350	What are some causes of facial nerve paralysis?	Ramsay Hunt syndrome, otitis media, otitis externa, mastoiditis, Lyme disease, birth injury (traumatic forceps delivery), penetrating facial trauma, cerebrovascular accident, AIDS, diabetes mellitus, Mobius syndrome, skull base fracture, acoustic neuroma, meningioma, temporal bone malignancy, parotid malignancy, iatrogenic injury (partoidectomy, mohs surgery, mastoidectomy), amyloidosis, Wegener's granulomatosis, neurosarcoidosis, multiple sclerosis, Guillain-Barre syndrome, Bell palsy (idiopathic)
351	Describe the House-Brackmann grading scale for facial paralysis.	Grade I: Normal facial function Grade II: Complete eye closure, minimal asymmetry with facial movement Grade III: Symmetry at rest, complete eye closure with effort, slight mouth asymmetry with movement Grade IV: Symmetry at rest, incomplete eye closure, obvious asymmetry with movement Grade V: Asymmetry at rest, barely perceptible movement Grade VI: No facial movement
352	What physical examination findings are associated with facial paralysis?	Brow ptosis, upper eyelid ptosis, lagophthalmos, ectropion, increased scleral show, loss of midfacial width, effacement of nasolabial fold, collapse of external nasal valve, inferior position of oral commissure, jowling, synkinesis

353	Describe the role of electroneuronography (ENoG) in preoperative evaluation of facial paralysis.	ENoG measures the motor response of facial musculature to an electrical stimulus applied to the facial nerve near the ipsilateral stylomastoid foramen. Comparison is made between the paralyzed and non-paralyzed sides of the face. If the paralyzed side shows greater than 90% degeneration relative to the non-paralyzed side, the prognosis for return of satisfactory facial nerve function is poor.
354	What surgical options exist for the correction of brow ptosis resulting from facial paralysis?	Direct brow lift, midforehead brow lift, pretrichial brow lift, endoscopic brow lift, and coronal brow lift
355	What surgical options exist for the correction of ectropion resulting from facial paralysis?	Tarsorrhaphy, lateral tarsal strip procedure, canthoplasty, canthopexy, fascia lata sling, temporalis transfer, expanded-polytetrafluoroethylene (e-PTFE) sling, suborbicularis oculi lift
356	What surgical options exist for the correction of lagophthalmos resulting from facial paralysis?	Tarsorrhaphy, gold weight placement, placement of upper eyelid spring
357	What materials can be used to perform a static facial sling?	Fascia lata, temporalis fascia, acellular human dermal allograft, e-PTFE, and permanent suture
358	What are some potential complications of static sling placement for the treatment of facial paralysis?	Stretching of graft material and loss of correction, infection, extrusion of graft, allergic reation to graft, hematoma, skin necrosis
359	Describe the technique of direct VII–XII neuro-rrhaphy with parotid release for the treatment of facial paralysis.	A mastoidectomy is performed, and the vertical segment of the facial nerve is decompressed to the stylomastoid foramen and divided just distal to the second genu. The facial nerve is then released from the fibrous attachments at the stylomastoid foramen and followed to the pes anserinus. The posterior parotid is then released from the surrounding soft tissue, providing additional length. The hypoglossal nerve is then found near the submandibular gland and direct end-to-side neurorrhaphy of the facial and hypoglossal nerve is performed.
360	Describe the technique of cross-facial nerve grafting for the treatment of facial paralysis.	Recipient nerves are identified on the paralyzed hemiface and followed back to the pes anserinus. Next, the contralateral facial nerve is identified proximally and followed out to the terminal branches. Regions with redundant innervation are selected using facial nerve stimulation to minimize donor-site morbidity. A sural nerve or great auricular nerve graft is then harvested and interposed between donor and recipient nerve endings.
361	Describe the technique for temporalis muscle sling for the treatment of facial paralysis.	A curvilinear incision is extended superiorly from the helical root into the parietal scalp. Dissection is carried down to the deep temporalis fascia and the middle third of the muscle is incised, leaving an inferior pedicle. A subcutaneous tunnel is created from the oral commissure to the temporal region. The myofascial flap is brought through the subcutaneous tunnel, and the distal ends are secured to the superior and inferior orbicularis oris.

10 Facial Trauma

Ian J. Lalich, David J. Archibald, Kyle S. Ettinger, and Eric J. Moore

Trauma Evaluation

1	What is the first step in treating every trauma patient?	Ensure the patient has a safe and adequate airway (airway, breathing, circulation, or ABCs)
2	List the contraindications to cricothyrotomy.	Contraindicatioins include cricotracheal separation, laryngeal fracture, and young age. Children younger than 5 to 12 years of age should have needle cricothyrotomy or primary tracheostomy because of anatomical differences.
3	Describe the Glasgow Coma Scale (GCS) score scoring system. (► Table 10.1)	The GCS maximum score is 15, and the minimum score is 3. The GCS is based on the cumulative score from three categories: eye opening, verbal responses, and motor responses.

Table 10.1 Glasgow Coma Scale: the final score is determined by adding the values of each behavioral response (maximum score = 15).

Behavior	Best Response	Score
Eye opening	Spontaneous	4
	To verbal command	3
	To pain	2
	None	1
Verbal response	Oriented	5
	Confused, but coherent speech	4
	Inappropriate words	3
	Incomprehensible sounds	2
	No sounds	1
Motor response	Obeys commands	6
	Purposeful movement	5
	Withdraws in response	4
	Flexion in response to pain (decorticate posturing)	3
	Extension in response to pain (decerebrate posturing)	2
	No response	1

Data from Teasdale G, Jennet B. Assessment of coma and impaired consciousness: a practical scale. Lancet. 1974 Jul 13;2 (7872):81–84.

4	What measure is a good indicator of the resuscitation status of a trauma patient with significant blood loss?	Urine output
5	Based on the physiology of a 70-kg man, roughly how much blood loss must occur before hypotension results?	1.5 to 2 L

| 6 | In an adult patient who is unsure of his or her vaccination history, what tetanus prophylaxis should be provided after a deep cut to the hand with a rusty knife? (▶ Table 10.2) | Tetanus-diphtheria and tetanus immune globulin |

Table 10.2 Tetanus prophylaxis in routine wound management (TIG = tetanus immune globulin).

Tetanus/diphtheria vaccination history	Clean Wounds		All Other Wounds	
	Give vaccine*	Give TIG	Give vaccine*	Give TIG
Unknown or < 3 doses	Yes	No	Yes	Yes
≥ 3 doses	Only if last dose was received ≥ 10 years ago	No	Only if last dose was received ≥ 5 years ago	No

* The Advisory Committee on Immunization Practices has specific recommendations on use of vaccinations: DTaP for infants and children 6 weeks up to 7 years of age (or DT pediatric if pertussis vaccine is contraindicated); Td toxoid for persons 7 through 9 years of age; and ≥ 65 years of age; Tdap for persons 10 through 64 years of age if using Adacel or 10 years of age and older if using Boostrix, unless the person has received a prior dose of Tdap.
Data from U.S. Centers for Disease Control and Prevention: Vaccine Recommendations of the Advisory Committee for Immunization Practices (ACIP).

| 7 | What radiographic examination is most helpful in evaluating maxillofacial trauma? | Dedicated axial, sagittal, and coronal maxillofacial computed tomography (CT) with fine cuts (1 to 3 mm), including bone and soft tissue windows. Head and neck CT should also be obtained if there is concern for intracranial or neck/laryngeal injury. |

Soft Tissue Trauma

8	List the bacteria commonly present in dog bites.	*Pasteurella multocida*, *Staphylococcus aureus*, *Streptococcus viridans*, and oral anaerobes
9	As a general rule, how long after initial injury can simple lacerations be closed?	Up to 3 days
10	What are the benefits of applying a negative pressure wound VAC to a partial avulsion injury?	Application of subatmospheric pressure has been shown to decrease bacterial counts, promote granulation tissue formation, and improve the rate of contracture.
11	Cleaning soft tissue injuries with hydrogen peroxide, modified Dakin's solution, or povidone-iodine has been shown (in vitro) to be toxic to what cell types?	Fibroblasts and keratinocytes
12	Pigmented debris left in a wound bed may lead to what complication?	Traumatic tattooing
13	What is the mechanism of a pincushion (trapdoor) deformity after soft tissue trauma?	• When elevated or redundant tissue abuts a curvilinear-shaped scar • Most likely results from concentric wound contracture and lymphedema
14	Why should eyebrows be trimmed conservatively (not shaved) when treating patients with extensive facial trauma?	Regrowth of eyebrow hair may take as long as 6 months, and hair regrowth may be incomplete.
15	What suture technique is best for everting skin edges when closing a soft tissue laceration?	Vertical mattress
16	As a general rule, what suture type should be used to close the epidermis of young pediatric patients?	Absorbable suture is used because permanent suture will be difficult to remove in the office setting.

17	Which wound adhesive is approved by the Food and Drug Administration (FDA) for closure of skin?	Octyl-2-cyanoacrylate (Dermabond)
18	What is the mechanism of action of the tissue adhesive octyl-2-cyanoacrylate?	On exposure to moisture, octyl-2-cyanoacrylate undergoes an exothermic reaction as it polymerizes to form a strong tissue bond.
19	How does the location of a facial laceration influence whether or not wound exploration should be carried out for facial nerve neurorrhaphy?	Because of the extensive distal arborization of the facial nerve, injuries medial to the lateral canthus are unlikely to result in significant facial nerve deficits and generally do not warrant wound exploration.
20	What is the preferred management of a traumatically avulsed segment of the proximal extratemporal facial nerve?	Mobilization with primary (end-to-end) neurorrhaphy is preferred. If a tension-free anastomosis cannot be obtained, then an interposition cable graft using greater auricular nerve or sural nerve should be used.
21	What treatment options can be used to decrease the risk of sialocele after traumatic parotid duct transection?	Options include primary anastomosis over a stent, duct ligation, or fistulization of the duct into the oral cavity.
22	What length of the lower lip can be managed with primary closure without significant distortion or microstomia?	Loss of up to one-third, or even one-half, of the lower lip can be managed with primary closure without significant distortion or resultant microstomia.
23	How much of the eyelid can be closed primarily after an avulsion injury?	25%
24	What must be done to the avulsed segment of the auricle before its burial in a postauricular pocket for delayed reconstruction?	De-epithelialization of the avulsed segment
25	What antibiotic class should be used for injuries involving cartilage?	Fluoroquinolones should be used in adult and adolescent patients to adequately cover *Pseudomonas aeruginosa*. Fluoroquinolones represent the only oral antibiotic class with reliable activity against *Pseudomonas* spp. Parenteral anti-psuedomonal cephalosporins (ceftazidime and cefepime) should be used in children if perichondritis or chondritis is suspected.
26	What is the definition of a *first-degree burn*?	Damage no deeper than the epidermis, resulting in pain and erythema, but little or no permanent injury
27	What is the definition of a *second-degree burn*?	Injury involves the epidermis and a portion of the dermis (partial thickness) and is accompanied by pain, erythema, and blistering. The depth of dermal injury is used to further stratify second-degree burns as being either *superficial* or *deep*.
28	What is the definition of a *third-degree burn*?	Injury involves the epidermis and the full thickness of the dermis, destroying adnexal structures, blood vessels, and nerve endings.
29	The head and neck make up what percentage of the total body surface area (TBSA)?	9% The "rule of nines" for calculating TBSA: • Each leg = 18% TBSA • Each arm = 9% TBSA • Anterior trunk = 18% TBSA • Posterior trunk = 18% TBSA • Head and neck = 9% TBSA
30	What is the Parkland formula for fluid resuscitation of burn victims?	Total volume is administered in the first 24 hours of resuscitation (with lactated Ringer's solution) = 4 mL x weight (kg) x %TBSA burned. Half of the calculated volume is given over the first 8 hours, and the remaining volume is delivered at an even rate over the next 16 hours.

31	In addition to IV antibiotics, why are topical antibiotics recommended to prevent superinfection in burn patients?	Burn eschar has a poor blood supply, decreasing the likelihood that therapeutic levels of systemically delivered antibiotic will penetrate the wound bed.
32	When should burns involving the oral commissure be reconstructed?	Most surgeons recommend initial observation with conservative wound care and waiting to surgically intervene only after full scar maturation.
33	What treatment should be considered for patients with oral commissure electrical burns to decrease the risk of microstomia?	Oral appliance use is designed to splint the oral commissure.

Neck, Larynx, and Trachea Trauma

34	The Battle sign refers to what physical examination finding?	Postauricular ecchymosis that suggests a basilar skull fracture
35	After a head trauma, the patient experiences massive hemorrhage from the ear canal with postauricular ecchymosis. What is the next step in this patient's treatment?	Pack the ear canal to control bleeding, and perform an arterial angiogram to examine for petrous carotid injury.
36	Subcutaneous emphysema that extends from the neck into the face travels in what plane?	Along the platysma and subcutaneous musculoaponeurotic system (SMAS)
37	Describe the anatomical boundaries of the three zones of the neck used for the evaluation and treatment of penetrating neck trauma. (▶ Fig. 10.1)	• Zone I: Clavicle and sternal notch to cricoid cartilage • Zone II: Cricoid cartilage to angle of mandible • Zone III: Angle of mandible to skull base

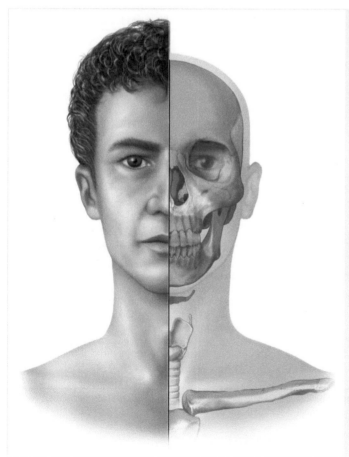

Fig. 10.1 Zones of the neck for evaluation of penetrating trauma. (Used with permission from Thieme Atlas of Anatomy: Head and Neuroanatomy, © Thieme 2007, illustration by Karl Wesker.)

38	With penetrating injuries to zone I of the neck, what structures are at risk of damage?	Aortic arch, carotid and vertebral arteries, subclavian vessels, innominate vessels, lung apices, esophagus, trachea, brachial plexus, recurrent laryngeal nerves, and thoracic duct are at risk.
39	With penetrating injuries to zone II of the neck, what structures are at risk of damage?	Common carotid artery with both internal and external branches, phrenic nerve, vagus nerve, hypoglossal nerve, internal jugular vein, larynx, hypopharynx, and proximal esophagus are at risk.
40	With penetrating injuries to zone III of the neck, what structures are at risk of damage?	Distal internal carotid artery, external carotid artery with major branches, vertebral artery, jugular vein with contributing venous drainage (retromandibular, facial, etc.), prevertebral venous plexus, parotid gland, and facial nerve are at risk.
41	Of the neck zones, which is the most surgically accessible?	Zone II
42	Describe the main factors that influence the injury incurred from ballistic strike.	Kinetic energy (KE) (velocity is more important than mass), design of projectile, composition of receiving tissue KE = $(\frac{1}{2})$ (mass) (velocity)^2
43	What commonly used radiographic technique has been shown to reduce significantly the number of negative surgical neck explorations in penetrating neck trauma?	CT angiography
44	When performing esophagography in a patient with penetrating neck trauma, why is it important to use a water-soluble contrast agent?	Extravasation of barium into the mediastinum can cause mediastinitis and fibrosis. This risk is mitigated by the use of water-soluble contrast agents (Gastrografin). However, barium is less toxic to the lungs if it is aspirated.
45	In penetrating neck trauma, which structure, if it is not violated, significantly decreases the probability of aerodigestive or vascular injury?	Platysma
46	Review the signs of carotid vascular injury after penetrating neck trauma.	Hematoma/ecchymosis, hypovolemic shock, external hemorrhage, absent carotid pulse, carotid bruit or thrill, diminished ipsilateral radial pulse, contralateral hemiparesis, and altered mental status
47	Review the signs of aerodigestive injury in penetrating neck trauma.	Dysphagia, hoarseness, subcutaneous emphysema/crepitus, hemoptysis, hematemesis, gas escape from neck wound, dyspnea, airway obstruction, and stridor
48	What are the indications for immediate surgical exploration after penetrating neck injury?	An unstable patient with significant hemorrhage, expanding hematoma, nonexpanding hematoma with hemodynamic instability, hemomediastinum, hemothorax, airway decompensation
49	What are common findings in blunt laryngeal trauma?	Subcutaneous emphysema, dysphagia, dysphonia, dyspnea, stridor, hemoptysis, neck swelling
50	Describe the Schaefer classification system of laryngeal injury.	• Group I: Minor endolaryngeal hematoma without detectable fracture • Group II: Edema, hematoma, minor mucosal disruption without exposed cartilage, nondisplaced fractures • Group III: Massive edema, mucosal disruption, exposed cartilage, vocal fold immobility, displaced fracture • Group IV: Group III with two or more fracture lines or massive trauma to laryngeal mucosa • Group V: Complete laryngotracheal separation
51	List conservative therapies that should be considered when treating a patient with a laryngeal fracture.	Voice rest, humidified blow-by, steroids, antibiotics, antireflux medications

52	Review the symptoms of laryngeal fracture.	Dysphonia, neck pain, odynophagia, dyspnea, dysphagia
53	Review the signs of laryngeal fracture.	Hemoptysis, neck tenderness, subcutaneous emphysema, anterior neck ecchymosis, laryngeal deviation, loss of laryngeal prominence, stridor
54	What is the most important imaging study for evaluating laryngeal trauma?	Fine-cut CT
55	Which age group tends to have the highest mortality after laryngeal trauma?	Patients older than 70 years of age
56	Describe the reasons why children rarely sustain laryngeal fractures.	Their larynx is situated higher in the neck and is therefore more protected by the mandible; cartilages are not ossified and therefore are more resistant to fracture.
57	Describe the mechanism of injury for laryngeal fractures.	Compression of the larynx between an intrusive object and the rigid cervical spine The degree of injury depends on the amount of compressive force and degree of cartilage ossification.
58	What is the preferred method of airway management for patients with advanced laryngeal trauma?	Awake tracheotomy in the operating room
59	List the potential pitfalls and complications associated with endotracheal intubation in patients with laryngeal trauma.	Cervical spine injuries, laryngeal lacerations and hemorrhage, displaced laryngeal architecture, and cricotracheal separation
60	Describe the steps to repair advanced laryngeal fractures.	Secure the airway with awake tracheotomy, direct laryngoscopy with rigid bronchoscopy, neck exploration, laryngotracheal/endolaryngeal repair, cartilage stabilization
61	How long are stents usually left in place after laryngeal fracture repair?	In general, 2 to 3 weeks
62	During an open laryngeal repair, a keel is useful in preventing what type of complication?	Anterior glottic web

Plating and Fixation

63	What are the general treatment goals of facial reconstruction following trauma?	Restoration of form (facial height, facial width, and facial projection) and function (airway, occlusion, mastication)
64	What must fracture fixation accomplish to allow for direct (primary) bone healing?	Fixation must overcome natural forces acting across the fracture site that would lead to mechanical instability and poor apposition of the fractured segments.
65	Name the two major types of plating materials.	• Metal • Resorbable
66	What material is most commonly used in metal plating systems?	Titanium alloy
67	How do the various trauma plate types differ?	• Alloy composition • Plate hole size • Screw head type
68	What is the importance of bone fragment contact in fracture healing?	Bone contact allows direct (primary) bone healing to occur at a fracture site. *Direct bone healing* is a combination of "contact healing" and "gap healing" in which there is no formation of an intervening callus during repair. *Indirect (secondary) bone healing* results from mechanical instability and lack of close apposition of bone segments at a fracture site. Secondary healing requires callus formation for bone healing to occur.
69	The term *miniplate* refers to what plate characteristic?	Plate thickness of 1.3 mm or less

70	What characteristic does a locking plate possess?	As the screws are tightened into the plate, the screw heads "lock" to the plate, thus stabilizing the segments without the need to compress the bone to the plate and does not require perfect contour with the underlying bone.
71	What is the purpose of a compression plate?	It enhances interfragmentary compression by drawing bone fragments together by using eccentric drill/screw placement. It should be noted that trends in fracture management are moving away from using dynamic compression plates because of the higher complication rates secondary to greater technique sensitivity.
72	What is the primary disadvantage of conventional trauma plates?	They require precise contouring of the plate to the underlying bone. If there are gaps between the plate and bone segments, tightening the screws will pull the bone segments toward the plate, which can alter reduction.
73	What is the potential disadvantage of bicortical screw placement?	Damage of deeper structures including tooth roots and underlying neurovascular structures
74	What are the two basic types of fracture fixation?	• Load-bearing: Fixation that provides sufficient strength to bear the entire physiologic load applied to the bone during function • Load-sharing: Fixation that relies on inherent bony buttressing on either side of the fracture line to share some of the load during physiologic function
75	When is load-bearing fixation necessary?	Fractures with missing fragments, comminuted fractures, and fractures with inadequate bone buttressing to allow for a load-sharing construct to be used (i.e., atrophic mandibular fractures)
76	When is load-sharing fixation used?	In simple linear fracture repair where two opposing bone fragments provide sufficient bony buttressing to allow for adequate sharing of the physiologic forces across the fracture site without leading to fracture dislocation
77	When applying a compression plate, what type of screw placement is required?	Eccentric drilling with the pilot hole away from the fracture site so that when the screws are tightened there is a vector that draws the bone fragments together
78	What are the two basic types of screws?	• Self-drilling: Possess a sharp tip and do not require a pilot hole. These screws require more force for initial placement, so they are less ideal for comminuted or very dense bone. • Self-tapping: Possess a blunt tip that requires an initial pilot hole. They do not require as much force for insertion as self-drilling screws.
79	What is an emergency screw?	An emergency screw is used when a standard screw strips (continues to turn and will not tighten). The shaft is fractions of a millimeter wider, increasing the chance of bone purchase in a hole that has previously stripped.
80	In general, what is the minimum number of screws that should be used on either side of a fracture fragment for load-sharing fixation?	At least two screws need to be used; however, three screws are desirable, particularly when using a single plate.
81	Define *rigid fixation*.	Any form of fixation that is strong enough to prevent interfragmentary motion across the fracture site when actively using the skeletal structure With true rigid fixation, direct (primary) bone healing occurs (i.e., without callus formation).

82	What are the goals of open reduction and internal rigid fixation?	• Accurate anatomical reduction • Atraumatic operative technique preserving the viability of bone and soft tissue • Rigid internal fixation that produces a mechanically stable skeletal unit allowing for early, active, and pain-free mobilization of the skeletal unit
83	Define *nonrigid fixation*.	Any form of fixation that permits interfragmentary movement Healing occurs from indirect (secondary) bone healing, which occurs via formation of a subperiosteal callus.

Mandible Fractures

84	Define *Angle class I molar occlusion*.	Mesiobuccal cusp of the maxillary first molar interdigitates with the mesiobuccal (central) groove of the mandibular first molar
85	Define the occlusal relationships of *overjet* and *overbite*.	• *Overbite* is the vertical distance that the incisal edges of the maxillary anterior teeth overlap the incisal edges of the mandibular anterior teeth in an inferosuperior direction. • *Overjet* is the horizontal distance that the incisal edges of the anterior maxillary teeth project beyond the incisal edges of the mandibular anterior teeth in an anteroposterior direction.
86	Define *crossbite*.	Under normal occlusal relationships, the maxillary dentition should be located in a position more buccal than the mandibular counterparts. For the anterior teeth (incisiors and canines), the maxillary teeth should be more anterior than the mandibular teeth. For the posterior teeth (premolars and molars), the maxillary teeth should be more lateral than the mandibular teeth. A crossbite is when these occlusal relationships are reversed.
87	Sublingual ecchymosis at the floor of the mouth after trauma usually indicates what type of injury?	Mandibular fracture
88	What nerve provides sensory innervation to the mandible?	The inferior alveolar nerve, a branch of the mandibular division of the trigeminal nerve (V3)
89	Which cranial nerve (CN) innervates the muscles of mastication?	Trigeminal nerve (CN V3)
90	List the muscles that insert into the mandible and their respective functions.	The digastric muscles and the geniohyoid extert posteroinferior pull on the mandible. The masseters, medial pterygoids, and temporalis muscles elevate the mandible. The lateral pterygoids cause translation of the condylar processes of the mandible and facilitate mandibular opening. The mylohyoid serves to elevate the tongue and floor of mouth and also has the ability to depress the mandible if the position of the hyoid is fixed.
91	Describe the embryologic development of the mandible	During the 4th week of embryologic development, the mandibular processes (first branchial arch derivatives) fuse in the midline. The mandibular processes then develop into the mandible and lower face.
92	What are the subsites of the mandible?	Symphysis, parasymphysis, body, alveolar process, angle, ramus, coronoid, and condyle
93	What are the two most common sites of mandibular fracture?	The mandibular condyle and the mandibular body

94	With respect to frequency, how common are mandible fractures compared with other facial trauma injuries?	Nasal fractures are most common, followed by mandible fractures. Mandible fractures are two to three times more common than midface fractures.
95	What constitutes a favorable or unfavorable fracture?	Fragments of the fracture are either pulled together (favorable) or apart (unfavorable) by the tension from the muscles of mastication.
96	Define the term *horizontally unfavorable* in the context of classifying mandibular fractures. (► Fig. 10.2)	A *horizontally unfavorable fracture* is one that is unable to resist the upward displacing forces on the mandible by the muscles of mastication when viewed in the horizontal plane. Muscles typically responsible for horizontally unfavorable fractures are the temporalis, masseter, and medial pterygoid.

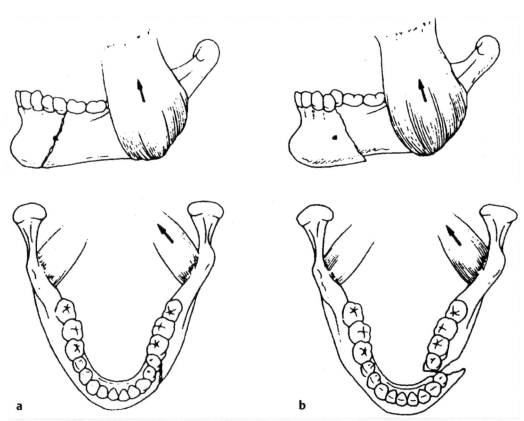

Fig. 10.2 Favorable (a) and unfavorable (b) mandibular fractures. Fragments of the fracture are either pulled together (favorable) or apart (unfavorable) by the tension from the muscles of mastication. (Used with permission from Papel ID, Frodel J, Holt GR, et al, eds. Facial Plastic and Reconstructive Surgery 3rd Edition. New York, NY: Thieme; 2009.)

| 97 | Define the term *vertically unfavorable* in the context of classifying mandibular fractures. | A *vertically unfavorable fracture* is one that is unable to resist medial displacing forces on the mandible by the muscles of mastication when viewed in a vertical plane. Muscles typically responsible for vertically unfavorable fractures are the medial pterygoids, the spurahyoid muscles, and the digastric muscles. |

98	Outline the dental classification for mandibular fractures.	• Class I: Teeth are present on both sides of the fracture line. • Class II: Teeth are present on only one side of the fracture line. • Class III: No teeth are in proximity of either side of the fracture line.
99	How would you manage a displaced fracture of the body of the mandible in a 5-year-old child?	Closed reduction with fixation using orthodontic splints
100	Review the complications associated with inter-maxillary fixation (IMF) of mandible fractures.	Dental injury, periodontal injury, potential for airway compromise, weight loss or malnutrition
101	List the contraindications to IMF.	Alcoholism, epilepsy, mental retardation, nutritional deficiency, advanced respiratory disease, psychosis, pregnancy, noncompliant patient
102	List the disadvantages of closed reduction repair of mandible fractures.	Fractures lines are not rigidly fixed, which leads to indirect (secondary) bone healing. Prolonged IMF may result in temporomandibular joint (TMJ) ankylosis, and IMF fixation renders oral hygiene and adequate oral intake difficult.
103	What are the primary reasons for pursuing early (within 24 to 36 hours) repair of mandible fractures?	Earlier return to function and to manage pain
104	Which mandible fracture has the highest incidence of infection?	Mandibular angle fractures
105	Review the primary indications for open reduction of mandible fractures.	• Unfavorable or unstable fractures • Concurrent comminuted facial fractures • Edentulous mandible with severe displacement • Delayed treatment with interposing soft tissue that prevents adequate closed reduction • Patients with contraindications to IMF
106	Describe the *Champy technique* of mandible fracture repair. (▶ Fig. 10.3)	Use of miniplate fixation in simple fractures along the ideal lines of osteosynthesis to form load-sharing or semi-rigid fixation constructs

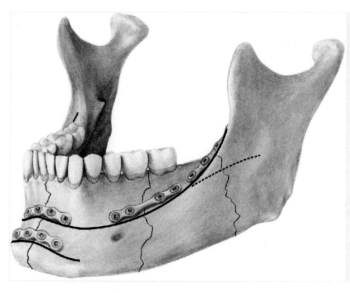

Fig. 10.3 Champy technique of plate placement along the ideal osteosynthesis lines of the mandibular body. (Used with permission from Haerle F, Champy M, Terry BC. Atlas of Craniomaxillofacial Osteosynthesis: Microplates, Miniplates, and Screws. New York, NY: Thieme; 2009.)

107	How should a lag screw be placed relative to a mandibular fracture?	Always place the lag screw perpendicular to the line of fracture to prevent fragments from overriding and displacement.
108	Review the indications for external pin-fixation repair of mandible fractures.	• Severely comminuted fractures • Pathological fractures • Grossly infected fracture sites or fractures with a high propensity for future infection (e.g., gunshot wounds) • Comminuted edentulous mandible fractures
109	Name the complications associated with open-reduction internal fixation of mandible fractures.	Osteomyelitis, plate infection/loosening/extrusion/failure, malunion, nonunion, malocclusion, trismus, scaring (external approach), paresthesia
110	What is the time period for primary bony healing to occur in facial fractures treated with open reduction and internal fixation?	Primary bony healing of repaired facial fractures takes place over 4 to 10 weeks. If healing does not take place by this time, the diagnosis of nonunion can be suspected.
111	What are the radiographic characteristics of nonunion (mandibular fractures) on panoramic X-ray?	• Sclerotic bone margins • Osteolytic changes within the bone adjacent to the fracture site • A persistent radiolucent gap where bone has not bridged the fracture site
112	What factors contribute to nonunion after mandible fracture repair?	• Inadequate immobilization • Incomplete reduction • Infection • Poor blood supply • Nutritional or metabolic alterations
113	What structure protects the coronoid process of the mandible when in occlusion?	The zygomatic arch
114	What muscular force tends to distract high condylar fractures out of alignment?	Medial displacement of the condyle by the pull of the lateral pterygoid muscle
115	Review the absolute indications for open reduction of condylar neck fractures.	Invasion of joint by foreign body Lateral extracapsular displacement Inability to achieve occlusion with closed reduction Involvement of the middle cranial fossa or external auditory canal
116	What is the most common subunit location of condylar process fractures?	Subcondylar > condylar neck > condylar head (intracapsular)
117	What is the immediate concern with bilateral condylar process fractures?	Airway compromise
118	Review the primary reasons to consider tooth extraction during repair of mandible fractures.	Evidence of periapical or gross periodontal infection, tooth preventing fracture reduction, root fracture, exposure of root apex after fracture reduction, teeth without adequate bone support, partially erupted third molars with evidence of active pericornitis

Maxillary Fractures

119	What is the definition of periodontal concussion?	Injury to the periodontium resulting in sensitivity to percussion without loosening or displacement of the tooth
120	What is the definition of *periodontal subluxation?*	Injury to the periodontium resulting in loosening of the tooth without tooth displacement
121	What is the definition of *periodontal luxation?*	Injury to the supporting structures of a tooth resulting in loosening and clinical or radiographic displacement Luxation can be extrusive, intrusive, mesial, distal, buccal, or lingual.

122	What is the most commonly avulsed tooth?	Maxillary central incisor due to its vulnerability as the most anteriorly positioned tooth in either arch (presuming a normal occlusal relationship)
123	What physiologically compatible solutions are best for storing avulsed teeth?	Hank's balance salt solution, ViaSpan, milk, saliva, saline
124	What arteries contribute to the primary blood supply of the maxilla?	• Internal maxillary artery • Ascending pharyngeal artery • Ascending palatine branch of the facial artery
125	What is the most common complication associated with maxillary fractures?	Hemorrhage, which may be self-limiting but may require nasal packing for control
126	What test should be performed in a patient who develops delayed intermittent epistaxis following severe midface trauma?	Angiography to evaluate for aneurysms or pseudoaneurysms that can result in immediate or delayed postoperative bleeding
127	Describe a *Le Fort I fracture*. (▶ Fig. 10.4)	A Le Fort I fracture is a horizontal fracture of the maxilla extending through the nasal septum, lateral nasal walls, lateral maxillary sinus walls, extending posteriorly to the pterygomaxillary junction. The fracture involves the nasomaxillary, zygomaticomaxillary, and pterygomaxillary vertical buttresses of the face.

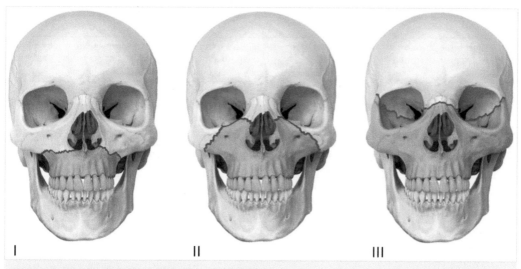

Fig. 10.4 LeFort classification of midfacial fractures. (Used with permission from Thieme Atlas of Anatomy: Head and Neuroanatomy, © Thieme 2007, illustration by Karl Wesker.)

128	Describe a *Le Fort II fracture*.	A *Le Fort II fracture* is a pryramidal fracture involving the nasofrontal suture, medial and inferior orbital walls, zygomaticomaxillary suture, lateral maxillary sinus walls, and the pterygomaxillary junction.
129	Describe a *Le Fort III fracture*.	A *Le Fort III fracture* is a craniofacial dysjunction; the fracture passes through the nasofrontal suture, frontal process of the maxilla, lacrimal bones, ethmoid sinus, and lamina papyracea. It then extends across the orbital floor to the inferior orbital fissure. From this point, it extends in three directions: across the lateral orbital wall through the zygomaticofrontal suture, through the zygomatic arch, and through the pterygoid plates.

130	Describe a *palatal split fracture*.	A *palatal split fracture* begins anteriorly at the anterior pyriform aperture and extends posteriorly to the posterior aspect of the hard palate. Palatal fractures are more likely to manifest as true sagittal palatal split fractures in pediatric patients because of an unfused midpalatal suture. Para-sagittal palatal fractures are more common in adults because this is the area where the palatal bone is the thinnest.
131	What is a *Gunning splint*?	A *Gunning splint* is a plate fabricated to the existing edentulous ridge with arch bars or suspension brackets used to establish intermaxillary fixation in edentulous or partially edentulous patients.
132	In complicated palatal fractures with bone loss or severe comminution, what can be used to maintain the palatal arch?	Dental splints created from premorbid impressions or dentures (in edentulous patients)
133	What structures make up the vertical buttresses of the midface?	• Three paired buttresses: Zygomaticomaxillary (lateral), nasomaxillary (medial), pterygomaxillary (posterior) • Single unpaired structure: Septovomerian buttress (midline)
134	What structures constitute the horizontal buttresses of the midface?	• Frontal buttress: Supraorbital rims • Zygomatic buttress: Infraorbital rims, body of the zygoma, and zygomatic arch • Maxillary buttress: Maxillary alveolus and palatine processes
135	What is the characteristic deformity associated with a midface fracture?	Midface retrusion and an anterior open bite resulting from the posterior and inferior traction of the medial and lateral pterygoids on the mobile maxillary fragment
136	How do you reduce an impacted maxilla after a midface fracture?	Early reduction may be performed using a Rowe or Hayton-Williams forceps. Delayed repair is more likely to require osteotomies and surgical down-fracture.

Nasal, Frontal, and Naso-Orbito-Ethmoidal Fractures

137	Why is nasal packing generally contraindicated in treating nasal bone fractures in young children?	Young infants are obligate nose breathers.
138	What landmark demarcates the transition point between the thicker nasal bone superiorly and the thinner bone inferiorly?	Intercanthal line Most nasal bone fractures occur below this level.
139	What role does age play in the pathophysiology of nasal trauma?	Younger patients are more likely to sustain cartilaginous injuries and greenstick fractures because of the greater proportion of nasal cartilage and incomplete ossification of nasal bones. Older patients generally have greater degrees of comminution.
140	What is the most common cause of facial fractures in children over the age of 5 years?	Motor-vehicle accident
141	What are the complications associated with failure to identify a septal fracture when evaluating a patient with nasal bone fractures?	Decreased projection, septal deviation, septal hematoma
142	What other associated injuries may occur with nasal bone fractures?	Epiphora, fractures of the lacrimal bones and ethmoid complex, widening of intercanthal distance (NOE fracture), malocclusion and open bite deformity (Le Fort fracture), frontal sinus fracture, cribriform plate fracture, dural tears leading to pneumocephalus and CSF rhinorrhea

143	In addition to a history and physical examination, what other social history should be obtained in patients who sustain a blunt facial trauma?	Is the patient a victim of domestic abuse? About 30% to 60% of women with facial trauma from assault are victims of domestic violence.
144	What are the potential causes of hyposmia after nasal bone fractures?	• Nasal obstruction secondary to edema, septal dislocation, epistaxis, brain contusion or shearing of olfactory filaments • Up to two-thirds of patients with severe head trauma experience some degree of olfactory dysfunction.
145	What effect does telescoping of the bony or cartilaginous fragments after nasal bone fracture have on the nasolabial angle?	It increases the nasolabial angle.
146	Regardless of trauma history, what percentage of patients will have a clinically apparent septal deviation on nasal examination?	Approximately 80%
147	Why is it difficult to distinguish old fractures from new ones on plain films?	Only 15% of nasal bone fractures heal by ossification.
148	When is the optimal window of time to perform closed reduction of a nasal bone fracture?	If it is not performed immediately after the injury (before edema occurs), then it is best to wait 2-10 days after the injury to allow swelling to subside. The development of fibrous connective tissue within the fracture decreases the likelihood of optimal fracture reduction. This occurs 10 to 14 days after the injury.
149	What is the mechanism of septal perforation after a hematoma?	Septal cartilage receives its vascular supply from the mucoperichondrium. Septal hematoma results in subperichondrial dissection, which deprives the cartilage of blood supply and results in ischemic necrosis.
150	Describe the potential complications of infected septal hematoma (abscess).	Necrosis and subsequent perforation, contiguous spread or retrograde thrombophlebitis leading to osteomyelitis, orbital and intracranial abscess, meningitis, and cavernous sinus thrombosis
151	What is the gold standard for establishing the diagnosis of CSF leak?	β2-transferrin
152	What is the natural history of most CSF leaks after nasal trauma?	More than 50% resolve spontaneously within 1 to 2 weeks with conservative management, including bed rest, head elevation, and stool softeners to reduce strenuous valsalva. Coughing, sneezing, and nose blowing should be avoided.
153	What can be instilled into the frontal sinus to assess patency of the nasofrontal recess?	Methylene-blue or fluorescein
154	What is an alternative to open reduction and internal fixation of moderately displaced anterior table frontal sinus fractures?	Endoscopic reduction with miniplate fixation or fracture camouflage with porous polyethylene sheets (MEDPOR, Porex Surgical, Inc., Newnan, GA) or hydroxyapatite placement
155	Anterior frontal sinus wall fractures are typically not aesthetically noticeable if they are displaced less than _____?	2 mm
156	When performing open-reduction internal fixation of a frontal sinus fracture via a coronal approach, it is important to preserve a vascularized pericranial flap because it might be used for what purpose, if necessary?	For dural repair, as a tissue filler for frontal sinus obliteration and as a tissue barrier for isolation of the neurocranium from the nasophyarynx during frontal sinus cranialization

157	The blood supply to the pericranium comes from what three sources?	Vessels arising from the underlying cranial bones, deep branches of the superficial temporal, supratrochlear, and supraorbital vessels, and interconnecting vessels arising from superficial branches
158	What percentage of patients with a nondisplaced posterior table frontal sinus fracture with a confirmed CSF leak will have the leak resolve spontaneously with observation?	50%
159	Moderate to severe comminution involving greater than 25% of the posterior table is generally considered an indication for what type of repair?	Frontal sinus cranialization, particularly if there is comminution of the floor of the sinus.
160	What are the treatment options for traumatic nasofrontal recess injury?	For mild injuries, endoscopic surgical exploration or observing for the development of frontal sinusitis and/or mucocele can be considered. For severe injury, frontal sinus obliteration should be considered.
161	As a general rule, why are displaced fractures of the posterior table of the frontal sinus explored?	Depressed fragments may cause intracranial hemorrhage or CSF leak, and there is possibility of mucocele formation.
162	Why is it necessary to remove all the mucosa of the frontal sinus before adipose tissue obliteration when treating severe frontal sinus fractures?	To decrease risk of mucocele/pylocele formation
163	What are the potential sequelae of trauma-related frontal sinus mucoceles?	Secondary mucoceles may enlarge and erode bone with invasion of the orbit or intracranial space. If the mucoid contents of the mucocele become infected (mucopyocele), orbital abscess, osteomyelitis of the frontal bone, epidural abscess, meningitis, or brain abscess may occur.
164	What are the primary vertical and horizontal buttresses of the NOE complex?	• Vertical: Frontal process of the maxillary bone • Horizontal: Superior and inferior orbital rims
165	What is a normal intercanthal distance?	Approximately 30 to 35 mm or one-half the interpupillary distance or the width of the alar base
166	What are the typical facial deformities seen in patients with acute NOE fractures?	Nasal dorsum flattening, traumatic telecanthus, increased nasal tip rotation, and decreased nasal projection
167	What is the best management of epiphora in a patient with an obstruction distal to the common canaliculus of the lacrimal drainage system?	Endoscopic dacryocystorhinostomy
168	Describe the classification system of NOE fractures. (▶ Fig. 10.5)	Markowitz classification: • Type 1: A single, noncomminuted central fragment without medial canthal tendon (MCT) disruption. • Type 2 fractures: Comminution of the central fragment, but the MCT remains attached to a definable segment of bone. • Type 3 fractures: Severe central fragment comminution with disruption of the MCT insertion

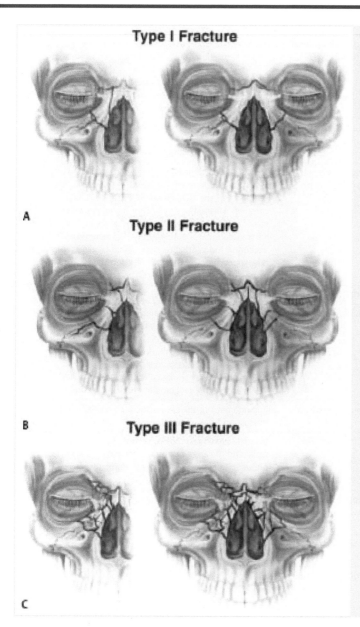

Type I Fracture

A

Type II Fracture

B

Type III Fracture

C

Fig. 10.5 Markowitz classification of naso-orbito-ethmoid complex fractures. (Used with permission from Papel ID, Frodel J, Holt GR, et al, eds. Facial Plastic and Reconstructive Surgery 3rd Edition. New York, NY: Thieme; 2009.)

---

169   Describe the treatment of type 1 NOE fractures.

- *Nondisplaced fractures* without an increase in intercanthal distance may be observed; however, development of delayed telecanthus may still occur.
- *Displaced fractures* require open reduction and internal fixation, which can be accomplished via coronal, transconjunctival, sublabial, or external eyelid approaches. Existing lacerations may also be used. Because type 1 fractures are noncomminuted by definition, one-, two-, or three-point fixation can often be utilized. Three-point fixation will require plating at the nasofrontal, nasomaxillary, and infraorbital buttresses. Often, for type I NOE fractures, a coronal approach is not necessary to obtain adequate exposure.

170	What is a common complication of malpositioned transnasal wire placement when treating NOE fractures?	Placement of transnasal wires anterior to the lacrimal fossa results in rotation of the central fragment laterally, resulting in iatrogenic telecanthus. The wires should be placed posterior and superior to the lacrimal fossa. Wire placement should also be placed below the frontoethmoid suture line to avoid intracranial injury.
171	What examination findings are characteristic for avulsion of the medial canthal tendon?	• Absent bowstring sign • Proptosis • Rounding of the medial canthal angle
172	Describe the technique of transnasal canthopexy for repair of an avulsed medial canthal tendon.	Transnasal canthopexy is typically accomplished after open reduction and internal fixation of the fractured bony segments of the NOE complex. The medial canthopexy is completed using the wire anchor technique with or without use of a transcaruncular barb. Canthal dissection is required if a transcaruncular barb is not used. Once secured, the wire anchoring the canthal tendon should be directed posteriorly, superiorly, and medially and secured to a titanium plate along the medial wall of the orbit.

Zygomaticomaxillary Complex and Orbital Fractures

173	A ZMC ("tripod") fracture involves which structures?	Tripod fracture is a misnomer because a ZMC fracture involves four sites (tetrapod fracture is a more accurate description): • Temporal bone (zygomaticotemporal suture) • Maxilla (zygomaticomaxillary suture) • Frontal bone (zygomaticofrontal suture) • Sphenoid bone (zygomaticosphenoid suture)
174	In ZMC fractures, what usually causes restricted mandibular opening?	Impingement of the zygomatic arch on the coronoid process and temporalis muscle
175	List surgical complications associated with ZMC fracture repair.	Lid malposition (ectropion, entropion), persistent diplopia, facial and malar asymmetry, plate palpability, malunion/nonunion, enophthalmos, cheek numbness (V2), and blindness (extremely rare)
176	What approaches are the most appropriate for an isolated zygomatic arch fracture with no comminution?	Gilles approach or Keen approach
177	What is the most prominent portion of the ZMC, and where is it located?	Malar eminence located 2 cm inferior to the lateral canthus

178	Describe the Zingg classification of ZMC fractures.	• Type A: Isolated to one segment of the ZMC
		  ○ A1: Zygomatic arch
		  ○ A2: Lateral orbital wall
		  ○ A3: Inferior orbital rim
		• Type B: Classic tetrapod fracture involving all four processes of the zygoma
		• Type C: Complex fracture with comminution of zygomatic bone

179	Name the weakest bone involved in the ZMC fracture.	Orbital floor
180	Rotation of the ZMC is due primarily to the pull of which muscle?	The masseter muscle
181	What is the gender distribution of ZMC fractures?	Male-to-female: 80%:20%
182	Name the common approaches to the zygomaticofrontal buttress.	• Lateral brow incision • Upper blepharoplasty incision • Hemicoronal incision • Existing lacerations

183	What contraindications exist for the immediate repair of orbital floor fractures?	• Globe rupture • Hyphema • Retinal detachment • Traumatic optic neuropathy • Involvement of the patient's only seeing eye (relative contraindication)
184	What physical examination findings would necessitate urgent surgical intervention of an orbital floor fracture?	Muscular entrapment (particularly in children), soft tissue herniation with nonresolving oculocardiac reflex, significant soft tissue emphysema leading to increased intraocular pressure, and visual impairment
185	How should traumatic retrobulbar hematoma with vision loss initially be managed?	Lateral canthotomy and inferior cantholysis
186	What pharmacologic agents can be used to help manage high intraocular pressure?	IV mannitol, acetazolamide, corticosteroids, ophthalmic β-blockers, ophthalmic α-agonists, cholinergic medications
187	What are common findings associated with retrobulbar hematoma?	Eye pain, proptosis, chemosis, diplopia, increased intraocular pressure, tense globe, decreasing visual acuity, loss of direct pupillary light reflex and ophthalmoplegia, papilledema
188	What is the gold standard for diagnosis of inferior rectus or oblique muscle entrapment after orbital floor fracture?	Forced duction test
189	What is the gold standard test to confirm carotid-cavernous fistula after orbital trauma?	Angiogram
190	Describe the hydraulic and buckling theories with respect to the pathogenesis of orbital floor fractures.	• *Buckling theory*: Fracture occurs as result of transmission of force directly to the orbital floor via the orbital rim. • *Hydraulic theory*: Fracture occurs due to transfer of kinetic energy to the orbital floor via the noncompressible orbital soft tissue.
191	V2 division trigeminal nerve paresthesia is a common finding in which type of facial fracture?	Orbital floor fractures
192	What is the most common complication of orbital floor fracture repair?	Inferior orbital nerve injury
193	Approximately what percentage of the orbital floor must be involved for enophthalmos to occur after orbital floor fracture?	More than 50%
194	Name the structures that pass through the superior orbital fissure.	Oculomotor nerve (III), trochlear nerve (IV), abducens nerve (VI), V1 divisions of the trigeminal nerve, ophthalmic vein
195	Describe the signs and the treatment of traumatic optic neuropathy.	• *Marcus Gunn pupil* (relative afferent pupillary defect), central scotoma, and decreased visual acuity • Steroids and/or surgical decompression is sometimes used, but a high rate of spontaneous recovery may obviate the need for intervention.
196	In the setting of traumatic optic neuropathy from orbital fracture, what fracture type is more favorable for visual recovery?	Absence of fracture (most favorable) > anterior orbital fracture > posterior orbital fracture (least favorable)
197	Describe common findings associated with *orbital apex syndrome*.	Ophthalmoplegia from damage to the oculomotor, trochlear, and/or abducens nerves (CN III, IV, and VI), mydriasis from damage to oculomotor nerve (CN III), pain/anesthesia of the eye and forehead from damage to the ophthalmic branch of the trigeminal nerve (V1), and decreased visual acuity from optic nerve dysfunction (CN II)

198	What is the *orbital septum*?	An extension of the periosteum at the orbital rim that forms the anteriormost border of the orbital contents. It blends with the levator palpebrae superioris in the upper lid, and the tarsal plate in the lower lid.
199	Describe common approaches to the inferior orbital rim and orbital floor. (▶ Fig. 10.6)	• *Transconjunctival approach*: An incision inferior to the tarsal plate for preseptal approach and incision just anterior to the fornix for postseptal approach. Carries risk for entropion • *Subciliary (blepharoplasty) approach*: An incision 1 to 2 mm below the gray line of the lower eyelid, high risk of ectropion, and greater technical difficulty • *Subtarsal/mid-eyelid approach*: Straightforward approach, direct access to floor, carries risk of ectropion, and has a visible scar • *Infraorbital approach*: Straightforward approach, most visible scar, associated with greater postoperative edema, and carries risk of ectropion. For the aforementioned reasons, the infraorbital approach has fallen out of favor compared with the first three orbital approaches unless an existing laceration is already present in this area.

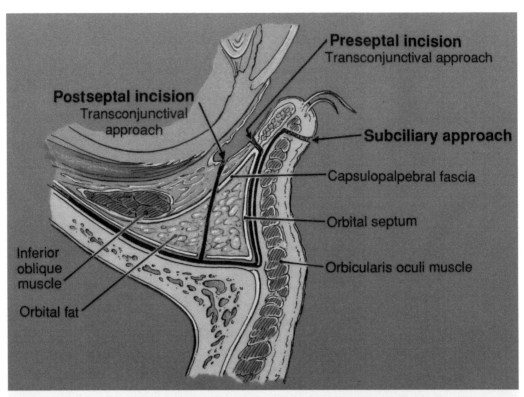

Fig. 10.6 Sagittal cross section of the lower eyelid demonstrating common surgical approaches to the inferior orbital rim and orbital floor. (Used with permission from Strong EB, Sykes JM. Zygoma complex fractures. Facial Plast Surg 1998;14(1):109, figure 7.)

11 Salivary Gland Disorders

Brian C. Gross, Amy C. Dearking, Brandon W. Peck, and Daniel L. Price

Overview

1	During what week of embryogenesis does the parotid gland develop?	The 7th embryonic week
2	Where does the parotid gland originate during development, and what is its relationship to the facial nerve?	The parotid gland originates at the site of the eventual duct orifice and grows in a posterior direction. The facial nerve develops in an anterior direction. The facial nerve eventually becomes surrounded by parotid gland tissue.
3	What are the different types of acini in the salivary glands?	There are three types: *serous acini* are found in the parotid, *mucous acini* in the sublingual and minor salivary glands, and *mixed acini*, which are found in the submandibular gland.
4	Describe the salivary gland duct system. (▶ Fig. 11.1)	An *acinus* is the main secretory component that is composed of a central lumen surrounded by acinar cells that produce saliva. Intercalated ducts form early connections between acini. Both acini and intercalated ducts are lined with myoepithelial cells that help to contract and propel saliva forward. Intercalated ducts feed into larger striated ducts and then into excretory ducts.

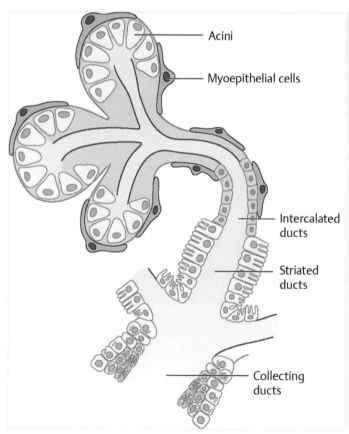

Acini

Myoepithelial cells

Intercalated ducts

Striated ducts

Collecting ducts

Fig. 11.1 Components of the salivary gland ductal system. (Used with permission from Bradley PJ, Guntinas-Lichius O, eds. Salivary Gland Disorders and Diseases: Diagnosis and Management. New York, NY: Thieme; 2011.)

5	What is the relationship of lymph nodes to the salivary glands?	Lymph nodes develop within the pseudocapsule of the parotid gland, leading to intraparotid lymph nodes. No other salivary gland has intraglandular lymph nodes.
6	Where are intraparotid lymph nodes typically located?	The parotid gland is the only salivary gland with lymph nodes actually within the gland. Most intraparotid lymph nodes lie within the superficial lobe, although they are present in both the superficial and deep lobes.
7	Describe the path of the Stenson duct (parotid duct).	It originates from superficial portion of parotid gland, travels anteriorly on the masseter muscle and buccinator fat pad, and then travels medially to pierce the buccinator muscle. The duct empties lateral to the second maxillary molar.
8	Where does the Wharton duct (submandibular duct) empty into the oral cavity?	The submandibular duct empties just lateral to the lingual frenulum.
9	What fascial layer forms the parotid fascia?	The parotid fascia is continuous with the superficial layer of the deep cervical fascia.
10	Describe the fascial connections of the superficial musculosaponeurotic system (SMAS) and its relationship to the parotid gland.	The SMAS gives support to the many muscles of facial expression. Over the parotid gland, it is located just superficial to the parotid fascia.
11	What is the autonomic nerve supply of the parotid glands?	The parasympathetic nervous system supplies the parotid gland via the glossopharyngeal nerve (cranial nerve IX). The sympathetic nervous system supplies the gland via the superior cervical ganglion.
12	Describe the path of the parasympathetic innervation of the parotid gland. (▶ Fig. 11.2)	Parasympathetics that are part of the glossopharyngeal nerve (tympanic branch) enter the middle ear through the tympanic canaliculus as the Jacobson nerve. They then exit the middle ear cavity and travel through the middle cranial fossa as the lesser petrosal nerve. The lesser petrosal nerve exits the skull base through the foramen ovale and travels to the otic ganglion. After synapsing in the otic ganglion, postsynaptic fibers are carried via the auriculotemporal nerve to the parotid gland.

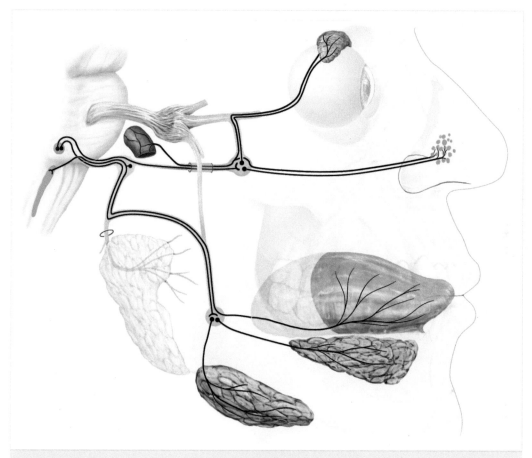

Fig. 11.2 Parasympathetic innervation of the major salivary glands. (Used with permission from Thieme Atlas of Anatomy: Head and Neuroanatomy, © Thieme 2007, illustration by Karl Wesker.)

13	Define *accessory parotid gland tissue.*	Accessory parotid tissue lies anterior to the main parotid gland between the skin and the masseter muscle.
14	What are important anatomical landmarks for identification of the facial nerve during parotidectomy?	The facial nerve can be located via its relationships to the tragal pointer, tympanomastoid suture line, and the attachment of posterior digastric muscle to digastric groove, or it can be identified distally and dissected in a retrograde fashion or drilled out from the mastoid bone and traced anterograde.
15	How does the parotid gland change histologically with age?	There is an increase in adipose cells in the parotid parenchyma with age.
16	In which anatomical triangle is the submandibular gland located, and what are its boundaries?	The submandibular triangle: its boundaries are the anterior and posterior bellies of the digastric muscle and the inferior aspect of the mandible.
17	What nerve carries the parasympathetic supply to the submandibular gland?	The chorda tympani carries parasympathetic fibers to the submandibular and sublingual glands via the lingual nerve.
18	Secretomotor function of the submandibular and sublingual glands is controlled by which nerve?	Parasympathetic contribution of facial nerve (nervus intermedius) via the chorda tympani

19	Where is the lingual nerve found during a submandibular gland excision?	The lingual nerve is found deep to the submandibular gland. With inferior retraction of the gland and anterior retraction of the mylohyoid muscle, the lingual nerve and the submandibular ganglion can be exposed.
20	What is the relationship of the lingual nerve to the submandibular duct in the floor of mouth? (▶ Fig. 11.3)	The lingual nerve courses from a posterolateral to anteromedial position, passing below the Wharton duct.

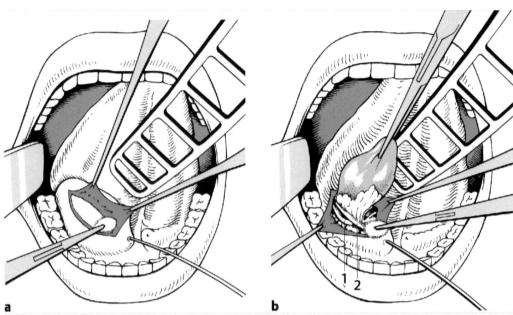

Fig. 11.3 (a) Transoral excision of a right floor of mouth ranula (b) demonstrating the course of the (1) lingual nerve traveling from a posterolateral to anteromedial position, passing below (2) Wharton duct. (Used with permission from Theissing J, Rettinger G, Werner JA. ENT–Head and Neck Surgery: Essential Procedures. New York, NY: Thieme; 2011.)

21	Where are the facial artery and vein found in relation to the submandibular gland?	The facial vein is found on the lateral surface of the submandibular gland; the facial artery is located on the posterior surface of the gland and is often ligated on both the superior and inferior aspect of the gland during submandibular gland excision.
22	Name the ducts through which the sublingual gland drains.	The sublingual gland drains into the mouth via the smaller duct of Rivinus (which empties into the floor of the mouth or into submandibular duct) and larger duct of Bartholin (empties into submandibular duct).
23	What structures border the sublingual gland?	The sublingual gland is bordered by the mandible, genioglossus muscle, and mylohyoid muscle.
24	What structures are important to be aware of during excision of the sublingual gland?	The lingual nerve and Wharton (submandibular) duct run between the sublingual gland and the genioglossus muscle.
25	Where are most minor salivary glands located?	The hard palate mucosa harbors most of the mouth's minor salivary glands.
26	What are the functions of saliva?	There are many functions of saliva, the most important being lubrication of food, buffering and prevention of caries, mineralization of teeth, antibacterial and bactericidal function, digestion, and taste.

27	List the order of salivary gland saliva production from most serous to most viscous.	In order from most serous to most viscous: parotid gland > submandibular gland > sublingual gland > minor salivary glands
28	What are the important physical examination findings to assess when evaluating a salivary gland mass?	One should appreciate the size of the mass, invasion of overlying skin, mobility versus fixation, tenderness to palpation, facial nerve function, trismus, pharyngeal fullness, and whether there is evidence of a primary skin or scalp lesion.
29	Typically, how large must a parapharyngeal mass be to visualize it intraorally?	Usually, a parapharyngeal mass must be at least 3.5 cm to visualize it intraorally.
30	Name the key surgical landmarks associated with the location of the facial nerve during parotidectomy?	• The facial nerve lies 1 to 1.5 cm deep and inferior to the tragal pointer. • The attachment of the posterior belly of the digastric muscle to the digastric ridge identifies the plane of nerve. • The nerve lies 6 to 8 mm deep to the tympanomastoid suture.
31	What is the pathophysiology of Frey syndrome after parotidectomy?	Postganglionic parasympathetic secretomotor fibers carried on the auriculotemporal nerve, which normally innervate the parotid gland tissue, aberrantly reinnervate sweat glands of the overlying skin.
32	Name an objective test for Frey syndrome.	The Minor starch-iodine test is an objective measure of gustatory sweating. The preauricular region is coated with iodine, allowed to dry, and then dusted with starch. The patient is then given a sialagogue, and a positive test (indicating Frey syndrome) results in dark blue spots where sweat has dissolved the starch and reacted with iodine.
33	What are the treatment options for Frey syndrome?	Treatment options are broad and depend on the patient's discomfort level. Options range from observation and use of antiperspirant, to medications such as glycopyrrolate, or more invasive therapy such as botulinum toxin injection or tympanic neurectomy.
34	What techniques can be used to reduce post-parotidectomy gustatory sweating?	The most important surgical techniques to prevent Frey syndrome are raising a thick skin flap and doing only a partial superficial parotidectomy.
35	What additional techniques are being used to try to reduce post parotidectomy gustatory sweating?	Rotational sternocleidomastoid flaps, fat transfer, Alloderm implants, and superficial musculoaponeurotic system interposition are all being used.

Benign Disorders

36	Which salivary gland is most susceptible to acute bacterial sialadenitis?	The parotid gland
37	Which population groups are most commonly affected by acute suppurative sialadenitis?	Patients who are medically debilitated, postoperative, and/or patients with severe dehydration
38	Which surgical patients are most commonly affected by acute suppurative sialadenitis?	Patients who have undergone major abdominal surgery and hip replacement/repair, likely a result of poor oral intake attributable to their debilitated state, are most commonly affected.
39	Why does the saliva produced by the parotid gland make this gland more prone to sialadenitis compared with the submandibular and sublingual glands?	Parotid saliva is mostly serous compared with the mucinous saliva produced by the submandibular and sublingual glands. Serous saliva lacks antibodies, acid, and enzymes with antimicrobial properties.
40	In hospitalized patients, what is the most commonly cultured organism in acute suppurative sialadenitis?	*Staphylococcus aureus*

41	When is imaging of acute suppurative parotitis recommended?	Imaging is indicated after failure to respond to antibiotics or if signs, symptoms, and physical examination raise concern for a parotid abscess.
42	What is the best initial treatment of acute suppurative sialadenitis?	Empiric antibiotics with both aerobic and anaerobic coverage, sialagogues, warm compresses, parotid massage, pain medication, and rehydration
43	What is the recommended treatment of a parotid abscess?	Surgical drainage through a standard parotidectomy exposure is recommended. When making incisions in the parotid fascia, it should be done parallel to facial nerve branches to minimize risk of damage to the nerve.
44	What is the most common symptom that raises concern for sialolithiasis?	Pain and swelling of the salivary glands, especially associated with eating
45	Which salivary gland carries the highest risk for salivary calculi formation?	The submandibular gland is the most common location of salivary calculi as a result of increased calcium concentration, higher pH, more mucinous saliva, and potential anatomical factors (e.g., length, gravity).
46	What imaging options are available for diagnosis of sialolithiasis?	There are many choices. Plain X-ray offers little extra information other than the presence of a radiopaque stone. Sialography can give information on strictures, dilations, or filling defects of the ductwork. Ultrasound can be done if a radiolucent stone is suspected. CT often offers the most complete information.
47	Which salivary calculi are most often radiopaque on standard X-ray?	Submandibular stones. 80% of parotid stones are radiolucent.
48	What are the treatment options for sialolithiasis?	Conservative treatment is a valid option. This includes sialagogues, heat, massage, and increased hydration. For larger stones that will not pass with conservative measures, bedside sialotomy, sialendoscopy, or lithotripsy are options. Gland excision is final treatment option for refractory disease.
49	What is the number one cause of chronic sialadenitis?	Parotid duct obstruction secondary to sialolithiasis
50	What is the best treatment for chronic sialadenitis?	No treatment is consistently successful. Antibiotics, massage, warm compresses, and sialagogues may be tried. Ultimately, if conservative measures fail, the affected gland should be surgically resected.
51	Patients with chronic sialadenitis should be monitored for what serious condition?	Patients with chronic sialadenitis are at an increased risk for salivary duct carcinoma.
52	When should sialorrhea be managed as an abnormal condition in the pediatric population?	Sialorrhea is associated with the balance of oral control of secretions and swallowing. Up until about 18 months of age, sialorrhea is a normal event because of poor neuromuscular control. If it is still present by 4 years of age, a patient should undergo further workup.
53	What other medical conditions are associated with sialorrhea?	Conditions associated with poor neuromuscular control, which cause difficulty swallowing secretions, can be associated with sialorrhea, most commonly in children with cerebral palsy. It is also seen in adults with amyotrophic lateral sclerosis, Parkinson disease, and history of stroke.
54	How can sialorrhea be treated medically?	Anticholinergics such as oral glycopyrrolate and topical scopolamine can be helpful with careful consideration of the many side effects of these medications. Botulinum injections of the salivary glands are also used but require repeated injections.

55	Describe the side effects of anticholinergic medications.	Urinary retention, increased body temperature/decreased perspiration, tachycardia, xerostomia (increased risk of dental caries), vision changes, confusion, respiratory suppression, mydriasis, and constipation are all common side effects of anticholinergics.
56	What are the surgical options for treatment of sialorrhea?	Removal of salivary tissue can be done via bilateral submandibular gland excision and parotid duct ligation. Transection of the chorda tympani can also decrease salivary output. The submandibular and parotid ducts can be rerouted to decrease output into the oral cavity.
57	Define the difference between *sialorrhea* and *ptyalism*.	These terms are often used interchangeably. By strict definition, though, *sialorrhea* means excessive flow of saliva. Usually, it is secondary to administration of medications such as antipsychotics, anticonvulsants, anticholinesterases, or other parasympathomimetic medications. Excessive flow can also be related to medical conditions such as pregnancy, gastroesophageal reflux disease, and oral ulceration/irritation. *Ptyalism* is the act of drooling and the excessive production of saliva. Historically, it is most commonly used in pregnancy as *ptyalism of pregnancy*.
58	What is the most common cause of xerostomia?	By far, the most common cause is medication side effect.
59	What is one of the most important preventative treatments to reduce complications of xerostomia from head and neck radiation?	Topical fluoride and excellent oral hygiene are used to prevent the formation of dental caries because saliva is protective of the teeth.
60	What drug is used to treat xerostomia?	Pilocarpine, a parasympathomimetic drug that acts on the M3 acetylcholine muscarinic receptor
61	Describe the three stages of radiation-induced sialadenitis.	• Stage 1: Acute response of salivary glands to lower dose (20 to 30 Gy). Self-resolution is expected. • Stage 2: Functional loss of glandular tissue with higher doses (up to 75 Gy). Nonrestorative. • Stage 3: Chronic changes with high-dose radiation (> 75 Gy). Cirrhotic changes with complete glandular atrophy. Nonrestorative.
62	Describe *Mikulicz syndrome*.	*Mikulicz syndrome* involves bilateral salivary gland swelling that is not associated with another systemic disease. Specifically, it is distinct from salivary swelling associated with Sjögren syndrome.
63	What are the clinical signs and symptoms of sialadenosis?	Sialadenosis is characterized by bilateral, recurrent, painless parotid gland swelling, unrelated to food intake.
64	What are the histologic findings in sialadenosis?	On histology, one would expect to find enlarged acinar cells (up to three times normal), degenerative neural changes, and myoepithelial atrophy.
65	What are the three categories for the development of sialadenosis?	• Endocrine-related sialadenosis (e.g., diabetes mellitus, acromegaly, adrenal disorders, hypothyroidism, pregnancy) • Dystrophic-metabolic sialadenosis (e.g., pellagra, beriberi, kwashiorkor, anorexia nervosa, bulimia, alcoholism) • Neurogenic sialadenosis (e.g., anticholinergic medications)
66	What differentiates a *mucous retention cyst*?	It is a true cyst with a complete epithelial lining.
67	From what salivary gland does a ranula develop?	Ranulas are mucoceles that develop from the sublingual gland.

68	What is the common appearance of a ranula on physical examination?	Ranulas often appear as a bluish, translucent mass on the floor of mouth.
69	What is the difference between a *ranula* and a *plunging ranula*?	A *ranula* is extravasated mucus that forms a pseudocyst between the mucosa of the floor of mouth (superior border) and mylohyoid muscle (inferior border). A *plunging ranula* is a ranula that extends inferior to the mylohyoid muscle into the neck.
70	What are the routes in which a plunging ranula can pass to reach the neck?	Extravasated mucus from a ranula typically passes around the posterior border of mylohyoid or passes through dehiscent areas of the mylohyoid.
71	What are the prevalence and location of mylohyoid muscle dehiscence?	Studies show that up to 50% of mylohyoid muscles are dehiscent in the anterior two-thirds of the muscle.
72	What are the treatment options for ranulas, and which is most successful?	Conservative treatment options include injection of sclerosing agents, intraoral marsupialization, or excision of the ranula alone. The most effective treatment, with a recurrence rate of 1 to 2%, is excision of the sublingual gland and ranula together.
73	Name the most common cause of nonsuppurative acute parotitis?	The mumps virus is the most common cause of nonsuppurative acute parotitis.
74	The virus that causes mumps is in what family?	Paramyxovirus (RNA)
75	What are the most common initial symptoms of mumps?	Children between the ages of 5 and 10 years have nonspecific symptoms of headache, fever, myalgia, and anorexia, followed by bilateral parotid gland swelling.
76	Name several viruses that have been associated with viral parotitis.	Influenza, coxsackievirus, echovirus, rabies, mumps, and hepatitis viruses can be associated with viral parotitis.
77	How is cat-scratch parotitis diagnosed?	Diagnosis is suggested by a history of exposure to cats and confirmed by elevated titers of *Bartonella henselae* immunoglobulin (Ig)G and IgM.
78	How is actinomycosis of the parotid gland diagnosed?	Diagnosis is achieved using FNA or tissue biopsy.

Manifestations of Systemic Disease

79	What is the pathophysiologic mechanism of Sjögren syndrome?	Autoimmune destruction of exocrine glands
80	What are the two broad classifications of Sjögren syndrome?	The two classifications are *primary* and *secondary* Sjögren syndrome. *Primary* cases involve only exocrine glands. *Secondary* cases involve exocrine glands and any additional connective tissue disease.
81	What are the common initial signs and symptoms of Sjögren syndrome?	Xerostomia, keratoconjunctivitis sicca, and parotid gland enlargement
82	Patients with Sjögren syndrome are at risk for developing what neoplasm?	Patients with Sjögren syndrome have a 44 times greater risk of lymphoma than do matched controls; 5% of patients with Sjögren syndrome develop lymphoma.
83	What autoimmune disease is associated with primary mucosa-associated lymphoid tissue, or MALT, lymphoma of the salivary glands?	Sjögren n syndrome
84	What are the risk factors for lymphoma development in Sjögren syndrome?	Risk factors include persistent enlargement of parotid glands, splenomegaly, lymphadenopathy, palpable purpura, leg ulcers, or a mixed monoclonal cryoglobulinemia.
85	Other than clinical history and laboratory workup, what in-office procedure can be performed to help establish the diagnosis of Sjögren syndrome?	Lower-lip minor salivary gland biopsy

86	What laboratory tests are most commonly ordered for suspected Sjögren syndrome?	A rheumatologic workup for Sjögren syndrome includes SS-A and SS-B, the most specific tests for Sjögren syndrome. Additional tests including antinuclear antibodies, rheumatoid factor, and sedimentation rates are also frequently obtained.
87	True or false. *Benign lymphoepithelial lesion of the salivary glands* is another name for *benign lymphoepithelial cysts of the salivary glands.*	False. Although often used incorrectly in the literature, the term *benign lymphoepithelial lesions of the salivary glands* are clinically and histologically distinct from *benign lymphoepithelial cysts.* Benign lymphoepithelial lesions are thought to result from an autoimmune condition related to other disease processes such as Sjögren syndrome, Hashimoto disease, chronic sclerosing sialadenitis, sarcoidosis, and HIV.
88	True or false. Patients with benign lymphoepithelial lesions of the salivary glands are at increased risk for malignancy.	True, unlike benign lymphoepithelial cysts, benign lymphoepithelial lesions are at increased risk for lymphoma transformation.
89	A patient with multiple parotid cysts should be tested for what disease? (▶ Fig. 11.4)	HIV

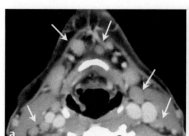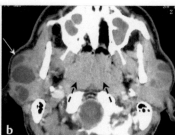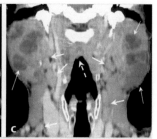

Fig. 11.4 HIV infection with nodal and parotid gland involvement. (a) Contrast-enhanced axial CT images at the level of the infrahyoid neck, (b) suprahyoid neck, and (c) coronal view demonstrating multiple enlarged, homogeneously enhancing nodes (arrows), enlarged adenoid tissue (dashed arrows), and bilateral lymphoepithelial cysts in the parotid glands (thin arrows), consistent with HIV infection. (Used with permission from Mafee MF, Valvassori GE, Becker M. Imaging of the Head and Neck 2nd Edition. New York, NY: Thieme; 2005.)

90	What are the initial symptoms of Kimura disease?	Diffuse lymphadenopathy, salivary gland swelling (parotid or submandibular), red cutaneous nodules on the head and neck, as well as pigmented, coarse, pruritic skin overlying glandular swelling
91	What is the population most commonly affected by Kimura disease?	Young males in their 20s and 30s from Southeast Asia
92	What inflammatory cell is most commonly elevated in Kimura disease?	Eosinophils (both peripheral eosinophilia and intralesional eosinophilia).
93	Aside from a CBC, what other blood tests should be ordered in a patient with Kimura disease?	Blood urea nitrogen (BUN), creatinine, and urinary protein to rule out nephrotic syndrome
94	What are the treatment options for Kimura disease?	Surgical resection has been considered the treatment of choice. Observation can be offered if the patient is asymptomatic. Medical treatment includes steroids and immunosuppressants.
95	What is the most common initial manifestation of necrotizing sialometaplasia?	Ulcer on the posterior hard palate is the most common symptom. The lesions of necrotizing sialometaplasia heal spontaneously in 5 to 9 weeks; thus, the only treatment required is supportive care.

96	In a patient with hard palate ulceration, what conditions should be considered in the differential diagnosis?	Aphthous ulcer, trauma, malignancy such as mucoepidermoid carcinoma or squamous cell carcinoma, necrotizing sialometaplasia
97	What are the initial symptoms of a patient with adenomatoid hyperplasia of a salivary gland?	Painless swelling of the oral mucosa, suggestive of neoplasia, is usually seen; pathology reveals benign salivary tissue.
98	Heerfordt syndrome is an extrapulmonary form of what systemic disease?	Sarcoidosis
99	What are the characteristics of Heerfordt syndrome?	Heerfordt's syndrome, also know as uveoparotid fever, presents with uveitis, non-suppurative parotitis, and in 50% of the patients, facial palsy.
100	How is uveoparotid fever treated?	Heerfordt syndrome, also known as uveoparotid fever, initially manifests with uveitis, nonsuppurative parotitis, and facial palsy. Treatment for Heerfordt syndrome includes systemic steroids and eye care.
101	What are the treatment options for benign lymphoepithelial cysts associated with HIV?	Cysts in such cases can be treated with observation, repeated aspiration, and antiretroviral medication such as zidovudine, sclerosing agents, radiation, or surgery.
102	True or false. Benign lymphoepithelial cysts associated with HIV have malignant potential if not removed.	False. HIV-positive patients are at increased risk of malignancy, but no reports are documented that show malignant potential of benign lymphoepithelial cysts.
103	Rapid growth of a salivary gland in a patient with HIV is most concerning for what pathology?	Malignancy such as Kaposi sarcoma or lymphoma
104	When is surgery indicated for management of salivary gland enlargement associated with HIV?	When a gland undergoes rapid growth or other clinical indicators of malignancy, surgery may also be offered if conservative management fails and a patient is worried about cosmesis.
105	Apart from Heerfordt syndrome, how often does sarcoidosis affect the salivary glands?	About 5 to 7% of sarcoidosis patients have salivary gland enlargement.
106	How should extrapulmonary sarcoidosis with persistent parotid swelling be treated?	Oral steroids
107	What is the presentation of salivary gland involvement with Wegener granulomatosis?	It is a rare association, but patients with Wegener granulomatosis and parotid involvement most often have painful parotid swelling. Biopsy shows necrotizing granulomatous changes and microabscesses.

Benign Tumors

108	What is the most common benign parotid tumor in children?	Hemangiomas or pleomorphic adenomas, depending on the series
109	What is the most common benign salivary epithelial tumor in children?	Pleomorphic adenomas
110	What is the relative incidence of benign to malignant lesions based on the salivary gland site of origin?	Of all lesions in each salivary gland, 75% of parotid masses are benign, more than 50% of submandibular masses are benign, but more than 80% of minor salivary gland masses are malignant.
111	What is the most common benign salivary tumor, and where is it most commonly found?	Pleomorphic adenoma (represents ~75% of benign salivary tumors) is most often found in the parotid gland.
112	What is the recommended treatment for pleomorphic adenoma?	Surgical excision along with a cuff of normal salivary tissue is recommended.
113	What is the risk of malignant transformation of an unresected pleomorphic adenoma?	Estimates of malignant transformation of a pleomorphic adenoma are 1.5% in the first 5 years and 10% after 15 years.

114	What risk factor is unique to Warthin tumor?	Smoking; no other salivary gland tumors are directly associated with a history of smoking.
115	Which benign salivary tumor is most often bilateral?	Warthin tumor of the parotid gland
116	The cells of a true oncocytoma contain an abundance of what organelle?	The cells of an oncocytoma contain a very large number of mitochondria.
117	Where are salivary monomorphic adenomas most commonly located?	The most common presentation is of minor salivary glands on the upper lip.
118	What are some of the histologic types of mono-morphic adenomas?	*Monomorphic adenoma* is a term that refers to a set of rare salivary gland tumors. They include basal cell adenoma, canalicular adenoma, clear cell adenoma, glycogen-rich adenoma, and myoepithelioma.
119	What is the most common location of a benign salivary canalicular adenoma?	Salivary canalicular adenomas are most commonly found in minor salivary glands of the upper lip.

Malignant Tumors

120	What is the most common salivary gland malig-nancy in children?	Mucoepidermoid carcinoma
121	True or False. A history of radiation therapy to the head and neck is a risk factor for future develop-ment of salivary gland tumors.	True. A history of radiation therapy at any age and any dose increases the risk for development of salivary gland tumors.
122	List the risk factors associated with salivary gland cancer.	Previous radiation exposure, history of head and neck skin cancer, Epstein-Barr virus, HIV infection, Hodgkin disease, industrial exposure to rubber manufacturing or nickel compound, or employment in a beauty salon are risk factors.
123	What are clinical signs and symptoms of salivary gland malignancy?	Pain, fixed lesion, invasion of overlying skin, rapidly growing mass, facial nerve palsy, and cervical lymphadenopathy
124	True or false. In general, the best radiologic study to evaluate a malignant salivary gland mass is CT with contrast.	False. Although CT provides useful information, MRI is the preferred imaging modality for parotid gland lesions. MRI provides superior detail regarding invasion of surrounding structures and type of pathology.
125	True or False. FNA biopsy of salivary gland malignancies has high sensitivity but low specificity.	False. The sensitivity is fairly low, whereas the specificity is quoted to be greater than 90% in most studies.
126	Define the *T stages* for the Tumor, Node, Metas-tasis (TNM) classification for major salivary gland malignancies.	(▶ Table 11.1)

Table 11.1 AJCC tumor (T) staging of salivary gland malignancies.

Stage	Description
T1	≤ 2 cm
T2	> 2 cm and ≤ 4 cm
T3	≥ 4 cm and/or extraparenchymal extension
T4a	Invades skin, mandible, ear canal, or facial nerve
T4b	Invades skull base, pterygoid plates, or encases carotid artery

Data from Edge SB, Byrd DR, Compton CC, Fritz AG, Greene FL, Trotti A, eds. AJCC Cancer Staging Manual 7th Edition. New York, NY: Springer; 2010.

127	Define the *N stages* for the TNM classification for major salivary gland malignancies.	• Nx: Regional lymph nodes cannot be assessed. • N0: No regional lymph nodes • N1: Single ipsilateral node, 3 cm or smaller • N2a: Single ipsilateral node 3 to 6 cm in diameter • N2b: Multiple ipsilateral nodes; none larger than 6 cm • N2c: Bilateral or contralateral nodes, none larger than 6 cm • N3: Any lymph node larger than 6 cm in diameter
128	Define the overall staging (I through IV) for major salivary gland malignancies.	• Stage I: T1N0M0 • Stage II: T2N0M0 • Stage III: T3N0M0 or T1–3N1M0 • Stage IVA: T1–3N2M0 or T4aN0–2M0 • Stage IVB: T4bN1–3M0 or T1–4N3M0 • Stage IVC: M1
129	What is the incidence of malignancy in tumors of the major salivary glands?	About 15 to 32% of parotid tumors are malignant, 41 to 45% of submandibular tumors are malignant, and 70 to 90% of sublingual gland tumors are malignant.
130	What is the incidence of cervical lymph node metastasis in a primary submandibular neoplasm?	30%
131	What is the most common histologic subtype of malignant salivary gland tumors?	Mucoepidermoid carcinoma is the most common malignant salivary gland tumor, followed by adenoid cystic carcinoma, and then adenocarcinoma.
132	Grading of mucoepidermoid carcinoma is critical to prognosis and management. What is the histologic appearance of low-grade mucoepidermoid carcinoma?	Low-grade mucoepidermoid carcinoma is more cystic with little atypia and low mitotic activity. High grade is more solid.
133	What is the prognosis of mucoepidermoid carcinoma?	Patients with low-grade and intermediate-grade carcinoma with no regional or distant metastases have an excellent prognosis, with 5-year survival greater than 90%. High-grade tumors have a lower 5-year survival of around 50%.
134	What is the recommended treatment for low-grade and high-grade mucoepidermoid carcinoma?	Low-grade carcinoma requires removal of the salivary gland with a margin of healthy tissue, but elective neck dissection is not necessarily required. High-grade carcinoma requires total excision and elective or therapeutic neck dissection and often adjuvant radiation.
135	Describe the natural history of adenoid cystic carcinoma.	Adenoid cystic carcinoma is difficult to cure. Its course is slow and prolonged; it commonly has perineural invasion at manifestation; and despite excision, it frequently recurs.
136	Which salivary gland malignancy has the highest rate of distant metastasis?	Adenoid cystic carcinoma. About 30% to 50% of patients develop metastasis, most commonly to the lungs.
137	What are the 5- and 10-year survival rates for patients with acinic cell carcinoma?	Acinic cell carcinoma is a relatively low-grade cancer with a 5-year survival rate ranging from 75 to > 90% and a 10-year survival rate ranging from 60 to 75%.
138	What are the two main subtypes of malignant mixed tumor?	Carcinoma ex-pleomorphic adenoma and carcinosarcoma (rare)
139	True or False. With complete surgical excision, patients with salivary gland carcinosarcoma have good long-term survival.	False. Death from disease often occurs within 3 years of diagnosis even with complete surgical excision.
140	What is the most common presentation of carcinoma ex-pleomorphic adenoma?	A male patient in his 60s to 70s with a long-standing parotid mass that suddenly increases in size over several months
141	What is the most common manifestation of a polymorphous low-grade adenocarcinoma?	The most common initial manifestation is an asymptomatic mass of the hard palate present for months to years.

142	Describe the clinicopathologic features of poly-morphous low-grade adenocarcinoma.	Slow growth, indolent behavior, and almost exclusively involves minor salivary glands with an infiltrative growth pattern and perineural invasion
143	What other cancer does salivary duct carcinoma histologically resemble?	High-grade ductal carcinoma of the breast
144	What is the most important diagnosis to rule out when squamous cell carcinoma is found in the parotid gland?	Other primary (e.g., skin) carcinomas with metastasis to the parotid must be ruled out. This situation is much more common than primary parotid squamous cell carcinoma.
145	Which cancer most commonly metastasizes to the parotid lymph nodes?	Skin cancer of the head and neck
146	Although this topic is debated, what are the general indications for total parotidectomy in a patient with parotid malignancy?	• Benign tumors in the deep lobe • Malignant tumors in the deep lobe • High-grade parotid tumors, even if in superficial lobe • Parotid malignancy with cervical lymph node metastasis • Any tumor that metastasizes to parotid gland
147	In general, what is the management of salivary gland malignancy with cervical lymph node metastasis?	If a parotid gland malignancy has cervical metastases, an ipsilateral modified radical or select neck dissection is recommended.
148	True or False. Patients with node-negative (N0) necks and parotid malignancies < 4 cm should undergo prophylactic neck dissection.	False. Although the topic is debated, most of the literature shows that tumors with larger than 4-cm extraparotid tumor extension and higher-risk histologic types (undifferentiated carcinoma, squamous cell carcinoma, high-grade mucoepidermoid, adenocarcinoma not otherwise specified, carcinoma ex-pleomorphic adenoma, and salivary duct carcinoma) are the only parotid tumors that warrant prophylactic neck dissection.
149	What type of neck dissection should a patient with a node-negative (N0) neck and high-grade salivary gland malignancy have?	In general, selective neck dissection: levels I through IV for a parotid primary and levels I through III for submandibular primaries
150	What are the indications for adjuvant radiation therapy for salivary gland malignancies?	Adjuvant radiation is indicated in cases of advanced stage, positive margins after resection, high-grade tumor, perineural invasion, or bony invasion.
151	What is the most common tumor type of the minor salivary glands?	When combining all tumor types, malignant tumors are more common than benign tumors in the minor salivary glands, with mucoepidermoid carcinoma the most common malignant tumor.

12 Endocrine Disorders

Brian C. Gross, Amy C. Dearking, Brandon W. Peck, and Benzon M. Dy

Parathyroid Overview

| 1 | How common is a supernumerary parathyroid gland, and where is the supernumerary gland most likely to be found? (► Fig. 12.1) | The incidence of a supernumerary parathyroid gland is up to 15%. They are most often found in the thymus, thyrothymic tract, and carotid sheath. |

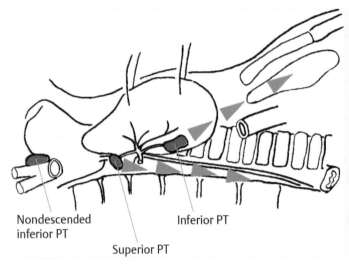

Fig. 12.1 Most common locations of the superior and inferior parathyroid glands and the course of their embryological migration. (Used with permission from Gemsenjaeger E. Atlas of Thyroid Surgery: Principles, Practice, and Clinical Cases. New York, NY: Thieme; 2009.)

Nondescended inferior PT

Inferior PT

Superior PT

2	Where do the superior and inferior parathyroid glands obtain their blood supply?	Most of the blood supply comes from the inferior thyroid artery, although occasionally the superior glands may get their blood supply from the superior thyroid artery (in 15% of cases).
3	What options are available for minimally invasive parathyroidectomy?	Minimally invasive parathyroidectomy is gaining popularity among surgeons. Typically, a technetium-99 sestamibi scan preoperatively determine a single hyperfunctioning parathyroid adenoma, and exploration of that gland alone is done using intravenous (IV) sedation and intraoperative parathyroid hormone assay monitoring.
4	When conducting a subtotal parathyroidectomy, what tissue should be left behind?	Approximately three and one-half glands should be excised and the remaining half of a gland left to its blood supply. Most prefer to leave a portion of an inferior parathyroid gland because there would less risk to the recurrent laryngeal nerve.
5	How can PTH levels be used intraoperatively to determine the completeness of a parathyroidectomy?	PTH has a half-life of 2–5 minutes, so PTH levels can be drawn from the patient before incision and then 5 to 10 minutes after excision. If there is at least a 50% decrease in the PTH level, into the normal or near normal range, the excised gland was likely the offending gland.
6	What structures have been described as landmarks to identify the superior parathyroid gland?	About 80% of superior parathyroid glands are found on the posterior aspect of the thyroid gland within a 1-cm diameter centered 1 cm superior to the intersection of the recurrent laryngeal nerve and inferior thyroid artery.

7　What branchial pouch gives rise to the superior and inferior parathyroid glands? (▶ Fig. 12.2)

The fourth branchial pouch gives rise to the superior parathyroid gland and C cells. The third branchial pouch gives rise to the inferior parathyroid gland and thymus.

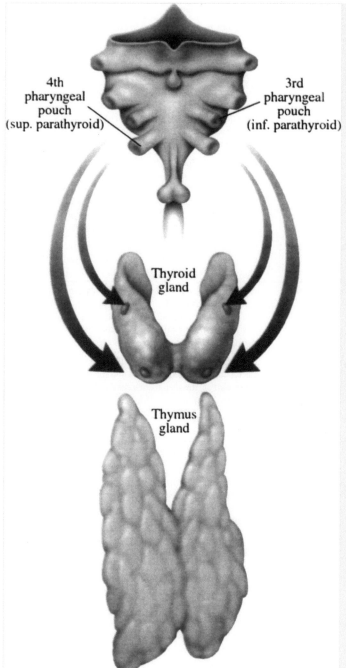

4th pharyngeal pouch (sup. parathyroid)

3rd pharyngeal pouch (inf. parathyroid)

Thyroid gland

Thymus gland

Fig. 12.2 The embryologic origin of the parathyroid glands. (Used with permission from Terris DJ, Gourin CG, eds. Thyroid and Parathyroid Diseases: Medical and Surgical Management. New York, NY: Thieme; 2009.)

8	How does PTH maintain calcium levels?	PTH increases calcium absorption from the gut, mobilizes calcium from the bones, inhibits calcium excretion from the kidneys, and stimulates renal hydroxylase to maintain activated vitamin D levels.
9	What is the most potent regulator of PTH release?	Serum calcium levels
10	Where can one find PTH receptors, and what downstream effects do they have in each location?	PTH binds to PTH receptors in two locations: bone and kidney. In bone, PTH receptors on osteoblasts cause release of receptor activator of nuclear factor-κ ligand, which then activates osteoclasts, which break down bone to increase serum calcium. In the kidney, PTH binds to renal tubule cells and induces reabsorption of calcium and decreases reabsorption of phosphate from the filtrate. It also induces the expression of an enzyme that converts the inactive form of vitamin D (25-hydroxyvitamin D) to the active form (1,25-dihydroxyvitamin D).
11	When monitoring total calcium levels in a patient, what factor do you also need to note?	Albumin level. Total calcium can vary with albumin level. In a patient with normal albumin, total calcium can be monitored. In a patient with abnormal albumin levels, the corrected total calcium can be calculated (total serum calcium decreases by 0.8 g/dL for every 1-g/dL decrease in albumin), or the ionized calcium level can be followed.
12	What test results support the diagnosis of familial hypocalciuric hypercalcemia?	Hypercalcemia with 24-hour urinary calcium:creatinine clearance ratio below 0.01, as well as one or more first-degree relatives with hypercalcemia
13	What are common symptoms of chronic hypercalcemia?	The symptoms of chronic hypercalcemia can be remembered by the mnemonic "bones, stones, abdominal groans, and psychiatric moans," referring to renal calculi, bone pains, abdominal pain, and depression, anxiety, cognitive dysfunction or other psychiatric problems.
14	What testing is necessary to diagnose primary hyperparathyroidism?	Elevated albumin-corrected serum calcium or ionized calcium and elevated PTH. Imaging serves as an adjunct but is not part of the diagnostic criteria of primary hyperparathyroidism.
15	Name the most common cause of hypercalcemia in an outpatient clinic setting.	Parathyroid adenoma
16	Name the most common cause of hypercalcemia in an inpatient hospital setting.	Underlying malignancy
17	A patient has hypercalcemia and low or undetectable PTH levels. What is the likely diagnosis?	Primary hyperparathyroidism is ruled out by the low or undetectable PTH level. This patient likely has a paraneoplastic-induced hypercalcemia mediated by PTH-related protein.
18	What is the incidence of primary hyperparathyroidism in Western countries?	22 cases per 100,000 persons per year The incidence has increased since the 1970s because of increased detection of asymptomatic patients with elevated calcium levels. In postmenopausal women, the most common demographic, the incidence may be as high as 1 per 1,000/year.
19	What are the different types of parathyroid hyperplasia?	Parathyroid hyperplasia is predominantly caused by proliferation of the chief cells within the gland. Very rarely, water clear cell hyperplasia, which is a proliferation of vacuolated water clear cells, can be found. The water clear cell variant is clinically more severe and predominantly occurs in females.

20	Describe the typical patient population with primary hyperparathyroidism.	Most cases occur in women (74%); incidence peaks in the seventh decade of life. Before age 45, incidence in men and women is similar.
21	What causative factors are associated with primary hyperparathyroidism?	• Head and neck radiation in childhood • Long-term lithium therapy • Genetic predisposition
22	What are the guidelines for surgical treatment (parathyroidectomy) in an asymptomatic patient with primary hyperparathyroidism?	Despite being devoid of classic symptoms, some patients should be treated for hyperparathyroidism, including those with serum calcium greater than 1.0 mg/dl above the upper limit of the normal reference range, those with a calculated creatinine clearance less than 60 ml/minute, those with bone mineral density T score less than –2.5 at any site or previous fragility fracture. Patients younger than 50 years should also be considered to prevent long-term damage from elevated calcium.
23	What are the typical laboratory values of calcium, PTH, and phosphate in secondary hyperparathyroidism?	In secondary hyperparathyroidism, one would expect low-normal calcium and elevated PTH. Phosphate levels vary based on the etiology (high in renal insufficiency, low in vitamin D deficiency).
24	What are some possible causes of secondary hyperparathyroidism?	Secondary hyperparathyroidism can occur from renal failure, which causes a decline in the formation of activated 1,25 vitamin D and calcium absorption in the gut. Phosphate excretion is also impaired, which together cause low serum calcium. It can also result from low vitamin D levels in the setting of adequate renal function, such as in cases of dietary insufficiency. In addition, patients with short gut syndrome or a history of gastric bypass surgery are at risk for secondary disease resulting from malabsorption of both calcium and vitamin D. In all cases, low serum calcium triggers secretion of PTH and growth of the parathyroid glands.
25	What is the treatment of secondary hyperparathyroidism?	• Correction of the underlying cause, such as renal transplant in patients with renal failure or vitamin D therapy in vitamin D deficiency • Patient symptoms from secondary disease may improve with medications such as cincalcet or bisphosophate therapy. • There is a role for subtotal parathyroidectomy if medical management fails.
26	What is tertiary hyperparathyroidism?	Tertiary hyperparathyroidism is a state of excess secretion of PTH after long-standing secondary hyperparathyroidism. Phosphate levels in tertiary hyperparathyroidism are decreased; however, renal dysfunction may lead to hyperphosphatemia despite elevated PTH levels. A classic example is hyperparathyroidism persisting after renal transplantation.
27	What is the pathophysiology of tertiary hyperparathyroidism?	The hypertrophied parathyroid glands become autonomous in their function and hypersecrete PTH, leading to hypercalcemia despite withdrawal of calcium and calcitriol. High calcium levels can cause diffuse calcinosis.
28	What is the treatment of tertiary hyperparathyroidism?	Total parathyroidectomy with autotransplantation or subtotal parathyroidectomy (3 and ½ gland resection)
29	What are the components of hyperparathyroidism-jaw tumor syndrome?	Recurrent parathyroid adenomas, fibroosseous tumors of the mandible, and Wilms tumors

30	How do the symptoms of *acute* and *chronic* hypoparathyroidism differ?	*Acute* hypoparathyroidism, such as after surgery, can cause dramatic hypocalcemia and associated paresthesias, muscle spasms, tetany, and seizures. The hypocalcemia induced by *chronic* hypoparathyroidism is gradual in onset and may not present until the patient develops blurry vision from cataracts.
31	What are the most common causes of hypoparathyroidism?	By far, the most common cause of hypoparathyroidism is iatrogenic, by either treatment of hyperparathyroidism or injury during thyroid surgery. The next most common causes are congenital, when the third and fourth branchial arches fail to develop properly.

Parathyroid Tumors

32	What is the histologic description of a parathyroid adenoma?	A parathyroid adenoma appears as a hypercellular gland consisting of chief and oncocytic cells with decreased intercellular fat.
33	What are some intraoperative techniques used to identify a parathyroid adenoma?	Localization of an adenoma can be assisted by preoperative injection of methylene blue, which stains abnormal parathyroid glands preferentially. Preoperative injection of sestamibi in conjunction with intraoperative gamma probes can also be used to identify a parathyroid gland.
34	What is the most sensitive imaging study for identifying the location of a parathyroid adenoma?	Technetium-99 m sestamibi with single-photon emission CT (or SPECT; sensitivity from 70 to 100%). Ultrasound imaging is reported to be successful in localization in 50 to 90% of cases but is highly user dependent. 4D CT scan is an emerging technology, but the localization success rate remains to be determined.
35	How frequently is primary hyperparathyroidism caused by a single adenoma versus four-gland hyperplasia?	A single parathyroid adenoma is the cause in 80 to 85% of cases and four-gland hyperplasia in 10 to 15% of cases. Other causes of primary hyperparathyroidism include double adenomas (5%) and parathyroid carcinoma (<1%).
36	What features of a patient with hypercalcemia and elevated PTH are more concerning for a parathyroid carcinoma compared with benign parathyroid adenoma?	Aside from a palpable neck mass, other features worrisome for parathyroid carcinoma include markedly elevated serum calcium levels (>14), markedly elevated PTH, concomitant renal and bone disease, symptoms consistent with severe hypercalcemia, and evidence of invasion such as recurrent laryngeal nerve palsy.
37	What proportion of primary hyperparathyroidism is caused by parathyroid carcinoma?	About 0.1 to 1% of persons with primary hyperparathyroidism have a parathyroid carcinoma.
38	What are the incidence and prevalence of parathyroid carcinoma?	Parathyroid carcinoma is one of the rarest of all human cancers, with an incidence of 0.015 per 100,000 population and a prevalence of 0.005% in the United States.
39	How does the patient population with parathyroid carcinoma compare with patients with parathyroid adenoma?	There is an even distribution of males and females with parathyroid carcinoma, whereas there is female predominance in parathyroid adenoma. Patients on average are younger with parathyroid carcinoma (average age in 40s) compared with parathyroid adenoma (average age 50 to 60s).
40	What feature on physical examination is most concerning for parathyroid carcinoma?	A palpable neck mass (reported in 30 to 76% of patients with parathyroid carcinoma), which is rarely associated with a benign adenoma
41	What is the gross pathologic description of a parathyroid carcinoma compared with a benign adenoma?	Benign adenomas are generally soft, round, or oval and reddish brown. Parathyroid carcinoma is frequently a large, lobulated, and firm to stony-hard mass, with a grayish white capsule that is frequently adherent or invasive to surrounding tissues.

42	What is the American Joint Committee on Cancer (AJCC) staging system for parathyroid carcinoma?	There is no AJCC staging system for parathyroid carcinoma because of its low incidence.
43	What is the most common cause of death in patients with parathyroid carcinoma?	Patients often die from the effects of excessive PTH secretion and uncontrolled hypercalcemia rather than growth from tumor mass.
44	What is the best prognostic factor in parathyroid carcinoma?	Early recognition and complete surgical resection at initial operation offer the best prognosis.
45	Describe the prognosis for parathyroid carcinoma.	Surgical cure and survival can be achieved in patients undergoing an R0 (complete) resection. Patients with recurrent disease can be palliated with aggressive surgical therapy and calcimimmetic medications such as cincalcet.
46	What is the preferred treatment approach to parathyroid carcinoma?	Parathyroid carcinoma should be aggressively treated with en bloc resection of the tumor, ipsilateral central neck components, including thyroid lobectomy, tracheoesophageal soft tissue, and central lymph node dissection.
47	What is the most common pattern of malignant spread of disease in parathyroid carcinoma?	Parathyroid carcinoma is generally indolent with local recurrence and involvement of contiguous neck structures representing the most likely pattern of spread.
48	What is the rate of recurrence in parathyroid carcinoma?	About 40 to 60% of patients have a postsurgical recurrence, which usually occurs 2 to 5 years after surgery.
49	In a patient with recurrent and widely disseminated parathyroid carcinoma, surgical resection is no longer effective. Therapeutic goals should be control of hypercalcemia and decreasing bone resorption. How can this be treated medically?	Aggressive hydration restores fluid volume and increases urinary calcium excretion. Loop diuretics increase calciuresis. Bisphosphonates interfere with osteoclast-mediated bone resorption.
50	What is the pattern of metastatic disease in parathyroid carcinoma?	Late metastases occur via both lymphatic and hematogenous spread with the most common site being the lungs.

Thyroid Overview

51	From what branchial structures does the thyroid develop?	The thyroid develops from an endodermal diverticulum of the floor of the primitive pharynx. The medial primordia is derived from the first and second pharyngeal pouches. The lateral primordia is derived from the fourth and fifth pharyngeal pouches.
52	The ultimobranchial bodies develop into what structures?	Ultimobranchial bodies derive from the fourth pharyngeal pouch neural crest cells and give rise to parafollicular cells (C cells) of the thyroid, which release calcitonin.
53	What is the relationship of the ultimobranchial bodies to the thyroid gland?	The ultimobranchial bodies fuse with the thyroid gland during its descent, consistently in the middle to upper thirds of thyroid gland.
54	What is the most common pattern of descent of the thyroid gland in relation to the hyoid bone? (▶ Fig. 12.3)	The thyroid gland descends anterior to the hyoid bone during gestational weeks 4 through 7.

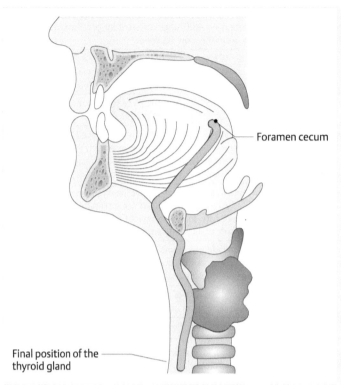

Fig. 12.3 The pathway of descent of the thyroid gland during development. (Used with permission from Mafee MF, Valvassori GE, Becker M. Imaging of the Head and Neck 2nd Edition. New York, NY: Thieme; 2005.)

Foramen cecum

Final position of the thyroid gland

55	What is the most common location of ectopic thyroid tissue?	As the thyroid forms from an endodermal diverticulum of the pharynx, the most common location of ectopic thyroid tissue is found in the base of tongue (*lingual thyroid*).
56	What does the proximal portion of the thyroglossal duct form?	Foramen cecum of the tongue
57	What does the caudal remnant of the thyroglossal duct form?	Pyramidal lobe of the thyroid, which is present in 40 to 55% of patients
58	What is the recommended surgical treatment for a thyroglossal duct cyst?	The Sistrunk procedure, which includes complete removal of the thyroglossal duct along with a portion of the central hyoid bone
59	What is the most common path of the right and left recurrent laryngeal nerves?	The right recurrent laryngeal nerve wraps around and passes deep to the right subclavian artery. It then travels in a more oblique path to enter the larynx just posterior to the cricothyroid joint. The left recurrent laryngeal nerve wraps around and passes deep to the arch of the aorta. The nerve then travels in a more medial path within the tracheoesophageal groove.
60	What does the recurrent laryngeal nerve innervate? (▶ Fig. 12.4)	The intrinsic muscles of the larynx and sensory innervation of the glottis (shared innervation with internal branch of superior laryngeal nerve) and subglottis

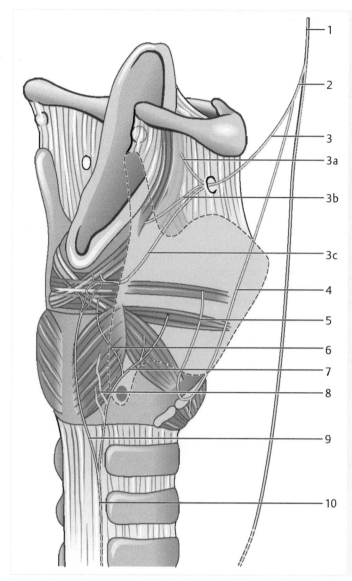

Fig. 12.4 Innervation of the larynx. 1, Vagus nerve; 2, superior laryngeal nerve (SLN); 3, internal branch of the SLN; 3a, superior branch of the internal SLN; 3b, middle branch of the internal SLN; 3c, inferior branch of the internal SLN; 4, external branch of the superior laryngeal nerve; 5, ventricular branch of the external SLN; 6, posterior branch of the recurrent laryngeal nerve; 7, anterior branch of the recurrent laryngeal nerve; 8, branches to the posterior cricoarytenoid muscle; 9, ansa galeni to the inferior branch of the internal SLN and branches to the interarytenoid muscle; 10, recurrent laryngeal nerve. (Used with permission from Behrbohm H, Kaschke O, Nawka T, Swift A. Ear, Nose, and Throat Diseases: With Head and Neck Surgery. New York, NY: Thieme; 2009.)

61	What is the relationship of the recurrent laryngeal nerve and the cricothyroid joint?	The recurrent laryngeal nerve enters the larynx posterior to the cricothyroid joint.
62	What does the external branch of the superior laryngeal nerve innervate?	The cricothyroid muscle
63	What is the function of the cricothyroid muscle?	The cricothyroid increases tension on vocal cords, inducing a higher pitch when vocalizing, and is innervated by the superior laryngeal nerve.
64	What does the internal branch of the superior laryngeal nerve innervate?	The internal branch of the superior laryngeal nerve pierces the thyrohyoid membrane to enter the larynx. The superior laryngeal nerve provides sensation to the supraglottic structures and shares sensation of the glottis with the recurrent laryngeal nerve.

65	Where does the superior laryngeal nerve branch off from the vagus?	Immediately below the nodose ganglion (inferior ganglion) of the vagus nerve, which is located just inferior to the jugular foramen
66	Where does the thyroid gland obtain its blood supply?	Typically from the superior and inferior thyroid arteries but occasionally from a thyroid ima artery
67	What is the name of the prelaryngeal lymph node?	Delphian node
68	What are the boundaries of the level VI cervical lymph nodes?	Level VI represents the central neck compartment and is bordered by the hyoid bone superiorly, the brachiocephalic (innominate) vein inferiorly, and the carotid arteries laterally.
69	What is the name of the naturally occurring thyroidal enlargement on the lateral portion of the gland?	The tubercle of Zuckerkandl
70	What is the name of the posterior suspensory ligament of the thyroid?	Berry ligament
71	Define the borders of the Simon triangle.	The Simon triangle is defined as the space between the esophagus medially, the carotid artery laterally, and the inferior thyroid artery superiorly.
72	Define the borders of the Joll triangle.	The Joll triangle is defined as the space between the inferior pharyngeal constrictor and cricothyroid muscle medially, the sternothyroid muscle laterally, and the superior thyroid pole inferiorly.
73	Which is the active form of thyroid hormone?	Triiodothyronine (T_3). Thyroxine (T_4) must be deiodinated to T_3 to act on peripheral tissue.
74	Describe the internal regulatory pathway of thyroid hormonogenesis.	Hypothalamus releases thyroid-releasing hormone (TRH). TRH binds a receptor in the anterior pituitary that increases production and release of thyroid-stimulating hormone (TSH). TSH stimulates the release of stored T_3 and T_4, increases production of T_3 in relation to T_4, and increases the production of thyroglobulin and thyroperoxidase (TPO). The entire system is controlled by negative feedback by downstream hormones.
75	What is the Wolff-Chaikoff effect?	The Wolff-Chaikoff effect describes decreased thyroid hormone production as a result of excess iodine ingestion such as with Lugol iodine administration in patients with Graves disease.
76	What hormones are produced by the thyroid gland?	The thyroid produces T_3 and T_4. These are made by iodinating the amino acid tyrosine.
77	Thyroid storm is a medical emergency. What medications are the mainstay of treatment in the acute setting?	Propranolol to control tachyarrhythmias, and methimazole to reduce thyroid hormone production. An hour after methimazole has been given, potassium iodide can be given to decrease hormone release and vascularity of the thyroid gland if surgery is considered.
78	What are the key components of thyroid hormone?	Thyroglobulin and iodine represent the key components to make and store thyroid hormone.
79	What is the name of the key enzyme required for thyroid hormonogenesis?	TPO, an enzyme that performs the iodination of thyroglobulin and coupling of monoiodotyrosine and diiodotyrosine to form T_3 and T_4
80	What is the most common cause of unilateral proptosis?	Graves' ophthalmopathy, which results in deposition of glycosaminoglycans and lipogenesis in the orbit.

81	What are the two ways in which amiodarone can cause hyperthyroidism?	• Type 1 amiodarone-induced thyrotoxicosis: Excess iodine (amiodarone is 37% iodine) causes excessive thyroid hormone production and is best treated with thionamides and discontinuation of amiodarone. • Type 2 amiodarone-induced thyrotoxicosis: Amiodarone-induced thyroiditis causes a destructive thyrotoxicosis and is best treated with prednisone. Amiodarone use can continue.
82	Describe the preferred treatment for subacute (de Quervain) thyroiditis in the hyperthyroid stage.	Symptomatic treatment with β-blockers and NSAIDs is the standard treatment. Severe cases are treated with high-dose prednisone.
83	A rare cause of thyrotoxicosis is a hydatidiform mole. What is the mechanism?	Hydatidiform moles, a form of gestational trophoblastic disease, produce chorionic gonadotropin, which has TSH-like activity.
84	Where is a hormone-producing focus of metastatic follicular carcinoma typically found on radioactive body scan?	Usually in the lungs or bone
85	In a nongravid woman with thyrotoxicosis, radioactive iodine uptake is found in the pelvis. What is the diagnosis?	Struma ovarii, a teratoma of the ovary that contains functional thyroid tissue
86	What findings indicate a diagnosis of thyrotoxicosis factitia?	Thyrotoxicosis factitia is a disorder in which a patient takes exogenous thyroid hormone surreptitiously, typically for weight loss. Typical findings are a suppressed TSH, low thyroglobulin, high T_4 and T_3, a negative radioactive iodine uptake level, and absence of a goiter.
87	Name the four main classifications of hypothyroidism.	• Primary hypothyroidism is the result of a dysfunctional thyroid gland. • Secondary hypothyroidism is caused by a dysfunctional pituitary gland. • Tertiary hypothyroidism results from hypothalamic dysfunction. • Finally, peripheral hypothyroidism is caused by hormone receptor resistance.
88	What is the most common cause of hypothyroidism in the world?	Iodine deficiency
89	What is the most common cause of hypothyroidism in the United States?	Hashimoto thyroiditis
90	What is the cause of myxedema coma?	Myxedema coma is an extreme hypothyroid state that is typically brought on by some systemic stress, often infection, in a hypothyroid patient.
91	Why should head and neck cancer patients have thyroid function closely monitored?	Hypothyroidism is common in patients with head and neck cancer after surgery and particularly after radiation therapy. Patients should have thyroid function tests drawn after 6 weeks of intervention and then every 6 to 12 months thereafter.
92	What is the recommended starting dose of levothyroxine for young healthy adults with hypothyroidism, and how is this different for older adults with underlying ischemic heart disease?	• For young adults, the typical starting dose is 1.6 μg/kg and adjusted depending on the TSH level after 6 to 12 weeks on a stable levothyroxine dose. • For those with known ischemic heart disease or arrhythmias or for elderly adults, the typical starting dose is 25 μg daily with 25 μg increases every few weeks.
93	Approximately how long does the hypothyroid phase of thyroiditis last?	Thyroiditis typically produces a transient hyperthyroid state and then either recovery or a transient hypothyroid state. When it occurs, the hypothyroid state typically lasts 2 to 8 weeks.

94	What is the likely cause of subacute granulomatous thyroiditis (de Quervain thyroiditis)?	Most likely a viral illness is the cause. Common associations include mumps, influenza, coxsackievirus, and adenovirus. Some believe it is more likely a result of a postviral inflammatory response than of viral infection itself.
95	What laboratory values are elevated in patients with Hashimoto thyroiditis?	TSH (evidence of primary thyroid disorder), antimicrosomal antibodies (anti-thyroperoxidase antibodies), and anti-thyroglobulin antibodies are usually elevated. However, 10% of patients with clinical Hashimoto thyroiditis may be antibody negative.
96	What causes the initial hyperthyroid state in some patients with Hashimoto thyroiditis?	Transient release of stored thyroid hormone from damaged thyroid cells (hashitoxicosis) causes a temporary surge in serum thyroid hormone.
97	What is the relationship between Hashimoto thyroiditis and thyroid cancer?	Patients with Hashimoto thyroiditis have a slightly increased incidence of papillary thyroid carcinoma compared with the general population.
98	What are the indications for surgery in a patient with Hashimoto thyroiditis?	Large goiter with obstructive symptoms, cosmetic concerns, or worrisome nodularity
99	Is subacute thyroiditis always painful?	No. Painless thyroiditis is sometimes seen. The inflammatory component may be mild and not require therapy.
100	What are the characteristic physical examination findings of Riedel thyroiditis?	Rock-hard, fixed, painless goiter. Compressive symptoms including dysphagia, dysphonia, cough, and dyspnea may also occur.
101	What organisms most commonly cause acute suppurative thyroiditis?	*Staphylococcus aureus*, *Streptococcus pneumoniae*, β-hemolytic streptococci are the most common offenders. Occasionally, it can be caused by *Fusobacterium* and *Haemophilus* species as well.
102	What criteria for a thyroid FNA must be met in order to be considered diagnostic?	The presence of at least six follicular cell groups, each with at least 10 cells, that are derived from at least two aspirates of the cyst or nodule.
103	Why is FNA of cystic thyroid nodules of low diagnostic yield?	FNA of cystic nodules often yield nondiagnostic findings because of the scant cellularity of fluid and the difficulty in obtaining a biopsy of the very thin cyst wall.
104	What are the false-negative and false-positive rates of thyroid nodule FNA?	For thyroid nodules, FNA is a sensitive and specific test. The false-negative rate is approximately 1 to 6%, and the false-positive rate is less than 5%.
105	When should a benign (based on results of previous FNA) thyroid nodule undergo rebiopsy?	When it changes significantly in size, a cyst recurs, or the nodule changes texture
106	What is the Pemberton sign?	Distension of the jugular veins, facial edema or erythema when a patient extends both arms above the head, indicating cervicothoracic inlet obstruction seen in patients with a substernal goiter
107	What is the Chvostek sign?	The Chyostek sign is seen in cases of hypocalcemia and is positive when tapping a finger on a patient's cheek over the course of the facial nerve results in contraction of the ipsilateral facial muscles.
108	What is the Trousseau sign?	The Trousseau sign is seen in cases of hypocalcemia, where inflation of a blood pressure cuff above systolic blood pressure for 3 minutes results in ipsilateral spasm of the wrist and hand muscles.

109	What are the main complications of thyroid surgery?	Major complications include hematoma, infection, superior laryngeal nerve injury (most common nerve injured), recurrent laryngeal nerve injury, and hypocalcemia.
110	Name the four main types of thyroid surgeries, and define each one.	• Thyroid lobectomy: Removal of a single lobe with or without the isthmus • Subtotal thyroidectomy: Incomplete removal of thyroid tissue, leaving more than 1 g of thyroid remaining • Near-total thyroidectomy: Incomplete removal of thyroid tissue, leaving behind a small amount of tissue adjacent to the recurrent laryngeal nerve • Total thyroidectomy: Removal of all grossly visible thyroid tissue
111	Name some disease-specific risk factors for permanent recurrent laryngeal nerve injury during thyroidectomy.	Recurrent thyroid carcinoma, substernal goiter, and thyroiditis
112	At what point in the thyroid dissection must one be aware of the superior laryngeal nerve?	The external branch of the superior laryngeal nerve, which supplies the cricothyroid muscle, lies near the superior pole vessels. Special care should be undertaken during division of the superior pole to protect the superior laryngeal nerve.

Thyroid Tumors

113	How common are thyroid nodules?	Thyroid nodules are common; incidence is 50% in adults.
114	What is the most common pathology of a thyroid nodule?	Benign follicular adenoma
115	Why are thyroid nodules often found during pregnancy?	The incidence of thyroid nodules during pregnancy is 5 to 20%. Increased hormones and relative iodine deficiency may be associated with increased thyroid nodularity.
116	How often are thyroid nodules cancerous?	Approximately 5% are cancerous.
117	Is a thyroid cyst benign?	Not always. Malignancies such as papillary thyroid carcinoma and parathyroid carcinoma can be cystic.
118	What are the factors that increase suspicion of malignancy in a patient with a thyroid nodule?	Age younger than 20 years, male sex, family history of thyroid cancer, pheochromocytoma, hyperparathyroidism, Gardner syndrome, Cowden disease, and a history of head and neck radiation
119	Are thyroid nodules more likely to be malignant in adults or in the pediatric population?	Pediatric. Approximately 5% of adult thyroid nodules are malignant and 20 to 50% of pediatric thyroid nodules are malignant.
120	What is the most common cause of a thyroid nodule in the pediatric population?	Follicular adenoma, just as it is with adults
121	What signs and symptoms in a patient with a thyroid nodule are worrisome for cancer?	• Rapid growth, a solid and fixed lesion, lymphadenopathy, pain, or compressive symptoms such as dysphagia or stridor • In addition, dysphonia may be secondary to compressive symptoms or invasion of the recurrent laryngeal nerve.
122	What is the most common presentation of a patient with thyroid cancer?	Nontender, palpable thyroid mass
123	What are the ultrasound imaging characteristics of a lymph node that are concerning for metastatic thyroid cancer?	Loss of the fatty hilum, increased vascularity, rounded node configuration rather than ovoid, hypoechogenicity of a solid nodule, microcalcifications, and peripheral vascularity

124	What is the value of PET imaging in thyroid cancer?	PET imaging allows for initial staging of poorly differentiated thyroid cancer and tumor surveillance after treatment of more advanced/metastatic thyroid cancer; it also offers prognostic data for patients with known metastasis.
125	What are the subtypes of well-differentiated thyroid cancer?	Papillary thyroid cancer, follicular thyroid cancer, and Hürthle cell thyroid cancer are all considered well-differentiated.
126	What are the most common staging systems available for well-differentiated thyroid cancer?	AJCC tumor node metastasis (TNM) classification system, AMES (age, metastasis, extent of disease, size), AGES (age, grade, extent of disease, size), MACIS (metastasis, age, completeness of surgical resection, invasion, size), Ohio State University, and Memorial Sloan-Kettering Cancer Center
127	Which tumor staging system for thyroid cancer includes gross resection of tumor in its prognostic calculation?	Specimen size is included in the MACIS score, calculated by the following formula: 3.1 (patient age < 40) or 0.08 x age (patient ≥ 40) + 0.3 x tumor size (cm) + 1 (if extrathyroidal extension) + 1 (if incomplete resection) + 3 (if distant metastasis)
128	How does extrathyroidal extension impact thyroid cancer staging?	• T3: Any extrathyroidal extension • T4a: Extrathyroidal invasion of subcutaneous soft tissue, larynx, trachea, esophagus, or recurrent laryngeal nerve • T4b: Invasion of prevertebral fascia or encasement of the carotid artery or mediastinal great vessels
129	How is age used in the AJCC TNM stage classification for thyroid cancer? (▶ Table 12.1; ▶ Table 12.2; ▶ Table 12.3; ▶ Table 12.4)	There are different staging systems for patients younger than 45 years compared with those who are 45 years old or greater. Patients over the age of 45 years generally have a greater (worse) stage of disease than younger patients with similar disease characteristics.

Table 12.1 Thyroid Cancer Staging: Primary Tumor (T)

Stage	Description
TX	Primary tumor cannot be assessed
T0	No evidence of primary tumor
T1	Tumor ≤ 2 cm in greatest dimension limited to the thyroid
T1a	Tumor ≤ 1 cm, limited to the thyroid
T1b	Tumor > 1 cm but ≤ 2 cm in greatest dimension, limited to the thyroid
T2	Tumor > 2 cm but ≤ 4 cm in greatest dimension, limited to the thyroid
T3	Tumor > 4 cm in greatest dimension limited to the thyroid or any tumor with minimal extrathyroid extension (e.g., extension to sternothyroid muscle or perithyroid soft tissues)
T4a	Tumor of any size extending beyond the thyroid capsule to invade subcutaneous soft tissues, larynx, trachea, esophagus, or recurrent laryngeal nerve
T4b	Tumor invades prevertebral fascia or encases carotid artery
cT4a	Intrathyroidal anaplastic carcinoma
cT4b	Anaplastic carcinoma with gross extrathyroid extension

Data from Edge SB, Byrd DR, Compton CC, Fritz AG, Greene FL, Trotti A, eds. AJCC Cancer Staging Manual 7th Edition. New York, NY: Springer; 2010.

Table 12.2 Thyroid Cancer Staging: Regional Lymph Nodes (N).

Stage	Description
NX	Regional lymph nodes cannot be assessed
N0	No regional lymph node metastasis
N1	Regional lymph node metastasis
N1a	Metastases to Level VI (pretracheal, paratracheal, and prelaryngeal/Delphian lymph nodes)
N1b	Metastases to unilateral, bilateral, or contralateral cervical (Levels I, II, III, IV, or V) or retropharyngeal or superior mediastinal lymph nodes (Level VII)

Data from Edge SB, Byrd DR, Compton CC, Fritz AG, Greene FL, Trotti A, eds. AJCC Cancer Staging Manual 7th Edition. New York, NY: Springer; 2010.

Table 12.3 Thyroid Cancer Staging: Distant Metastasis (M).

Stage	Description
M0	No distal metastasis
M1	Distal metastasis

Data from Edge SB, Byrd DR, Compton CC, Fritz AG, Greene FL, Trotti A, eds. AJCC Cancer Staging Manual 7th Edition. New York, NY: Springer; 2010.

Table 12.4 Thyroid Cancer Staging: Anatomic Stage/Prognostic Groups.

Stage	T	N	M
Papillary or follicular (differentiated)			
younger than 45			
I	Any T	Any N	M0
II	Any T	Any N	M1
45 and older			
I	T1	N0	M0
II	T2	N0	M0
III	T3	N0	M0
	T1	N1a	M0
	T2	N1a	M0
	T3	N1a	M0
IVA	T4a	N0	M0
	T4a	N1a	M0
	T1	N1b	M0
	T2	N1b	M0
	T3	N1b	M0
	T4a	N1b	M0
IVB	T4b	Any N	M0
IVC	Any T	Any N	M1

Stage	T	N	M
Medullary carcinoma (all age groups)			
I	T1	N0	M0
II	T2	N0	M0
	T3	N0	M0
III	T1	N1a	M0
	T2	N1a	M0
	T3	N1a	M0
IVA	T4a	N0	M0
	T4a	N1a	M0
	T1	N1b	M0
	T2	N1b	M0
	T3	N1b	M0
	T4a	N1b	M0
IVB	T4b	Any N	M0
IVC	Any T	Any N	M1
Anaplastic carcinoma			
IVA	T4a	Any N	M0
IVB	T4b	Any N	M0
IVC	Any T	Any N	M1

Data from Edge SB, Byrd DR, Compton CC, Fritz AG, Greene FL, Trotti A, eds. AJCC Cancer Staging Manual 7th Edition. New York, NY: Springer; 2010.

130	In which types of thyroid cancer are there different staging systems based on age of the patient?	Papillary thyroid carcinoma and follicular carcinoma have separate staging criteria based on age. Medullary and anaplastic carcinoma do not.
131	What is the most significant predictor of overall prognosis for well-differentiated thyroid cancer?	Distant metastasis is the most significant prognostic factor.
132	Review low-, intermediate- and high-risk features of well-differentiated thyroid carcinoma.	• Low risk: Localized disease without aggressive histologic subtypes or vascular invasion; all macroscopic disease removed at first surgery; no postoperative I-131 uptake outside thyroid bed • Intermediate risk: Microscopic tumor invasion outside the thyroid bed, positive cervical lymph nodes, aggressive histologic subtype or vascular invasion, and I-131 uptake outside thyroid bed • High-risk: Macroscopic extrathyroidal invasion, distant metastasis, incomplete surgical resection, and elevated postoperative thyroglobulin
133	Which risk factor most significantly increases the risk of thyroid carcinoma?	Exposure to ionizing radiation, especially as a child or adolescent
134	What is the recommended surgical treatment for patients with well-differentiated thyroid cancer?	Total thyroidectomy is recommended in cases of well-differentiated thyroid carcinoma except in cases of papillary thyroid carcinoma of low risk and < 1 cm in size. In this case, a thyroid lobectomy is considered sufficient treatment by many surgeons.

135	How should local invasion of the esophagus by thyroid carcinoma be treated?	Local invasion of the pharynx or esophagus by thyroid carcinoma should be resected and then repaired by primary closure of the defect.
136	What adjuvant forms of treatment exist for well-differentiated thyroid carcinoma?	TSH suppression with exogenous thyroid hormone, radioiodine ablation, or external beam radiation. Other treatments such as tyrosine kinase inhibitors may delay disease progression but have not been proven to increase survival.
137	What is TSH suppression?	Increased thyroxine levels administered to decrease the concentration of TSH released by the pituitary gland. Side effects of TSH suppression include bone loss, cardiac arrhythmias, and symptoms of hyperthyroidism.
138	Why is radioiodine ablation treatment used after surgery?	To destroy microscopic residual disease
139	How does radioiodine ablation assist in long-term management of well-differentiated thyroid carcinoma?	Complete removal of microscopic and macroscopic disease by surgery and adjuvant radioiodine ablation allows for closer management of recurrence or persistent disease with thyroglobulin measurements and whole-body radioiodine scans.
140	What are the complications of radioiodine ablation?	Sialadenitis, dental caries, nasolacrimal duct obstruction, xerostomia, and rarely secondary malignancies
141	What is the recommended treatment for well-differentiated thyroid carcinoma found in a thyroglossal duct cyst?	A Sistrunk procedure is adequate in cases in which clinical and radiologic examinations demonstrate normal thyroid and regional lymph nodes. Proceeding with total thyroidectomy should be considered in high-risk patients, as defined by age greater than 45 years, tumor diameter greater than 4 cm, extracapsular spread, regional or distant metastasis, or clinical or radiologic evidence of disease in the thyroid gland or regional lymph nodes.
142	How often do patients with thyroglossal duct cyst carcinoma have concurrent intrathyroidal cancer?	Based on a Mayo Clinic study from 1997, 33% of patients with thyroglossal duct cyst carcinoma had concurrent intrathyroidal malignancy.
143	What is the recommended treatment for a pregnant woman with well-differentiated thyroid carcinoma?	Surgical excision is recommended, either during the second trimester or after delivery.
144	Does thyroid cancer discovered during pregnancy behave differently from disease found in non-pregnant females?	No, there is no difference.
145	What are the recommendations for radioiodine ablation in regard to women of childbearing age?	Pregnancy should be avoided for 12 months after radioiodine ablation.
146	What is the treatment for locoregional metastatic well-differentiated thyroid carcinoma?	Ideally, surgical excision. Radioiodine ablation, external-beam radiation, or clinical trials, if available, may be considered.
147	What is the treatment for well-differentiated thyroid carcinoma with tracheal invasion?	Complete surgical resection is the best treatment. It may include shaving tumor from the trachea or esophagus, segmental tracheal resection and reanastomosis, or laryngopharyngectomy.
148	As a general rule, what is the best treatment for well-differentiated thyroid carcinoma with pulmonary metastasis?	I-131 radioiodine ablation therapy
149	In a case of well-differentiated thyroid cancer, how should involvement of the recurrent laryngeal nerve be managed?	If preoperative vocal cord function is normal, the nerve should be left intact if at all possible.

150	What are the two most sensitive tests for tumor surveillance after treatment of well-differentiated thyroid carcinoma?	Blood thyroglobulin levels and neck ultrasound. Thyroglobulin is a reliable marker in patients who do not produce anti-thyroglobulin antibodies, as its production is a marker for functioning thyroid tissue.
151	How might anti-thyroglobulin antibodies affect posttreatment thyroglobulin levels?	The antibodies can produce a falsely low level of thyroglobulin and its utility as a tumor marker becomes invalid.
152	Describe the role of chemotherapy in treating well-differentiated thyroid malignancies.	In well-differentiated thyroid cancers, there are no data to support the use of adjunctive chemotherapy, but doxorubicin may be used as a radiation sensitizer in patients undergoing external beam radiation therapy. Also, tyrosine kinase inhibitors have been used to improve progression-free survival but do not have a synergistic effect with radiation.
153	Which age group most commonly has cervical and distant metastases in papillary thyroid carcinoma: adults or children?	Children more commonly manifest with advanced disease.
154	What is the current recommended treatment for papillary thyroid microcarcinoma (< 1 cm) isolated to one lobe without extracapsular extension, positive lymph nodes, or distant metastasis?	Thyroid lobectomy
155	What should the detectable level of thyroglobulin be after total thyroidectomy and postoperative radioactive iodine therapy for advanced papillary carcinoma?	The goal is for an undetectable thyroglobulin level.
156	What histologic features are unique to papillary thyroid carcinoma? (▶ Fig. 12.5)	Psammoma bodies, which are concentric calcified structures, "Orphan Annie" eyes from large nuclear inclusions and nuclear grooves

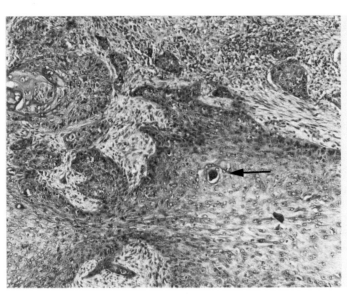

Fig. 12.5 Psammoma body (*black arrow*) in papillary thyroid carcinoma (H&E, × 100). (Used with permission from Donald PJ, ed. The Difficult Case in Head and Neck Cancer Surgery. New York, NY: Thieme; 2010.)

157	In regard to papillary thyroid carcinoma, which pathological variants carry a worse prognosis?	Tall cell variant, columnar cell variant, and diffuse sclerosing variants of papillary thyroid carcinoma carry a worse prognosis.
158	What type of thyroid cancer is most common in the pediatric population?	Papillary thyroid carcinoma

159	How is papillary thyroid microcarcinoma defined?	Papillary thyroid carcinoma measuring 1 cm or smaller irrespective of extrathyroidal extension, lymph node metastasis, or distant metastasis
160	How does papillary thyroid carcinoma tend to spread?	Papillary carcinoma has a predilection for spreading via lymphatic channels within the thyroid gland, leading to frequent multifocal disease, as well as to local lymph nodes in the paratracheal and cervical regions.
161	Is cervical lymph node metastasis more common in papillary or follicular thyroid carcinoma?	Papillary thyroid carcinoma. Cervical lymph node metastases are present in 30 to 70% of patients.
162	What is the effect of cervical lymph node metastasis on the prognosis of papillary thyroid cancer?	Currently, this topic is debatable, but most contend that there is no decrease in survival with local lymph node involvement. However, there is an increased risk of recurrence after surgical treatment.
163	How is a follicular thyroid adenoma differentiated from follicular thyroid carcinoma?	Surgical pathology is required to make the differentiation, as carcinomas have capsular or vascular invasion. Follicular thyroid carcinoma cannot be diagnosed with fine needle aspiration.
164	Are patients with follicular adenomas most commonly hyperthyroid, hypothyroid, or euthyroid?	Euthyroid
165	Is distant metastasis more common in papillary or follicular thyroid carcinoma?	Follicular thyroid carcinoma because it spreads via hematogenous dissemination
166	Name the three categories of follicular thyroid carcinoma.	• Minimally invasive: Displays invasion of capsule but does not invade through the capsule • Moderately invasive: Has angioinvasion with or without capsular invasion • Widely invasive: Has invasion into extrathyroidal tissue
167	For thyroid lobectomies with preoperative FNA results of "indeterminate" or "follicular neoplasia suspected," what percentage of final pathology results come back positive for follicular carcinoma?	Approximately 15 to 20%
168	What is the significance of a pathology report indicating aneuploid follicular carcinoma?	Aneuploid follicular carcinomas are more aggressive in their behavior compared to other follicular carcinomas.
169	Describe the histopathologic findings of Hürthle cell tumors (oncocytic neoplasms).	• Predominance of Hürthle cells, which are large, granular, eosinophilic cells • Malignancy is determined by the presence or absence of extracapsular spread, lymphovascular invasion, or presence of metastases.
170	How do Hürthle cell carcinomas respond to radioiodine therapy?	Hürthle cell carcinomas tend to be aggressive and have decreased iodine uptake; thus, they are resistant to radioiodine therapy.
171	Medullary thyroid carcinoma accounts for what percent of all thyroid malignancies?	Approximately 5%
172	Medullary thyroid carcinoma originates from what cell type?	Parafollicular cells (C cells) of the thyroid gland, which produce calcitonin and are of neuroendocrine origin
173	What laboratory abnormalities are associated with medullary thyroid carcinoma?	Elevated calcitonin and often elevated CEA
174	What is the most common manifestation of medullary thyroid carcinoma?	• Patients with sporadic tumors usually have an enlarging palpable neck mass and cervical lymphadenopathy. • Patients with familial disease are often diagnosed in a presymptomatic state as a result of early screening.
175	What is the most important prognostic factor in patients with medullary thyroid carcinoma?	Stage is the most important prognostic factor, followed by age.

176	How does radioiodine affect medullary thyroid carcinoma?	Medullary thyroid carcinoma does not take up radioiodine because it originates from the parafollicular cells, which are not involved in production of thyroid hormone.
177	What is the recommended treatment for patients with medullary thyroid carcinoma?	Minimum total thyroidectomy and central compartment neck dissection are recommended. For patients with lateral cervical node involvement or primary tumors larger than 1 cm, an ipsilateral level II through V neck dissection should also be performed.
178	What is the standard treatment for medullary thyroid carcinoma?	Total thyroidectomy with regional cervical lymph node dissection. In patients with tumors greater than 1 cm, an ipsilateral modified radical neck dissection should be considered. Chemotherapy and radiation are not effective treatments for medullary thyroid carcinoma.
179	How common is anaplastic thyroid carcinoma?	It is the rarest form of thyroid cancer, representing less than 5% of thyroid malignancies.
180	What is the age range of patients affected by anaplastic thyroid cancer?	Most are over 70 years old, and rarely do patients younger than 50 years have anaplastic thyroid carcinoma.
181	What are common initial symptoms of anaplastic thyroid carcinoma?	It is a rapidly enlarging neck mass, often associated with dyspnea, dysphagia, hoarseness, and pain.
182	What is the relationship between anaplastic thyroid cancer and well-differentiated thyroid cancer?	In some cases, anaplastic thyroid carcinoma may develop from a long-standing well-differentiated thyroid malignancy such as papillary thyroid carcinoma.
183	What is the prognosis for anaplastic thyroid cancer?	It is almost universally fatal within 6 to 12 months of diagnosis.
184	What is an indication for surgery with anaplastic thyroid cancer?	Although controversial, tumor debulking for palliation can be considered. In addition, small, contained cancers may be approached with intent to cure.
185	What is a currently accepted protocol to treat anaplastic thyroid cancer?	Chemotherapy with doxorubicin, hyperfractionated radio-therapy, and surgical debulking.
186	In what type of thyroid cancer is external-beam radiation used most commonly?	External-beam radiation has been used with limited success in anaplastic carcinoma as a neoadjuvant therapy in surgically unresectable cases.

Multiple Endocrine Neoplasia Syndrome

187	Which of the MEN subtypes includes involvement of the parathyroid glands?	MEN 1 patients have multiglandular disease requiring subtotal parathyroidectomy. MEN-2A patients have a para-thyroid adenoma or multiglandular disease and primary hyperparathyroidism. There is no parathyroid involvement in MEN-2B or familial non-MEN medullary thyroid carcinoma.
188	How does hyperparathyroidism manifest in patients with MEN-2A?	About 15 to 30% of patients with MEN-2A develop primary hyperparathyroidism, which is typically mild or asymptomatic clinically. It can manifest as single parathyroid adenoma or multiple gland hyperplasia. The average age of onset is age 38 years, and it is usually present many years after diagnosis of medullary thyroid carcinoma.
189	Which subtype of medullary thyroid carcinoma is more common, sporadic or familial?	Sporadic cases represent 75% of medullary thyroid carcinomas.
190	What are the different subtypes of familial medullary thyroid carcinoma?	MEN-2A and MEN-2B. Additionally, there are several rare types of familial non-MEN medullary thyroid carcinoma.
191	What conditions are associated with MEN-2A syndrome?	Medullary thyroid carcinoma, pheochromocytoma, and parathyroid hyperplasia

192	What conditions are associated with MEN-2B syndrome?	Medullary thyroid carcinoma, pheochromocytoma, marfanoid body habitus, and mucosal neuromas
193	What is the inheritance pattern of familial medullary thyroid carcinoma?	Autosomal dominant
194	What gene mutation(s) are responsible for familial medullary thyroid carcinoma?	Gain of function mutations of the RET proto-oncogene
195	What is the most common subtype of familial medullary thyroid carcinoma?	MEN-2A is most common, followed by familial non-MEN and then MEN-2B.
196	Which form of medullary thyroid carcinoma is the most aggressive?	MEN-2B is most aggressive, followed by sporadic cases, then MEN-2A, then familial non-MEN, which has the best prognosis.
197	What is the recommended treatment for patients with a RET mutation and/or a family history of medullary thyroid carcinoma?	For children, prophylactic thyroidectomy is the recommended treatment. In general, early intervention improves outcome by preventing metastases. In MEN-2A, thyroidectomy is recommended in pre-teenage patients, whereas in MEN-2B, resection is recommended in infancy, often before the age of 1 year.
198	What gene is involved in MEN-2?	MEN-2 has three clinical subtypes: MEN-2A, MEN-2B, and familial medullary thyroid carcinoma (FMTC). All are associated with mutations in the RET proto-oncogene.
199	What endocrine neoplasms are associated with MEN-2A?	Medullary thyroid carcinoma, pheochromocytoma, and primary hyperparathyroidism (parathyroid adenoma)
200	How frequently do individuals with MEN-2A develop the various clinical manifestations of this syndrome?	About 70 to 95% develop medullary thyroid carcinoma, 50% develop pheochromocytoma, and 15 to 30% develop primary hyperparathyroidism.
201	What is the typical presentation of medullary thyroid carcinoma in individuals with MEN-2A?	In patients with MEN-2A, medullary thyroid carcinoma typically presents with a neck mass or neck pain, usually before age 35 years. Other symptoms include diarrhea or gastrointestinal disturbance.
202	How frequently are cervical lymph node metastases present on presentation of medullary thyroid carcinoma in MEN-2A?	Up to 70%
203	What are the clinical findings associated with MEN-2B?	Medullary thyroid carcinoma (particularly aggressive form), pheochromocytoma, mucosal neuromas, marfanoid body habitus, and diffuse ganglioneuromatosis of the gastrointestinal tract. There is no clinically significant involvement of the parathyroid gland in MEN-2B.
204	Describe the natural history of medullary thyroid cancer in MEN-2B and its recommended treatment.	Almost all patients develop an aggressive form of medullary thyroid carcinoma, with a high rate of metastases before age 10 years. Often, patients will even have microscopic disease present before the first year of life. Prophylactic total thyroidectomy is recommended as soon as the infant is able to tolerate surgery, ideally before age one. In the past, the average life expectancy was 21 year, before when prophylactic thyroidectomy was recommended.
205	Describe the distinctive facial features of MEN- 2B.	Mucosal neuromas on the dorsal surface of the tongue, palate, or pharynx; prominent "blubbery" lips; submucosal nodules on the vermillion border of the lips; and eyelid neuromas.
206	Describe the distinctive body habitus associated with MEN-2B.	Around 75% of individuals with MEN-2B have a marfanoid body habitus: tall and lanky, kyphoscoliosis or lordosis, joint laxity, and proximal muscle wasting.

207	What is the incidence of pheochromocytoma in MEN-2B?	50%; approximately half are bilateral.
208	What defines the clinical diagnosis of familial medullary thyroid carcinoma?	Historically, it is diagnosed in families with four or more cases of medullary thyroid carcinoma without pheochromocytomas or parathyroid adenoma or hyperplasia. The RET oncogene is associated with FMTC, so FMTC may be viewed as MEN-2A with reduced organ-specific penetrance.
209	Describe the age of onset and penetrance of medullary thyroid carcinoma in FMTC syndrome compared with MEN-2A and -2B.	Medullary thyroid carcinoma has a later age of onset in FMTC and decreased penetrance compared with MEN-2A and -2B.
210	What is the pattern of inheritance in MEN-2 syndromes?	The RET proto-oncogene is inherited in an autosomal dominant pattern for all MEN-2 syndromes (MEN-2A, -2B, and FMTC). However, 50% of individuals with MEN-2B have a de novo germline mutation.
211	What is the recommended primary preventative measure in an individual with an identified germline RET mutation?	Prophylactic thyroidectomy
212	What is essential before surgery in any patient with MEN-2A, MEN-2B, or medullary thyroid carcinoma?	Screening for the presence of a functioning pheochromocytoma. Adrenalectomy should be performed before thyroidectomy in any patient with a pheochromocytoma to avoid intraoperative hypertensive crisis. Calcium and parathyroid levels should also be checked for possible primary hyperparathyroidism.
213	What is the rate of recurrence of medullary thyroid carcinoma in individuals with MEN-2 who have undergone total thyroidectomy and cervical lymph node dissections?	Approximately 50%
214	In individuals with MEN-2 who have undergone prophylactic thyroidectomy, what is the recommended screening protocol for medullary thyroid carcinoma?	Annual serum calcitonin levels

13 Odontogenic Disorders

David G. Stoddard, Brian C. Gross, W. Jonathan Fillmore, and Daniel L. Price

Overview

1	What germ layers and which branchial arch give rise to the teeth?	• Ectoderm • First branchial arch as well as ectomesenchyme from the neural crest and mesoderm
2	Name the muscles of mastication.	• Masseter muscle • Medial pterygoid muscle • Lateral pterygoid muscle • Temporalis muscle
3	Name the teeth from lateral to medial.	• Molars: Third (wisdom tooth), second, first • Premolars: Second bicuspid/premolar, first bicuspid/premolar • Canines: Cuspid • Incisors: Lateral incisor, central incisor
4	Number the teeth according to the universal numbering system. (► Fig. 13.1)	Count maxillary teeth from right to left: • No. 1: Right maxillary third molar • No. 16: Left maxillary third molar • No. 17: Mandibular left third molar • No. 32: Mandibular right third molar

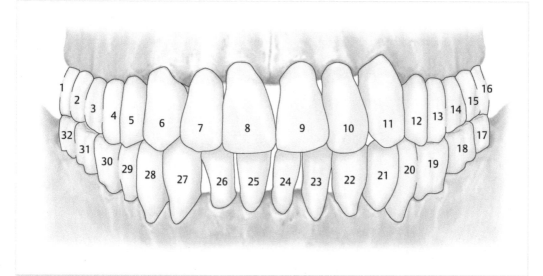

Fig. 13.1 Universal teeth numbering system. (Used with permission from Thieme Atlas of Anatomy: Head and Neuroanatomy, © Thieme 2007, illustration by Karl Wesker.)

5	Name the origin, insertion, and function of the lateral pterygoid muscle.	• *Origin*: Superior head, greater wing of sphenoid; inferior head, lateral aspect of lateral pterygoid plate • *Insertion*: Superior head, articular disk; inferior head, condylar neck • *Function*: Opens and protrudes jaw

| 6 | Name the main components of the temporo-mandibular joint (TMJ) within the joint capsule from superior to inferior. (▶ Fig. 13.2) | • Glenoid fossa
• Superior joint space
• Articular disk
• Inferior joint space
• Head of mandibular condyle |

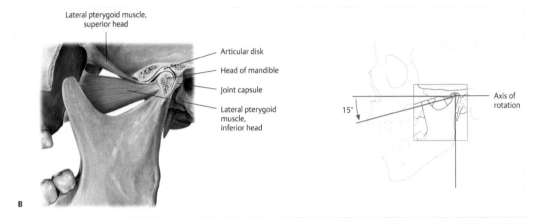

Fig. 13.2 Components of the temporomandibular joint. (Used with permission from Thieme Atlas of Anatomy: Head and Neuroanatomy, © Thieme 2007, illustration by Karl Wesker.)

| 7 | Describe the various surfaces of the teeth. (▶ Fig. 13.3) | • *Mesial*: Toward the midline
• *Distal*: Away from the midline
• *Facial*: Toward the cheek or lips
• *Labial*: Toward the lips (anterior teeth)
• *Buccal*: Toward the cheeks (posterior teeth)
• *Lingual*: Toward the tongue
• *Incisal*: Toward the biting surface (anterior teeth)
• *Occlusal*: Toward the biting surface (posterior teeth)
• *Apical*: Toward the apex or tip of the root |

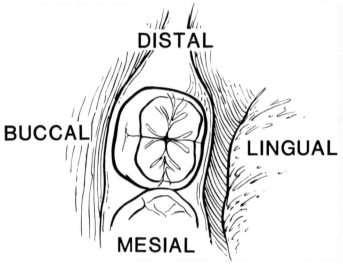

Fig. 13.3 Surfaces of the tooth. Mesial = toward the dental midline (the space between the central incisors); distal = away from the dental midline; buccal = adjacent to the cheek; lingual = adjacent to the tongue. (Used with permission from Edelstein DR, ed. Revision Surgery in Otolaryngology. New York, NY: Thieme; 2009.)

8	Describe the sensory innervation to the TMJ.	The masseteric, deep temporal, and auriculotemporal nerves (all branches of cranial nerve [CN] V3) supply the joint capsule.
9	What are the three main layers of a tooth? (▶ Fig. 13.4)	• Enamel • Dentin • Dental pulp

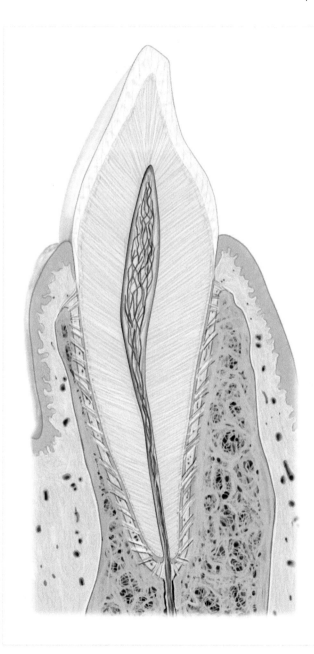

Fig. 13.4 Longitudinal section of a tooth and its layers. (Used with permission from Thieme Atlas of Anatomy: Head and Neuroanatomy, © Thieme 2007, illustration by Karl Wesker.)

10	What are the functions of the posterior teeth?	The premolars and molars grind food as well as establish a vertical dimension of occlusion.
11	What are *bone morphogenic proteins (BMPs)*?	Proteins that are osteoinductive and are instrumental in regulating bone and cartilage development and formation
12	Describe the Angle classification of dental relationships. (▶ Fig. 13.5)	• Class I: Normal occlusion, mesiobuccal cusp of the maxillary first molar aligns with the buccal groove of the mandibular first molar • Class II: Distoclusion (retrognathism), mesiobuccal cusp of the maxillary first molar mesial to the buccal groove • Class III: Mesioclusion (prognathism), mesiobuccal cusp of the maxillary first molar distal to the buccal groove

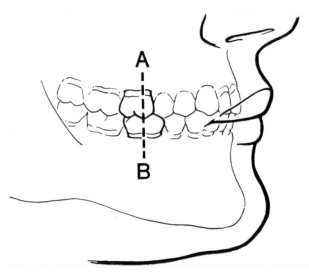

Fig. 13.5 Angle's classification of occlusion: Class I (normal). The mesiobuccal cusp of the maxillary 1st molar aligns with the buccal groove of the mandibular first molar. (Used with permission from Donald PJ. The Surgical Management of Structural Facial Disharmony: A Self-Instructional Package. Washington, DC: American Academy of Otolaryngology–Head and Neck Surgery; 1985:13,14,15.)

13	Describe the evaluation of a panoramic radiograph (orthopanotomogram).	Evaluation should include the teeth and any evidence of dental caries or periapical pathology, the alveolar and basal bone of the jaws, the inferior alveolar nerve canal, ramus and condyles, and maxillary sinuses; account for any impacted or missing/supernumerary teeth.
14	Describe the radiologic findings common to benign odontogenic tumors.	Common findings include radiolucency, often multilocular, and a propensity to expand the cortical boundaries of the jaw and push the inferior alveolar nerve inferiorly. Cortical margins are typically intact. Teeth may be displaced or roots resorbed (more aggressive malignancy will often show the whole root and a "tooth floating in space").
15	Which anatomical regions are best visualized by standard dental X-rays?	Tooth-bearing regions of the maxilla and mandible are well demonstrated by dental films; the ramus, condylar region, and inferior aspect of the mandible are usually missed by most dental films (periapical and bitewing films). Panoramic radiographs show the jaws and the condyle more completely, but they are less accurate in diagnosing dental disease. Panorex is often distorted in the midline.
16	Describe the causes of osteoradionecrosis (ORN) of the mandible.	Radiation therapy results in endarteritis and fibrosis with resulting tissue becoming hypocellular, hypovascular, and hypoxic. ORN may develop spontaneously or even after minor trauma. Typical radiation thresholds for risk are 50 to 60 Gy.

17	How long after radiation does ORN typically develop?	Onset is bimodal and peaks at both 3 months and 5 years after radiation. It can occur as early as 2 months and as late as 15 years.
18	What are some signs and symptoms of mandibular ORN?	Deep bone pain, exposed bone with or without super-infection, trismus, fistula, halitosis, dysgeusia, pathologic fracture, paresthesia, anesthesia, and edema
19	What is the mechanism of bisphosphonate-related osteonecrosis of the mandible?	Bisphosphonates downregulate osteoclast function, resulting in impaired bone turnover and bone repair. They have also been found to inhibit angiogenesis. After even minor dentoalveolar trauma, affected bone has a limited capacity to heal and may develop osteonecrosis. Intravenous (IV) bisphosphonate use results in a significantly higher risk for development of osteonecrosis of the jaw.

Temporomandibular Joint

20	Name the two descriptive categories of TMJ disorders. Which is most common?	*Extra-articular* disorders and *intra-articular* disorders. Extra-articular disorders are far more common.
21	Contrast the findings in TMJ osteoarthritis and TMJ synovitis.	*Osteoarthritis* is a degenerative disease in the TMJ, as it is in other joints in the body. It is caused by a loss of articulating tissues and can be described as a mechanical, noninflammatory disease with bone-on-bone contact. By contrast, TMJ *synovitis* is definable by its inflammatory nature. Inflammatory mediators may accumulate secondary to trauma, disk malfunction, or parafunctional habits.
22	What is the best imaging modality for the TMJ?	Disk displacement and internal derangement of the TMJ are best imaged using MRI. Bony diseases such as ankylosis or degenerative joint disease are best evaluated using CT. Panorex may be used as to screen for fracture, condylar resorption, or large pathology.
23	How is TMJ internal derangement classified?	The Wilkes classification • Stage 1: Asymptomatic, painless clicking; mild disk displacement with reduction • Stage 2: Occasional painful clicking or locking; mild disk displacement and deformity • Stage 3: Joint pain with functional changes (limited opening); nonreducing disk with deformity • Stage 4: Chronic pain and functional deficit, degenerative osseous changes, and disk deformity • Stage 5: End stage with crepitus, degenerative joint disease (DJD), and disk perforation or loss
24	Name the two categories of TMJ disk displacement.	• Disk displacement *with* reduction (often heard as popping or clicking) • Disk displacement *without* reduction (usually no associated noise) *Note*: Often, displacement with reduction leads to displacement without reduction, which limits range of motion. This may be reversed with conservative therapy or with arthrocentesis or arthroscopy.
25	In the case of anterior disk displacement with or without reduction, what are the indications for intervention?	Pain, impaired mobility (especially acute closed lock), joint locking, failure to respond to conservative therapy Asymptomatic joint noise is common (in up to 35% of Americans).

26	How does osteoarthritis of the TMJ manifest?	Degenerative joint disease or arthritis of the TMJ most commonly affects the elderly population, but it can affect all ages. Painful motion and joint loading are the hallmarks, along with CT findings of DJD. Myofascial pain symptoms must be ruled out. Unless related to ankylosis, it will not vastly reduce range of motion.
27	What are the risk factors for septic TMJ arthritis?	History of trauma, burn, surgery or dental work, and systemic factors such as autoimmune disease, diabetes, immunosuppression, sexually transmitted infection, or prolonged steroid use
28	What is the most common systemic inflammatory condition to affect the TMJ?	Rheumatoid arthritis. Traditional rheumatologic laboratory studies in addition to MRI are useful for establishing a diagnosis.
29	What radiographic findings are expected in acute posttraumatic TMJ arthralgia?	Widening of the joint space might be seen, but radiographs may also be entirely normal.
30	How should trismus be clinically evaluated in a patient with head and neck cancer who has undergone radiation?	Objectively measure the mouth opening (opening < 35 mm is generally considered restricted) and compare with subjective assessment of restriction as well as its effect on daily functions. Assess for pain on opening or other symptoms besides simple restriction of opening from fibrosis.
31	What is the best initial therapy for postradiation trismus?	Stretching exercises, including insertion of stacked tongue blades or use of a commercial device such as Therabite. This requires multiple daily treatments over a period of months.
32	How should ankylosis of the TMJ be managed?	Many algorithms have been described, but most include a description of resection of the ankylotic mass with ipsi-lateral coronoidectomy. Reconstruction is often with costochondral grafting, with or without an interpositional temporalis myofascial flap. Early and rigorous physiotherapy is imperative.
33	Auriculocondylar syndrome is thought to develop from abnormalities in which branchial arches and which craniofacial bones are most commonly affected?	Known also as Goldenhar syndrome, hemifacial micro-somia, and branchial arch syndrome, it affects the first and second branchial arches. There is high variability of expression and may affect the mandible, condyle, maxilla, zygoma, orbit, and temporal bones.
34	Describe the clinical features of auriculocondylar syndrome.	• Auricular abnormalities (question-mark ear with con-stricted middle to lower thirds of the pinna, auricular cleft) • TMJ/condylar abnormality (mandibular hypoplasia, con-dylar hypoplasia, or dysmorphism) • Facial asymmetry with chin deviation toward the affected side • Micrognathia • Microstomia
35	Describe the clinical features of mandibular con-dylar hypoplasia.	Usually unilateral with mandibular deviation toward the affected side and severe malocclusion.
36	Define the condition of *mandibular condylar hyperplasia*.	• Excessive, progressive unilateral growth of mandibular condyle resulting in aesthetic and functional problems such as facial asymmetry, occlusal disturbance, and joint dysfunction • Imaging must distinguish condylar hyperplasia from osteochondroma. • Condylar hyperplasia may also be described in terms of hemimandibular hypertrophy and hemimandibular elon-gation

37	How does bone single-photon emission CT scan aid in the diagnosis of mandibular condylar hyperplasia?	Technetium-99 radioisotope uptake is increased in the hyperplastic condyle, which is indicative of unilateral condylar activity. This is sensitive but nonspecific. Uptake is also increased with inflammation, infection, and neoplasia. Results should be interpreted along with clinical presentation.
38	Define *myogenous temporomandibular disorders.*	Pain and dysfunction of the TMJ area that results from abnormal function or disease processes of the muscles of mastication. It is also known as *masticatory myalgia* and includes the following subtypes: myofascial pain, myositis, muscle spasm, and muscle contracture.
39	What features characterize myofascial pain dysfunction syndrome (MPD)?	MPD is a dull, aching pain in the mandible, temple, or face that is associated with specific trigger points and can usually be reproduced by palpation of trigger points. Pain is typically located over the muscles of mastication or neck musculature rather than over the joint proper. MPD may be with or without concurrent intra-articular disease.
40	What features characterize myositis of the masticatory musculature?	Diffuse, continuous pain over the entire muscle that may limit range of motion and cause swelling. Inflammation of the muscle is secondary to injury or infection, and pain worsens with muscle use.
41	Describe the initial steps to treat masticatory myalgia.	Rest the jaws and muscles by adhering to the following: soft diet, avoiding caffeine, using heat or ice, take NSAIDs, avoid parafunctional habits, avoid sleeping on the stomach, and avoid excessive or prolonged jaw opening.
42	How is a patient with complex myogenous masticatory pain treated after conservative measures have failed?	A pain clinic or pain team is most useful. Physical therapy, along with pharmacologic and lifestyle interventions, are helpful, as comprehensive treatment offers the best chances of success.
43	What differentiates *masticator muscle contracture* from *muscle contracture associated with masticator muscle spasm*?	Chronicity. Masticator muscle contracture is a chronic condition with continued muscle shortening, whereas masticator muscle spasm is an acute condition that is often accompanied by pain.
44	Describe lateral pterygoid spasm. (▶ Fig. 13.6)	• Acute, involuntary contracture of the lateral pterygoid muscle

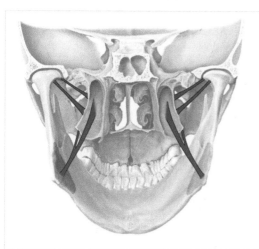 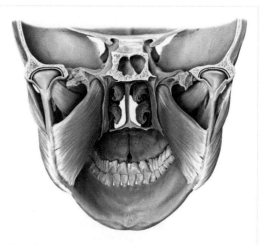

Fig. 13.6 Muscles of mastication, highlighting pterygoid function. (Used with permission from Thieme Atlas of Anatomy: Head and Neuroanatomy, © Thieme 2007, illustration by Karl Wesker.)

		• The muscle is shortened and produces decreased jaw mobility (often acute open lock) and accompanying localized pain.
45	What differentiates *myofascial pain dysfunction syndrome* from *fibromyalgia*?	These may share underlying disease processes and are along the same spectrum. In general, fibromyalgia is notable for more diffuse muscle pain, greater association with sleep disorders, and depression. Myofascial pain is influenced more by regional factors (posture, parafunctional habits, trauma, etc.).
46	What reconstructive options are available for TMJ arthroplasty?	The mainstay for modern arthroplasty is total and hemijoint prostheses. Autogenous grafts, such as costochondral grafts, may also be used. Gap arthroplasty may be augmented with a temporalis myofascial flap. Conchal cartilage has also been used as a disk replacement.
47	How often is surgery indicated for disorders of the TMJ, and what are the absolute indications?	Only 5% of cases require surgical intervention. Absolute indications include treatment of neoplasia, joint ankylosis, or congenital/growth abnormalities that could alter maxillofacial growth.
48	Name the different surgical interventions for TMJ disease.	Arthrocentesis, arthroscopy, modified condylotomy, and open joint surgery (including disk repair, repositioning, diskectomy, eminectomy, and joint replacement).
49	A significant complication of open TMJ surgery is damage to the facial nerve. Which branch of the facial nerve is most commonly injured?	The temporal division of the facial nerve; temporary weakness is present in 5% of cases, and permanent weakness is reported in up to 1% of cases. Other complications include hemorrhage, occlusal changes, persistent change, heterotopic bone formation, and fibrous adhesion formation.

Cysts

50	What is the most common type of odontogenic cyst, and does it affect vital or nonvital teeth?	Periapical (radicular) cyst, which affects only nonvital teeth It is primarily the manifestation of a small chronic dental abscess.
51	How does a lateral *periodontal* cyst differ from a *periapical* cyst?	Lateral periodontal cysts are developmental, arising from the epithelial rests of Serres or Malassez, and are most commonly found lateral to premolars and canines. Periapical cysts are found associated with any tooth and are found apically in the setting of chronic infection.
52	What is the preferred management for the most common type of odontogenic inflammatory cyst?	• The most common type of odontogenic inflammatory cyst is a radicular or periapical cyst. • Management may include extraction of the infected tooth and enucleation of the cyst. In many cases, root canal treatment may be indicated over extraction, depending on symptoms, chronicity, and prognosis of the tooth.
53	What odontogenic cyst develops in the place of absent teeth?	• Primordial cysts, which are the rarest of all odontogenic cysts • History is important in this instance to ensure that the tooth has not simply been removed at an earlier date, which would indicate a residual cyst or dentigerous cyst.
54	Are dentigerous cysts associated with erupted or unerupted teeth, and where are they most likely to be found?	Unerupted or impacted teeth, found with mandibular third molars, maxillary third molars, and maxillary canines (in decreasing order of frequency)
55	How common are dentigerous cysts, and what association do they have with odontogenic carcinoma?	Dentigerous cysts are the second most common odontogenic cysts. Up to 25% of odontogenic malignancies are thought to have transformed from an associated dentigerous cyst.

56	How can *botryoid odontogenic* cysts be distinguished from *lateral periodontal cysts*?	Both cysts manifest preferentially in the same alveolar process locations (namely, the lateral surface of teeth, usually the mandibular premolar or canines). However, the botryoid cyst is multilocular, as its name indicates, and this is reflected histologically and radiographically. Botryoid cysts have a higher incidence of recurrence.
57	What are the components of Gorlin syndrome (Gorlin-Goltz or basal cell nevus syndrome)? (▶ Fig. 13.7)	Diagnosis requires two major criteria or one major and two minor criteria. Major criteria: (1) excessive basal cells or basil cell carcinoma earlier than age 20; (2) odontogenic keratocyst when younger than 20; (3) palmar or plantar pitting; (4) lamellar calcification of the falx cerebri; (5) medulloblastoma, typically desmoplastic; (6) first-degree relative with basal cell nevus syndrome. Minor components: (1) rib anomalies (e.g., bifid rib); (2) skeletal malformations and radiologic changes (i.e., vertebral anomalies, kyphoscoliosis, short fourth metacarpals, postaxial polydactyly); (3) macrocephaly; (4) cleft lip/palate; (5) ovarian/cardiac fibroma; (6) lymphomesenteric cysts; (7) ocular abnormalities (i.e., strabismus, hypertelorism, congenital cataracts, glaucoma, coloboma)

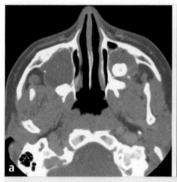 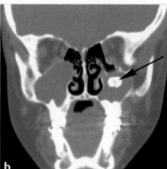 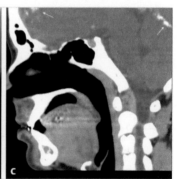

Fig. 13.7 Odontogenic keratocysts in 14-year-old with basal cell nevus syndrome. Axial (a), coronal (b), and sagittal (c) CTs, demonstrating an unerupted tooth entrapped in a odontogenic keratocyst invading the maxillary sinus (*black arrow*). (Used with permission from Wetmore RT, Muntz HR, McGill TJ, eds. Pediatric Otolaryngology: Principles and Practice Pathways 2nd Edition. New York, NY: Thieme; 2012.)

58	Describe the manifestation of odontogenic keratocysts.	Odontogenic keratocysts occur in any jaw location, although they are most commonly noted in the posterior mandibular body and in the ramus. They are frequently noted in association with the crown of an unerupted tooth or near the tooth root. Recurrence is common (between 5 and 60%).
59	What are the histologic features of a "ghost cell," and with what odontogenic cyst is this most commonly associated?	Ghost cells are large, eosinophilic epithelial cells that lack a nucleus and are most commonly associated with calcifying odontogenic (or Gorlin) cysts. These ghost cells may later become calcified and may cause a foreign-body reaction that gives rise to the cyst. Ghost cells are also occasionally seen in odontomas, ameloblastic fibro-odontomas, and ameloblastomas.
60	What is the preferred management for extraosseous calcifying odontogenic cysts (Gorlin cyst)?	Simple lesion removal. These cysts account for up to 25% of all Gorlin cysts and are often seen within the gingiva in patients in their sixth decade of life or later, and they are often seen in association with other odontogenic tumors.

61	What is the preferred management for calcifying odontogenic cysts (Gorlin cysts)?	If the cyst is unilocular, enucleation is preferred. Multilocular lesions often require bony curettage.
62	Describe the clinical features of glandular odontogenic cysts.	Rare and recently described, glandular odontogenic cysts (sialo-odontogenic cysts) may clinically resemble a low-grade central mucoepidermoid carcinoma. They appear anywhere in the jaw but favor the anterior regions. They may be multilocular with epithelial lining including eosinophilic columnar or cuboidal cells.
63	What is the preferred management for an infant with an eruption cyst?	Expectant management; no intervention is necessary.
64	What distinguishes a cyst from a pseudocyst?	Odontogenic cysts comprise an epithelial-lined pathologic cavity, usually fluid or semisolid filled. Pseudocysts lack epithelial lining.
65	What are the clinical features of nasopalatine duct cysts, and in what gender and age of patient do they most often occur?	Nasopalatine duct cysts are classically well-circumscribed, heart-shaped, anterior midline palate masses. They are most commonly seen in men (twice as common as in women) and appear in the fourth to sixth decades.
66	What are the clinical features of nasolabial cysts, and in what gender and age of patient do they most often occur?	These cysts manifest with painless swelling of the labial vestibule and/or nasal floor and are seen more commonly in women (three times as common as males) in the fifth decade of life.
67	What is the favored management of traumatic bone cysts?	Surgical exploration. Traumatic bone cysts are more common in young patients, found primarily in the mandible, and are pseudocysts because they do not contain an epithelial lining. As such, there is nothing to excise surgically. However, by opening the cavity and inducing hemorrhage, surgical exploration induces granulation tissue formation, which resolves the lesion.
68	What are Epstein pearls, what is their source, and how should they be managed?	Epstein pearls are midline palatal inclusion cysts of white/yellow vesicles comprising rests of epithelial tissue trapped in the median raphe of the palate or the hard/soft palate junction. They are self-limited and require no intervention.
69	What are Bohn nodules, what is their source, and how should they be managed?	Bohn nodules are round, whitish papules commonly found along the alveolar ridge in infants in their second to fourth months of life. The papules contain keratin, are more commonly found in the maxilla than the mandible, and are thought to arise from minor salivary glands. They are self-limited and require no intervention.
70	What is pathophysiologic basis for Stafne bone cysts?	Stafne bone cysts are not true cysts but rather a depression in the lingual surface of the mandible. A pathognomonic finding is an ovoid radiolucency inferior to the inferior alveolar canal in the region of the second or third molar. Most often, this depression is filled with an accessory lobe of the submandibular gland, although adipose or lymphoid tissue may also be found.

Tumors

71	What clues at initial manifestation may signify increased concern for a malignant versus benign odontogenic tumor?	Pain, paresthesia, trismus, and rapid onset of malocclusion are associated with increased risk of malignancy.
72	What are the important aspects of the history of a patient with a possible odontogenic mass?	Onset and duration/progression of the mass, complete dental history including any previous surgical intervention, erupted teeth, paresthesia, loose or displaced teeth, malocclusion, pain or absence thereof, trauma, and systemic symptoms

73	What are the most common sites for odontogenic tumors?	Mandibular molars and maxillary cuspids
74	Name the different types of odontogenic malignancies.	Malignant ameloblastoma, ameloblastic carcinoma, primary intraosseous squamous cell carcinoma, clear cell odontogenic carcinoma, malignant calcifying epithelial odontogenic tumors, odontogenic ghost cell carcinoma, ameloblastic fibrosarcoma
75	What are the most common sites of metastasis for malignant odontogenic tumors?	Lungs are most common, followed by regional lymph nodes.
76	Describe the classification system for primary intraosseous carcinomas of the jaw presented by Elzay in 1982.	• Type I: Arising from exodontogenic cysts (e.g., squamous cell carcinoma) • Type II: Odontogenic carcinomas (e.g., ameloblastic carcinoma) • Type III: Arising de novo (e.g., squamous cell carcinoma) • Type IV: Sarcomas (e.g., myoepithelial carcinoma)
77	What is the recommended treatment for odontogenic malignancies?	Because of the extreme rarity of these cancers, no definitive diagnostic algorithm has been developed. In general, wide surgical excision is the treatment of choice.
78	How should a biopsy be undertaken for suspected intraosseous odontogenic tumors?	Depending on patient tolerance and anticipated procedure, anesthesia may be local only or any form of sedation or general anesthesia. Typically, mucosal incision takes place in an uninvolved area that can be easily closed. Aspiration is advised to rule out vascular lesions, after which safe entrance through the bone is undertaken. Specimens should include any areas of radiologic variation to ensure adequate sampling. Excisional biopsy is appropriate for cysts that are small and do not appear malignant on imaging. Incisional biopsy is warranted for larger lesions concerning for malignancy as a precursor to more definitive resection.
79	What aspects of an odontogenic tumor are most important to management decision-making?	Although histology is useful in distinguishing these lesions from one another, it is less important in terms of management. Intervention should be dictated by the behavior of the lesion itself, with particular attention given to the extent of local invasion, disruption of nearby anatomical structures, and destructiveness of the lesion.
80	What are common risk factors for malignancies originating from odontogenic cysts and tumors?	Many odontogenic carcinomas are found in sites of prior cysts, (more commonly than odontogenic tumors), and many are noted in edentulous sites on the mandible/maxilla. Dentigerous cysts are the source of transformation in as many as 25% of cases.
81	Describe the clinical presentation of ameloblastoma. (▶ Fig. 13.8)	Ameloblastomas manifest in a wide range of ages, with peak in the third and fourth decades of life. Patients have a slow-growing, painless bony mass, usually in the posterior mandible, although both jaws may be affected. The tumor is locally invasive, and malignant transformation is rarely noted. The tumor may recur with inadequate resection, especially the solid variant. Radiology is notable for expansive radiolucent lesions that can be unilocular or multilocular and have a characteristic "soap bubble" or "honeycombed" appearance.

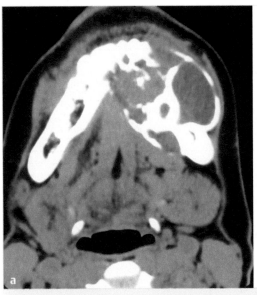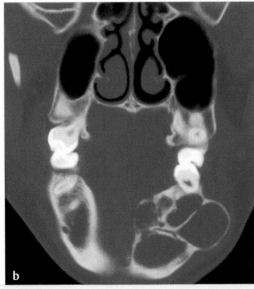

Fig. 13.8 Ameloblastoma of the left mandible. Axial (a) and coronal (b) CTs demonstrating an expansile lesion in the body of the left mandible. (Used with permission from Mafee MF, Valvassori GE, Becker M. Imaging of the Head and Neck 2nd Edition. New York, NY: Thieme; 2005.)

82	What is the most common odontogenic tumor?	Ameloblastoma
83	Compare and contrast *ameloblastoma* with *calcifying epithelial odontogenic tumors* (CEOT; Pindborg tumors).	Both are highly infiltrative and destructive epithelial-derived tumors, presenting as a radiolucent, slow-growing, and painless mass. CEOTs are much less common than ameloblastoma and histopathologically show evidence of scattered calcification with concentric rings known as Liesegang rings. Unlike ameloblastoma, CEOT has large areas of eosinophilic tissue that stain positive for amyloid with Congo red.
84	What is the difference between *malignant ameloblastoma* and *ameloblastic carcinoma*?	Malignant ameloblastoma is characterized by benign-appearing histology but distant metastasis. Ameloblastic carcinoma has the basic ameloblastoma pattern but is dedifferentiated with atypia, hypercellularity, and mitoses, with or without regional or distant metastasis.
85	How can malignant ameloblastoma be distinguished from ameloblastoma or ameloblastic carcinoma?	Malignant ameloblastoma is identified by the presence of metastasis, most often to the lungs. Local invasion is frequently aggressive, similar to ameloblastoma. Histology is notable for similar appearance to the primary ameloblastoma, but the hallmarks of malignancy (invasion of surrounding structures, frequent mitotic figures) are seen in ameloblastic carcinoma. Resection of the tumor is recommended in all cases, and although controversial, adjuvant treatment with radiation or chemotherapy is sometimes warranted.
86	Why is the adenomatoid odontogenic tumor known as the "two-thirds tumor"?	Adenomatoid odontogenic tumors occur in the second and third decades of life, two-thirds of the time in females. Two-thirds are associated with an unerupted/impacted tooth (usually a cuspid), two-thirds of which are a canine, two-thirds of the time in the maxilla.
87	What are *mesenchymal odontogenic neoplasms* (no epithelial component)?	Odontogenic myxoma, cementoblastoma, central and peripheral odontogenic fibromas

88	Compare and contrast *odontogenic myxoma* with *ameloblastoma*.	Both tumors are similar in terms of clinical and radiographic presentation in that both are slow growing and usually asymptomatic, both can be quite destructive (displacement/absorption of tooth roots), both manifest preferentially in the posterior mandible, and both do not impact sensation. However, myxomas frequently appear earlier (in the third decade vs. the fourth for ameloblastoma), and ameloblastomas originate from the epithelium, whereas myxomas are mesenchymal. Both demand excision with a wide margin of tissue.
89	What distinguishes a *cementoma* from other benign odontogenic tumors?	*Cementoma* is an outdated term used to indicate a tumor producing cementum (a calcified substance covering the tooth root). There are three different entities previously associated with the term *cementoma*: periapical cemento-osseous dysplasia, cementoblastoma, and ossifying fibroma.
90	What clinical features define ameloblastic fibroma?	Ameloblastic fibromas are found primarily in younger patients (seldom over age 40 years), usually in the posterior mandible. They present as a painless, radiolucent mass that often overlies an unerupted tooth.
91	What is the natural history of most osteomas of the jaws?	Osteomas are benign hamartomatous bony proliferations, and are made up of compact bone found either on the surface of the jaws in the case of periosteal osteoma or within the bone in endosteal osteomas. An association between multiple osteomas and familial adenomatous polyposis is described in Gardner syndrome.
92	What is the cause of mandibular tori?	It is probably multifactorial, with a possible autosomal dominant inheritance. They may also be a result of bone stress.
93	What is the recommended treatment for torus palatinus?	Observation, unless there is need for a denture, recurrent traumatic ulceration, or a change in speech
94	Describe the presentation and management of central giant cell lesions.	Central giant cell tumors are benign, but locally aggressive lesions affecting the long bones can also occur in the jaws, particularly the anterior mandible. The first through the third decades are most common, and they manifest as an asymptomatic, painless swelling, although pain or numbness is occasionally noted. Curettage is typically an effective treatment, although recurrence should prompt wider resection. Medical interventions have also been described as having some success, notably steroids, interferon, and calcitonin. Bisphosphonate therapy has also been advocated.
95	Why is the name *aneurysmal bone cyst* a misnomer?	Aneurysmal bone cysts are not cysts at all because they lack any endothelial or epithelial lining. Rather, they are expansile osteolytic bone lesions that fill with blood. They are thought to be a variant of giant cell tumor or develop within these tumors.
96	Describe the natural history of ossifying fibroma.	Ossifying fibromas are benign growths that stem from mesenchymal cells. They occur most often in the tooth-bearing jaws and are more common in women. They can become quite large but respond to enucleation and curettage if detected early (under 2 to 3 cm). Larger masses require resection, although a large margin is unnecessary as they are unlikely to recur. They progress from radiolucent to mixed to radio-opaque.
97	What is the cause of fibrous dysplasia?	Fibrous dysplasia is a genetic condition in which medullary bone is replaced by immature bone and fibrous tissue. It most commonly affects one bone (monostotic—90%) but can be seen in multiple bones (polyostotic), most notably in McCune-Albright syndrome.

| 98 | Describe the findings in McCune-Albright syndrome. (▶ Fig. 13.9) | Patients with McCune-Albright syndrome commonly have at least two of the following: hyperfunction of endocrine glands (often manifest with precocious puberty), cafe-au-lait spots (unilateral), and polyostotic fibrous dysplasia (which can manifest in the mandible/maxilla, among many other locations). |

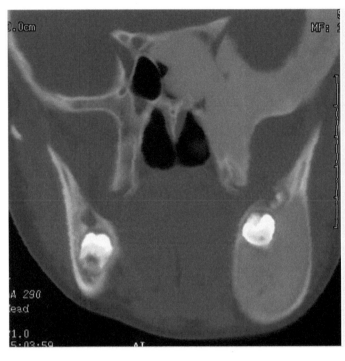

Fig. 13.9 Polyostotic fibrous dysplasia. Coronal CT showing fibrous dysplasia involving the left sphenoid bone and left hemimandible. (Used with permission from Mafee MF, Valvassori GE, Becker M. Imaging of the Head and Neck 2nd Edition. New York, NY: Thieme; 2005.)

| 99 | What pathologic change gives rise to the characteristic mandibular swelling in cherubism? | In cherubism, bone in the mandible (and occasionally maxilla) is gradually replaced by multilocular cysts comprising vascular fibrous tissue with multinucleated giant cells. It is symmetric and usually self-limited and will frequently regress with the onset of puberty, often with total involution. Surgery is rarely warranted to treat ophthalmologic or orthodontic complications. Inheritance is autosomal dominant, with near complete penetrance in males. |

| 100 | Describe the pathophysiology of osteitis deformans (Paget disease), and how is diagnosis made? | Paget disease arises from increased bone formation and resorption. Dense, sclerotic pagetoid bone will be disorganized and weak and may bend or fracture in earlier stages. Diagnosis is often delayed by the fact that patients are asymptomatic. Eventually, deep bone pain or characteristic enlargement of the skull, bowing of the legs, hearing loss, or fractures may bring the disease to the attention of the patient or clinician. Diagnosis is confirmed by radiographs, which demonstrate polyostotic or mosaic-patterned bone. Elevated serum alkaline phosphatase and urine hydroxyproline from increased bone turnover are also useful. |